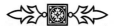

HEALTH POLITICS
AND POLICY

TO
Brenda Litman and Charles Backstrom
whose patience, emotional support, and encouragement
sustained us in this endeavor

Online Services

Delmar Online
To access a wide variety of Delmar products and services on the World Wide Web,
point your browser to:
    http://www.delmar.com/delmar.html
    or email: info@delmar.com

thomson.com
To access International Thomson Publishing's
home site for information on more than 34 publishers
and 20,000 products, point your browser to:
    http://www.thomson.com
    or email: findit@kiosk.thomson.com

A service of **I(T)P**®

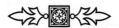

HEALTH POLITICS
AND POLICY

3rd edition

Theodor J. Litman Ph.D.
Professor
Program in Healthcare Administration
University of Minnesota
Minneapolis, Minnesota

Leonard S. Robins, Ph.D.
Professor
Public Administration Program
Roosevelt University
Chicago, Illinois

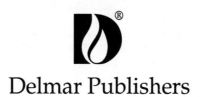

Delmar Publishers

an International Thomson Publishing company

Albany • Bonn • Boston • Cincinnati • Detroit • London • Madrid
Melbourne • Mexico City • New York • Pacific Grove • Paris • San Francisco
Singapore • Tokyo • Toronto • Washington

Notice to the Reader

Publisher does not warrant or guarantee any of the products described herein or perform any independent analysis in connection with any of the product information contained herein. Publisher does not assume, and expressly disclaims, any obligation to obtain and include information other than that provided to it by the manufacturer.

The reader is expressly warned to consider and adopt all safety precautions that might be indicated by the activities herein and to avoid all potential hazards. By following the instructions contained herein, the reader willingly assumes all risks in connection with such instructions.

The publisher makes no representation or warranties of any kind, including but not limited to, the warranties of fitness for particular purpose or merchantability, nor are any such representations implied with respect to the material set forth herein, and the publisher takes no responsibility with respect to such material. The publisher shall not be liable for any special, consequential, or exemplary damages resulting, in whole or part, from the readers' use of, or reliance upon, this material.

Cover Design: *Carol D. Keohane*
Delmar Staff
Publisher: *William Brottmiller*
Editor: *Bill Burgower*
Assistant Editor: *Hilary A. Everson-Schrauf*
Project Editor: *Judith Boyd Nelson*
Production Coordinator: *James Zayicek*
Art and Design Coordinator: *Carol D. Keohane*

COPYRIGHT © 1997
By Delmar Publishers Inc.
a division of International Thomson Publishing Inc.

The ITP logo is a trademark under license.

Printed in the United States of America

For more information, contact:

Delmar Publishers Inc.
3 Columbia Circle, Box 15015
Albany, New York 12212-5015

International Thomson Editores
Campos Eliseos 385, Piso 7
Col Polanco
11560 Mexico D F Mexico

International Thomson Publishing Europe
Berkshire House 168-173
High Holborn
London, WC1V 7AA
England

International Thomson Publishing GmbH
Konigswintrer Strasse. 418
53227 Bonn
Germany

Thomas Nelson Australia
102 Dodds Street
South Melbourne 3205
Victoria, Australia

International Thomson Publishing Asia
221 Henderson Road
#05-10 Henderson Building
Singapore 0315

Nelson Canada
1120 Birchmont Road
Scarborough, Ontario
Canada, M1K 5G4

International Thomson Publishing—Japan
Hirakawacho Kyowa Building, 3F
2-2-1 Hirakawacho
Chiyoda-ku, Tokyo 102
Japan

All rights reserved. No part of this work covered by the copyright hereon may be reproduced or used in any form or by any means—graphic, electronic, or mechanical, including photocopying, recording, taping, or information storage and retrieval systems—without the written permission of the publisher.

1 2 3 4 5 6 7 8 9 10 XXX 03 02 01 00 99 98 97

Library of Congress Cataloging-in-Publication Data

Health politics and policy / [edited by] Theodor J. Litman, Leonard S.
   Robins. — [3rd ed.]
       p.   cm. — (Delmar series in health services administration)
       Includes bibliographical references and index.
       ISBN 0-8273-6776-7
       1. Medical policy—United States.   2. Medical care—Political
   aspects—United States.   3. Public health—Political aspects—United
   States.   I. Litman, Theodor J.   II. Robins, Leonard S.
   III. Series
       [DNLM: 1. Health Policy—United States.   2. Politics—United
   States.   WA 540 AA1 H48 1997]
   RA395.A3H4257   1997
   362.1'0973—dc21
   DNLM/DLC   96-39278
   for Library of Congress   CIP

INTRODUCTION
TO THE SERIES

This Series in Health Services is now in its second decade of providing top-quality teaching materials to the health administration/public health field. Each year has witnessed further strengthening of the market position of each of the principal books in the series, also reflecting the continued excellences of the products. Each author, book editor, and contributor to the series has helped build what is widely recognized as the top textbook and issues collection of books available in this field today.

But we have achieved only a beginning. Everyone involved in the series is committed to further expansion of the scope, technical excellence, and usability of the series. Our goal is to do more for you, the reader. We will add new books in important areas, seek out more excellent authors, and increase the physical attributes of the books to make them easier for you to use.

We thank everyone, the authors and users in particular, who have made this series so successful and so widely used. And we promise that this second decade will be dedicated to further expansion of the series and to enhancement of the books it contains to provide still greater value to you, our constituency.

Stephen J. Williams
Series Editor

DELMAR SERIES IN HEALTH SERVICES ADMINISTRATION

Stephen J. Williams, Sc.D., Series Editor

Ambulatory Care Management, second edition
Austin Ross, Stephen J. Williams, and Eldon L. Schafer, Editors

The Continuum of Long–Term Care
Connie J. Evashwick, Editor

Health Care Economics, fourth edition
Paul J. Feldstein

Health Care Management: Organization Design and Behavior, third edition
Stephen M. Shortell and Arnold D. Kaluzny, Editors

Health Politics and Policy, third edition
Theodor J. Litman and Leonard S. Robins, Editors

Introduction to Health Services, fourth edition
Stephen J. Williams and Paul R. Torrens, Editors

Motivating Health Behavior
John P. Elder, E. Scott Geller, Melbourne F. Hovell, and Joni A. Mayer, Editors

Really Governing: How Health System and Hospital Boards Can Make More of a Difference
Dennis D. Pointer and Charles M. Ewell

Strategic Management of Human Resources in Health Services Organizations, second edition
Myron D. Fottler, S. Robert Hernandez, and Charles L. Joiner, Editors

Financial Management in Health Care Organizations
Robert A. McLean

Principles of Public Health Practice
F. Douglas Scutchfield and C. William Keck

The Hospital Medical Staff
Charles H. White

Essentials of Health Services
Stephen J. Williams

Essentials of Health Care Management
Stephen M. Shortell and Arnold D. Kaluzny, Editors

Health Services Research Methods
Leiyu Shi

SUPPLEMENTAL READER:

Contemporary Issues in Health Services
Stephen J. Williams

CONTRIBUTORS

Gary L. Albrecht, Ph.D.
Professor, Health Policy and Administration
School of Public Health
University of Illinois–Chicago

Charles H. Backstrom, Ph.D.
Professor
Department of Political Science
University of Minnesota

Morris L. Barer Ph.D.
Director, Centre for Health Services and
    Policy Research and Professor
Department of Health Care and Epidemiology
University of British Columbia

Roger M. Battistella, Ph. D.
Professor, Health Policy and Management
Sloan Program in Health Services Administration
Department of Policy Analysis and Management
Cornell University

Robert J. Blendon, Sc.D.
Professor, Health Policy and Political Analysis
Harvard School of Public Health and
The Kennedy School of Government

Dana Burr Bradley, Ph.D.
Adjunct Assistant Professor, Gerontology
University of North Carolina–Charlotte

William P. Brandon, Ph.D.
Metrolina Medical Foundation
Distinguished Professor of Public Policy
University of North Carolina–Charlotte

Mollyann Brodie, Ph.D.
Senior Researcher and
Director of Special Projects
Henry J. Kaiser Family Foundation

Robert G. Evans, Ph.D.
Professor
Department of Economics and
Centre for Health Services and Policy Research
University of British Columbia

David Falcone, Ph.D.
Professor
Department of Health Administration and Policy
College of Public Health
University of Oklahoma

Rashi Fein, Ph.D.
Professor, Economics of Medicine
Department of Social Medicine
Harvard Medical School

Paul J. Feldstein, Ph.D.
Professor and Robert Gumbiner Chair
Health Care Management
Graduate School of Management
University of California–Irvine

Irene Fraser, Ph.D.
Director, Center for Organization and
    Delivery Studies
Agency for Health Care Policy and Research

Lynn C. Hartwig, D.P.H.
Director, Center for Community Health
Health and Human Services Division
University of Southern Mississippi

Bette Hill, Ph.D.
Associate Professor
Department of Political Science
Buchtel College of Arts and Sciences
The University of Akron

Katherine A. Hinckley, Ph.D.
Associate Professor
Department of Political Science
Buchtel College of Arts and Sciences
The University of Akron

William W. Lammers, Ph.D.
Professor
Department of Political Science
University of Southern California

Donald W. Light, Ph.D.
Professor, Comparative Health Care Systems
University of Medicine and Dentistry of
   New Jersey and
Adjunct Senior Fellow
Leonard Davis Institute of Health Economics
University of Pennsylvania

Debra J. Lipson, MHSA
Associate Director
Alpha Center
Washington, D.C.

Theodor J. Litman, Ph.D.
Professor
Division of Health Management and Policy
University of Minnesota

Theodore R. Marmor, Ph.D.
Professor, Public Policy and Management
Yale School of Management

James Morone, Ph.D.
Professor
Department of Political Science
Brown University

Keith J. Mueller, Ph.D.
Director, Center for Rural Health Research
Department of Preventive and Societal Medicine
University of Nebraska Medical Center

Barry G. Rabe, Ph.D.
Associate Professor
Department of Health Management and Policy
School of Public Health
University of Michigan

Leonard S. Robins, Ph.D.
Professor
Public Administration Program
Roosevelt University

David A. Rochefort
Professor
Department of Political Science
Northeastern University

Frank J. Thompson, Ph.D.
Professor and Dean
Graduate School of Public Affairs
Nelson A. Rockefeller College of Public Affairs
   and Policy
State University of New York–Albany

CONTENTS

LIST OF
FIGURES AND TABLES

FOREWORD

S tanding apart from other industrial nations, the United States has no public or private program or combination of programs designed to assure all residents access to health care services or to protect all residents from the economic burdens of ill health. Nevertheless, like other societies, America does have a long and rich history of central, state, and local government involvement in health care and health policy. At the federal level, one is reminded of the U.S. Public Health Service, which is almost two hundred years old; the Pure Food and Drug Act, passed in 1906; the Marine Hospital Services Hygienic Laboratory, reorganized into the National Institute of Health in 1930; the Medicare and Medicaid amendments to the Social Security Act, enacted and signed into law in 1965. These, and countless other specific pieces of legislation and regulatory initiatives, bespeak a public concern with the funding and provision of health care services, the training of health care professionals, the underwriting of biomedical research, as well as inspecting, testing, and other activities designed to assure safety and quality. As with the federal government's involvement with the health care sector, so, too, has been that of other levels of government.

I mention this in order that we be reminded that the intimate relationship between government and the health sector and the frequent calls for even greater public-sector involvement long predate the most recent attempt, in the early 1990s, to enact universal insurance protection. Furthermore, the concerns about new legislation and the need for new regulations to meet newly emerging issues, concerns that extend far beyond issues of budget and payment for medical care services, continue. They do so and will do so even in spite of the fact that the reforms called for by President Clinton died (and not with a bang, but with a whimper). The reminder about the continuing relationship between the public sector and the health of the public alerts us to the significance of this volume. The failure to enact the Clinton health program may gladden some and sadden others. Yet none should conclude that it equates with or portends a fundamental break in the federal government's long-standing concern with and interest in the development of health policy (though, of course, it does portend a different near-term agenda and a search for new approaches to long-standing problems).

Health policy will continue to be debated at all levels of government. Health issues and health policy will remain on the public-sector agenda. This is the case not solely because America remains the "odd man out"—the only Western industrial nation without a system that substantially protects all individuals and families from the financial repercussions of illness. Government will remain involved with health care even if we do not soon return to a debate about extending health insurance to millions of Americans without insurance and government's concerns will extend far beyond a traditional concern with containment of communicable disease and control of epidemics.

Furthermore, government will remain involved with health care even though the American health sector is undergoing rapid change as health care delivery is restructured with calls for decline in government regulatory efforts accompanied by a much greater emphasis on private-sector competitive behavior. It is true that the various changes emphasize the creation and strengthening of private competitive markets as the mechanism designed to further efficiency, contain rising costs and expenditures, and provide for increased consumer rather than government control. Yet even if the balance between government regulation and competitive market competition shifts, government will remain active in the health enterprise.

Why, in spite of widespread skepticism about government's responsiveness and ability to attain agreed-upon goals with some attention to efficiency, will government remain heavily involved? There is more to the answer than the simple (and simplistic) response that large bureaucratic institutions seldom turn existing responsibilities over to others or let programs, already in place, expire. Inertia is a powerful force, but a richer explanation is warranted.

That explanation can be found in this volume. The essays contained herein help answer the question readers might ask: Why, even in the United States, a nation long characterized by skepticism, cynicism, and antipathy toward the "feds," will government continue to develop public policy responses (admittedly of varying efficacy) to perceived medical care needs? The essays, written by a group of distinguished contributors who have studied the role of politics and health care, provide answers to our question by placing public interventions into the historical setting of the world of health and health care, as well as into the historical development of the world of politics and policy.

Thus, as the Table of Contents suggests and as a reading of the essays makes clear, the volume moves well beyond the generalizations that might be presented as part of a keynote address at this or that symposium or conference. Such keynotes are useful in that they help "set the stage," but the success of the meeting depends crucially on what follows, that is, on the play itself. In this volume the authors have the time and space to present their texts, permitting us to judge what they say and how the various monologues or soliloquies hang together as a drama.

It surely does not come as a surprise that I find the play impressive indeed. Of course, one welcomes the individual essays and would do so even if they stood alone and had been published in one or another peer-reviewed journal—and we can be certain they would have been accepted and published. But the whole is more than the sum of its parts.

In no small measure, this is due to the editors' vision that moves the essays—and, ipso facto, the reader—in Part One from a general overview through the beginnings of an explanatory and zeroing-in process that places health, government, and politics in the uniquely American context. Still, proceeding, as it were, from the macroscopic to the microscopic, Part Two calls our attention to the particular roles of the executive and legislative branches of the federal government, to the role of states, and to the important, but often neglected, process (and challenge) of *implementation*. I emphasize the importance of the latter as a reminder of the significance of the questions "But, will it work?" and "What is the error rate?"—vital matters, regrettably not of particular interest to some of the disciplines that contribute to policymaking.

The essays in Part Three, designed to peel away additional layers of the onion, focus on and provide a rich discussion of variables at work in influencing the political process: public opinion and health interest groups. Again, we benefit from the movement from the abstract to the concrete, from theory to practice.

In Part Four, we encounter nine "case studies" that apply the knowledge already gained to specific health policy issues and target populations. It would be a pity, indeed, if readers interested in one or another specific issue—AIDS, or rural health care, or mental health—read only the chapter that discusses that particular subject. The analyses of the relationship among politics, health issues, and health policy have a cumulative effect and an impact that extends beyond the particular area under examination.

The message is clear: the American health enterprise touches every resident and does so in ways that extend far beyond the financial considerations that have been (and, legitimately, will continue to be) one of the foci of attention. Medical care has long been considered a "necessary": the kind of things that, as Adam Smith put it over two centuries ago, include not only items necessary for life itself, but others that common decency and custom require be available to all. Medical care is special because we, you and I, are offended when we see unnecessary pain, suffering, and early death—pain, suffering, and death that could have been prevented, but for inability to pay, lack of access, or discriminatory behavior.

The phrases "common decency and custom" and "we, you and I" should be read as implying something more than individualism and individual actions. The market (presumably) imparts coherence to the countless individual buy, sell, and other decisions. But a society is more than a collection of competitive (and other) markets and, as the individual is more than just a collection of organs, so the community is more than just a collection of individuals. So it is that we turn, as we have and as we must, to instruments and institutions through which we can act in collective fashion. One such instrument—indeed, the most inclusive one—is government.

Certainly, as this volume illustrates, government processes, politics, and policy need improvement. But no criticisms should lead to the view that we can do without the institution called "government." Reading this volume will remind us of some important process and outcome failures (and successes). It will acquaint us with some of the reasons for those various outcomes. I believe the awareness of failure should not lead us to abandon the struggle for better government and a better and more equitable health care system, but to work harder at it. I rather suspect the editors and authors will not be troubled if others share that conclusion and if that turns out to be one more of the contributions of this volume.

Rashi Fein, Ph.D.

Professor, Economics of Medicine
Department of Social Medicine
Harvard Medical School
Boston, MA

PREFACE

A short time before his untimely death from cancer, former Vice President Hubert H. Humphrey noted that the moral test of a government—and, we would add, a nation—is how it treats those who are in the dawn of life, its children; those who are in the twilight of life, its aged; and those who are in the shadow of life, its sick, needy, and handicapped. For a government (society), he went on to observe, that can neither educate its children, care for and sustain its elderly, nor provide hope and meet the needs of its infirmed sick, poor, and disabled, is a government without compassion and a nation, we would argue, without a soul.

The resolution of such issues, more often than not, tends to be a political one, arrived at in the political arena as part of a political process. It is toward understanding the process and the context within which such decisions are made vis-à-vis health and health care that this book is addressed. It is intended to provide interested students and faculty in the health sciences, government, and public administration with a comprehensive analytical overview of the politics of health. Through an examination of the historical and contemporary involvement of government and politics in the organization, financing, and delivery of health care both here and abroad, it attempts to underscore the important role political factors play in the development of health policy.

While there has been considerable speculation—if not actual sharp intellectual debate—over the years among political scientists specializing in the study of the politics of health as to whether there is something analytically unique from a political science perspective about health politics other than its subject matter, we would tend to concur with Falcone[1] that the politics of health is not *theoretically* different from the politics of other policy areas, such as defense, welfare, and education, but that there are aspects of health politics that, although individually not unique, need to be presented in overview form to help the reader understand developments in the various areas of health politics discussed by the contributors to this volume.

Health politics, for example, is usually conducted in a favorable political climate. The notion of health is a popular one: the public, for good or ill, remains convinced of the efficacy of medicine in promoting and maintaining it and believes that future medical advances guarantee less sickness and longer life. This results in strong popular support for spending money in all fields of health, especially biomedical research and medical care

---

[1]Falcone, David. (1980–81). Health policy analysis: Some reflections on the state of the art. *Policy Studies Journal, 9* (Special No. 1), 188–197.

services. The only important constraint is, obviously, budgetary; that is, people do not want their taxes raised or the budget unbalanced.

Other fields are not so fortunate when they enter the political arena. Welfare spending, for example, is not merely opposed because of possible adverse tax or spending consequences, but there are important segments of the public that oppose welfare spending in principle. They believe that it is worse than doing nothing, because it encourages laziness and dependency on the part of those receiving welfare. And while there is more support for spending on national defense, even here, the public does not want to spend more than is deemed necessary to defend the nation's vital interests.

It would be a mistake, however, to assume that all health policies have the same type of politics. Lowi,[2] for example, describes three major patterns of political conflict that are said to be associated with three different types of public policies—distributive, regulative, and redistributive.[3] It is clear, however, that actual policies are never as distinct as Lowi's typology suggests. All public programs redistribute resources, but most are not primarily attempts to do so. Likewise, all government programs depend on an ultimate capacity to regulate the conduct of citizens, but most do not make such regulation their prime object. And almost all government programs involve the distribution of goods and services among different groups, though the question of which county or which social class should receive them is not always the key issue.

Given the debate surrounding Lowi's and others' attempts to identify policy arenas and the politics associated with them precisely, no one typology can be presented as being definitive. It is important, however, to recognize that the politics of obtaining funds for biomedical research is not the same as the politics of drug regulation and that neither is the same as the politics of national health insurance.

What remains to be explained, however, is why until recently health and health care have received relatively little attention in political science as a policy domain in comparison with other fields such as education, law enforcement, and defense. Despite both its practical implications and potential theoretical relevance, the politics of health has been a generally neglected area of inquiry among political scientists. In contrast with their counterparts in sociology and economics, political scientists—with the notable exceptions of Garceau's[4] classic pioneering exposition on the political life of the AMA, Eckstein's[5] landmark analysis of pressure group politics in the British Medical

---

[2]Lowi, Theodore. (1964). American business, public policy, case studies, and political theory. *World Politics, 16*, 677–715.

[3]Distributive policies that parcel out public benefits to interested parties provoke a stable alliance of diverse groups that seek portions of the pork barrel. Regulative policies, which constrain the relationships among competing groups and persons, provide incentives for shifting coalitions, pluralistic competition, and the standard forms of compromise. Redistributive policies, on the other hand, reallocate benefits and burdens among broad socioeconomic population groups and foster polarized and enduring conflict in which large national pressure groups play central roles. (see Lowi, note 2).

[4]Garceau, Oliver. (1941). *The Political Life of the American Medical Association*, Cambridge, MA: Harvard University Press.

[5]Eckstein, Harry. (1960). *Pressure group politics: The case of the British Medical Association.* Palo Alto, CA: Stanford University Press.

Association, and Glaser's[6] penetrating look at doctors and politics—up until fairly recently, have evidenced little interest or involvement in the study of health politics.

The minimal role political science has played in the development of the study of health policy appears to be the result of a variety of factors. Weller,[7] for example, has attributed the discipline's limited contributions in this area to its relatively narrow focus, concentrating on too few groups or too narrow a set of issues, that is, the physician and the medical profession; an overreliance on case studies confined to either a particular group, issue, or piece of legislation; a disciplinary boundary problem over whose purview health policy belongs, that is, political science, public administration, social welfare, or something else; the complex nature of the health field; and the belief on the part of some political scientists, at least, that the pressure group approach exhausts the possibilities for the political analysis of health.

Other explanations include the general paucity of available research support for the study of such a "politically sensitive" subject as the *politics* of health and the historically "private" character of health care delivery in the United States. In the case of the latter, although it can persuasively be argued that politics occurs in nearly all endeavors in life, political scientists have traditionally and still primarily do emphasize those political phenomena that essentially relate to government. Thus, whereas the vast bulk of taxing, spending, and employment in the fields of education, law enforcement, and defense have been in the public sector, that for health, at least up to the first half of this century, was ostensibly a private endeavor and as such held little fascination or interest for political scientists.

With the passage of Medicare and Medicaid, however, along with the other legislative initiatives in the 1960s and later, the degree of public involvement in health has increased dramatically as has the need for political research and analysis to guide the development of health policy. Thus there is reason to believe that health politics will assume a far greater research significance than it has had within the discipline of political science.

But if political science has been found wanting as far as its contribution to the politics of health is concerned, the field of health and medical care has been equally remiss in its lack of knowledge and understanding of the political environments within which it operates. For instance, a 1988 study by the Institute of Medicine[8] on the future of public health reported that not only are many public health professionals either ignorant or disdainful of politics, but eschew a role for themselves in the political process. Similarly, a survey of the catalog listings of each of the nation's accredited schools of public health by McFarlane and Gordon[9] found that although twenty of the twenty-four

---

[6]Glaser, William A. (1960). Doctors and politics. *American Journal of Sociology, 66,* 230–345. See also bibliographic references at the end of this volume.

[7]Weller, G. R. (1977). From pressure group politics to medical industrial complex: The development of approaches to the politics of health. *Journal of Health Politics, Policy and Law, 1,* 444–470.

[8]Institute of Medicine Committee for the Study of the Future of Public Health. (1988). *The future of public health,* Washington, D.C.: National Academy Press.

[9]McFarlane, Deborah R., & Larry J. Gordon. (1992). Teaching health policy and politics in U.S. schools of public health. *Journal of Public Health Policy, 13* (Winter), 428–434.

schools offered courses in health policy and politics as part of their curricula (fourteen offered one to three courses in the area and six offered four or more), most public health students were not required to take such coursework as part of their professional training. Moreover, although there was considerable variation in the content offered, only a handful of the courses surveyed focused on government institutions and political processes. Rather, most of the courses offered were presented within the context of health care delivery. Such ignorance or neglect of political factors in the organization, financing, and delivery of health care services omits a critical element in the potential resolution of health care problems. For, like it or not, health and health care have become so deeply enmeshed in the body politic that in order to achieve success within it, there is a need for health care administrators and practitioners to learn to understand it, adjust to it, and turn it to their advantage.

Toward this end, the following developments would seem to bode well for the future:

1. The formation of the Committee on Health Politics in the early 1970s by a group of interested faculty members in political science departments and health services administration programs.
2. The establishment of the *Journal of Health Politics, Policy and Law.*
3. The introduction of courses and seminars on the politics of health in programs in health administration, schools of public health, and nursing and other health professional schools. A 1992–93 survey of the nation's fifty-six graduate-level health administration programs by Borisoff and Showalter,[10] for instance, found that twenty-six of the thirty-two responding programs indicated that they offered some type of health politics and policy course, as either an elective or as the required capstone course in the last semester in the final year of their master's degree program. In the case of the latter, however, the focus of the course was usually on health policy decision making within a health care organization or agency, whereas where it was offered as an elective, broader policy issues were addressed. Finally, most such course offerings were presented in a seminar form, involving class discussions, student projects, and the use of guest speakers (60%), for example, lobbyists, politicians, legislative staff, and policy analysts, to enhance and bring real-life experiences to the class.
4. The publication of Marmor and Durham's[11] penetrating exploration of the role and limits of the application of political science to the field of health and health care.
5. The call by the Institute of Medicine's Committee for the Study of the Future of Public Health[12] for an increase in that professions' awareness, knowledge, understanding, and facility to use and work within the political arena.

---

[10]Borisoff, Mindy J., & J. Stuart Showalter. (1994). Health politics and policy: Survey of U.S. health administration courses. *Journal of Health Administration Education, 12* (Spring), 215–219.

[11]Marmor, Theodore R., & Andrew B. Dunham. (1982). Political science and health. In Thomas Choi & Jay N. Greenberg (Eds.), *Social sciences approach to health services research* (pp. 58–80). Ann Arbor, MI: Health Administration Press.

[12]Institute of Medicine Committee for the Study of the Future of Public Health (note 8).

6. The establishment of the Robert Wood Johnson Foundation's 1993 Scholars in Health Policy Research and 1996 Investigator Awards in Health Policy Research programs that enable a select number of scholars to undertake and pursue research in health policy, including the interplay among the social, economic, and political forces that have shaped health, health care, and health policy in this country.

When the first edition of this book was written, it was at the onset of the Reagan presidency. A number of leading academicians and practitioners in the field were invited to prepare original expositions on the politics of health and health care. In the ensuing years, the U.S. health care system has seen many dramatic changes, the most important of which have been: (1) the growing advocacy of free market competition as the solution to the problems of financing and the delivery of services; (2) the introduction, paradoxically, by the Reagan administration of the most intrusive regulatory control over the health care system in the nation's history, with the adoption of DRG-based prospective payment to hospitals under Medicare; (3) the limitation that the nation's fiscal and budgetary policies have placed on the federal government's potential for initiatives in health and health care; (4) the nation's brief flirtation with the possible enactment of national health care reform during the first two years of the Clinton administration; (5) the Republican takeover of both houses of Congress following the 1994 midterm elections and their efforts to overturn and dismantle much of the social-welfare legislation of the previous sixty years.

The latter two developments and their aftermath presented both a challenge and opportunity to putting the current volume together, as we and our contributors were confronted with the need to contemplate, interpret, and respond to the virtual paradigm shift that took place in health policy in the little over two years that transpired between the time that the new edition was contracted for and its final submission to the publisher. Thus, whereas the nation appeared to be poised on the threshold of adopting some form of national health care reform when our contributors agreed to join us in this endeavor, a little over a year later following on the heels of the Republican revolution, legislation calling for profound changes in the nature of Medicare and Medicaid, the role of the states, and the future of a host of regulatory agencies dominated the legislative agenda.

That our contributors were able to develop and adapt their pieces under such changing social-political circumstances, much less speculate on the future, is a tribute to their skill and expertise, a task that was not made any easier by the prolonged impasse over the 1996 budget between the Republican Congress and the Democratic president.

Like its two predecessors, the content of the book is organized around four major themes—health politics and policy in perspective, health policy and the political structure, the role of public opinion and interest groups in health policy, and health policy and the political process—and seeks through a series of original readings by some of the nation's foremost scholars and writers in the field to provide the reader with a greater knowledge and understanding of the political process and the role government and politics play in the formulation of health care policy.

But while following the general framework of its earlier counterparts, in response to suggestions and feedback from the field, several substantive changes have been made in the present edition. A number of new authors and chapters have been added: Fein (Forward), Blendon and Brodie (Public Opinion), Marmor and Barer (Universal Health Insurance), Morone (Gridlock and Breakthrough in American Health Politics), Albrecht (The Politics of Disability), Rochefort (Mental Health Care), Mueller (Rural Health), and Rabe (Environmental Health); and others retained and updated: Litman (Introduction), Battistella with Ostrick (The Political Economy of Health Services), Light (the Restructuring of the American Health Care System), Lammers (Presidential Leadership), Falcone and Hartwig (the Congress and Health Policy), Lipson (the Role of the States), Thompson (Bureaucratic Implementation), Feldstein (Health Interest Groups and the Demand for Legislation), Hinkley with Hill (the Strategic Choices of Health Interest Groups), Evans (Health Care Finance), Fraser (Access), Brandon and Bradley (the Elderly) and Robins and Backstrom (AIDS). The book concludes with an Epilogue followed by a chronology of capsule highlights of the involvement of government in health and health care in this country and an extensive research bibliography.

Finally, no endeavor such as this could be successfully accomplished without the aid and assistance of others. In addition to our contributors, a special note of gratitude and appreciation is owed our assistant editor Hilary Schrauf for her patience and forbearance as well as the staff at Delmar Publishers, the Division of Health Management and Policy and the University of Minnesota School of Public Health, our student research assistant, Karen Yuille and most of all, our secretaries, Shirley Fernandez and John Benda, without whom, along with the added assistance of Jarrod Davis and Brenda Litman, the final preparation of this compendium would not have been possible.

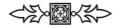

PART ONE

HEALTH POLITICS AND POLICY
IN PERSPECTIVE

To a large extent, each nation's health care system is a reflection as well as the product of its own social, political, economic, and cultural history and tradition. In his introductory chapter on the relationship of government and politics to health and health care, the senior editor provides a sociopolitical overview of the American experience, noting its evolutionary development and the nation's continuing struggle to determine the proper role, if any, government should play in this sphere of American life. The chapter concludes with a summary list of lessons to be learned from previous such entreaties both here and abroad.

Donald Light then examines the historical and contemporary forces that have led and now shape the restructuring of the American health care system, followed by James Morone's critical analysis of the demise of the Clinton health reform plan and the consequences of the increasing corporatization of American medicine that it inadvertently spurred.

Finally, Roger Battistella, with the assistance of John Ostrick, concludes this section with an incisive review and assessment of the major ideological influences—normative, rationalist, neoconservative and Neo-Marxist—that have shaped the health policy debate in this country, and the growing threat that rising costs pose for the future of government entitlement programs not only in the United States but in every major industrialized nation in the world, where each is in the process of rethinking its social agenda in the face of an increasingly competitive global economy.

CHAPTER

The Relationship of Government and Politics to Health and Health Care— A Sociopolitical Overview

Theodor J. Litman

When the Eighty-ninth Congress adjourned in 1966, its record of legislative accomplishments made it the most health-minded Congress in U.S. history.[1] Not only had more national health legislation been enacted into law during its first session than had been passed in both sessions of all Congresses in the past decade, but it had appropriated more money for health in the final two years of its term than its predecessors had in the previous 168 years. Never before had one session of Congress produced legislation of such far-reaching implications for the health, education, and socioeconomic welfare of the American people than had been enacted in 1965 (Gardner et al., 1967). So extensive was the legislative activity in terms of the number and scope

---

[1] A total of fifteen pieces of legislation that had direct and far-reaching impact on health services were enacted: the most publicized were Medicare and Medicaid, Titles XVIII and XIX of the 1965 amendments to the Social Security Act. Others included: PL 89-239—Heart Disease, Cancer and Stroke amendments of 1965 (Regional Medical Program); PL 89-74—Drug Abuse Control amendments of 1965; PL 89-92—Federal Cigarette and Labeling and Advertising Act; PL 89-105—Mental Retardation Facilities and Community Mental Health Centers Construction Act amendments of 1965; PL 89-109—Community Health Services Extension amendments of 1965;

PL 89-115—Health Research Facilities amendments of 1965; PL 89-134—Water Quality Act of 1965; PL 89-272—The Clean Air Act amendments and Solid Waste Disposal Act of 1965; PL 89-290—Health Professions Educational Assistance amendments of 1965; PL 89-292—Medical Library Assistance Act of 1965; PL 89-4—The Appalachian Regional Development Act; PL 89-73—The Older Americans Act; PL 89-333—The Vocational Rehabilitation Act amendments of 1965; PL 89-117—The Housing and Urban Development Act of 1965. A sixteenth bill (PL 89-749—Comprehensive Health Planning) was passed in 1966.

of health actions taken that one observer depicted the period as a turning point in health law (Forgotson, 1967).

As far as health care financing was concerned, the issue was no longer one of public versus private enterprise. According to Anne Somers, that issue had seemingly been settled in favor of the nation's or the United States' unique pluralistic health care economy with its programmatic amalgamation of public and private activities. What had changed was the nature of the mix, which seemed to lean markedly in favor of the public sector (Somers, 1966). Moreover, with the passage of the National Health Planning and Resources Development Act (PL 93-641) in 1974 (Rubel, 1975), the question of the federal government's right to interfere in the private practice of medicine appeared to be decided, for all intents and purposes, in favor of government.

The role of the federal government in the organization, financing, and delivery of health care services in the United States, then, seemed assured, and the prospects for adoption of some form of national health insurance seemed imminent, if not a foregone conclusion. But if the federal initiatives in health during that period had been seen by many as a sociopolitical watershed in which the powers and machinery of government were mobilized to improve access to services, to further distributive justice and equity, and to redress social and economic wrongs (Fein, 1980), times and circumstances change, new problems arise, and events often overcome good intentions.

Thus some thirty years later, in the wake of the demise of President Clinton's heralded health care reform plan and the subsequent Republican takeover of the House and Senate following the 1994 off-year congressional elections, the nation found itself once again in the throes of intense political debate over what role, if any, the federal government should play in health and health care, as the very nature and viability of two of the cornerstones of President Johnson's Great Society, Medicare and Medicaid, came under Republican assault in the 104th Congress.

That the Clinton plan failed in its initial foray through the legislative labyrinth, or that Medicare and Medicaid became the subject of congressional scrutiny by the new Republican majority should not have come as any great surprise. Major changes in health policy, Fuchs (1991, p. 16) has noted, like those in any area, are political acts undertaken for political purposes. In an earlier article (1976), Fuchs offered four reasons why the United States has been the last major industrialized nation to provide universal health insurance coverage to its citizens: distrust of government, its heterogeneous population, a robust voluntary sector, and a lessened sense of noblesse oblige.

Successful efforts at big, bold policy reforms such as that attempted here, Heclo (1995, p. 87) reminds us, are historically rare in this country. By constitutional design, he notes, political power in the United States is structurally fragmented, favoring incremental action or inaction. As a result, ever since the issue was raised by Theodore Roosevelt in his 1912 presidential campaign, the notion of federally supported national health insurance has been a recurring, if intermittent, item on the nation's policy agenda (Heclo, 1995, p. 95).

Seven times over the course of the twentieth century—during the Roosevelt, Truman, Kennedy–Johnson, Nixon, Ford, Carter and most recently, Clinton administrations—major legislative initiatives were considered or launched to attain some form of comprehensive universal national health insurance in this country. Only once, however, did such efforts succeed, with the passage of Medicare and Medicaid in the mid-1960s, and only then after the death of a popular president (Kennedy) and the landslide election victory of his successor (Johnson over Barry Goldwater) in 1964 (Skocpol, 1995, p. 80; Steinmo & Watts, 1995; Blumenthal, 1995). Few remember that legislation to provide medical care coverage for the elderly had been the subject of political debate over three elections (1960, 1962, and 1964) and had failed twice, first as the Forand and later as the King–Anderson bills, to attain congressional approval.

Moreover, despite immense personal and political popularity, Democratic majorities in both houses of Congress and a wide mandate to promote progressive social reform, even President Roosevelt (FDR) chose not to pursue enactment of national health insurance in the 1930s in the face of the hostile reception it would likely receive at the hands of key southern Democratic committee chairs, the hospital and insurance industries, and the American Medical Association, fearing that such a proposal would jeopardize passage of Social Security and the rest of the New Deal agenda (Steinmo & Watts, 1995, pp. 339–340).

The failure of the Clinton plan has been attributed by critics and supporters alike to a number of structural, strategic, and tactical factors (Fuchs, 1991; Steinmo & Watts, 1995; Starr, 1995; Blumenthal, 1995; Skocpol, 1995; also see Johnson & Broder, 1996) including the following:

- The forces actively opposed were strong and well organized, with a clear sense of what they did not want, whereas those actively in favor were relatively weak, disorganized, and frequently at odds over the best way to attain reform (Fuchs, 1991; Hage & Hollingsworth, 1995).
- Institutional fragmentation in Congress and ideological differences between the president and his own party caused problems (Weir, 1995).
- Due to a fragmented committee structure and a lack of consensus on the part of the majority party, the president's proposal had to run the gauntlet of five different House and Senate committees, each with its own political agenda and point of view.
- The plan itself was too complex and bureaucratic.
- The plan's overlapping objectives, that is, universal coverage and cost control, did not translate into an easily understood call to action (Blumenthal, 1995), readily subjecting it to distortion by its opponents.
- The plan's drafters were academically talented but politically naive and inexperienced in the "ways of Washington" (Hage & Hollingsworth, 1995).
- Although the administration consulted widely, its deliberations and decisions were made in secret in order to produce a coherent, integrated plan. This in turn diminished the prospects of educating the major stakeholders—Congress, opinion leaders, and the public—about the difficult trade-offs that would be required as well as precluded any prenegotiated arrangements with potential allies (Heclo, 1995).
- The administration took too long to introduce its plan, which allowed opponents to gather momentum and the legislation to fall victim to the time pressures at the end of the session (Blumenthal, 1995).
- The decision to emphasize access and universal coverage rather than cost control was not a fortuitous one (Hage & Hollingsworth, 1995).
- Other events, both domestic (e.g., the North America Free Trade Agreement [NAFTA]) and foreign (e.g., Bosnia, Somalia), diverted the president's attention.
- The president's political base of support was extremely narrow; he had come into office on only 43 percent of the popular vote.
- The president had a well-known penchant for vacillation and compromise.
- The plan's core reform was directed at a politically weak constituency and opposed by well-financed special interests.
- There was a lack of an institutional or ideological infrastructure on which to build grassroots support (Skocpol, 1995).
- The media treated the issue as a political horse race rather than focusing on the adequacy and substance of the proposals (Skocpol, 1995).
- The plan failed because of Republican obstructionism in the House and the decision by party leaders to abandon bipartisanship in order to gain political advantage in the coming off-year congressional elections (Talbott, 1995).
- An improved economy coupled with a moderation in premium charges (in part precipitated by the threat of passage of the Clinton plan) lessened a sense of urgency to act.
- The plan promised too much cost-cutting regulation and not enough reward to organized groups and the middle class (Skocpol, 1995).

Such reasons aside, even more disturbing from the standpoint of advocates of health care reform was the decision by the White House, after all the hype surrounding its introduction, to summarily abandon its initiative when it faltered in Congress and not choose to pursue it either as a campaign issue in the fall off-year elections or include it as part of its legislative agenda for the 104th Congress. As a consequence, another opportunity for attaining genuine health care reform in this country was lost, leaving the United States along with South Africa as the only major industrialized nations in the world without some form of government-assured universal health care coverage, with the prospects for such adoption before the turn of the century seemingly slim indeed.

The seeds of the so-called Republican revolution of 1994 and its assault on the Medicare and Medicaid programs, on the other hand, lay in the election of President Ronald Reagan in 1980. The heady optimism and faith in the unbridled growth and beneficent intervention of the federal establishment of the 1960s, had given way to the disillusionment and distrust of government of the 1970s, as the new president entered office.

In the area of health care, despite a number of notable accomplishments—such as demonstrated gains in access to care and in health status among the poor and the elderly (Mooney, 1977), greater rationalization of the health planning process, and increased production of health personnel—skepticism and dissatisfaction with such initiatives began to grow in the face of rising costs, economic stagflation, limited revenues, diminished financial resources, programmatic cutbacks, indifferent if not hostile administration, and bureaucratic insensitivity to the infringement of federal policies, directives, and regulations on state and local prerogatives.

The response was sudden and pointed. The new chief executive, who had ridden to victory on a promise to get government off the backs of the American people, moved quickly and decisively. Within six months of taking office, through the deft and imaginative use of the budgetary process and with the support of a group of conservative Democrats (known as the Boll Weevils) who were ideologically closer to the Republican Party than their own, the president succeeded in gaining congressional approval of a package of budget cuts that repealed and modified scores of programs that had become integral parts of the nation's social and economic fabric, as he sought to reverse the federal expansion of the previous half century and reduce the size and scope of government.

When he left office eight years later, the impact his administration had on the nation's health care system was judged by some to be greater than that of any of his predecessors since Lyndon Johnson. In contrast with the expansionist policies of Johnson's Great Society, however, the Reagan years were marked by a reductionist effort to cut health care costs and shift responsibility for many programs from the federal government to the states and private sector (Sorian, 1989). The Reagan strategy to defederalize health care in the United States, Rabe (1987) has noted, followed three general lines of attack: (1) decentralization, that is, the transfer of authority to the states by the dismantling of existing federal categorical programs and consolidation of others into block grants; (2) deregulation through the abolition or weakening of regulations, appointment to leadership positions of individuals who were opposed or unsympathetic to the basic mission or purpose of certain bureaus or agencies, and a reduction in funding; and (3) redistribution, that is, proposed reductions in, or elimination of, direct forms of government assistance to individuals through entitlement programs such as Medicare. All of which served as the mantra and formed the cornerstone for the legislative agenda of the new Republican majority in the 104th Congress.

Whether the aftermath of the 1994 congressional elections and the attendant Republican attack on the twin pillars of President Johnson's Great Society and other entitlement programs of the New Deal mark the century's third great upheaval in social welfare policy in this country, as Samuelson (1995, 1996) has contended, signaling a major shift in sociopolitical thought vis-à-vis the relationship of government to the individual and his or her health care, or is merely an aberrational interlude in the nation's continuing flirtation with the adoption of some form of universal health insurance, remains to be seen. Suffice it to say that the answer is likely to lie in an understanding of the peculiar role government and politics play in American life, with the decision reached being the product of a deliberative political process.

GOVERNMENT AND HEALTH IN THE UNITED STATES

A number of years ago, the noted British social historian T. H. Marshall observed that no modern government could disdain responsibility for the health of its people nor would it wish to do so. Policies, he noted, differ not so much in the aims pursued as in the methods adopted in pursuit of them (Marshall, 1965). But although the notion of a national system of health services has long been a well-established fact in much of the rest of the world, it has been slow to take hold in the United States. Since the first government system of health care was established in Germany under Bismarck in 1883, the provision of health and medical care to an entire population on a nationwide basis through some form of national health service or insurance mechanism has been adopted in nearly half of the world's sovereign nations, including most of those in Western Europe. On the whole, this development has generally come about through an evolutionary rather than revolutionary process, a function of the social, cultural, political, and economic fabrics of the various countries involved. In most cases, government programs for the financing of health care services have evolved as part of a broader system of social benefits.

To a large extent, each nation's health care system is a reflection of its own particular legacy of traditions, organization, and institutions, and the American experience has been no exception (Litman & Robins, 1971).

In contrast with other advanced countries, for instance, as Tallon and Nathan (1992) have noted, the United States lacks any unifying plan for government action in the field of health, tending to "eschew or limit governmental authority and avoid centralizing power at either the federal or state level," with the net effect being "a patchwork of federal and state health functions decided ad hoc as each issue is addressed—not unlike American government as a whole" (Tallon & Nathan, 1992, pp. 8–9). As a result, government health policies and programs at the federal level have generally evolved in a piecemeal manner, usually in response to needs unmet by either the private sector or by state and local governments. The making of health policy in this country, Lee and Estes (1983) remind us, is a complex process encompassing both the private and public sectors, including multiple levels of government, involving:

- the relationship of the government to the private sector
- the distribution of authority and responsibility within a federal system of government

- the relationship between policy formulation and implementation
- a pluralistic ideology as the basis of politics
- incrementalism as the strategy for reform (Lee & Estes, 1983, p. 88)

Thus, to understand where the United States is and may be heading, it is necessary to know something about the past and the nature of the government system.

The U.S. System of Government

As most students of government are aware, ours is a limited system of federalism predicated on the notion of representative government with an emphasis on minority rights, majority rule, and the preservation of individual liberty. Historically, the American conception of freedom has taken the guise of rights to be protected from restraint, rather than duties to be performed, and a suspicion of established authority. Thus, largely in response to government oppression experienced in Europe, the framers of the Constitution provided an extensive system of checks and balances on the federal establishment. Although Madison and others recognized the need for national supremacy—earlier attempts to rest sovereignty in the state or colonial legislatures as called for under the original Articles of Confederation had proven unsuccessful—they were also aware of the need for protection from the arbitrary use of power by the national government. To pit sovereignty against sovereignty, however, was seen as a formula for disaster.

The solution was outlined in *Federalist Paper* No. 5:

> In the compound republic of America, the power surrendered by the peoples, is first divided between two distinct governments, and then the portion allotted to each, subdivided among distinct and separate departments. Hence a double security arises to the rights of the people. The different governments will control each other at the same time that each will be controlled by itself (Hamilton, Madison, & Jay, 1981).

As set forth under Article I, Section 8 of the Constitution, the relationship between the states and the federal government was fairly well drawn, with the federal government given certain prescribed, delegated powers;

other powers were reserved for the states; still others were to be exercised jointly.[2]

But the framers were also farsighted and realized that the United States was bound to change over time. As a result, the Constitution was envisioned to be a flexible document, confined to neither time nor place. Thus, the role of government in American life has evolved over the past two hundred years or so in large part through judicial interpretation and response to executive initiatives and legislative action.

Federalism and the Constitutional Relationship between the National Government and the States

The question of the proper role of government in general, as well as the relative distribution of powers among the national, state, and local governments in particular, has been the subject of prolonged philosophical debate in the United States, with the line in any given controversy ultimately drawn by the courts. Such deliberations have ranged from Marshall's Doctrine of National Supremacy (*McCulloch v. Maryland*)[3] to the Doctrine of Dual Federalism of the Taney Court (*Cooley v.*

Board of Wardens),[4] with the states having concurrent powers in those matters considered to be truly local in character, to the Cooperative Federalism of the Cardozo Court (Steward Machine Company case)[5] to the concept of Creative Federalism under President Johnson[6] and the New Federalism[7] and the new, New Federalism of the Nixon and Reagan administrations.

Before the 1930s, both federal and state legislation in the field of social welfare was invalidated by the courts on the basis of the due process clause.[8] In 1937, however, the Supreme Court reversed itself (*West Coast Hotel Company v. Parrish*) and repudiated the old doctrine that the due process clause could be used to crush social welfare legislation. Nevertheless, it was Marshall's interpretation of the commerce clause and the supremacy of the central government that served as the basis for much of the legislative initiatives of the New Deal (Roosevelt), the Fair Deal (Truman), the New Frontier (Kennedy), and the Great Society (Johnson).

STATE–FEDERAL REGULATIONS

The role of the states in the U.S. political system has changed dramatically over the past two hundred years as events and trends have altered the fiscal, functional, and political balance within the federal system and rekindled debate over the proper division of powers and responsibilities among the constituent units (Advisory

---

[2]Significantly, the Constitution did not specify the functions and powers of the states, nor were the lines between national and state powers precisely drawn. Consequently, in order to maintain supremacy of the national government over the constituent states in any conflict of authority, the original framers took the following steps: (1) they included a supremacy clause in the Constitution that made the Constitution, federal laws, and treaties of the United States binding on the judges in all states; (2) they required all state officers and judges to take an oath to support the U.S. Constitution, including the supremacy clause; (3) they provided for a national guarantee of a republican form of government in each state, which implied the right of the national government to intervene in state governments; and (4) they provided for judicial review of state legislative acts in federal courts. Finally, no state was permitted to nullify or obstruct the acts of the national government (Anderson, 1955).

[3]Chief Justice John Marshall proclaimed that the U.S. government was one of enumerated powers derived from those specifically delegated to it by the Constitution; that is, Article I, Section 8, sets forth seventeen enumerated powers, plus those implied from the "necessary and proper clause." Later, in *Gibbons v. Ogden,* Marshall held that Congress's power over commerce was plenary, absolute, and complete, subject to no limitations except those expressly stated by the Constitution. The power to regulate was the power to prescribe rules by which commerce was governed.

---

[4]This doctrine upheld state action in interstate commerce via the state's police powers. Within the powers reserved by the Tenth Amendment, the states were sovereign, with final determination of the scope of state powers to rest with the national judiciary. Taney allowed for concurrent regulation by the state while acknowledging both state and national government powers. It permitted state action where the federal government failed to act.

[5]This case envisioned cooperation between the two levels of government.

[6]The expression was used by President Johnson in 1964 in a speech given in Ann Arbor, Michigan, and referred to an improved system of federal relations with state and local governments in connection with the transfer of federal funds for a variety of programs and purposes to local governments. It had been used earlier in conjunction with state and federal sharing arrangements, such as federal grants-in-aid, interstate compacts, and revenue sharing under the Eisenhower administration.

[7]This term is epitomized in the use of block grants.

[8]For example, *Lochner v. New York* (attempted state restrictions on working hours), *Adkins v. Children's Hospital* (minimum wage law), and *Hamner v. Dagenhardt* (attempt to restrict child labor in manufacturing).

Commission on Intergovernmental Relations, 1980; Stenberg, 1980; Lee & Estes, 1983).

The expansion of the federal government's role in American life, however, was neither a historical accident nor an altogether noxious historical legacy, but came about for good historical reasons (Kennedy, 1981). The Constitutional Convention of 1787, for example, was called largely to cure the crippling chaos of decentralized government under the old Articles of Confederation. In his well-known *Federalist Paper* No. 10, Madison argued that a federal government, presiding over the large and disparate polity, would be proof against "faction" or the monopoly of political power by a small group. A corollary is that only the central government, by virtue of its aloofness from local passions, is equipped to lift the nation above the petty parochialisms and prejudices of local interests (Kennedy, 1981).

Beginning under Roosevelt's New Deal and continuing under the Democratic administrations of the 1960s, a fairly broad agreement was reached in Congress that the federal government should play an active role in areas traditionally within the province of state and local governments, particularly regulation where state laws were either nonexistent or failed to conform to one another. There was also broad agreement that the federal government should have a role in providing financial assistance to states and localities for a variety of purposes, such as fighting poverty, pollution control, local law enforcement, and housing. The issue was no longer legitimacy of whether the federal government should be involved in such areas but rather how it should go about assisting the state and local governments (*Congressional Quarterly*, 1972; Lee & Estes, 1983).

Under both the Nixon and Reagan-Bush administrations, as well as among congressional Republicans, however, increasing concern has been expressed as to how large the federal government's role should be in its relations with its state and local counterparts. The answer has been caught up in philosophical differences that separate not only Democrats from Republicans but also conservatives from liberals within each party (*Congressional Quarterly*, 1972).

Traditionally, federal assistance has been in the form of categorical grants-in-aid made to a variety of government and other public and private entities for specific purposes. Such grants-in-aid enable state and local governments to preserve their autonomy within a framework of federal assistance to assure minimum levels of services regardless of income inequities among states and localities, and to help achieve national objectives that states and localities may be unwilling or unable to pursue as well as stimulate, through federal matching, increased investment of state and local funds. Moreover, since federal taxes are generally more progressive than their state and local counterparts, federal grants help reduce interstate inequities in both the level of government services and the tax burden. As a matter of fact, one of the major reasons for the proliferation of categorical grants programs was that not only could the federal government tap far more revenue sources than the states and localities, but also the latter officials could not or would not provide funds to deal with certain problems (*Congressional Quarterly*, 1972).

On the other side of the coin, the expansion of federal power at the expense of state and local governments is inherent in such revenue-sharing mechanisms, leading to federal domination or control. It was in reaction to just such concerns, as well as the trend toward centralization of government authority in Washington, D.C., that the concept of block grants was developed. Block grants, which are federal payments to state or local governments for specified purposes such as health, education, or law enforcement without rules restricting the latter's authority, have been pushed by Republicans in Congress and the executive branch since the 1960s as a way of returning federal decision making to state and local officials. In contrast to categorical grants, which can only be used for specific programs directed by Congress, block grants allow state or local officials to make the decisions on how the money is used within the general program area (*Congressional Quarterly*, 1981).

Whereas proponents of block grants argue that categorical funding forces local programs into a one-size-fits-all national model, subordinates local needs to uniform federal requirements, slows innovation, and imposes excessive administrative costs on local agencies, critics worry that under such grants funding is likely to be less dependable, susceptible to the vagaries and caprice of state politics, vary widely among the states, and due to their diffuse purposes are more vulnerable in Congress than categorical programs, which often develop their own constituencies that will fight for their support (Brown, 1996). As a rule of thumb, categorical funding has long been favored by Democrats and Big City mayors whereas block grants have been supported by Republicans and the states' governors.

The New Federalism

The debate continued with President Reagan's efforts to return many government programs to the states. However, his proposal, although clothed in the mantle of "New Federalism," represented less a sorting out of functions among the various levels of government than opposition of fiscal conservatives to large-scale public-sector spending on particular domestic activities regardless of the level of government (Falkson, 1976).[9] Moreover, although the Reagan proposal to return power and responsibilities to the states was viewed by some as a watershed in the history of U.S. federalism, critics saw the president's New Federalism and Economic Recovery Act as devices to reduce federal expenditures for key domestic activities, and as an abandonment of the national commitments to certain costly social programs, involving the transfer of responsibility to the states and their political subdivisions without adequate funding (Stavisky, 1981).

And, as Nexon (1987, p. 80) observed, "with no specific services provided by the federal government, no clearly identifiable needs to which funds were targeted, and no constituency for the funds beyond state health officials," the administration hoped that not only would congressional interest in the block grant program be

small but that the "life of the new blocks would be short."

Such criticisms aside, however, the president's initiative in this area, like that of his predecessor, Nixon, was directed at a number of real and purported deficiencies associated with the federal government's expanded domestic role in the 1960s and 1970s. Among these were:

1. the inefficiency, complexity, and inequity of categorical grants
2. the vesting of policymaking and control in quasi-independent agencies, unaccountable to any constituency, that is, the voters, nor responsive to local needs and priorities, that is, local health service agencies (HSAs)
3. the distortion of state and local priorities through the stifling of local initiative and taxing ability, forcing local governments to structure themselves around categorical programs rather than their own needs
4. the imposition and enforcement of stereotyped, inflexible solutions for local recipients by federal bureaucrats, out of touch and unaccountable to the public
5. maldistribution of federal funds to those who master the grants application procedure rather than those who have the greatest need (Penchansky & Axelson, 1974; Richardson, 1973)

The Reagan proposal also seemed to strike a responsive chord with the American public. Although the public was concerned about the impact of such a program on their state and local taxes and the ability of states and cities to serve the needs of the disadvantaged through block grants, as well as uneasy about the complexity of transferring responsibility from the federal to the state governments, an October 18, 1981 Gallup Poll revealed initial public support, at least in principle, for the president's overture (Gallup, 1981).

As states and local units of government were forced to struggle with the need to provide more human services in the face of ever-diminishing financial resources in the 1980s, proposals to return such functions to their control, without a commensurate transfer of funds, tended to lose much of their aura and appeal. The

---

[9]The New Federalism proposed by President Reagan should not be confused with that advocated under the Nixon administration a decade or so earlier. The latter embodied a broad spectrum of sociopolitical philosophies advocated by people who shared a common background in state and local government, as well as federal service, and a common belief in the need for reforming the structure of domestic policymaking and program implementation. Although both the New Federalists and fiscal conservatives are generally concerned about the growth of federal power, only the latter have sought total cessation of public-sector spending on social programs (Falkson, 1976).

movement toward shifting more power and authority over federal programs to the states, however, gained renewed momentum during the debate over the Clinton health care reform plan, and came to full fruition with the Republican takeover of both houses of Congress along with a majority of the state houses, following the 1994 elections.

The new members of Congress—many (including seventy-three Republican freshmen) swept into office on a platform (the "Contract with America") calling for "devolution," the transfer of power and money from Washington to the state capitols, and sympathetic to the pleas of the states for relief from the burden of unfunded mandates and overly restrictive federal regulations as well as for greater flexibility in the administration of federal health and welfare programs—responded by pro-posing to convert Medicaid into a block grant program. Their proposal, however, quickly became embroiled in political controversy. In addition to a dispute between high- and low-growth states over the formula to be used to distribute money to the states, the question of how much federal control should be retained to protect the needs of children, the poor, and the elderly found the Republican-controlled Congress pitted against the Democratic president, leading to legislative gridlock and a series of shutdowns of the federal government at the end of 1995 and early 1996, as the debate over the proper role government should play in American life continued.

Representative Government, Interest Group Politics, and Legislative Process

The political process in the United States revolves around two complementary but at times conflicting themes—participatory democracy and representative government. To many, the quintessence of the U.S. government system is found in Madison's *Federalist Paper* No.10:

Extend the sphere, and you take in a greater variety of parties and interests, you make it less probable that a majority of the whole will have a common motive to invade the rights of other citizens or if such common motive exists, it will be more difficult for all who feel it to discover their own strengths and to act in unison with each other (Hamilton, Madison, & Jay, 1981).

From this flows the electoral system of "single-member" districts, a citizen Congress composed of members elected on the basis of state and local areas, and a theory of public interest representation. The framers of the Constitution carefully set forth a tripartite structure of government involving an intricate system of checks and balances and a separation of powers among the three branches—the legislative, executive, and judicial.

LEGISLATIVE PROCESS

The power of Congress to legislate is defined in Article I, Section 1 of the Constitution. In addition to writing federal laws, Congress has the power to conduct investigations; monitor federal agencies; impeach federal officials (including the president); declare war; approve treaties; raise or lower federal taxes; appropriate money; and approve appointments to federal agencies, the judiciary, and the armed forces. It may also override a presidential veto with a two-thirds majority vote in each chamber, or delay or subvert a president's legislative initiatives by the use of the filibuster (requiring sixty votes to invoke cloture) or the deft use of a lesser known parliamentary device, the senatorial hold.[10]

The legislative process is a slow and deliberate one, especially in the case of controversial issues. A wide diver-

---

[10]Unlike the House, where a simple majority is all that is needed for passage of a piece of legislation, quite a different calculus and set of roadblocks need to be overcome in the Senate. In contrast to the lower chamber, Senate rules allow for unlimited debate. As a result, a member may delay or prevent action from being taken on a proposed bill by literally talking it to death. This tactic, known as the filibuster, allows a single lawmaker to derail the will of the Senate majority. A fixture of the Senate from almost its beginning, the rules governing its use have been modified twice. In 1917, the Senate in special session adopted Rule XXII (cloture), which provided that debate could be cut off by a two-thirds vote of the membership. Later, in response to the use of the manuever by southern lawmakers in the 1960s to prevent civil rights legislation from becoming law, the rule was modified to further reduce the requirement to shutoff debate to a three-fifths vote or sixty of the one hundred senators. Still the filibuster remains a vexing tactic that disrupts the legislative process. For not only does it take sixty votes to break it (an extremely difficult task to achieve), but the mere threat of evoking such a manuever is often enough to sidetrack a piece of legislation or a presidential nominee. Moreover, the sixty-vote requirement, in effect, means that all legislation must achieve a supermajority to pass, heightening the prospects of

sity of political views and regional interests, coupled with political caution, serve to deter change. As a result, Congress is more prone to following trends than creating them (Fuchs & Hoadley, 1987, p. 215; Sheler, 1985, p. 46).

Committee System

At the heart of the legislative process is the congressional committee system that has existed in the House and Senate since 1789 and allows for a division of work as well as an orderly consideration of legislation. There are some seventeen Senate and twenty House standing committees plus a host of special, select, and ad hoc committees and subcommittees (National Health Council, 1993). Moreover, under Democratic control during the 1980s and early 1990s, the numbers of committees and subcommittees were allowed to proliferate, giving each and their respective chairs their own place in the sun. As a matter of fact, over the course of a sixty-year period, since 1930, the size of congressional staffs increased from 1,425 in 1930 to 6,255 in 1960 to 20,000 by 1990 (Phillips, 1994). Such structural diffusion, makes enactment of controversial legislation such as health care reform more complicated and difficult to achieve. For instance, no less than sixteen committees alone sought hearings or jurisdiction over the Clinton proposal, each advocating their own version of health care reform.

In the aftermath of the 1994 off-year elections, however, which saw the Republican Party gain control over the House for the first time in forty years, came a number of major changes in how the lower chamber conducts its business, including the elimination of three full committees (Postage and Civil Service; District of Columbia; and Merchant Marine and Fisheries), reduction in the number of select and special committees, cuts in both the budgets and number of professional staff by one-third, a ban on the multiple submissions of legislative proposals, and limitation on the tenure of the speaker to four consecutive terms (though granting him unilateral discretion in the selection of committee chairs).

Committee assignments are generally allocated in proportion to the representation of the majority and minority party's membership in each chamber, and up until 1995 on the basis of seniority when the new speaker (Newt Gingrich [R-GA]) appointed several Republican freshmen to key House committees. While members generally want to be on committees related to their personal interests and backgrounds and the economic interests of their districts or state, some committees are more powerful than others. Among the latter are the Senate and House Appropriations Committees, which control the flow of money to programs authorized by other committees; the Senate Finance and House Ways and Means Committees, which consider tax legislation; and the House and Senate Budget Committees, which establish national priorities through the preparation of the national budget.

Health and the Committee Structure

Although the word "health" does not appear in the official title of any congressional committee, at least fourteen committees and subcommittees in the House and twenty-four in the Senate along with over sixty other such legislative panels have been identified as having some direct or oversight responsibility or influence on health legislation (Lewis, 1976; National Health Council, 1993). Of these, six committees—three in the House and three in the Senate—control much of the legislative activity in Congress.

The House committees are as follows:

The Ways and Means Committee. The most influential by virtue of its power to tax, it was the launching pad for much of the health financing legislation passed in the sixties and early seventies under the chairmanship

---

legislative gridlock. Nevertheless, since 1990, the Senate has averaged at least fifteen filibusters a year, more than in all the previous 140 years (Haas, 1993; *USA Today,* 1994).

A much lesser known parliamentary device to delay or divert legislative action in the upper body is the "senatorial hold," a procedural maneuver that allows senators to keep bills from coming to the floor without identifying themselves, by requesting additional time for review and evaluation of a piece of legislation before voting on it. During the 1996 session, it was used by a coterie of Senate conservatives to hold up a bipartisan bill authored by Senators Kassebaum (R-KS) and Kennedy (D-MA) and opposed by the health insurance industry that would help persons between jobs maintain their health insurance coverage (portability) and limit the ability of insurers and employers to deny coverage because of preexisting conditions (guaranteed issue) (Schmickle, 1996).

of Representative Wilbur Mills (D-AR). In addition to sole jurisdiction over Medicare Part A, Social Security, unemployment compensation, public welfare, and more recently health care reform, it shares jurisdiction over Medicare Part B with the House Commerce Committee.

The Commerce Committee. This committee, formerly Energy and Commerce, has jurisdiction over Medicaid, Medicare Part B, matters of public health, mental health, health personnel, health maintenance organizations, food and drugs, the Clean Air Act, the Consumer Protection Safety Commission, health planning, biomedical research, and health protection.

The Committee on Appropriations. Appropriations and its subcommittee on Labor, Health and Human Services, Education and Related Agencies, holds the power of the purse strings, allocating and distributing federal funds for individual health programs.

The Senate committees are as follows:

The Committee on Labor and Human Resources. This committee has jurisdiction over most health bills referred to it, including the Public Health Service Act, the Federal Drug and Cosmetic Act, health maintenance organizations, health personnel, and mental health legislation (e.g., Community Mental Health Centers Act). This committee formerly included a subcommittee on Health and Scientific Research, which was used by its then chairman Senator Edward Kennedy (D-MA), as a forum for debate on national health insurance. When the full committee came under Republican control in the 1980s, the subcommittee was abolished.

The Committee on Finance and Subcommittee on Health. Like the Ways and Means Committee in the House, the Senate Finance Committee has jurisdiction over taxes and revenues, including matters related to Social Security, Medicare, Medicaid, national health insurance, and Maternal and Child Health (Title V). It is responsible for many of the Medicare and Medicaid amendments, such as professional services review organizations (PSROs), prospective reimbursement, and controlling hospital and nursing home costs.

In 1989, ostensibly in an effort to ease its heavy workload and keep all its members happy, the Finance Committee decided to split its health subcommittee in two, with responsibility for Medicaid policy and the problems of making health insurance available to the uninsured assumed by the subcommittee on Health for Families and the Uninsured, and oversight of Medicare and the search for ways to cover the high cost of long-term nursing home care to be dealt with by the subcommittee on Medicare and Long-term Care.

The Committee on Appropriations and Subcommittee on Labor, Health and Human Services, Education and Related Agencies. Like their counterparts in the House, these committees allocate and distribute federal funds for individual health programs.

It has been estimated that although the tax committees (House Ways and Means and Senate Finance) have jurisdiction over only 15 percent of all health program legislation, they control about 70 percent of all federal health dollars expended. The two principal authorizing committees, on the other hand—the House Committee on Energy and Commerce and the Senate Committee on Labor and Human Resources—review approximately 70 percent of all federal health program legislation but directly affect only 15 percent of the total health dollars (Schmidt, 1980). Interestingly enough, at a time when considerable attention has been focused on constraining the federal budget, it is sobering to note that only 6 percent of the Department of Health and Human Services budget can be cut at the discretion of the appropriation committees, with the rest devoted to entitlements (e.g. Medicare, Medicaid, and Social Security).

Finally, although not health committees per se, two others, the Senate and House Budget Committees, because of their significant power over authorization and appropriations, play an important role in the health legislative process as well. Created by the Congressional Budget and Impoundment Control Act of 1974 (PL 93-3411), the Budget Committees set limits on all federal spending and some twenty "functional" categories, specify the minimum revenues to be raised, estimate the resulting deficit, set limits for the authorization committees, and routinely review operations of the Congressional Budget Office. They also draft early versions of the reconciliation bill as called for in the 1974 act, which requires that spending and tax bills comply with the budget resolutions, including instructing the authorizing committees to cut spending in specific programs (National Health Council, 1993).

Problem of Turnover

Once considered stable legislative bodies, with long tenure for members and a committee seniority system that ensured enduring power to multiterm members, especially committee chairs, the House and Senate in recent years have been plagued by high membership and staff turnover, overlapping jurisdictions, and changes in rules that have significantly increased the independence of individual members at the expense of party discipline, institutional accountability, and legislative efficiency.

Of particular concern, as far as it affects the development of congressional policy on health and medicine, has been the high turnover rate among members and their aides who have had a special interest or involvement in these areas. Between 1977 and 1981, for example, while the turnover rate among members in both houses of Congress approximated 40 percent, and for their aides, nearly 90 percent, membership changes in the 6 key committees and subcommittees that deal with most health legislation were massive, that is, 66 percent, and nearly 90 percent for their staff. Moreover, of the 435 representatives and 100 senators who had voted on the Medicare and Medicaid legislation 16 years earlier, only 68 (13%) of the former and 13 (13%) of the latter still remained in office in 1981. Similarly, a survey of the personal aides and professional staffs serving the 6 legislative committees that organized and funded these programs and continue to have jurisdiction over them revealed not a single staff member remained who had played a significant role during that period (Grupenhoff, 1982).[11] And the pattern continues unabated, as contrary to the proponents of term limits, a combination of long hours, increased partisan bickering, disillusionment, expensive and negative campaigns, and voter anger has served to drive an increasing number of House and Senate members to retirement, either voluntarily or at the will of the electorate, over the past few years. For instance, the huge influx of new members (110 in the House and 11 in the Senate) in 1993, followed by the dramatic Republican takeover of both chambers in 1995 marked the largest turnover of Congress in nearly 50 years. Moreover, the impact was particularly pronounced in the House Ways and Means Committee where over half of the members on the Health subcommittee had departed (Peterson, 1993).

The same has been true with respect to the congressional staff, where low wages, huge workloads, demanding bosses, poor working conditions (up until recently, i.e., the 104th session, Congress did not have to abide by fair labor standards), and a lack of job security have been accompanied by a 40 percent turnover of staff (Wolfe, 1992), a situation further exacerbated by the one-third cut in staff mandated by House Republicans in 1995. Whatever the benefits accrued by such downsizing, the downside is that in the absence of experienced staff, there is a serious loss of institutional memory. As a result, Congress has been left with a huge vacuum in terms of knowledge and expertise at the very time it must grapple with major initiatives designed to alter greatly health care and related programs.

Role of the Executive Branch

Despite Congress's predominant role in the legislative process, the executive branch is not without its resources. In addition to proposing, lobbying, and vetoing legislation, including as of 1996 the power to reject specific spending items or special tax breaks (the line item veto), it can effectively thwart, if not emasculate, legislative intent by withholding or rescinding funds through the Office of Management and Budget (OMB),[12] weaken en-

---

[11]A similar concern has been voiced by Levine (1984) at the state level, where continuing budget crises, inadequate compensation, competition from the private sector, the rise of single-issue politics, and legislative burnout have eroded the legislative and bureaucratic infrastructure of state government at the very time the federal government has proposed returning to states more responsibility for the implementation of human service programs. While such turnover may provide a means of bringing new ideas and people into government, new members are largely the least effective and most poorly informed (Hanson, 1987).

[12]The OMB has been likened to a shadow government (Downey, 1975). Just as Congress has relied on the power of the purse strings to wend its will, so too has the OMB, especially under the directorship of David Stockman in the Reagan administration. Stockman, through his deft use and mastery of the budgetary process, was far more powerful and had a much greater impact on public policy, although less publicly accountable, in his role as director of OMB than in his former role as congressman from Michigan, where he was but one voice among 535 (see *Congressional Quarterly*, 1986).

forcement by nominating or not nominating agency heads or appointing persons unsympathetic or antagonistic to direct the program involved,[13] or delay implementation by not issuing necessary regulations.[14]

Moreover, it should be noted that the president's role in the legislative game and the attendant calculus guiding it tend to vary depending on the nature of party control over both houses of Congress and the White House. For instance, in contrast to his predecessors Nixon, Ford, Reagan, and Bush, who effectively wielded the veto to thwart the will of the Democratic majority in Congress by mobilizing the support of one-third of the membership in either house plus one, to prevent adoption of the latter's legislative agenda, President Clinton found himself confronted by the need to obtain at least sixty votes in the Senate in order to assure floor action on his health care reform initiative—a much more daunting task.

INTEREST GROUP POLITICS AND HEALTH

The efforts of organized interest groups to influence government policy in the United States are an inherent part of the political process and, in large measure, rest on First Amendment guarantees of free speech and the people's right to petition government for a redress of grievances. The increasing complexity of modern life and the attendant increase in the role of government in the everyday lives of its citizens have tended to heighten such organizational activity as part of the political process. Thus, as power has moved toward the federal government, there has been a proliferation of interest group activity (in both number and variety) at the national level. Each year hundreds of such organized interest groups attempt to wield considerable influence over government policy, constituting what has been referred to as the Washington Lobby[15] (*Congressional Quarterly*, 1972; also see Drew, 1967; Felicetti, 1975; Hixson, 1976; Milbrath, 1964; Redman, 1974). It has been estimated by the National Health Council, a clearing house for health care advocates, that the number of health care organizations maintaining offices in the nation's capital or employing lobbyists grew from 117 in 1979, to 502 in 1986, to over 740 in 1992 (Ettorre, 1992).

In their efforts to gain results, such organizations, often directed by professionals in the art of government, tend to direct their focus at key points in the decision-making and policy implementation process. If unsuccessful in Congress, for example, a group may continue to pursue its aims in the agency charged with responsibility for its execution. The legislative game, then, does not end with congressional passage of a bill and its subsequent signature into law; rather, the entire thrust of a piece of legislation may be muted, if not reversed, in the writing of the regulations or administration of the act.

In addition to attempting to influence the views of individual representatives and senators or key members of the executive branch on specific issues, many organized interest groups take an active part in the elective process itself, contributing large sums of money to the campaign coffers of individual candidates as well as those of the political parties themselves (in many cases hedging their bets by contributing to the candidates on both sides of the political aisle).

Since 1979, for instance, more than 370 insurance, pharmaceutical, and health care industry political action

---

[13]The latter was epitomized by the controversy in the Reagan administration over the management of the so-called Superfund and the Environmental Protection Agency (EPA) under the direction of Anne Gorsuch Burford. Burford, who resigned her position under fire in March 1983, had earned a reputation as a staunch opponent of environmental protection laws while she was a member of the Colorado state legislature before appointment to head the EPA.

[14]As was the case with the nursing home reform provisions of the 1987 Omnibus Budget Reconciliation Act (OBRA-87), which was designed to overhaul federal oversight of the nation's nursing home industry and provide residents a "bill of rights." Five years after it was signed into law by President Reagan, five of the seven enabling regulations had not been issued by the Health Care Financing Administration (Migdail, 1992). Moreover, efforts by House Republicans in 1995 to scuttle the entire package of federal nursing home regulations were only headed off by the intervention of a coalition of moderate Republicans led by Senator William Cohen (ME) and Senate Democrats (Eisler, 1995; also see Rovner, 1995).

[15]Especially noteworthy in the area of health was the role played by Mary Lasker (Drew, 1967; Redman, 1974). An equally if not more important influence on government is that wielded by the large think tanks such as The Brookings Institution, the American Enterprise Institute for Public Policy Research, the Urban Institute, and the Rand Corporation (Guttman, 1976; Federation of American Hospitals, 1979).

committees (PACs) have contributed over $150 million to congressional campaigns, with much of this directed at members of key legislative committees—that is, Senate Finance, House Ways and Means, and House Commerce (formerly Energy and Commerce)—incumbents, and members of the majority (nominally the Democratic) party (Makinson, 1992, pp. 128, 131). In the wake of the 1994 congressional elections, however, the health care industry, like many other special interest groups, switched their political generosity from the Democrats to the Republicans. The managed care industry, for example, which gave 56.4 percent of its PAC money to Democrats in 1993–94, gave 74.9 percent of its financial largess in 1995 to Republicans (Public Citizen's Congress Watch, 1995). Similarly, AMPAC, the political action committee for the American Medical Association that had directed 56 percent of its 1993–94 war chest to House and Senate Republicans, increased this percentage to 95 percent in 1995. Prime beneficiaries of the health industry's financial favors were the new Republican leaders of the House and Senate. For instance, Speaker of the House Newt Gingrich, who had received $16,000 from health-related industries as a Georgia congressman in 1993, saw this amount soar to $70,500 in 1995. The same was true of the new chair of the House Ways and Means Committee's subcommittee on health, Representative William Thomas (CA), who in the first six months of 1995 received $66,500 from health-related sources compared to only $26,300 in 1993 (Colford, 1995).

Moreover, both the level and pace of such activity have continued relatively unabated, according to the Washington-based trade group Citizen Action, which has traced the financial involvement of health care political action groups for nearly twenty years. Leading the way during the 1993–94 election cycle, as it has since Citizen Action began keeping records, was the American Medical Association,[16] whose total contribu-

tions of $2,562,368 far exceeded those of all other health care and insurance PACs, followed by the American Dental PAC ($1,394,451), American Nurses Association ($1,226,598), American Hospital Association ($1,120,540—double that given during the previous two-year cycle), American Academy of Ophthalmology ($863,355), American Optometric Association ($660,230), American Chiropractic Association ($597,118), Independent Insurance Agents of America ($552,171), American Society of Anesthesiologists ($513,700), and American Health Care Association ($497,217) (Weissenstein, 1995).

Over the course of the past few years, considerable concern has been raised over the rise of single-issue interest groups and their power to wield a disproportionate influence on the legislative elective process through the creation of lavishly funded political action committees (*Congressional Quarterly*, 1972).

While traditionally interest group activity in the United States has involved groups of individuals representing similar economic or social interests (e.g. labor unions, business, farmers, etc.), as the federal government broadened its sphere of activities, a new type of pressure group developed—a coalition of diverse economic and social interests brought together by concerns over a single issue (*Congressional Quarterly*, 1988). Moreover, in the case of highly charged political controversies, given the heightened nature of the rhetoric and the euphemistic characterization of the opposing sides, it is often difficult to discern the players without a score card as this excerpt of a letter, written by then Surgeon General C. Everett Koop, which accompanied his report to the president on the health effects of abortion on women, clearly attests:

> It is difficult to label the opposing groups in the abortion controversy. Those against abortion call themselves pro-life. On the other hand, those who are not pro-life say they are not pro-abortion; rather, they refer to themselves as pro-choice and are supportive of women's right to choose abortion.
>
> It is true that some who are pro-choice are personally opposed to abortion. It is not clear to them where the lines should be drawn between the rights of the fetus and the rights of the mother. So the pro-choice forces are not monolithic.

---

[16]According to data compiled by the Federal Election Commission, over the course of the fourteen year period, 1979–93, the American Medical Association through its political action committee contributed some $15,016,193 to members of Congress, followed by the National Association of Life Underwriters ($7,702,144), the American Dental Association ($6,002,861), the Independent Insurance Agents of America ($4,370,458), and the American Hospital Association ($525,957) (Lewis, 1993).

Nor are the pro-life forces monolithic. Many ardent pro-life individuals who are dedicated to preserving the life of the fetus do not consider contraception to be ethically, morally, or religiously wrong. But others in the pro-life camp do; indeed, some equate contraception with abortion (Shannon, 1989).

For the most part interest groups tend to gear their operations to the power structure and procedures of Congress, with much of their efforts directed at the committee system. It has been estimated, for example, that about 90 percent of all legislation passed on the floor of either house was passed in the form previously reported by the committee having jurisdiction over it (*Congressional Quarterly,* 1972).

The power of committees to draw up and prevent legislation as well as determine its nature makes them an inviting target for interest group activity. The Washington Lobby, for example, goes to great lengths to keep abreast of government developments that might have a bearing on the interests of its membership. It makes sure to know and watch the work of committees important to its interests, establish and maintain working relationships with key committee members and their staff, stay informed about potential or actual legislative developments, and provide testing and submit prepared statements setting forth its view before the committee (*Congressional Quarterly,* 1972).

On the whole, a group's power to influence legislation rests as much, if not more, on the size of its membership, the financial and personnel resources it can bring to bear on an issue, the astuteness of its representatives, and its political acumen and skills, as it does on the soundness or righteousness of the ideas or positions it expounds (*Congressional Quarterly,* 1988). As one observer has noted, "The majority of the American people are not members of special interest groups and hence are much less articulate on particular issues than are the interested minority whose affiliation with some active organization gives them a greater political leverage" (George B. Galloway, as quoted in *Congressional Quarterly,* 1972, p. 4).

Falik (1975) has argued that the power potential of health as a political issue is circumscribed by the equivocal nature of interest group politics. Although the politicization of health issues helps stimulate public debate, educate the public, and broaden the population base for affirmative legislative action on national health matters, it is equally true that political gamesmanship tends to give disproportionate advantage to those groups that are effectively organized for lobbying. In the health field, this has largely been representative of the medical-educational complex, that is, health professional schools, organized medicine, hospital industry, and third-party payers (Falik, 1975; Health Policy Advisory Center, 1968; also see Common Cause, 1991). Such vested interest group activity manifests itself in the currying of the support of elected officials in both the legislative and executive branches by representatives of major provider groups in order to gain protection and funding of their favorite programs, with most such activity and financial support directed more at preventing legislative action than enacting it (e.g., the health insurance industry's efforts to derail the Clinton plan).

According to the Center for Public Integrity (1994), more than $100 million was spent by health care-related special interests to defeat the Clinton health reform plan (60% on advertising, 40% on PACS), making it "the most heavily lobbied legislative initiative in recent U.S. history" (Selye, 1995). A comparison of the political positions taken by key participant groups during the legislative battle over the Clinton proposal and that of Medicare thirty years earlier is informative, revealing that as times and circumstances change, so do political alignments and positions of special interests.

Thus in contrast to the early 1960s, when debate centered on both the need for and the legitimacy of a federal role in providing medical care for the elderly, thirty years later there was fairly general consensus that something needed to be done to reform the nation's health care system. Even the American Medical Association and the Chamber of Commerce, longtime foes of federal intervention, initially endorsed the idea.[17] Far

---

[17]The Association dropped its unequivocal and universal condemnation of government intervention in health care in 1990 and in a remarkable May 1991 issue of its official publication, the *Journal of the American Medical Association* (*JAMA*), urged the federal government to guarantee basic medical insurance to all Americans, stating that it was "no longer acceptable morally, ethically or economically" for the 31 million to 37 million of the nation's citizens to live with inadequate or nonexistent health insurance. At a news conference unveiling the May 12–17 issue, the journal's editor, George Lundberg, explained the Association's changed position: "If the Iron Curtain can be lifted, the Warsaw Pact dissolved, and East and West Germany politically

less clear, however, was how it should be done, with support for the Clinton plan narrow and thin, and that of its opponents broad and intense.

As for the roles played by the various interest groups involved, the five-year struggle for the passage of Medicare (see Anderson, 1968; Harris, 1967) found the American Hospital Association (AHA), the Blue Cross Association led by President Walter J. McNearney,[18] the American Nurses Association (ANA), organized labor (ostensibly the powerful AFL-CIO and United Auto Workers), the liberal and moderate wings of the Democratic Party, the American Public Health Association (APHA), the American Public Welfare Association, the National Association of Social Workers, the National Council of Churches, the National Council of Jewish Women, the National Council of Senior Citizens (a surrogate of organized labor), the Farmers Union, the Physicians Forum, and the Physicians Committee for Health Care for the Aged through Social Security, pitted against the formidable opposition of the American Medical Association, the U.S. Chamber of Commerce, the National Association of Manufacturers (NAM), the American Dental Association, most large and small businesses, the Republican Party, and conservative southern Democrats in the House and Senate.

Although the legislative order of battle thirty years later remained pretty much the same, the positions taken and alignments of a number of the participants had changed.

Among the organizations and groups supporting the president's plan were the following:

• the Alliance for Managed Competition, comprised of a number of the nation's largest health insurers and

health plans, for example, Aetna, Prudential, Travelers, Metropolitan Life, Cigna (all of whom pulled out of HIAA), and Blue Cross who saw a role for them to play in the regional alliances called for in the Clinton plan (Pear, 1992).

• the twenty-four-member Corporate Health Care Coalition, mostly comprised of Fortune 100 companies such as Dupont and IBM, who already provided relatively generous benefits to their workers (Firshein, 1994).

• the National Leadership Coalition for Health Care Reform, a bipartisan group chaired by former Democratic Congressman Paul Rogers (FL) and former Iowa Republican Governor Robert Ray, which included the Big Three automakers and several steel companies (Firshein, 1994)

• the Ad Hoc Business Group on Health Care Reform, comprised of 120 large companies, many of which also belonged to the National Leadership Coalition, including Bethlehem Steel, Chrysler, Ford, and Giant Food

• the 77,000-member American College of Physicians, representing many primary care providers

• the American Dental Association, which fought against capping the tax deductibility for health insurance but sought expanded coverage for preventive dental services

• AHA

• APHA

• ANA

• the National Council of Jewish Women

• Families USA

• the Health Care Reform project, a coalition of seventeen medical, consumer, business, and labor groups comprised of members spanning the ideological spectrum, including the American Association of Retired Persons (AARP),[19] all of whom contributed $5,000 each to fight for comprehensive health reform

• a weakened labor movement that has seen its percentage of the nation's workforce drop from 25 percent in 1950 to 16 percent in the 1990s and preferred a single-payer plan

---

reunited, all quite rapidly, because it was the right thing to do . . . surely we can provide basic medical care to all of our people now, because it too is the right thing to do and the time has come" (*Star Tribune*, 1991). Similarly, a 1993 Times Mirror nationwide telephone survey of 408 physicians found that almost two-thirds (64%) agreed that the U.S. health care system needed fundamental change (Times Mirror, 1993).

[18]The decision by AHA and Blue Cross as well as that of the American Nurses Association earlier to break organized medicine's solid front against the involvement of the federal government in the provision of health insurance for the aged is considered to mark one of the major turning points in the long battle over the passage of Medicare, for no longer could the AMA portray itself as the sole spokesman for the health care field (see Harris, 1967).

---

[19]Who otherwise stood on the sidelines after being burned over its support of the earlier ill-fated Catastrophic Coverage Act.

- a splintered Democratic Party, with its liberal wing spearheaded by Senator Paul Wellstone (D-MN) pushing for a single-payer system

Arrayed against the Clinton initiative were the following:

- the Health Insurance Association of America (HIAA), representing 275 small and medium-sized insurance firms and best known for its $16 million advertising campaign featuring a series of "Harry and Louise" television commercials attacking the Clinton plan
- the National Association of Life Underwriters (NALU), which included the 10,000-member Association of Health Insurance Agents and the Independent Insurance Agents of America, representing some 280,000 agents and their employees who saw the proposed health alliances as a threat to their livelihood (Kent, 1994)
- the Council for Affordable Health Insurance, an organization representing thirty small indemnity insurers catering to individuals
- the National Association of Manufacturers (NAM), representing 125,000 members, nearly all of which employed fewer than 500 workers, 95 percent of whom pay for their workers' insurance coverage (Firshein, 1994)
- the National Federation of Independent Businesses (NFIB), representing some 607,000 small businesses, concentrated in the rural south and west; about 2 percent or 11,400 of its members are insurance agents; this group feared the imposition of an employer mandate.
- the U.S. Chamber of Commerce, representing 220,000 small businesses. After initially (March 1993) indicating its support for the concept of "shared responsibility," it reversed its position under intense pressure from its membership a year later (February 28, 1994) and came out in opposition to employer mandates (*Medicine & Health,* 1994).
- the Business Roundtable, representing two hundred of the nation's largest companies. It initially supported reform, but pushed by its insurance-dominated health subcommittee, abandoned its support on a split vote in favor of Representative Jim Cooper's (D-TN) plan.
- Association of Private Pensions and Welfare Plans (APPWP), representing 470 large and small compa-

nies, many of which are benefit consulting firms. Like both the Chamber of Commerce and the Business Roundtable, it initially supported the concept of "shared responsibility" in which both employer and employee would contribute to the purchase of coverage, but backed away from the Clinton plan due to its call for an employer mandate and a weakening of business's control over benefits and costs.

- AMA. The unquestioned leading force in the battle over Medicare, the Association took a more conciliatory and less contentious role in the debate over health care reform. After initially calling for a federal guarantee of basic medical insurance for all in the May 15, 1991 issue of its official publication, the *Journal of the American Medical Association* (*JAMA*), it later backed off support of the Clinton plan at the urging of its more conservative members over the latter's emphasis on managed care (*Star Tribune,* 1991).
- the Pharmaceutical Manufacturers Association, which feared control over drug prices
- the American Farm Bureau
- the Christian Coalition
- anti-abortion groups concerned over the possible coverage of abortion
- conservative talk show hosts (e.g., Rush Limbaugh)
- the Republican Party, which at the urging of its political consultant William Kristol saw opposition to the Clinton plan as a campaign issue for the 1994 off-year election

Also aligned against the Clinton plan were a host of other sound-alike "grassroots" coalitions with noble-sounding names, often the creations of one or more of the larger interest groups, including:

- the Coalition for Equal Access to Medicine, financed by the Pharmaceutical Manufacturers Association
- the Health Equity Action League, spearheaded by the National Federation of Independent Business, which opposed the requirement that employers pay the bulk of the cost of their workers' coverage

Such permutations and combinations, in addition to illustrating that politics often makes strange bedfellows and tenuous alliances, also lends support to Feldstein's thesis (see Chapter 10 in this volume) of the importance economic self-interest plays in the demand for legislation.

PARTICIPATORY DEMOCRACY AND HEALTH

Public involvement in the determination of health policy in this country has not been confined to organized interest group activity, but has taken other forms as well, including community participation, initiative, and referendum.[20] Whereas community participation represents an extension of America's democratic heritage and has been seen as a means to perfect the democratic process (Burke, 1968), initiative and referendum constitute a basic right accorded at the state and local levels for the exercise of direct public control over legislation (Roemer, 1965).

Community Participation and Health

Historically, participation of the public in the making of health policy decisions was subsumed in the involvement of the community power structure in institutional governance—a pluralistic, class-based system. A series of classic studies (Elling & Lee, 1966; Belknap & Steinle, 1963; Holloway et al., 1963) has described the relationship between community influentials and voluntary and official health and welfare institutions and its impact on organizational decision making (Elling, 1968). Riska and Taylor (1978), on the other hand, have noted that not only are such board members recruited from a very narrow segment of the population, but they also share a narrow view of health policy that may be at variance with that of those whom they purport to serve, that is, their consumers.

The opportunity for full community or citizen participation in the determination of health policy was institutionalized under the provisions of the model cities (PL 88-164) and health planning legislation (PL 89-

[20]The initiative is an electoral device that empowers the people to propose legislation; the referendum is an electoral mechanism that accords the people the power to approve or reject legislation enacted by their representatives (Roemer, 1965).

749) of the Johnson administration. The movement toward broader participation in human service decision making, including health, has been attributed to diverse factors such as dissatisfaction with professional dominance in the area and a growing recognition of the political nature of decision making regardless of professional input (Silver, 1973). Not surprisingly, the application of the concept has resulted in a collision between what Geiger (1969) has termed "community insistence and professional resistance" and has led in some cases, unfortunately, to a politicization of the health care delivery system over the issue of who truly represents the community and what "participation" and "community" really mean (Geiger, 1969; Bellin, 1969, 1970; Brandon, 1977; Gordon, 1969; Moore, 1971; Thompson, 1974; Feingold, 1973).

Initiative and Referendum

Finally, a note should be added concerning the use of initiative and referendum in health. Unfortunately, the experience of the scientific communities with such extralegislative devices has been anything but promising. The submission of health issues to public referendum, for example, has produced mixed, if not discouraging, results. By far the most extensively studied case has been that related to the fluoridation of water. Of the six hundred referenda held on the issue during the 1950s and 1960s, despite widespread endorsement by the health care community, over 60 percent were rejected (Crain et al., 1968). Similar experiences were reported by Isman (1981), who found that of about nineteen referenda held on the issue in the United States in the first six months of 1980, seventeen ended in defeat. More recent attempts, on the other hand, in the 1990s, to restrict smoking, limit the distribution of cigarettes to minors, and even give terminally ill adults the right to "die with dignity" (Oregon) through the use of initiative/referenda have proven somewhat more successful, although a 1994 proposition that would have made California the first state to have a single-payer system was soundly (72%–28%) rejected at the polls.

Although a number of reasons have been offered to explain the failure of such proposals at the hands of voters, including ignorance, voter apathy, a growing distrust of government, and the health care establishment (Isman, 1981; Marmor et al., 1960; Gamson, 1961), it is sufficient to conclude as follows:

The submission of controversial health-related issues for voter approval is risky and should be entered into with great caution.

Reliance on the rationality of the voter, the persuasiveness of scientific evidence, the righteousness of the issues, the prestige of the health professions, and the implausibility of the charges of the opposition is presumptuous at best, if not self-defeating.

The successful undertaking of such an endeavor requires considerable political skills, extensive knowledge of the community, and mobilization of broad-based, community-wide support.

THE GROWTH OF THE GOVERNMENT IN HEALTH AND HEALTH CARE IN THE UNITED STATES: EVOLUTION, NOT REVOLUTION

It has long been a truism of U.S. political life that government is only permitted to do that which private institutions either cannot or are unwilling to do. The basic economic justification for government intervention, Blumstein and Zubkoff (1973) note, is as a remedy for some market failure. In essence, the traditional basis for government involvement has been a remedial one, when, for whatever reason, the market does not achieve an efficient allocation of resources.

In the area of health and welfare, this view was perhaps best expressed by a 1965 U.S. Chamber of Commerce Task Force on Economic Growth and Opportunity recommendation on the role of government: "Government programs should be used to help the sick, disabled and aged only if voluntary and private means—truly tried and tested—cannot adequately meet society's needs" (U.S. Chamber of Commerce, 1965).[21]

A related corollary to the above would add that with the exception of those powers delegated to it by the Constitution, the growth of the federal government's involvement has generally come about in those areas in which the states have also been found wanting. The Interstate Commerce Act of 1887, for instance, was passed only after the states had failed to control the spiraling interstate railroad networks, and enactment of the New Deal came after four years of economic collapse that found the states broke, with only seventeen having old age pension plans, most which were woefully underfunded (Kennedy, 1981).

The expansion of government or public intervention in health and health care in the United States has essentially been one of evolution rather than revolution, a function of social, economic, and political forces as well as judicial interpretation.

Constitutional Base

The bases for government involvement in health and health care at the state and federal levels rest on quite different constitutional principles. In the case of the states, this has been through the police powers[22] to "enact and enforce laws to protect the health, safety . . . and general welfare" of the public. The states, for example, have rather broad, comprehensive legal authority to regulate or affect virtually every aspect of the health care system within their boundaries (Grad, 1973; Wing, 1976). Such intervention, even by compulsion as in the case of immunization against communicable diseases, has been sustained by the courts (*Jacobson v. Massachusetts,* 197 U.S 11 [1905]) even in the face of a constitutional challenge to its abridgment of the exercise of First Amendment rights to the free expression of religion (Blumstein & Zubkoff, 1973).[23]

---

[21]Stevens (1982) has noted that government hospitals in the United States were established only where community need was self-evident and private efforts were unavailable—for example, to safeguard merchant seamen, protect

the general public from infectious and contagious diseases, isolate and treat the mentally ill, and provide care and shelter to the poor.

[22]The police power of the state is much broader than that of any power of the national government. It is a power that was reserved to the states and never given up by them.

[23]Compulsory fluoridation of water extends the concept of permissible infringement of personal freedom to include protection against a noncommunicable, non-life-threatening condition.

Federal involvement, on the other hand, has rested on judicial interpretation of the welfare clause and, in the case of drugs and medications, the commerce clause,[24] which has been honed and expanded over the past forty years. Historically, for example, the definition of commerce has varied widely and Congress's power in this area has vacillated between restricted regulation and a broad grant of power, subject to judicial interpretation. During periods such as 1880 to 1936, for example, when business has been dominant, the courts have tended to keep government under close rein through a narrow interpretation of the commerce clause. On the other hand, during periods in which the government is paramount, such as the past sixty years, the courts have given a rather broad interpretation to the word "commerce."

Historical Development

Over the course of the past two hundred years, the role of government in the organization, financing, and delivery of health care services in the United States has evolved from that of a highly constricted provider of services and protector of public health to that of a major financial underwriter of an essentially private enterprise whose policies and procedures have increasingly encroached on the autonomy and prerogatives of the providers of care, as he who pays the piper calls the tune.

Although extensive and, at times, seemingly pervasive, such growth has come about neither capriciously nor because legislators or bureaucrats have had any great desire to interfere in this area of endeavor, but rather because the parties primarily involved—the providers (with the notable exception of organized medicine), consumers, insurance carriers, and politicians—came to recognize the need for assistance and government involvement.

Government's role in health and medical care in the United States has thus evolved over time.[25] In the early days of the Republic, for example, there were few organized government health programs at either the state or national level (Lee, 1968). There were no state Health Departments. Foreign quarantine was the responsibility of each port. Programs for communicable disease control and environmental sanitation were the responsibility of local government. Government intervention in health generally was confined to protecting society from the common risks, such as epidemic disease, and to meeting the essential needs of the poor and the destitute—a heritage from the Elizabethan poor laws. This was coupled with support provided by religious and other charitable agencies, fraternal societies, lodges, and clubs organized by immigrant groups (Falk, 1967b).

For the most part, the federal government's role in matters of health could be characterized as paternalistic, custodial, and, most of all, minimal, consisting essentially of responsibility for the care and treatment of merchant seamen and members of the armed forces—past, present, and future (Falk, 1967b). As a matter of fact, the first major involvement of the national government with illness and the provision of medical care for other than the military services began with the Marine Hospital Service Act in 1798 to provide for sick or disabled seamen.[26] Later this was extended to include American Indians who were held in protective custody on reservations as wards of the state. Out of this developed the Indian Health Service, which in 1976 was the object of a major resolution of the Alaska Medical Society calling for its dissolution as inimical to the private practice of medicine.

Throughout much of early U.S. history, health and medical care was considered essentially a private and personal matter—a pattern that continued relatively unchanged for almost eighty years. It remained as such until the 1920s, when, with the passage of the Sheppard–Towner Act on Maternity and Infancy in 1921, the federal role in health and medical affairs began to

---

[24]"The Congress shall have power to regulate commerce with foreign nations, and among the several States, and with the Indian tribes."

[25]In addition to the specific sources cited, we have also drawn on the following references: Falk, 1967b; Foltz & Brown, 1975; Foltz, 1975; Jackson, 1969; Clarke, 1980; Rosen, 1974; Mustard, 1945; Russell & Burke, 1978. For a more detailed outline of the key social, political, and legislative developments that underscored the evolution of the government's role in health and health care in the United States, see the Appendix.

[26]It is interesting to note that the origin of most of the major national health care systems in the world can be traced to the assumption by government of the responsibility for the medical care of merchant seamen and the maritime trades that were considered crucial to the lifeblood of the nation, dependent as they were on import–export trade (Straus, 1950, 1965).

take on its modern form. This act established the first continuing program of federal grants-in-aid to state health agencies for the direct provision of services to individuals, the forerunner of the present-day maternal and child health program. The act, however, largely through the action of the AMA, was allowed to die in 1929 (Schlesinger, 1967; Chapman & Talmadge, 1970, 1971).

The enactment of the Social Security Act in 1935, which marked the beginning of the U.S. system of social welfare, provided the next major development in the growth of federal involvement in matters of health. From this legislation two concepts of social welfare emerged: (1) social insurance for the working population, that is, unemployment insurance, workers' compensation, and guaranteed retirement benefits; and (2) public assistance, that is, direct financial aid provided by the states for those unable to work.

Although not intended as a medical insurance program for recipients of categorical assistance (considered too costly and neither the time nor the place by President Roosevelt), this precedent-setting law provided for federal grants to the states for public health, maternal and child health, and services for crippled children, as well as for public assistance for the aged, blind, and families with dependent children.

Another early federal initiative was the medical care programs of the Farm Security Administration from 1935 to 1947. Perhaps one of the earliest, most extensive, and most comprehensive federal endeavors in health care delivery in this country, the programs incorporated such contemporary precepts as consumer participation; decentralization of care; centralization of payment source; emphasis on prevention and health education; the use of nurse clinicians; salaried physicians; and administrative controls on referrals and hospitalization to serve low-income farmers, sharecroppers, and migrant workers. At its peak, more than 650,000 poor farmers and a million migrants were enrolled in medical care cooperatives or farm labor clinics in a third of all rural counties in the country. According to Grey (1994), it was the largest government-sponsored program in the nation dedicated to providing medical care for a specified civilian group until the passage of Medicare and Medicaid. Although strongly opposed by or-

ganized medicine, these programs received substantial physician support at the local grassroots level, driven by humanitarian and economic concerns. An improvement in physician income and the decline in the rural population, coupled with ideological conflict between the government and the medical program over federal intervention in medical care following the Second World War all contributed to the plans' eventual demise (Grey, 1994).

It is interesting to note that while initially invoked and promoted on largely humanitarian grounds, the passage of many pieces of social health legislation in this country, ostensibly those dealing with occupational safety and rehabilitation, rested essentially on utilitarian or pragmatic grounds, that is, returning people to the workforce and investing in the future—a reflection of Americans' reliance on and belief in the Protestant ethic.

The passage of the Hill–Burton Construction Act in 1946, on the other hand, which provided federal assistance to the hospitals whose physical plants had grown increasingly worn and obsolete following the Depression and World War II, served as a prototype for federal involvement in health care. In addition to establishing the principles of local initiative, state review, and federal support sharing, it also called for, via congressional mandate, at least the first vestiges of planning, that is, a state plan. Federal support was further extended to medical education and research in the 1950s and early 1960s, often over the bitter opposition of organized medicine (Anderson, 1966, 1968a; Carter, 1958; Harris, 1967; Hyde & Wolff, 1954; Rayack, 1967).

It remained, however, for the Eighty-ninth Congress under the Johnson administration to bring the federal role in health care to full fruition with the passage in 1965–66 of legislation providing for the establishment of regional medical programs, comprehensive health planning, extensive aid to medical and other related health profession education, and Titles XVIII and XIX of amendments to the Social Security Act of 1965—Medicare and Medicaid.

Certainly the sleeper here was the Medicaid bill, which was an extension and purported improvement of the earlier Kerr–Mills program and, like its predecessor, relied on the existing welfare system. The Medicaid bill was quickly passed as part of a political compromise to appease conservatives; its architects neither delineated clear goals nor came to grips with the problems inherent in the entire welfare system—particularly the determination of eligibility, which was left to the states. Moreover, as Medicaid began, policymakers had little if any sense of the potential costs of the program nor the impact of pumping vast sums of federal dollars into the private medical market (Friedman, 1977a, 1977b; Davis, 1974, 1975a, 1975b, 1976a, 1976b; Lewis et al., 1976; Stevens & Stevens, 1970; Stevens & Stevens, 1974; Weikel & Leamond, 1976).

Like the Kerr–Mills program before it, Medicaid tended to epitomize the problems inherent in reliance on the states and a states' rights approach to handling broad social programs. In attempting to retain state autonomy and decision making under the program, for example, the rich states tended to get richer whereas the poor states either took no action or had minimal participation in the program. Moreover, despite the offer of federal assistance, many states, especially in the South, were either unwilling or unable to expend the funds. As a result, there was a considerable lack of uniformity both between and within states, which became even further exacerbated in the face of a decline in the economy. Thus, a number of states encountered excessive costs brought on by an explosion of claimants as a result of the 1970 recession and were forced to cut back severely on their programs or, as was the case of New Mexico, pull out of the program altogether.

In addition, in return for the preservation of local control and the determination of local needs, such programs were subjected to the petty political jealousies and idiosyncratic administrative behavior of local welfare officials and county boards. Moreover, like much of President Johnson's War on Poverty and the welfare system itself, Medicaid proved to be an administrative nightmare. In contrast to Medicare, which had the advantage of being a completely new program administered solely at the federal level by a well-established and accepted entity in the Department of Health, Education, and Welfare, using the private sector and the insurance industry as fiscal intermediaries, a major debate soon arose as to whether Medicaid was an income-maintenance or health service program and whether it should be administered by the

welfare administration or the Public Health Service—a debate finally resolved in favor of welfare.

Growing concern on the part of the federal and state governments over the administration of the program, however, led to the enactment of several provisions to improve its management. These included the establishment of federal guidelines requiring that the states review on a continuing basis the cost, administration, and quality of the health care services rendered under their programs, including stricter standards to ensure quality care and periodic review of nursing homes.

In 1967, Congress mandated expansion of the program to include early and periodic screening diagnosis and treatment of children and youth under the age of twenty-one eligible for Medicaid. As a result, not only was the health of low-income children considered a major program priority, but the states were expected to administer and the federal government to oversee a program for direct provision of health care services (Foltz & Brown, 1975; Foltz, 1975). The program was expanded again in 1990 with the enactment of the Omnibus Budget Reconciliation Act of 1990, which extended Medicaid coverage to all children in poverty.

Nevertheless, continued frustration and disenchantment with the program were reflected in the repeated efforts under the Nixon, Ford, Carter, Reagan–Bush, and Clinton administrations as well as by congressional Republicans to constrain costs by reducing services and transferring more of the financial burden back to providers and their patients.

NATURE OF THE GOVERNMENT'S ROLE IN HEALTH AND HEALTH CARE IN THE UNITED STATES

Both traditionally and historically, responsibility for the medical care of recipients of public assistance, veterans with service-connected disabilities, and other special populations such as Indians and the armed forces and for public health in the United States has rested with government, whereas responsibility for the cost of facility construction and health personnel training has been shared among various levels of government and the private sector. The provision of direct personal health services, on the other hand, is and has been essentially a private endeavor.

According to Falk (1967a), government intervention in the U.S. health care system has tended to embrace the following features:

1. financial underwriting in order to assure the availability to all in the population through either contributory insurance (e.g., Medicare), general tax revenues (e.g., Medicaid), or both
2. the development and establishment of various standards and procedures to safeguard the quality of services financed through public funds
3. the provision of services wherever possible through nongovernment practitioners and institutions
4. extension toward comprehensiveness in publicly financed services
5. direct financial support for the modernization, construction, and equipment of health care facilities and for the education and training of needed personnel

Similarly, Brown (1989, p. 2), in an insightful piece prepared for the Ford Foundation, has noted that the federal government in this country as well as central governments in many comparable countries, intervene in the health care system with four objectives in mind and rely on four main policy strategies to achieve them. For instance, in addition to (1) efforts to influence the supply of health care services and resources via subsidized grants and assistance to providers and institutions, government may seek to (2) influence the demand for health care among all or part of its population—usually through the financing of a health insurance program created under public auspices; (3) alter the organization of the health care system by building new structures to serve special population groups (e.g., the VA health care system and the National Health Service Corps) or advance some larger goal such as improving access to care or contain costs through adoption or support of HMOs; and (4) influence the behavior of providers with respect to the use, price, and quality of services, as well as the size, location, and equipment of facilities through major regulatory programs such as peer review organizations, health system agencies and prospective payment.

The ownership, financing, and operation of the health services system in this country, Anderson (1968a, 1968b) has observed, is diffuse, with a wide dispersion of sources of funds and decision-making units. It is a pluralistic system in which the public and private sectors find themselves in what he has termed "uneasy equilibrium," with the various sectors negotiating with and accommodating one another.[27] As a matter of fact, the coexistence within the U.S. health care system of a wide variety of providers, organizational forms, and funding sources has been viewed by many as a positive attribute that contributes to the rapid diffusion of new technology, the enhancement of quality of care, and the capacity of the system to innovate and adapt to change (National Center for Health Services Research, 1977).

The flow of government funds to voluntary hospitals has a long and venerable history in the United States. According to Stevens (1982), state funding of voluntary general hospitals prior to the Depression was generally on a selective, ad hoc, individualized basis, often in response to specific requests from influential local groups. Government aid to hospitals at the local level, on the other hand, was determined by a combination of local political conditions, common sense, the strength of local interest groups, and the taxing structures of the respective states. This "distinctive American practice," as Goldwater (1909) termed it, that is, the appropriation of public funds for the support of hospitals managed by private benevolent corporations, is attributed by Stevens (1982) to the lack of distinction that has existed between public and private functions in the development of U.S. charitable institutions.

Federal Role

As indicated earlier, the federal role in health throughout much of U.S. history has tended to be a

---

[27]In contrast to many of its European counterparts, much of the health care delivery system in the United States is in the private sector. As a result, government is forced to bargain because it neither owns the facilities nor hires the personnel (Anderson, 1968b). The request in early 1983 by the Reagan administration for hospitals to reserve beds for use in a possible nuclear attack is a case in point.

constrained one, limited to crisis intervention (Falk, 1967a), the control and prevention of disease in public health. Typically, as Blumstein and Zubkoff (1973) have noted, federal intervention in the health arena has been on an ad hoc basis without an overall plan, formulation of objectives, or theoretical underpinning. Moreover, in the absence of any specific formulation, national health policy in the United States has been more or less an amorphous set of health goals, derived by various means within the federal structure (Finch, 1970), with little overall concordance or coordination.

Health Policy at the Federal Level

For the most part, the legislative initiatives in health at the federal level over the past thirty or so years, as Battistella reminds us in Chapter 4, rested on a set of assumptions and presumptions, many of which were well meaning and seemed to embrace the conventional wisdom of the period but have proven to be overly optimistic, idealistic, or unfounded.

To a large extent, according to Brown (1978), federal health care policy in the United States has tended to embrace two essentially antithetical models or approaches that are "nurtured in tension." Thus, while "mainstream" equalizing programs continue to receive strong public support, they are challenged by a set of federal proposals based largely on "revisionist" premises concerning constraints on supply and demand for services. As a result, U.S. health care policy has tended to be discontinuous, inconsistent, and, at times, contradictory. Brown goes on to note that by avoiding hard choices and by reconciling in public policy such seemingly contradictory models, we have tended to institutionalize our ambivalence—both preserving the claims of equality of medical services and delimiting its scope.

Role of the States

In contrast to their federal counterpart, whose influence over health stems in large measure from enormous fiscal power, the states have rather broad, comprehensive legal authority for a wide variety of programs. As a result, their role in health has taken a number of forms: (1) financial support for the care and treatment of the poor

and chronically disabled, including the primary responsibility for the administration of the federal and state Medicaid program; (2) quality assurance and oversight of health care practitioners and facilities (e.g., state licensure and regulation); (3) regulation of health care costs and insurance carriers; (4) health personnel training, that is, states provide the major share of the cost for the training of health care professionals; and (5) authorization of local government health services (Clarke, 1980).[28]

Although historically the power of the governor has been limited—a throwback to the colonists' distrust of the royal governor in the area of public taxation—the states' chief executive appears to exert considerable influence in determining health policy via the power of appointment. A review of the statutory authority governing public health decision making in the fifty states (Gilbert et al., 1983; Gossert & Miller, 1973), for instance, found the governor responsible for the appointment of about 91 percent of the 427 positions on the states' board of health. In eleven states, the members of the board sit at the pleasure of the governor.

In terms of their legislative structures, states vary widely in their size, how frequently and long they meet, the compensation they pay their legislators, and the size and expertise of their staffs, as well as the rules that govern their proceedings.

Finally, not only do they vary in terms of their health needs and financial resources, per capita spending on health, insurance coverage, and outcome measures (e.g., low birth weight babies, infant mortality, etc.), but each has its own Medicaid program, no two of which have the same benefits, levels of subsidy, or providers (Verhovek, 1995).

State Expenditures for Health

State spending and responsibility in health have traditionally been directed toward broad public health activities, institutional care of the mentally ill, and the purchase of health care services for the economically disadvantaged. During the past thirty-five years, state spending in health and other human services has been

---

[28]Local governments ultimately derive their powers from the states.

increasingly shaped by federal prescriptions and initiatives, including a variety of apportionment formulas and project grants. As a matter of fact, a familiar characteristic of the U.S. federal system is that many of the programs that carry out national policies are created and operated by the states under rules established by federal legislation and regulations. Moreover, variable methods of federal funding related to purpose, budgetary limits, formulas, and duration impose similar variability on the states' application of funds to the counties (Kramer, 1972; Davidson, 1978).

Like their federal counterparts, state expenditures for health are provided through direct provision of services and indirect purchase of services and have been the subject of considerable political debate over the scope, cost, level of funding, and appropriateness of such expenditures. For all this costs money, and the funds may not be readily available in times of economic recession. Thus many states found themselves with expanding treasuries during the late 1960s and early 1970s, fueled by inflation and aided and abetted by increased federal revenue sharing and a thriving economy, in the face of a serious economic downturn nationally, declining state revenues, reduced federal aid, rising costs, a heightened demand for health and welfare services, threatened taxpayer revolts, and bulging budget deficits,[29] they were forced to cut back greatly on their programs and allow more and more of the burden to fall on their local counterparts, a pattern that may well be repeated in the 1990s (Sheler, 1989).

The Impact of Federal Initiatives in Health on States and Localities

Finally, although the evidence on the extent of the impact of federal initiatives on state and local priorities in health is limited, the key to understanding the ways in which federal aid influences state health goals and

programmatic activities appears to lie in the political environment of the state. A study of six states and four public health programs (Buntz et al., 1978) found that although federal programs facilitate rather than inhibit the attainment of state health goals, federal influence tends to be secondary to that of the state's political environment. A federal program, they note, may elevate an issue to the state's active policy agenda but need not necessarily lead to formulation of a state policy or goals unless interests within the state are receptive. Moreover, the federal influence on state health policy appears to be both state- and program-specific, reinforcing changes supported at the state level and altering state goals at the margin. Such changes in state goals, however, are likely to occur only when the political environments of states are receptive to change. For although the federal government has the power to force states to pay attention to certain national goals, it cannot force them to shift their goals in any fundamental way or to accept those goals as legitimate.

According to Lehman (1987), a major effect of the Reagan administration's policies on state and local governments was the creation of a fiscal environment that forced state and local officials to rely more on their own—at times, inadequate—resources. This came about in several ways. First, federal aid as a percentage of total state–local outlays dropped from 25 percent in 1981 to around 19 percent in 1987, reversing a twenty-year trend from the 1950s to 1978. Second, in contrast to the practice under previous administrations, the federal government did not provide compensatory aid to states and localities hard hit by the economic downturn of the 1980s. As a result, many states created so-called rainy day funds to protect themselves should their economies suffer a serious downturn. Third, the Reagan administration continued the traditional federal policy toward the poorest states, that is, no special aids, forcing many to let programs formerly paid for by the federal government die. Finally, Reagan, like his predecessors, and with the help of Congress, increased the number of federally mandated but underfunded programs, requiring state and local governments to deliver more services in such areas as mental health and drug treatment, without additional funds to pay for them.

---

[29]Unlike the federal government, states are prevented by law from operating with a budget deficit. In the first part of 1983, for instance, forty states reportedly had experienced budget problems as a result of the recession. In the case of California, the government was forced to issue script, that is, IOUs, to creditors until a mutually acceptable budget balancing bill could be worked out between California's governor and the legislature.

PUBLIC AND PRIVATE FINANCING OF HEALTH CARE IN THE UNITED STATES

In contrast to most other industrialized nations in the world, which concentrate their resources in one health insurance system that provides universal or nearly universal coverage to their populations, the United States relies on an often diffuse, uncoordinated system of private and public providers of care and financing mechanisms to serve the health and medical care needs of its citizens. The nature of this system, or non-system, if you will, has been shaped, according to Iglehart (1993, p. 963), by a variety of factors, including pragmatism, political imperatives, periodic crises, a strong belief in limited government, individual freedom, science and technology, and an aversion to paying higher taxes.

Although initial consideration of the adoption of some form of national health insurance in the United States occurred at about the same time as in Europe (at the turn of the century) and in reaction to similar forces (industrialization, urbanization, the demise of the extended family, and employment practices and policies that heightened the threat of work-related injuries and disease as well as unemployment), unlike in Europe, the implementation of Social Security in the United States came about through selected income maintenance programs and the preservation of the voluntary sector (Blanpain, 1978).

Moreover, our devotion to economic individualism and a moralistic punitive stance toward the poor, Brown (1990) has noted, set us apart from Europe, Canada and other nations, where the "right to health care" is accepted as a kind of civic axiom. As a result, whereas in Europe national health insurance was built on a universal consensus that health care is a right, such protection in the United States has essentially revolved around work-related insurance in the private sector, leaving government a gap-filling role and from 10 percent to 15 percent of the population without any such coverage. All this led Brown (1989, p. 51) to observe that "in the United States, health care is a fringe benefit for most of the population, an entitlement qualified by categorical criteria for many, a matter of chance and charity for some."

Thus, the provision of third-party health insurance coverage in the United States developed primarily on a voluntary basis through Blue Cross and Blue Shield and the commercial insurance industry. The attendant mixture of approaches resulted in a complex pattern of health care financing in which (1) the employed are predominantly covered by voluntary insurance provided through contributions made by their employers and themselves; (2) the aged are insured through a combination of coverages financed out of Social Security tax revenues and voluntary insurance for physician and supplementary coverage; (3) the health care of the poor is covered through Medicaid via federal, state, and local revenues; and (4) special population groups, such as veterans, merchant seamen, Indians, members of the armed forces, Congress, and the executive branch, have coverage provided directly by the federal government (National Center for Health Services Research, 1977).

Private health insurance in this country, Kramer (1972) noted, primarily has been a collection of payment mechanisms that support and reinforce existing patterns of health services. Government spending for health, on the other hand, has been largely confined to filling the gap in the private sector, that is, environmental protection, preventive services, communicable disease control, care of special groups, institutional care of the mentally and chronically ill, provision of medical care to the poor, and support for research and training. The high cost of public medical care programs, she reminds us, owes its genesis to the unique division of risk taking and responsibility between the public and private sectors that has thrust upon government the cost of caring for those segments of the population with the highest incidence of illness and greatest need for care, that is, the aged, poor, mentally ill, retarded, chronically ill, and disabled.

In the absence of government action and given our penchant, as a nation, for private-sector solutions, we have relied heavily on employment-based, employer-provided health insurance as a means of providing coverage to the population, including even proposing to mandate such coverage as part of health care reform at both the state (e.g., Massachusetts, Minnesota, Washington) and national (Clinton) levels. The growth and development of such arrangements were stimulated by the incorporation of health insurance benefits as part of collective bargaining during the Second World War when wages and prices were frozen and by the favorable tax treatment they received. For unlike money wages, they were not deemed subject to either income or Social Security taxes for the worker, and could be deducted as a business expense by the employer.

Whereas over 80 percent of the workforce has access to health insurance through their place of employment and more than half of all Americans are covered by employment-based health insurance, reliance as a nation on such arrangements is not without its problems, chief among which are the following:

- It fails to assure universal coverage, applying only to those who are in the full-time workforce and possibly their dependents.
- Adequacy and extent of coverage are dependent on the generosity or power of the sponsors (i.e., employer or union vis-à-vis negotiation with third-party payers).
- Continuity of coverage is compromised, if not deterred, due to a lack of portability of benefits that do not transfer with a change in jobs—the focus of the bipartisan initiative introduced in the 104th Congress by Senators Kassebaum (R-KS) and Kennedy (D-MA).
- Both the cost of such coverage and its availability depend to a large extent on the size of the firm and type of industry, its union status, and the percentage of low wage earners on its payroll.
- Although originally provided by industry (big business) at a relatively low cost in lieu of wages, it has come to constitute a major drain on company revenues, especially that provided for retirees.
- Small businesses generally oppose mandated coverage, claiming that they cannot afford it, threatening to cut jobs or turn to part-time workers if forced to provide it—undercutting their competitors that do offer such coverage and making the playing field uneven.
- Due to their size, small businesses are discriminated against in the health insurance marketplace—paying more for coverage and subject to sharp increases in premiums or termination of coverage if one or more employees is at high risk because risk cannot be spread over a sufficiently large number of workers.
- Many businesses or occupations have been the subject of redlining (i.e., refused coverage due to presumed high risk) by the insurance industry.
- Many large industries have avoided state mandates and regulation under ERISA by self-insuring, again unbalancing the playing field.

The coexistence within the American health care system of a wide variety of providers, organizational forms, and financing sources has long been viewed as a positive attribute that has contributed not only to the innovation and rapid diffusion of new technology, but to the enhancement of quality care and the capacity of the system to adapt to change. Moreover, the use of fiscal stimuli through grants-in-aid, the commitment of major financing programs to retrospective reimbursement of costs on a fee-for-service basis, and reliance on peer review for quality assurance reflect a preference for the achievement of public objectives through strategies that offer inducements, persuasion, and positive rewards to providers for compliance rather than impose penalties or costs for failure to comply (National Center for Health Services, 1977; Anderson, 1968b). Such strategies, however, are and have been inherently expansive and expensive, tending to minimize the need for deliberate allocative choices by increasing the flow of resources into the health care system. Once costs rise and revenues become short, however, such choices no longer can be put off and questions of constraint and costs are raised.

Government Financing of Personnel Training: The Case of Medical Education

Before the enactment of the Health Professions Educational Assistance Act in 1963, the financing of graduate education in general and health professions in particular was traditionally within the purview of state government, students, or their families. The provision of direct financial aid from the federal government to medical schools in the 1960s and early 1970s to encourage biomedical research and expanded enrollments, bypassing the more traditional intergovernment transfer approach to funding aid, has been depicted by Millman (1980) as "private federalism."

At the state level, medical education tends to be addressed in the context of higher education rather than as part of health policy, and in response to state and local needs rather than to those of the nation as a whole; the opposite is true of federal endeavors. As the federal government has assumed an increasing role in the financial support of biomedical research and physician training—to the point where any given medical condition from prickly heat to cancer had its own congressional advocate for federal funding—an unduly large proportion of such support tended to be diverted from a focus on primary care to research and specialty training, distorting the teaching function of the educational institutions and perverting the long-standing reliance of public institutions on the largess of the state legislatures. So entwined had medical school financing become with federal funding for research and training that the state legislators and policymakers ended up on the outside looking in (Rogatz et al., 1970; Bloom & Martin, 1976). But if medical school dependence on federal financial support had become manifest over a twenty-five-year period, there was a point beyond which medical faculties were unwilling to go. This was reached in the late 1970s, when, in return for continued federal funding under the Health Professions Educational Assistance Act of 1976 (PL 94-484), Congress mandated that medical schools provide training for U.S. students studying abroad. Following the lead of two private institutions, Yale and Northwestern, along with the University of Indiana, U.S. medical schools, citing the abridgment of the right of educational institutions to determine their own admission policy, announced their refusal to go along with such a directive even if it cost them the price of federal support. In the face of such opposition, Congress "blinked" and the requirement was withdrawn.

The heyday of federal funding of health personnel training, however, appears to have been reached. So active and effective were such efforts that by the end of the past decade, the nation found itself with potentially more physicians and hospital beds than it needed. As a result, beginning in the mid-1970s and escalating

rapidly during the Reagan–Bush and Clinton administrations, federal goals have moved from a position of fostering a larger supply of health professionals to reducing sharply tax-based support for this purpose, leaving health professional schools and their students caught in the squeeze of rising educational costs, declining federal support, and reduced state revenues (Lewin & Derzon, 1981). In addition, Congress has sought to use its power over the purse strings to seek redress of the imbalance between specialist and generalist physicians through alteration of the General Medical Education (GME) formula used by Medicare to reimburse teaching hospitals.

THE PROBLEM OF COST VERSUS SERVICES IN GOVERNMENT PROGRAMS

The amount of money that a nation spends for its health services, as Anderson and Newhauser (1969) noted, tends to be a product primarily of a political process arrived at by implicit and explicit public policy decisions within the body politic. An equally appropriate maxim, however, is that whatever government giveth, it can taketh away. In other words, public programs are often initially enacted on essentially altruistic grounds, that is, to increase accessibility to health care services by removing the financial barriers to care and defraying the costs over a wide segment of the public. Once this is done, however, and the cost increases that were originally borne by patients, their families, or the private sector are now assumed by government, there is a strong tendency for the latter to cut back on its commitment by reducing the amount of coverage and increasing the amount paid by those who use the service.

Thus, as costs rise, the tendency is to cut back on the coverage especially if the constituency being served is not a very powerful or influential one, such as the poor, the socially and economically disadvantaged, and, up until the 1960s, the elderly.[30] For as commendable and

---

[30]Historically, considered politically impotent by politicians and political scientists alike, the aged, stimulated by their success in the battle over Medicare, have become an extremely potent electoral force in U.S. political life, heightened by their proclivity to vote. In contrast with those under twenty-five years of age, elderly voters consistently exhibit higher rates of electoral participation (Donahue & Tibbits, 1962).

needed a service may be and as legitimate as government involvement is, the question ultimately gets down to a fundamental economic one: the cost of the service given the limited funds (however defined) available for it.

And so, beginning in the latter part of the 1960s and early 1970s, the federal government and the states, confronted by escalating costs and depleted resources, began to cut back on the Medicare and Medicaid programs. Thus, in contrast to when the dual programs were first enacted and the primary policy concern was increased access to health care services for more U.S. citizens, ostensibly the aged and economically disadvantaged, the programs were so successful that the budget soon became incapable of containing them. As a result, the policy has taken a 180-degree turn,[31] going, in David Mechanic's (1986) terms, from one of advocacy to allocation and greater restriction and control, with the adverse effects on access and quality of care, in many cases a reflection of the admonition "penny cheap and pound foolish" (Roemer et al., 1975).

Case of Medicaid

This conflict between costs and services has been especially true of the Medicaid program, whose expenditures tend to be particularly susceptible to the forces of unemployment and inflation. For not only does the size of its clientele, that is, recipients of public assistance and "the medically indigent," vary with the level of unemployment, but the services it renders are purchased in the general medical marketplace and are susceptible to the impact of inflation. In addition, the negative effect of reduced tax receipts on state and local revenues as a result of a national economic recession tends to place both levels of government in a whipsaw as the demand for services on them rises because of heightened unemployment while their capacity to pay for them diminishes.

Moreover, not all states experience the impact of the burden equally. Since the federal contribution to Medicaid expenditures in a state historically depended on its per capita income relative to the national average two years earlier, the federal share has been relatively insen-

sitive to the distribution of the burden of the recession among the states or the mobility of welfare recipients between and within states (Davis, 1974, 1975a, 1976b).

At any rate, in the face of ever rising costs, fueled in part by the burden of unfunded federal mandates and diminished state revenues, state budgeting responses have taken on one or more of the following forms (Stone, 1992; Nye, 1991; Brown & Dallek, 1990), as our admonition on costs versus services tends to prevail:

1. reductions in the levels of eligibility, usually by lowering the income ceiling and thereby cutting down the number of potential recipients. In the case of the medically indigent, states had wide discretion in their determination of eligibility.
2. placement of limitations on the types and amount of services covered, that is, what and how much. This has generally taken the form of limitations on inpatient hospital services, that is, number of days per spell of illness or per year, cutbacks on optional services (other than those specifically mandated under the law), and reduction in services to the medically indigent.
3. reductions in the amount of provider reimbursement; placement of ceilings on maximal allowable profit; suspension of payments to providers, that is, physicians, hospitals, and nursing homes, sometimes arbitrarily determined; and, after the services have been rendered, leaving the patients to pay out of pocket, if they could, or the provider to absorb the cost—all of which has created considerable bitterness between patients and providers, as well as between providers and government. In fact, a major criticism leveled at the program by physicians and health care institutions has been its inadequate reimbursement and excessive red tape. This has led many providers to opt out of the program, leaving recipient patients to fend for themselves, avoid care, rely on an increasingly limited number of overworked private practitioners who would see them or on the services of notorious "Medicaid mills," seek care from the hard-pressed public hospitals, or make up the loss of income by excess visits, overuse of diagnostic lab work, and various forms of creative billing (Fever Chart, 1976).

---

[31]An interesting by-product of this new calculus was and has been the ascent of the role and involvement of the health economist and relative decline of that of the medical sociologist in health policy formulation and analysis.

4. the establishment of requirements for prior authorization or approval before treatment could be rendered as well as restrictions on where services could be obtained.

5. making it more difficult for nursing home patients to "spend down" by transferring their assets to their children or grandchildren in order to get the state to pay for the patients' care.

6. the use of deductibles and co-payment provisions in order to force recipients to share in the cost of the services by increasing their out-of-pocket expenses, which in turn, it has been argued, not only discourages use but helps offset or reduce the cost to government.[32]

7. increased use of managed care programs which restrict the sources of care beneficiaries may go to for service to those that afford the lowest cost to government. Some forty states, for instance, have "freedom of choice" waivers.

8. Medicaid maximization, that is, shifting such state-related health and social service programs as mental health, mental retardation, and some maternal and child health programs into Medicaid in order to obtain federal matching funds.

9. increased use of provider taxes and donations, intra- and intergenerational transfers, and disproportionate share hospitals (DSH) programs.

10. increasing cigarette taxes and earmarking any revenue gained to pay for health care.

11. conversion of the program to a block grant.

Finally, the willingness and ability of states to take such action are tempered by the fact that as a federal–state match program, Medicaid constitutes both an expenditure and revenue source for the state. As a result, any cutbacks in the program may be offset by an equal reduction in federal matching funds.

Case of Medicare

The situation has been much the same with the federally run Medicare program as the government has sought to recoup or reduce its costs, while reneging on its promises. Thus, beginning with the Nixon and Ford administrations and continuing under the succeeding Republican and Democratic administrations, attempts have been made to reduce the costs of the program by placing curbs on provider reimbursement and making the elderly assume more of the costs themselves by increasing the size of the deductible, the amount of co-payment required, and the premium for Part B, Supplementary Physician Coverage (e.g., from an initial $3.00 per month in 1966 to $46.10 in 1995 and projected to go even higher by the end of the decade), culminating in a proposal by the Reagan administration in early 1983 that called for the imposition of a "means test" on program beneficiaries.[33] Such provisions not only are a perversion of the original intent of the Medicare legislation (to relieve the elderly of the fear and heavy financial burden of the high cost of health and medical care while

---

[32]Such political-economic rhetoric and, perhaps, conventional wisdom aside, experience with such cost-sharing measures in the private sector, at least as far as inpatient hospital care is concerned, has proven to be far less cost-effective in reducing costs while often denying care for those most in need, delaying the need of more extensive services when such patients are ultimately admitted (*Blue Cross Perspectives,* 1972). Moreover, such devices focus primarily on the patients rather than the physicians who, through both their gatekeeping and decision-making roles, constitute the primary generators of costs in the institution. The reluctance, on the other hand, of politicians and government officials to impose controls on health care providers is a function of the essentially private character of the U.S. health care system. Thus, drafters of the Medicare and Medicaid legislation were wary of placing onerous restrictions on providers lest they withhold their services or fail to participate in the programs, fearing a possible replication of Canada's experience with a physicians' boycott in Saskatchewan (Tollefson, 1964). As a result, reliance was placed on the good faith of the medical profession and the provision of financial incentives to hospitals and third-party carriers for cooperation (Feingold, 1966; Marmor, 1973; Skidmore, 1970).

---

[33]In contrast to the infamous requirement of a pauper's oath to determine eligibility under the old Kerr–Mills program in the early 1960s, which was considered to be particularly demeaning by the elderly, most of whom had lived through the Depression and had taken pride in their independence and unwillingness to accept charity, the Reagan proposal sought to reduce the payment of benefits to the more affluent by placing an upper income limit on eligibility. The eventual result, however, would have been the same, that is, the conversion of the program from an earned entitlement available to all to an income-based benefit program limited to just some. The notion of tying the monthly premium the elderly would need to pay for Medicare Part B physician coverage to the size of their income reemerged again during the 1995–96 battle over the budget between the Republican-dominated 104th Congress and President Clinton.

allowing them to retain their sense of dignity through the mechanism of social insurance), but stand in direct contradistinction to the recommendations of almost every government and nongovernment advisory group and study commission appointed to look at the program over its first two and a half decades, including the 1971 and 1981 White House Conferences on Aging.

Such arguments aside, however, in the face of a growing budget deficit and rising health care costs, the above movement appeared to come to full fruition with the passage of the Catastrophic Coverage Act in 1988, which for the first time required that the cost of the program be borne by the recipients themselves through the imposition of a self-financing provision tied to a progressive tax structure, with income to be used as a determinant of the level of payment rather than as a basis of eligibility. But while perhaps justifiable on economic grounds, permitting an expansion of the Medicare program and an extension of benefits without an adverse effect on the federal budget, it evoked an immediate negative response from many of the nation's middle- and upper-income elderly, who bombarded their elective representatives with demands to repeal the act, rescind its income-related payment features, and return the benefits to entitlement status.

Finally, while all such cost-containment measures may well make public officials and their statistics look good,[34] they offer little solace to those who, in many cases through no fault of their own, are in need of care but are ineligible to receive it. Moreover, shifting the cost of such services to those who use them neither solves the problem nor removes the burden, but merely shifts it back onto those least able to bear it.

Thus, given the central focus cost containment has come to assume in government health and social programs, the ultimate question the United States must come to grips with is how much deterrence because of cost is both tolerable and permissible and in what areas. Again, it is the constituency with the least political power—the poor and socially disadvantaged—who are the most likely to feel the brunt of such cuts.

---

[34]To some, the "cheapest program" of all is the one in which no expenditures are made even though the cost of doing nothing ultimately may be higher.

A Case for a Federal Presence in Health and Health Care

The growth in the federal government's role in health and health care in the United States has not been without its problems and negative consequences, such as escalating costs, bureaucratic inflexibility, excessive regulation, red tape and paperwork, arbitrary and, at times, conflicting public directives, inconsistent enforcement of rules and regulations, fraud and abuse, inadequate reimbursement schedules, arbitrary denial of claims, insensitivity to local needs, consumer and provider dissatisfaction, and charges that such efforts tend to promote dependence rather than work.

Among the arguments cited for decentralizing such programs are the following:

- Our distrust of centralized government in general and lack of faith in the federal government as an administrator in particular (Morone, 1995; Tallon & Nathan, 1992; Grogan, 1993, p. 756) .
- The federal government has grown too large, intrusive, and paternalistic.
- The federal government is too impersonal, distant, and unresponsive.
- State and local governments are closer to the people and more familiar with local needs; therefore, they are more accessible and accountable to the public and better able to develop responsive programs than are federal agencies (Fein, 1980).
- National standards reduce flexibility and seriously constrain the ability of states to experiment and innovate. Nye (1991, p. 28), for instance, has noted that the often criticized lack of uniformity in Medicaid rates, benefits, and eligibility among the states allows them to respond more flexibly to local interests and concerns.
- In contrast to thirty years ago, states are better equipped to take on such functions (i.e., more full-time legislators, more professional staffs and bureaucrats) (Sparer, 1995).
- States are more likely to implement and enforce programs of their own making.
- States have served as important laboratories for testing different structures, approaches, and programs

and providing insight into the political and technical barriers encountered in enactment and implementation (Barrand & Schroeder, 1994).

- States respond to crises faster (Riley, 1995).
- It is easier to change a state law than a federal one (Riley, 1994).
- States are more willing to take risks (Sommerville, 1994).

Such problems and criticisms aside, the reason for a national endeavor in this area is not only that more funds are available and collectible at the federal level, but also and more important, there is an implied national commitment to action and resolution of the problem.[35] Illness and disease, for example, do not recognize jurisdictional boundaries and are nationwide in scope. Chronic disease, alcoholism and drug abuse, hypertension and stroke are as much a threat to the suburban as the inner-city population. Moreover, worldwide transportation and communication systems make a disease anywhere a potential problem everywhere, as exemplified by the various versions of the Asian flu in the 1970s and AIDS in the 1980s and 1990s. Thus, although health and human service programs may well be more administratively amenable to state and local control, the latter's track record in this area has been anything but impressive.

While the states, with the prompting of the U.S. Supreme Court in the early 1960s, have tended to improve greatly their administrative and legislative structures, which were the objects of allegations of incompetence and insensitivity to the needs of the socially and economically disadvantaged just a generation ago, they still possess a number of inherent weaknesses that severely deter their ability and willingness to assume a more extensive role in the organization, financing, and delivery of health and human services. Among these are the unpredictability and instability of state revenues, ideological inflexibility, and a bias and aversion to re-

distributive programs that benefit the poor (Sparer, 1995); an antigovernment political climate that has seen voters in some two dozen states impose term limits on their state legislators and place restrictions on the length of time lawmakers meet and the size of their operating budgets (Kent, 1995); and a lack of adequate data collection systems, much less analytic expertise to take on such a daunting task as health care reform (Holmes, 1994).

Furthermore, in addition to being unequal in financial ability, states differ widely in their needs for services and financial capacity to provide them. As a result, they are vulnerable to interstate competition over which state can provide the lowest amount of services to the fewest numbers in order to offer or maintain the most attractive business tax climate, that is, the race to the bottom. Similarly, states tend to be parochial in outlook and ready to pursue and preserve their own self-image in competition with other states in regard to population, industry, and the welfare burden, which leads to serious inequities in the assumption and delivery of services. Although innovative and at times ahead of their national counterparts, state actions tend to be piecemeal and lacking in uniformity. Fifty governors, fifty legislatures, and a host of laws, rules, and regulations for insurance all contribute to a patchwork system that poses a major headache to businesses that operate across state lines (Friedman, 1994; Barrand & Schroeder, 1994). Nor can states alone assure continuity of coverage (portability) for workers who move from state to state (Findley & Loranger, 1995, p. 36). Finally, state regulation of nursing homes, health insurance, pollution control, and so on, has often proven to be weak, episodic, and susceptible to industry capture.

In addition to the above, a further impediment to state health care reform has been the Employee Retirement Income Security Act (ERISA). Enacted in 1974 to protect the financial solvency of workers' pensions and health benefits, ERISA was intended to protect beneficiaries and pension plans from fraud and mismanagement and to give employers and unions greater flexibility in providing benefits to their employees. A key provision of the law, however, Section 514, precludes states from regulating employee benefits, leaving

---

[35]Nevertheless, as Clarke and others have aptly observed, although federal health policy may constitute a national consensus to do something, the actual implementation of such policy is often dependent on the influence of the "political environment" of the states (Clarke, 1981; Buntz et al., 1978; Altenstetter & Bjorkman, 1978).

them powerless to regulate firms that self-insure (more than half of the nation's insured population is covered by such plans), unless they can obtain a federal waiver. State efforts to do so, however, have been deterred by opposition from organized labor and large employers, who cite the difficulty of doing business in fifty states with fifty different sets of rules and the loss of flexibility to meet workers' needs and contain costs (Firshein, 1994).

Finally, while states can and do act as crucibles of innovation and serve as laboratories of experimentation, their reproducibility and ability to sustain such efforts in the face of economic distress remain open to question. Thus whereas in the absence of federal action in the late 1980s and early 1990s, some forty-four states, squeezed by recession and spiraling health care costs, had moved or enacted legislation that would reform the way health care is paid for and provided inside their borders, following the demise of the Clinton plan and the 1994 off-year elections the ardor for such reform waned. Oregon and Massachusetts, for example, postponed requiring employer contributions. Minnesota delayed implementing a key part of the program, establishment of integrated networks. Washington's and Vermont's efforts at reform ended in defeat at the hands of their state legislatures. Even Hawaii, long heralded as the first state to enact comprehensive health care reform legislation in 1974, in the face of ballooning enrollments in its Health Quest Program, began tightening its eligibility requirements in 1995 (*State Initiatives,* 1995; *State Health Watch,* 1995).

A similar situation exists at the local level. Often plagued by antiquated administrative structures, a lack of legal authority, insufficient financial resources, and a dearth of qualified personnel, local efforts frequently have been susceptible to petty conflicts of interests such as rural–urban or urban–suburban differences, racial and economic discrimination, and lack of uniformity in the provision of services or the requirements for eligibility. In some southern and rural counties, county welfare officials in the 1960s and 1970s waged deliberate campaigns to encourage families on relief to go to the more industrialized states or cities of the Northeast and Midwest where welfare payments were higher—even providing one-way tickets so as to reduce their own expenditures for welfare.

Many county officials, moreover, prefer local determination in deciding who should get benefits, regardless of the provisions of the law vis-à-vis eligibility. Some years ago (1968) at a joint meeting on legislative affairs put on by Minnesota's Health and Welfare Departments, a county commissioner from one of the state's southern rural areas was heard to say how he liked to know who was on welfare and determine for himself whether they *really* belonged there and needed what they claimed. "You know, when you live out there, you kind of get to know who should and shouldn't be on the welfare rolls." Federal or state rules and regulations aside, his role, as he perceived it, was that of a self-proclaimed judge and jury.

Similarly, many county boards, in the face of angry taxpayers and disgruntled voters (the taxpayers' revolt), tend to be particularly tightfisted with regard to expenditures for such services, often with self-defeating results. Several years ago, for example, an orthopedic patient at the Kenny Rehabilitation Institute in the Twin Cities would have been able to return home and lead a fairly productive life if the county had agreed to purchase a wheelchair. The county refused to do so, however, on grounds that such an expenditure was a luxury, resulting in a medically unnecessary and prolonged high-cost hospital stay at the county's expense.

Finally, the heavy reliance of local government on the property tax makes the provision of such services extremely difficult. This is especially so in view of the regressive nature of the tax as well as the fact that those who tend to benefit the most from such services or use them disproportionately more are the very ones—the poor and the elderly—who are the hardest hit by the tax and most resistant to increases in it, even to pay for the very services they rely or depend on. And so, given that many of our problems of health and health care are not restricted to or confined by city, county, township, or state lines and can effectively be resolved only on a broader geographic basis, we have tended to opt for a more global approach. As Anderson (1955) and others have noted, when problems tend to be national in scope, they call for national solutions. And over time, it has been the federal rather than constituent states who have had to act—sometimes alone, sometimes with the aid of the states, and sometimes in the aid of states. It has done so, moreover, consonant with the values and structure of the U.S. social, political, and economic system.

Conclusion

The growth in government's involvement in health has been an evolutionary one, responding to changes in times and circumstances. Over the past forty years, there have been major shifts in the role and posture of the federal government in the organization, financing, and delivery of health care services and its relationship with the states, in which the following have occurred:

1. The traditional federal role of sharing the cost of health care gradually has been expanded to include programs of care purchased by the government itself as well as the use of federal funding to initiate and develop new forms of delivery, such as, neighborhood health centers and health maintenance organizations (HMOs) (Penchansky & Axelson, 1974).
2. An increased use of categorical and project grants in health found the federal government involved in the budget funding of local programs and bypassing local governments considered unresponsive to the needs of the poor (Penchansky & Axelson, 1974).
3. The federal focus has shifted from encouraging the expansion of state programs to assuring their integrity and from concern over improving access to services to control over their costs, with both patients and providers often caught in the middle.

The progression in such involvement has been a slow and steady one, a function of the nature of the nation's political process and social and economic systems. Incrementalism, rather than fundamental changes in the structure of the health care delivery system, has been the hallmark of federal policies (Falik, 1975). What has evolved, then, as Anderson (1968a) has aptly observed, has been a partnership—sometimes rather tenuous and strained—between government (federal and state) and the voluntary system, working together, not as rivals but as partners—not necessarily equally or smoothly, but as partners nevertheless.

At a time when the nation is in the throes of reassessing its sociopolitical policy agenda, it may be useful to briefly review some of the lessons that can be learned from the experience of this and other countries with various government entreaties in health and health care.

1. Each nation's health care system is unique, based on its own social, political, cultural, and economic history and foundation.
2. All modern national health care systems, predicated as they are on sophisticated technology, are inherently costly (Anderson & Newhauser, 1969).
3. There is a significant positive correlation between a country's national per capita income and the share of that income devoted to health care (Evans, 1986, p. 87).
4. A striking feature of the international experience is the association of universal coverage with substantially lower expenditures for health services (Evans, 1986).
5. All countries, regardless of the percentage of their gross national (domestic) product (GNP) spent on health services, feel that such services are impinging on other priorities (Anderson, 1995, p. 10).
6. National health services, publicly owned and managed, have more direct control over expenditures, more equitable distribution of services, resources, and allocative efficiency, and lower out-of-pocket costs than a Social Security-type system (Elola et al., 1995).
7. No system of health care financing is free of problems or easily administered. Rather, all involve a trade-off between what a nation wants and what it can afford (Marmor, 1991, p. 5).
8. No nation has ever enacted a comprehensive health insurance program over the determined and united opposition of its medical profession without negotiating concessions and winning the relevant acquiescence of some factions (Glaser, 1994, p. 706).
9. Due to the inability of government-financed systems to respond to the many nuances of need and demand perceived by the public, every country with government and universal health insurance has a private medical sector, access to which a segment of the population is willing to pay or purchase insurance in order to increase their entry options (Anderson, 1995, p. 29).

10. Reform of the health care system in the United States is likely to be incremental, the result of a compromise involving the resolution of a number of competing interests.

11. Politics will always dominate policy analysis in the legislative process (Hadley, 1995, p. 128).

12. The formulation and enactment of health policy are influenced more by partisan politics and political ideology than the results of health services research.

13. Efforts to attain health care reform are more likely to succeed when couched in terms of cost containment (an economic, business, and middle-class concern) than improved or expanded access (a social justice, liberal, labor, low-income issue).

14. All third-party coverage, whether private or public, such as Medicare and Medicaid, contributes to inflation (Davis, 1974).

15. Open-ended reimbursement to providers on the basis of cost is inflationary, whereas inadequate, unrealistic, persistently lower payments or picayune controls tend to be self-defeating, leading providers to increased cost shifting or opting out of the system, leaving recipients a limited range of care choices.

16. An open-ended system of health care financing invites uncontrolled expenditure growth. The provision of "à la carte" financing in which each service component (i.e., hospital, physician, nursing home, home health care) is purchased separately from the same or different providers, and in which each provider is then paid for each service, is inherently inflationary, since vendors have a financial incentive to maximize the use of their services and thereby increase their own revenues, regardless of budgetary constraints on individual patients or the overall health care system (Waters & Tierney, 1984, p. 1251).

17. An inherent danger in constraining program expenditures is impaired access to and quality of care for beneficiaries, especially the more vulnerable segments of society—the poor, the old, and the infirm. As a result, careful monitoring is necessary to safeguard their interests (Sisk et al., 1987).

18. Health policy decision making in this country, over the past six administrations, has been dominated by the tyranny of the budget (Feldman, 1988).

19. A conflict between cost and services is inherent in government programs.

20. Equality in financing is not sufficient to guarantee equal access to medical care (Davis, 1974).

21. Access and cost control are complementary, not conflicting, goals. Government attempts to achieve universal access without containing costs are doomed to failure (McDonough, 1992).

22. Utilitarianism, that is, "put people back to work" and "get them off the welfare rolls and onto the taxpaying rolls," rather than humanitarianism and altruism, is the underlying motive for the ultimate adoption of most government human services programs.

23. While rising costs appear to be independent of type of ownership, source of funding, method of payment, or organization of delivery systems (Anderson, 1976), the ability to control such costs is not. For not only do industrialized Western nations with the greatest degree of government funding and administration of health services have the most extensive population coverage and the lowest administrative costs, but those in which the central government plays a major role in financing health services via general central taxation tend to have the greatest success in controlling health care expenditures (Navarro, 1985).

24. The maintenance of separate financing systems under a pluralistic system of health care financing leads to cost shifting, with each source of payment, public and private, seeking to protect itself at the expense of others by shifting costs to someone else. Such cost shifting may be minimized and financial responsibility for care fixed and apportioned through the adoption of an all payers system (Waters & Tierney, 1984).

25. Attempts by states to impose system-wide limits on health care spending or to control costs through some form of global budgeting, without nationally imposed ceilings applied to all states, risks being placed at a competitive disadvantage (Dukakis, 1992).

26. Application of cost controls to a narrowly defined population or set of services can result in or lead

providers to increase their charges to other population groups or services not subject to such constraints.

27. Government efforts to reduce expenditures for health services programs by transferring their costs, without appropriate financial safeguards, to lesser levels of government or recipients of services do not effectively reduce the overall costs of the services but merely shift the financial burden to those least able to bear it while depriving those most in need.

28. Once implemented, even well-designed public programs cannot be left unattended. Rather, they must be adapted to the changing conditions and needs of their beneficiaries (Schlesigner, 1988).

29. Any major domestic reform, especially one that imposes buyer costs, must enjoy a broad base of public support, especially among the middle class (Gergan & Slafsky, 1992).

30. While it is axiomatic in American politics that any major domestic reform, especially one that imposes higher costs, must enjoy a broad base of public support, especially among the middle class before Congress will act, high levels of favorable public opinion are not sufficient to guarantee passage. For example, over the course of the past sixty years, the percentage of persons expressing support for a greater government role in health care has ranged from 80 percent in 1937 to 74 percent in 1942; 67 percent in 1961; 63 percent in 1965; 66.7 percent in 1976; 61.3 percent in 1978; and 75 percent in 1992. Yet America is the last major industrialized nation in the world without a national health insurance system (Steinmo & Watts, 1995).

31. National programs require consideration of regional and local problems and needs.

32. Regional variations and the diversity and voluntary-private nature of the health care enterprise make the imposition of national fee schedules, reimbursement formulas, and facility guidelines difficult, if not impossible, to achieve.

33. States vary in their fiscal capacity and political willingness to organize and underwrite care, with often those in greatest need the least able (in terms of

fiscal resources) and least willing to do so. The same may be said at the local level.

34. The success of any national health care reform initiative is dependent on the widespread acceptance by the middle class that whatever its attendant risks and uncertainties, it is preferable to maintaining the status quo (Blumenthal, 1995).

35. While well-meaning and innovative, private charity may supplement and complement, but not substitute for, government programs. For not only are the needs too large and the resources too few, but the likelihood of their being reproducible on a large scale is questionable (Fein, 1988).

36. By themselves, the states cannot provide or assure universal access to health care at an affordable cost for all Americans (Dukakis, 1992).

37. Employment-related benefit programs, unless subsidized by government directly or indirectly (e.g., via tax credits), are unlikely to attain universal coverage due to the inability or unwillingness of small employers (i.e., less than one hundred employees) to offer such benefits because of uncertainty over those firms' fiscal stability and viability, significant start-up and potential termination costs associated with pension plans, and disproportionately high administrative costs.

38. Although any government system is likely ultimately to impose restrictions on the autonomy and prerogatives of providers, in a society such as the United States, where the private sector is dominant, such controls can neither be arbitrary nor capricious but should seek the cooperation of professional interests and the use of financial incentives and rewards.

39. In order for the states to make significant progress toward universal coverage, a combination of employer or individual mandates and subsidies along with federal assistance will be necessary (Lipson, 1994).

40. Protection against the financial burden of health and medical care is impossible without the placement of a ceiling on the patient's financial responsibility. Unless the family is guaranteed that its share of the cost of care will not exceed some reasonable

fraction of income, the goal of preventing or protecting against the financial burden of health care services cannot be achieved (Davis, 1974). But while the level of income or ceiling is open to debate, it should be noted that artificial financial barriers or income cutoffs tend to be highly susceptible to the tyranny of inflation; that is, as dollar amounts soar, real value and purchasing power decline.

41. The use of administrative and regulatory controls, such as Medicare's former requirement of a three-day hospital stay before a patient can be admitted to a nursing home, second opinion requirements, inadequate reimbursement to providers, reduction of the tax deduction for health and medical expenditures, and elimination of deductibility for health insurance premiums, rather than civil or criminal penalties, tend to be misdirected, self-defeating, and ultimately ineffective.

42. Programs covering only poor people must be carefully designed so as to avoid adverse incentives and inequities in which some people receive substantial assistance and others equally in need or deserving, that is, the near-poor or working poor, receive nothing or practically nothing.

43. Assumptions that the elderly are protected against the cost of long-term care by Medicare are ill-founded and in error. The only government-provided protection the elderly have against the cost of long-term chronic illness is Medicaid—a welfare program.

44. Pinning one's hopes or relying on an employment-based health care system is tenuous at best in both terms of access and cost containment, with those who have the weakest or least political and economic influence likely to be the least well served.

45. Universal coverage, regardless of its merits, cannot nor should be expected to alter basically the wide gaps in residential patterns and living conditions that separate the poor and the middle class (Ginsberg, 1994).

46. Government health care programs predicated on the virtues of competition and the free marketplace and a preferred single delivery system ignore the fact that one of the major sources of the high cost of hospital care in the United States has been the virtually unfettered, costly competition between health institutions for staff, equipment, and so on, which results in a duplication of services and minimizes the value of a diverse pluralistic system of delivery and the variable needs and demands of consumers as well as providers.

47. Despite claims to the contrary, there is no historical proof for the superiority of either government regulation or market competition in achieving optimal performance of the health care system (Schramm, 1986).

48. Legislative intent may often be thwarted, if not obviated, by the executive branch through the appointment of unsympathetic or even antithetical administrators, delay or failure to promulgate enabling regulations, issuance of contradictory orders, or failure to spend or rescind appropriated funds (e.g., OSHA, Environmental Protection, the Superfund, Family Planning and Abortion under the Nixon and Reagan administrations).

49. While governments are generally adept at creating and distributing benefits, whether in the form of direct subsidies or services, they are often woefully inexperienced and lack the political will to reduce or eliminate such benefits and services, particularly if they affect politically important constituencies (e.g., entitlement programs such as Medicare and Social Security and the aged) (Rabe, 1987, p. 40; Light, 1985).

50. Whatever the future role of government in health in the United States is to be, it will be the product of a deliberative decision made in the political arena and will likely embrace the unique features of the nation's social, political, economic, and health care system.

That some of these may seem contradictory is a reflection of the complexity involved in such endeavors in meshing the needs of the disparate parts of a pluralistic society such as ours, predicated and reliant as it is on the private sector for the provision of health care services.

And so the debate over the role of government in health and health care in this country goes on, and although it remains hazardous to guess where it will end, suffice it to say that given the predilection and expectations of the American public, one would expect that regardless of the mix, that is, government versus private:

- demand for quality services will remain high
- costs, if left unattended, will continue to grow—the question is, how much?
- each of the parties involved will seek to shift the burden of costs on to someone else
- demand for the imposition of some form of control, either explicit or implicit, will continue to be increasingly heard
- heralded new, innovative, miracle solutions will neither be new nor necessarily effective in stemming costs or impoving access, for the more things change, the more they stay the same

REFERENCES

Advisory Commission on Intergovernmental Relations. (1980). *The federal role in the federal system: The dynamics of growth.* Washington, D.C.: Advisory Commission on Intergovernmental Relations.

Altenstetter, Christa, & James Bjorkman. (1978). *State health politics and impacts: The politics of implementation.* Washington, D.C.: University Press of America.

Anderson, Odin W. (1966). Compulsory medical care insurance, 1910–1950. In Eugene Feingold (Ed.), *Medicare: Policy and politics.* San Francisco: Chandler Publishing Co.

Anderson, Odin W. (1968a). *The uneasy equilibrium, private and public financing of health services in the U.S. 1875–1965.* New Haven: College and University Press.

Anderson, Odin W. (1968b). Health services in a land of plenty. In William R. Ewald Jr. (Ed.), *Environment and policy: The next fifty years* (pp. 59–102). Bloomington: Indiana University Press. Also *Health administration perspectives, A7.* Chicago: University of Chicago Center for Health Administration Studies, Graduate School of Business.

Anderson, Odin W. (1976). All health care systems struggle against rising cost. *Hospitals, 50* (October 1), 97–102.

Anderson, Odin W. (1995). The health services establishment is becoming an independent variable: A life of its own. *Medical Care Research and Review, 52* (March), 6–33.

Anderson, Odin W., & Duncan Newhauser. (1969). Rising costs are inherent in modern health care. *Hospitals, 43* (February 16), 50–52.

Anderson, William A. (1955). *Nations and states: Rivals or partners.* Minneapolis: University of Minnesota Press.

Barrand, Nancy L., & Steven A. Schroeder. (1994). Lessons from the states. *Inquiry, 31* (Spring), 10–13.

Belknap, Ivan, & John G. Steinle. (1963). *The community and its hospitals: A comparative analysis.* Syracuse: Syracuse University Press.

Bellin, Lowell E. (1969). Medicaid in New York: Utopianism and bare knuckles public health. *American Journal of Public Health, 59,* 820–825.

Bellin, Lowell E. (1970). The new left and American public health—attempted radicalization of the American public health association through dialectic. *American Journal of Public Health, 60,* 973–981.

Blanpain, Jan, with Luc Delesie & Herman Nys. (1978). *National health insurance and health resources: The European experience.* Cambridge, MA: Harvard University Press.

Bloom, Bernard S., & Samuel P. Martin. (1976). The role of the federal government in financing health and medical services. *Journal of Medical Education, 51,* 161–169.

Blue Cross Perspectives. (1972). *7* (3), 1–5.

Blumenthal, David. (1995). Health care reform—past and future. *New England Journal of Medicine, 332* (February 16), 465–468.

Blumstein, James W., & Michael Zubkoff. (1973). Perspectives on government policy in the health sector. *Milbank Memorial Fund Quarterly, 51,* 395–431.

Brandon, William. (1977). Politics, administration and conflict in neighborhood health centers. *Journal of Health Politics, Policy and Law, 2,* 79–99.

Brown, E. Richard. (1996). Block grants and the public's health. President's Column. *The Nation's Health* (January), 2.

Brown, E. Richard, & Geraldine Dallek. (1990). State approaches to financing health care for the poor. *Annual Review of Public Health, 11,* 377–400.

Brown, Lawrence D. (1978). The scope and limits of equality as a normative guide to federal health care policy. *Public Policy, 26,* 481–532. Also The Brookings Institution General Series Reprint, No. 350, 1977.

Brown, Lawrence D. (1989). *Health policy in the United States: Issues and options* (Occasional Paper 4). New York: Ford Foundation.

Brown, Lawrence D. (1990). The deconstructed center: Of policy plagues on political houses. *Journal of Health Politics and Law, 15* (Summer), 427–434.

Buntz, C. Gregory, Theodore F. Macaluso, & Jay Allen Azarow. (1978). Federal influence on state health policy. *Journal of Health Politics, Policy and Law, 3,* 71–78.

Burke, Edmund. (1968). Citizen participation strategies. *Journal of the American Institute of Planners, 34,* 287.

Carter, Richard. (1958). *The doctor business.* New York: Doubleday and Co.

The Center for Public Integrity. (1994). *Well-healed: Inside lobbying for health care reform.* Washington, D.C.: The Center for Public Integrity.

Chapman, Carleton B., & John M. Talmadge. (1970). Historical and political background of federal health care legislation. *Law and Contemporary Problems, 35,* 334–347.

Chapman, Carleton B., & John M. Talmadge. (1971). The evolution of the right to health concept in the United States. *The Pharos, 34* (January), 30–51.

Clarke, Gary J. (1980). State government: Where the action is. *The Nation's Health* (April), 16.

Clarke, Gary J. (1981). The role of the states in the delivery of health services. *American Journal of Public Health, 71* (Suppl.), 59–69.

Colford, Steven W. (1995). Health care PACs favor Republicans. *USA Today* (November 30), A6.

Common Cause. (1992). The medical-industry complex and its PAC contributions to congressional candidates—January 1, 1981 through June 30, 1991: A common cause study. *Journal of Public Health Policy, 13* (Summer), 224–241.

Congressional Quarterly. (1972). Lobbies: The Washington lobby: A continuing struggle to influence government policy. *Congressional Quarterly guide: Current American Government.* Washington, D.C.: Congressional Quarterly, Inc., 1–4.

Congressional Quarterly. (1981). Block grants: An old Republican idea. *Congressional Quarterly* (March 14), 449.

Congressional Quarterly. (1982). Reconciliation's long-term consequences in question as Reagan signs massive bill. *Congressional Quarterly* (Spring), 55–60.

Congressional Quarterly. (1986). Budget Office evolves into key policy maker. *Congressional Quarterly Almanac* (Spring), 7–11.

Congressional Quarterly. (1988). Lobbies. The Washington lobby: A continuing effort to influence government policy. *Congressional Quarterly Almanac* (Spring), 83–87.

Crain, Robert L., Elihu Katz, & Donald B. Rosenthal. (1968). *The politics of community conflict—The fluoridation decision.* Indianapolis: Bobbs-Merrill Co.

Davidson, Stephen M. (1978). Variations in state Medicaid programs. *Journal of Health Politics, Policy and Law, 3,* 54–70.

Davis, Karen. (1974). Lessons of Medicare and Medicaid for national health insurance. The Brookings Institution General Series Report No. 295. Washington, D.C.: The Brookings Institution.

Davis, Karen. (1975a). Equal treatment and unequal benefits: The Medicare program. *Milbank Memorial Fund Quarterly/ Health and Society, 53,* 449–488. Also The Brookings Institution General Series Report No. 317, 1974.

Davis, Karen. (1975b). *National health insurance: Benefits, costs and consequences.* Washington, D.C.: The Brookings Institution.

Davis, Karen. (1976a). Medicaid payments and utilization of medical services by the poor. *Inquiry, 13,* 127–135.

Davis, Karen. (1976b). Achievements and problems of Medicaid. *Public Health Reports, 91,* 309–316. Also The Brookings Institution General Series Report No. 318, 1977.

Donahue, Wilma, & Clark Tibbits. (Eds.). (1962). *Politics of age* (pp. 36–47, 48–59, 63–74). Ann Arbor: Division of Gerontology, University of Michigan.

Downey, Gregg W. (1975). OMB, the secret of the secret agency. *Modern Health Care* (September), 23–27.

Drew, Elizabeth. (1967). The health syndicate—Washington's noble conspirators. *Atlantic Monthly, 220* (December), 75–82.

Dukakis, Michael S. (1992). The states and health care reform. *New England Journal of Medicine, 327* (October 8), 1090–1092.

Eisler, Peter. (1995). Plan severs federal ties to nursing homes. *USA Today* (September 25), A6.

Elling, Ray H. (1968). The shifting power structure in health. *Milbank Memorial Fund Quarterly, 46,* 119–144.

Elling, Ray H., & Ollie Lee. (1966). Formal connections of community leadership to health systems. *Milbank Memorial Fund Quarterly, 44* (Part 1, July), 294–306.

Elola, Javier, Antonio Daponte, & Vicente Navarro. (1995). Health indicators and the organizational health care systems in Western Europe. *American Journal of Public Health, 95* (October), 1397–1401.

Ettorre, Barbara. (1992). Is real reform possible? *Management Review* (July).

Evans, Robert G. (1986). Finding the levers, finding the courage: Lessons from cost containment in North America. *Journal of Health Politics, Policy and Law, 11,* 585–616.

Falik, Marilyn. (1975). Health as a political issue: The national foci. *Health politics, A Quarterly Bulletin, 5* (Summer), 12–17.

Falk, Isidore S. (1967a). Medical care in a university teaching program for hospital administration. *Medical Care, 5,* 6.

Falk, Isidore S. (1967b). Medical care and social policy. *Medical Care in Transition, 3* (PHS Publication No. 1128), 269–274.

Falk, Isidore S. (1977). National health insurance for the United States. *Public Health Reports, 92,* 399–406.

Falkson, Joseph. (1976). Minor skirmish in a monumental struggle: HEW's analysis of mental health services. *Policy Analysis, 2,* 93–119.

Federation of American Hospitals. (1979). Brookings and AEI: Testing grounds for "shadow cabinets" and policy ideas. *Review, 12,* 29–33.

Fein, Rashi. (1980). Social and economic attitudes shaping American health policy. *Milbank Memorial Fund Quarterly/Health and Society, 8,* 349–385.

Fein, Rashi. (1988). Toward adequate health care: Why we need national health insurance. *Dissent* (Winter): 98–104.

Feingold, Eugene. (1966). *Medicare: Policy and politics.* San Francisco: Chandler Publishing Co.

Feingold, Eugene. (1973). Citizen participation: A review of the issues. *The Citizenry and the Hospital,* 8–16. Duke Forum, Duke University.

Feldman, Roger D. (1988). Health care: The tyranny of the budget. In David Boaz (Ed.), *Assessing the Reagan years* (223–241). Washington, D.C.: CATO Institute.

Felicetti, Daniel A. (1975). *Mental health and retardation politics: The mind lobbies in Congress.* Lexington, MA: Lexington Books.

Fever Chart. (1976). *American Medical Association News* (March 22).

Finch, Robert. (1970). Testimony given before the United States Congress Senate Committee on Government Operations. *The federal role in health* (The Ribicoff Report) (Senate Report No. 809). Washington, D.C.: U.S. Government Printing Office.

Findlay, Steven, & Linda Loranger. (1995). Health reform 2. Should Congress look to the states? *Business and Health* (June), 28–38.

Firshein, Janet. (1994). Business retreats on comprehensive health reform. *Medicine and Health Perspectives* (August 22).

Foltz, Anne-Marie. (1975). The development of ambiguous federal policy: Early and periodic screening diagnosis and treatment (EPSDT). *Milbank Memorial Fund Quarterly/Health and Society, 53,* 35–64.

Foltz, Anne-Marie, & Donna Brown. (1975). State response to federal policy: Children, EPSDT and the Medicaid muddle. *Medical Care, 13,* 630–642.

Forgotson, Edward H. (1967). 1965: The turning point in health law—1966 reflections. *American Journal of Public Health, 57,* 934–946.

Friedman, Emily. (1977a). Medicaid: The promise path. *Hospitals* (August 16), 51–56.

Friedman, Emily. (1977b). The problems and promises of Medicaid. *Hospitals, 51* (Series April–November).

Friedman, Emily. (1994). Getting a head start: The states and health care reform. *Journal of the American Medical Association, 271* (March 16), 875–878.

Fuchs, Beth C., & John F. Hoadley. (1987). Reflections from inside the Beltway: How Congress and the president grapple with health policy. *PS, 20* (Spring), 212–220.

Fuchs, Victor. (1976). From Bismarck to Woodcock: The irrational pursuit of national health insurance. *Journal of Law and Economics, 19* (August), 347–359.

Fuchs, Victor R. (1991). National health insurance revisited. *Health Affairs, 10* (Winter), 7–17.

Gallup, George. (1981). Gallup poll: Transfer of power to states favored. *Minneapolis Tribune* (October 18), A26.

Gamson, William A. (1961). Social science aspects of fluoridation, a summary of research. *Health Education Journal, 19,* 159–169.

Gardner, John W., Wilbur J. Cohen & Ralph K. Huitt. (1967). *1965: Year of legislative achievements in health, education and welfare, health education and welfare indicators.* April 1965–February 1966. Washington, D.C.: U.S. Government Printing Office, IV. (Reprint)

Geiger, H. Jack. (1969). Community control—or community conflict? *NTRDA Bulletin* (November). (Reprint).

Gergan, David, & Ted Slafsky. (1992). Looking for leadership. *Health Management Quarterly, 14* (1), 5.

Gilbert, Benjamin, Merry K. Moos, & C. Arden Miller. (1983). State-level decision making for public health: The status of boards of health. *Journal of Public Health Policy, 3,* 51–63.

Ginsberg, Eli. (1994). Improving health care for the poor: Lessons from the 1980s. *Journal of the American Medical Association, 271* (February 9), 467.

Glaser, William. (1994). Doctors and public authorities: The trend toward collaboration. *Journal of Health Politics, Policy and Law, 19* (Winter), 706.

Goldwater, S. S. (1909). The appropriations of public funds for the partial support of voluntary hospitals in the United States and Canada. *Transactions of the American Hospital Association, 11,* 242–294.

Gordon, Geoffrey B. (1969). The politics of community medical projects: A conflict analysis. *Medical Care, 7,* 973–981.

Gossert, Daniel J., & C. Arden Miller. (1973). State boards of health, their members and commitments. *American Journal of Public Health, 63,* 486–493.

Grad, Frank. (1973). *Public health manual.* (3rd ed.). Washington, D.C.: American Public Health Association.

Grey, Michael R. (1994). The medical care programs of the Farm Security Administration, 1932 through 1947: A rehearsal for national health insurance? *American Journal of Public Health, 84* (October), 1678–1687.

Grogan, Colleen. (1993). Federalism and health care reform. *American Behavioral Scientist, 36* (July), 741–759.

Grupenhoff, John T. (1982). The Congress: Turnover rates of members and staff who deal with medicine/health/biomedical research issues. *Communications, 1.* Science and Health Communications Group.

Guttman, Daniel, & Barry Wittner. (1976). *The shadow government: The government's multi-billion dollar giveaway of its decision-making powers to private management consultants, experts and think tanks.* New York: Pantheon Books.

Haas, Cliff. (1993). The filibuster frustrates yet another chief executive: Drama has faded, but power of the tactic holds strong. *Star Tribune* (April 26), A7.

Hadley, Jack. (1995). Politics versus policy analysis. *Inquiry, 32* (Summer), 128.

Hage, Gerald, & J. Rogers Hollingsworth. (1995). *Clinton health care reform and the diminishment of the active state.* Paper presented at the 1995 annual meetings of the American Sociological Association, Washington, D.C., August.

Hamilton, Alexander, James Madison, & John Jay. (1981). *The federalist papers.* Baltimore, MD: Johns Hopkins University Press.

Hanson, Royce. (1987). Lawmaker turnover rate hurts. *Minnesota Journal* (July 21), 9.

Harris, Richard. (1967). *A sacred trust.* New York: New American Library.

Health Policy Advisory Center, Institute for Policy Studies. (1968). Medical empires: Who controls? *Health-PAC Bulletin, 1* (November/December), 3–6.

Heclo, Hugh. (1995). The Clinton health plan: Historical perspective. *Health Affairs, 14* (Spring), 86–98.

Hixson, Joseph. (1976). *The patchwork mouse: Politics and intrigue in the campaign to conquer cancer.* New York: Anchor-Doubleday.

Hollowy, Robert G., Jay H. Artis, & Walter E. Freeman. (1963). The participation patterns of economic influentials and their control of a hospital board of trustees. *Journal of Health and Human Behavior, 4* (Summer), 88–98.

Holmes, Alan. (1994). States' reform efforts directed by politics, lobbying and fear. *Medicine and Health Perspectives* (June 20).

Hyde, David R., & Payson Wolff. (1954). The American Medical Association: Power, purpose and politics in organized medicine. *Yale Law Journal, 63,* 938–1022.

Iglehart, John K. (1992). The American health care system: Introduction. *New England Journal of Medicine, 326* (April 2), 962–967.

Iglehart, John K. (1993). Health care reform: The labyrinth of Congress. *New England Journal of Medicine, 329* (November 18), 1593–1596.

Isman, Robert. (1981). Fluoridation: Strategies for success. *American Journal of Public Health, 71,* 717–721.

Jackson, Charles A. (1969). State laws on compulsory immunization in the United States. *Public Health Reports, 84,* 787–794.

Johnson, Haynes, & David Broder. (1996). *The system: The American way of politics at the breaking point.* Boston: Little, Brown.

Kaufman, Herbert. (1966). The political ingredient of public health services: A neglected area of research. *Milbank Memorial Fund Quarterly, 44,* 13–34.

Kennedy, David M. (1981). The federal role: It's still necessary. *Minneapolis Star and Tribune* (editorial page).

Kent, Christina. (1994). Insurance agents: They won the battle, but the war goes on. *Medicine and Health Perspectives* (October 10).

Kent, Christina. (1995). States eye reform: 1995. Is the glass half empty? *Medicine and Health Perspectives, 113* (January 9).

Kramer, C. (1972). Fragmented financing of health care. *Medical Care Review, 29,* 878–943.

Lee, Philip R. (1968). Role of the federal government in health and medical affairs. *New England Journal of Medicine, 279,* 1139–1147.

Lee, Philip R., & Carroll L. Estes. (1983). New federalism and health policy. *Annals, American Academy, Political and Social Sciences, 468* (July), 88–102.

Lehman, Tom. (1987). Federalism under Reagan: Has anything changed? *Humphrey Institute News, 10,* 25–26.

Levine, Peter B. (1984). An overview of the state role in the United States health scene. In Theodor J. Litman & Leonard S.

Robins (Eds.), *Health politics and policy* (pp. 194–230). New York: John Wiley & Sons.

Levinsky, Norman G. (1993). Lessons from the Medicare end-stage renal disease program. *New England Journal of Medicine, 329* (November 4), 1395–1398.

Lewin, Lawrence S., & Robert A. Derzon. (1981). Health professions education: State responsibilities under the New Federalism. *Health Affairs, 1,* 69–85.

Lewis, Charles, Rashi Fein, & David Mechanic. (Eds.). (1976). *A right to health: The problem of access to primary medical care.* New York: John Wiley & Sons.

Lewis, Neil A. (1993). Medical industry showers Congress with lobby money. *New York Times* (December 13).

Lewis, Ted, Jr. (1974). The incredible machine: How it grew. *Prism* (January), 17

Light, Paul. (1985). *Artful work: The politics of Social Security reform.* New York: Random House.

Lipson, Debra J. (1994). *Keeping the promise? Achieving universal coverage in six states.* Innovation in State Health Reform Series. Menlo Park, CA: Henry J. Kaiser Foundation.

Litman, Theodor J., & Leonard Robins. (1971). Comparative analysis of health care systems: A socio-political approach. *Social Science and Medicine, 5,* 573–581.

Makinson, Larry. (1992). Political contributions from the health and insurance industries. *Health Affairs, 11* (Winter), 129.

Marmor, Judd, Viola W. Bernard, & Perry Ottenberg. (1960). Psychodynamics of group opposition to health programs. *American Journal of Orthopsychiatry, 30,* 330–345.

Marmor, Theodore R. (1973). The politics of Medicare. London and Chicago: Aldine Publishing Co.

Marmor, Theodore R. (1991). Misleading notions, social, political and economic myths prevent us from learning from other countries' experiences in financing health care. *Health Management Quarterly, 13* (4), 5.

Marshall, T. H. (1965). *Social policy in the twentieth century.* Hutchinson University Library.

McDonough, John E. (1992). Mass retreat—the demise of Massachusetts hospital rate regulation. *Journal of American Health Policy, 2* (March/April), 40–44.

Means, James Howard. (1953). *Doctors, people and government.* Boston: Little, Brown.

Mechanic, David. (1986). *From advocacy to allocation: The evolving American health care system.* New York: The Free Press.

Medicine & Health. (1994). Chamber revises mandate policy. *Medicine & Health, 48* (March 7).

Merritt, Richard. (1981). State health reports. *The Nation's Health* (January), 5.

Migdail, Karen J. (1992). Nursing home reform: Five years later. *Journal of American Health Policy, 2* (September/October), 41–46.

Milbrath, Lester W. (1964). *The Washington lobbyists.* Chicago: Rand McNally.

Millman, Michael L. (1980). *Politics and the expanding physician supply.* Montclair, NJ: Allanheld, Osmun & Co.

Mooney, Anne. (1977). The Great Society and health: Policies for narrowing the gaps in health status between the poor and the nonpoor. *Medical Care, 15,* 611–619.

Moore, Mary L. (1971). The role of hostility and militancy in indigenous community health groups. *American Journal of Public Health, 61,* 922–930.

Morone, James A. (1990). *The democratic wish: Popular participation and the limits of American government.* New York: Basic Books.

Morone, James A. (1995). Nativism, hollow corporations, and managed competition: Why the Clinton health care reform failed. *Journal of Health Politics, Policy and Law, 20* (Summer), 391–398.

Mustard, Harry S. (1945). *Government in public health.* Boston: Commonwealth Fund.

National Center for Health Services Research. (1977). *Controlling the cost of health care.* (NCHSR Policy Research Report 1970–1977, DHEW Pub. No. [HRA] 77-3182). Hyattsville, MD: National Center for Health Services Research.

National Health Council. (1993). *Congress and health* (10th ed.). Washington, D.C.: National Health Council,

The Nation's Health. (1989a). New interest in a U.S. health plan but little movement in Washington. (February), 1.

The Nation's Health. (1989b). Congress facing catastrophic fallout; other issues. (February), 5.

Navarro, Vicente. (1985). The public–private mix in the funding and delivery of health services: An international survey. *American Journal of Public Health, 75,* 1318–1320.

Nexon, Davis. (1987). The politics of congressional health policy in the second half of the 1980s. *Medical Care Review, 44,* 65–88.

Nye, Christine H. (1991). Experience with Medicaid program offers lessons about the economics and politics of public-sector health insurance. *Health Management Quarterly, 13* (4), 25–28.

Pear, Robert. (1992). In shift, insurers ask U.S. to require coverage for all. *New York Times* (December 3), A1, A22.

Penchansky, Roy, & Elizabeth Axelson. (1974). Old values, New Federalism, and program evaluation. *Medical Care, 12,* 893–905.

Peterson, Mark A. (1993). Political influence in the 1990s: From iron triangles to policy networks. *Journal of Health Politics, Policy and Law, 18* (Summer), 395–438.

Phillips, Kevin. (1994). *Arrogant capital: Washington, Wall Street and the frustration of American politics.* New York: Little, Brown.

Public Citizen's Congress Watch. (1995). Managed care industry shifts campaign cash to Republicans. *Public Citizen 's Congress Watch* (September 29), as reported in *Medical Benefits* (November 30), 8.

Rabe, Barry G. (1987). The refederalization of American health care. *Medical Care Review, 44,* 37–63.

Rayack, Elton. (1967). The American Medical Association and the development of voluntary insurance. Parts 1, 2. *Social and Economic Administration* (April), 3–25; (July), 29–55.

Redman, Eric. (1974). *The dance of legislation.* New York: Simon & Schuster.

Richardson, Elliot L. (1973). The maze of social programs. *Washington Post and Times Herald, 96,* 3C, as reported in *Medical Care Review, 30,* 147.

Riley, Trish. (1995). Executive director of the national academy for state health policy as quoted in Emily Friedman. (1994). Getting a head start: The states and health care reform. *Journal of the American Medical Association, 271* (March 16), 875–878.

Riska, Elaine, & James A. Taylor. (1978). Consumer attitudes toward health policy and knowledge about health legislation. *Journal of Health Politics, Policy and Law, 3,* 112–123.

Roemer, Milton I. (1945). Government's role in medicine: A brief historical survey. *Bulletin of the History of Medicine, 18,* 145–168.

Roemer, Milton I., Carl E. Hopkins, Lockwood Carr, & Foline Gartside. (1975). Copayments for ambulatory care: Penny-wise and pound foolish. *Medical Care, 13,* 457–466. (See also comments by Chen, pp. 958–963; Dyckman, pp. 968–969; and authors' response, pp. 963–964.)

Roemer, Ruth. (1965). Water fluoridation: Public health responsibility and the democratic process. *American Journal of Public Health, 55,* 1337–1348.

Rogatz, Peter, Robert Bruner, & Donald Meyers. (1970). Health services working conference, Farleigh Dickinson University.

Rosen, George. (1974). *From medical police to social medicine.* New York: Science History Publications, Neale Watson.

Rovner, Julie. (1995). Nursing home standards: Flashpoint in federalism. *Medicine & Health Perspectives* (October 23).

Rubel, Eugene. (1975). Health planning act seen as declaration of federal role in health care system. *American Medical News* (July 7), 14.

Russell, Louise B., & Carol S. Burke. (1978). The political economy of federal health programs in the United States: An historical review. *International Journal of Health Services, 8,* 55– 77.

Samuelson, Robert J. (1995). RIP: The war on poverty. *Newsweek* (October 9), 59.

Samuelson, Robert J. (1996). *The good life and its discontents: the American dream in the age of entitlement 1945–1995.* New York: Times Books.

Schlesinger, Edward R. (1967). The Sheppard-Towner era—a prototype case study in federal–state relations. *American Journal of Public Health, 57,* 1034–1070.

Schlesinger, Mark. (1988). The perfectibility of public programs: Real lessons from large-scale demonstrations projects. *American Journal of Public Health, 78* (August), 899–902.

Schmickle, Sharon. (1996). Grams is latest senator to block vote on health bill opposed by insurers. *Star Tribune* (February 3), A12.

Schmidt, Terry L. (1980). The congressional process: An overview of how a bill becomes a law. *Group Practice Journal, 29* (January), 9–29.

Schramm, Carl J. (1986). Revisiting the competition/regulation debate in health care cost containment. *Inquiry, 23,* 236–242.

Selye, Katherine. (1995). Lobbyists are the loudest in the health care debate. *New York Times* (April 16), A1, A2.

Shannon, Iris. (1989). President's column. *The Nation's Health* (March 12), 2.

Sheler, Jeffery L. (1985). Congress' proud protection of its independence. *U.S. News and World Report* (January 23), 43–47.

Sheler, Jeffrey L. (1989). States and cited facing the budget music. *U.S. News and World Report* (May 29), 29.

Silver, George A. (1973). Participation and health resource allocation. *International Journal of Health Services* (3), 117.

Sisk, Jane E., Peter McMenamin, Gloria Ruby, & Ellen S. Smith. (1987). Analysis of methods to reform Medicare payment for physician services. *Inquiry, 24* (Spring), 36-47.

Skidmore, Max J. (1970). *Medicare and the American rhetoric of reconciliation.* Tuscaloosa: University of Alabama Press.

Skocpol, Theda. (1995). The rise and resounding demise of the Clinton plan. *Health Affairs, 14* (Spring), 66–85.

Somers, Anne R. (1966). Some basic determinants of medical care and health policy: An overview of trends and issues. *Health Services Research, 1,* 193–208.

Sommerville, Janice. (1994). State reform momentum builds. *American Medical News* (March 14), 3.

Sorian, Richard. (1989). A Reagan retrospective. *Medicine and Health Perspectives* (January 16).

Sparer, Michael. (1995). Great expectations: The limits of state health care reform. *Health Affairs, 14* (Winter), 191–201.

Star Tribune. (1991). AMA urges guaranteed basic health insurance. (May 14), A7.

Starr, Paul E. (1995). *Strategy and structure in health care reform.* Paper presented at the 1995 annual meetings of the American Sociological Association. Washington D.C.: August.

State Health Watch. (1995). Hawaii tightens eligibility for its public purchasing pool, cites ballooning enrollment, economic woes. (August), 3.

State Initiatives. (1995). Post-election review: States to move forward but strategies may change. (January/February), 4–5.

Stavisky, Leonard P. (1981). State legislatures and the New Federalism (book reviews). *Public Administration Review, 41,* 701.

Steinmo, Sven, & Jon Watts. (1995). It's the institutions, stupid! Why comprehensive national health insurance always fails in America. *Journal of Health Politics, Policy and Law, 20* (Summer), 329–372.

Stenberg, Carl W. (1980). Federalism in transition: 1959–79, Advisory Commission on Intergovernmental Relations. *Intergovernmental Perspective* (Winter), 4–9.

Stevens, Robert, & Rosemary Stevens. (1974). *Welfare medicine in America: A case study of Medicaid.* New York: The Free Press.

Stevens, Rosemary. (1982). A poor sort of memory: Voluntary hospitals and government before the Depression. *Milbank Memorial Fund Quarterly/Health and Society, 60,* 551–584.

Stevens, Rosemary, & Robert Stevens. (1970). Medicaid: Anatomy of a dilemma. *Law and Contemporary Problems,* 348–425.

Stone, Deborah A. (1992). Why the states can't solve the health care crises. *The American Prospect, 9* (Spring), 51–60.

Straus, Robert. (1950). *Medical care for seamen: The development of public medical services in the United States.* New Haven: Yale University Press.

Straus, Robert. (1965). Social change and the rehabilitation concept. In Marvin B. Sussman (Ed.), *Sociology and rehabilitation* (pp. 1–34). Washington, D.C.: American Sociological Association.

Talbott, Jeffery. (1995). Congressional partisanship and the failure of modern health care reform. *Journal of Health Politics, Policy and Law, 20* (Winter), 1033–1050.

Tallon, James R. Jr., & Richard P. Nathan. (1992). A federal/state partnership for health system reform. *Health Affairs, 11* (Winter), 7–16.

Thompson, Theodis. (1974). *The politics of pacification: The case of consumer participation in community health organizations.* Washington, D.C.: Howard University Institute for Urban Affairs and Research.

Times Mirror Center for the People and the Press. (1993). MDs seek less radical change. *USA Today* (April 14).

Tollefson, E.A. (1964). *Bitter medicine: The Saskatchewan Medicare feud.* Saskatoon, Saskatchewan: Modern Press.

U.S. Chamber of Commerce. (1965). *Poverty, the sick, disabled and aged* (1965 Task Force on Economic Growth and Opportunity Report). Washington, D.C.: U.S. Chamber of Commerce.

USA Today. (1994). Editorial: Rein in the power to shut down the Senate. (November 25).

Verhovek, Sam Howe. (1995). With power shift, state lawmakers see new demands. *New York Times* (September 24), 12.

Waters, William J., & John T. Tierney. (1984). Hard lessons learned. *New England Journal of Medicine, 311,* 1251–1252.

Weikel, M. Keith & Nancy A. Leamond. (1976). A decade of Medicaid. *Public Health Reports, 91,* 303–308.

Weir, Margaret. (1995). Institutional and political obstacles to reform. *Health Affairs, 14* (Spring), 102–104.

Weissenstein, Eric. (1995). Big health PACs bet heavily against reform. *Modern Healthcare* (August 2), 102.

Wing, Kenneth R. (1976). *The law and the public's health.* St. Louis: C.V. Mosby.

Wolf, Richard. (1992). Labyrinth of staffers on payroll. *USA Today* (October 1), A7.

CHAPTER

The Restructuring of the American Health Care System

Donald W. Light

The American health care system, one of society's largest and most influential institutions, is undergoing profound cultural and structural changes as large buyers of services wrest partial control from providers in order to restrain escalating costs. Major corporations and state health programs have awakened from the habit of passively paying medical bills and are aggressively pursuing ways to stop medical costs from continuing to rise at about twice the general rate of inflation (Burner et al., 1992). Government programs, especially Medicare and Medicaid but also the Veterans Administration, the armed services, and federal employee bene-

This essay is based on a policy research project analyzing the restructuring of American health care and its consequences for society. Support from The Twentieth Century Fund is gratefully acknowledged. I also wish to thank Howard Freeman, Sol Levine, Odin Anderson, Theodor Litman, and Adrian Wagner for their suggestions and critical remarks.

fit programs, are under constant pressure from Congress to keep costs down.

These large purchasers are buying medical services in volume at wholesale prices and even dictating terms, a radical change from the long-held custom of individuals or their insurers paying for their care retail on a case-by-case basis. Institutional buyers want to know what they are getting for their money—a simple question that has threatened the autonomy of physicians and hospitals to the core because the answers require detailed data, close scrutiny, and ultimately outside judgment of whether the services are worth their cost. The nature of insurance is being changed as buyers and insurers shift the risk of costs to patients and providers. Increasingly, the fiduciary relation between doctor and patient is stressed, perhaps even tainted, by competition for business and prepayment, while before it was compromised by paying physicians every time they carried out a procedure.

These fundamental changes—and the resistance to them—are easier to describe than to analyze. Our purpose here is to provide readers with a framework for understanding the current reconstruction of the American health care system. Central to that framework is new historical research showing that corporations and other institutional buyers were setting terms and contracting wholesale for medical services around 1900 as part of industrialization at that time. As a result, physicians were providing medical services for a fixed annual fee (capitation) or according to a discount fee schedule like today's preferred provider organizations. These buyers' markets were vigorously opposed through legal, economic, and political pressure by medical societies and suppressed until the late 1970s, when institutional buyers once again asserted themselves.

EARLY CORPORATE HEALTH CARE

During the nineteenth century, the corporate practice of medicine began in the railroad, mining, and lumber industries, where remote locations, high accident rates, and the growth of lawsuits by injured workers called for some corporate form of health care. These industries contracted for medical services on a retainer basis or on salary; some even owned hospitals and dispensaries for their workers. Some textile industries also established comprehensive medical services in mill towns. Thousands of doctors were involved in these contracts or worked on salary (Williams, 1932; Selleck & Whittaker, 1962).

By the end of the nineteenth century, however, more and more businesses with none of these special needs also began to contract on a competitive basis for the health care of their employees. For example, the Michigan State Medical Society reported in 1907 that many companies (of no particular size or reputation) were contracting for the health care of their employees (Langford et al., 1907). The Plate Glass Factory contracted with physicians and hospitals for all medical and surgical care of its employees and families for a dollar

per month apiece. The Michigan Alkali Company did the same, but did not include family members. Several other companies had contracts for the treatment of accidents and injuries. Commercial insurance companies of the day also got involved, putting together packages of services for a flat amount per person per year (capitation) or for a discounted fee schedule.

More widespread than early corporate health care plans were rapid comprehensive health care services offered for a flat subscription price per year to members of the fraternal orders that had proliferated rapidly during the same period. The national and regional orders of the Eagles, the Foresters, the Moose, and the Orioles as well as other national or regional fraternal associations offered medical care at deeply discounted prices through their local lodges (Ferguson, 1937; Gist, 1940). Various reports from medical societies and commissions in Louisiana, Rhode Island, California, and New York attest to the prevalence of such plans and of "contract practice," as competitive health care was then called. "[T]he growth of contract practice has been so amazingly great during the last twenty-five years as almost to preclude belief," reported a committee of physicians in 1916 (Woodruff, 1916, p. 508). "Practically all of the large cities are fairly honeycombed with lodges, steadily increasing in number, with a constantly growing membership."

The government also became heavily involved in organized buying near the turn of the century. Most of the more comprehensive reports on contract practice describe municipal, county, and state agencies putting out for bid service contracts for the poor, prisoners, and civil employees. At the federal level, the armed services and Coast Guard had long contracted for medical services at wholesale prices (Burrow, 1971; Richardson, 1945).

In response to these developments, more and more physicians competed to provide medical services at discount fees or for a low capitation fee. This greatly threatened independent practitioners, who were already facing keen competition from the glut of doctors being trained at proprietary medical schools, and from other kinds of providers such as homeopaths, osteopaths, naturalists, and chiropractors. Equally threatening to professional status, the institutions or organizations writing these contracts set the conditions under which medicine should be practiced.

SUPPRESSING CONTRACT MEDICINE

To battle contract medicine, county and state societies took a number of actions. They conducted studies and reported on the terrible conditions under which contract physicians worked. Strangely enough, however, the few times that remarks were published by physicians doing contract work, they said they liked the guaranteed income rather than having a quarter of their patients (on average) not pay their bills. They remarked on how they learned to handle hypochondriacs and other abusers of free medical care, and they pointed out that contract medicine was an excellent way to build up a private practice. Societies were also forced to acknowledge that a sizable proportion of their members actively bid for contracts and did contract work (Langford et al., 1907; Lytle, 1909; *Bulletin*, 1909; Haley et al., 1911; Woodruff, 1916).

To those leading this campaign, however, complicity appears to have been a good reason to redouble their efforts and save their colleagues from their own bad judgment. Some societies drew up lists of physicians known to practice contract medicine in order to embarrass them. Others drew up "honor rolls" of members who promised to swear off competitive contracts. Committee members would ferret out recalcitrant colleagues and make group visits to pressure them to abandon contract practice. Some societies threatened expulsion or censure of those members who did not cooperate in stamping out price-competitive medicine (Burrow, 1971).

These pressures worked much more effectively than they had in the nineteenth century, because medical societies succeeded in getting hospitals not to grant privileges to any physician who was not a member in good standing. The hospital had established itself as the center of modern medicine and professional status so that privileges became a powerful control mechanism. Mal-

practice insurance and other professional needs were contingent on membership too. More broadly, the success of practice depended on good relations with one's colleagues.

Although organized medicine never eliminated competitive contracts entirely, it greatly reduced their number. Fraternal orders did not want to cause a row with doctors and shifted their coverage to reimbursing medical bills rather than contracting for services. Reimbursement allowed doctors to set their own fees and eliminated any middlemen setting the terms of service. Several court decisions supported the profession's opposition to the corporate practice of medicine, even though its legal basis was (and is) weak. In a number of states, the medical profession persuaded legislators to pass legislation prohibiting the corporate practice of medicine or the practice of medicine by organizations run by nonphysicians. They also enabled other laws to be passed against the organized practice of medicine for profit. Medical societies meanwhile dusted off their old fee schedules and raised their prices to a professionally "respectable level" (Schwartz, 1965; Burrow, 1963; Rosen, 1983; Starr, 1982).

The goal of these and other efforts to gain control over the practice of medicine has never been to eliminate competition entirely but rather to keep outsiders (i.e., consumers and buyers) from setting terms, especially prices. As Max Weber (1968, p. 342) understood, guilds secured a monopoly over a domain and then let members compete freely *within* it. By the 1920s, the medical profession had contracts confined to a few industries with special needs, to group purchasing of services for the poor and the military, and to maverick experiments on the periphery of medicine (Williams, 1932).

MAKING INSURANCE PROVIDER-FRIENDLY

Although organized medicine had successfully opposed national health insurance, unpaid bills during the Great Depression made subscriptions and forms of prepayment appealing. Groups of physicians, county and state medical societies, individual hospitals, employers, and unions all began to experiment with prepaid contracts again. Although the American Medical Association (AMA) remained adamantly opposed to any such arrangement, especially if it placed a middleman between doctor and patient, the American Hospital Association (AHA) listened more sympathetically to the plight of member hospitals. Many could not meet payroll and had "payless days." An unknown but probably considerable percentage of them started to sell hospital days to one group or another on a prepaid basis of fifty cents per member month or a dollar per family month (Leland, 1932; Williams, 1932; Schwartz, 1965; Stevens, 1971; Rayack, 1967; Sigmond, 1989; Greenberg, 1971). Again the profession and now the hospital industry faced the threat of competition pitting one provider against another.

Out of this turbulence emerged what came to be known as Blue Cross. Few readers today realize that Blue Cross and Blue Shield formed as provider-controlled vehicles for pass-through insurance and that more cost-effective and comprehensive alternatives were passed up. Justin Ford Kimball is usually credited with having the genius to find the solution, because of his dynamic charisma and travels throughout the country advocating his hospital prepayment plan. In fact, however, Kimball's Baylor University Hospital was not the first to implement such a plan (it was Grinnell Hospital in 1917). Moreover, Kimball advocated competing hospital plans and opposed middlemen, such as Blue Cross would have to be, as the insurance administrators for multihospital plans. Instead, it was the soft-spoken, self-effacing Quaker, C. Rufus Rorem, along with a small group of colleagues, who realized that a prepaid hospital plan would have to include many or all of the hospitals in an area if the doctor and the patient were to have free choice like the multihospital plans that had arisen in Essex County, New Jersey, Sacramento, California, and West Virginia.

On other basics, Kimball and Rorem seemed to agree: the plan should be nonprofit and should not include doctors' services so as to avoid opposition from the AMA. They also understood that they were selling

the middle class access to semiprivate services (not necessarily semiprivate rooms) instead of the ward services they would get if they went to the hospital and were unable to pay. The genius of Rorem's vision lay in persuading state legislatures that in lieu of the sizable reserves required of insurance plans, hospitals could substitute guaranteed services. Indeed, the trick of early multihospital plan administrators was to negotiate a contract of payments with hospitals for their services that lay within the limits of the fifty cents to a dollar per month that subscribers were willing to pay.

Because prepaid hospital plans freed up patients' purses to pay doctors' fees, and because noncompetitive plans avoided the awkward problem of a doctor being affiliated with one hospital but his or her patient having a subscription with another, local physicians and medical societies backed Rorem's approach. Although many hospitals had at least one prepaid contract with a group, the idea quickly spread as a form of insurance that provided the working and middle classes with free choice and semiprivate services (Rorem, 1940; Reed, 1947; Rayack, 1967, Chapter 5).

From a comparative and historical point of view, Blue Cross is notable for providing only voluntary hospital insurance coverage for groups of workers who could afford the premium. Moreover, the special enabling legislation passed in many states to circumvent insurance laws required that hospital administrators, trustees, and physicians hold the majority of seats on the Blue Cross boards. Even though there was tension between Blue Cross plans and member hospitals in negotiating how much the plans would pay, from the start Blue Cross focused on what the profession valued most: hospital-based specialized care and surgery in the temple of medicine.

When the AMA and state and local medical societies decided a few years later that prepaid hospital plans were an idea worth imitating, they made Blue Shield even more provider-friendly by emphasizing payment for services rather than service contracts. This left the doctor free to bill as much as he or she wanted.

Instituting health insurance along professional lines and defeating prior efforts to legislate national forms of social insurance completed what Anderson calls "the health service infrastructure" (Anderson, 1991). The nature of that infrastructure is outlined in Figure 2-1 and could be characterized as a professionally driven health care system. At the heart of that system is the goal to provide the best possible clinical care to every sick patient where physicians choose to practice. Complementary goals include developing scientific medicine to its highest level and protecting the autonomy of physicians.

These goals asserted themselves at critical points in subsequent decades. When, after World War II, several proposals were made for government support of health care, ranging from national health insurance under President Truman to a GI bill for medical education, the AMA at the height of its power opposed all pro-

posals except the rebuilding of hospitals under the Hill–Burton Act and the support of national research institutes. As a result, over the next fifteen years, the American health care system became even more hospital- and subspecialty-based (Starr, 1982; Somers & Somers, 1961).

Then, when the pressure to insure the elderly and the poor became too great for the AMA to oppose in the mid-1960s, the AMA insisted that Medicare and Medicaid be structured as pass-through reimbursement of "usual and customary" fees with no interference (oversight) in the practice of medicine. The American Hospital Association insisted that debt service and a guaranteed surplus be built into the bed day-rate. This spawned a generation of debt-financed expansion of hospitals. Further, the rules for depreciation allowed ac-

FIGURE 2-1 Ideal Type of a Profession-Based Health Care System

Key Values and Goals	To provide the best possible clinical care to every sick patient (who can pay and who lives near a doctor's practice) To develop scientific medicine to its highest level To protect the autonomy of physicians and services To increase the power and wealth of the profession To increase the prestige of the profession	**Organization**	Centered on doctors' preferences of specialty, location, and clinical cases Emphasizes acute, high-tech interventions A loose federation of private practices and hospitals Weak ties with other social institutions as peripheral to medicine
Image of the Individual	A private person who chooses how to live and when to use the medical system	**Division of Labor**	Hierarchical, doctor-controlled Specialty-oriented
Power	Centers on the medical profession, and uses state powers to enhance its own	**Finance and Costs**	Private fees paid by individual to doctor when feasible Private, voluntary insurance as passive vehicle to pay bills Highly inflationary
Key Institutions	Professional associations Autonomous physicians and hospitals		

celerated depreciation on *replacement* cost, so that a hospital could depreciate the entire value of major equipment in less than three years while keeping it for seven to ten years and charging a fee every time it was used. A critic at the time called these provisions a "license to steal" (Somers & Somers, 1961).

The goals of a professionally driven health care system may be worthy in their own right, but one can see how they led to excesses and distortions that resulted in widespread discontent and revolt by consumers and buyers in the 1970s. One might call them the ironies of success. For example, professional goals lead to emphasizing state-of-the-art clinical interventions but ignoring primary care and prevention. Costs rise sharply, especially if reimbursed by provider-controlled insurance. Physician autonomy at the clinical level leads to fragmentation and underserved areas at the system level. An integrated delivery system that serves rural and inner-city patients as well as others would require a loss of individual autonomy.

As Figure 2-1 indicates, the resulting system consists of a loose federation of local offices and hospitals organized around physicians' preferences, with weak ties to other sectors such as the school or the workplace. Power centers on professional associations, which use the legal powers of the state to enhance their position but protest state interference in the practice of medicine. The American system differs from its counterparts in many other countries by the relative weakness of the state (Larkin, 1983; Willis, 1983; Coburn et al., 1983; Wilsford, 1987). Whereas the medical profession in those countries faced many similar issues of legitimacy and control, they worked with the state in matters of organization and financing.

CREATING A HAVEN FOR CAPITALISM

An ironic consequence of the American case is that the medical profession created protected markets where capitalism could flourish and eventually exert control over the profession itself. Although today we think of this happening with health care corporations, it was foreshadowed by the earliest and perhaps most important case of the medical profession harnessing the drug industry (Burrow, 1963; Rorem & Fischelis, 1932; Caplan, 1981).

As early as 1906, the AMA mounted a vigorous campaign against nostrums and patent medicine. Joined by druggists, who were also feeling the competition from patent medicine manufacturers, the AMA and some state medical societies sought to cordon off and control the sale of those drugs whose recipes were revealed, tested, and approved by the AMA. They succeeded and created a protected professional market of prescription drugs available only through physicians. Given that the profession opposed any state participation and that capitalism constituted the "natural" economic environment of the nation, it was inevitable that "ethical" drug companies (i.e., companies and drugs that conformed with AMA ethics) experienced tremendous growth and profits. What the profession did not anticipate is that these companies would soon influence professional judgment and make many facets of professional life dependent on them, not the least the AMA itself (Goldfinger, 1987; Lexchin, 1987; Mintz, 1967).

Corporations flourished in every other protected medical market—hospital supply, hospital construction, medical devices, laboratories, and insurance—until the only large sector left untouched was medical service itself. The profession somehow thought that it could allow corporations to dominate every other sector of medicine without their touching physicians. Meanwhile, professional judgments and decisions were being commercialized in numerous ways—by how insurance policies were written, by what medical devices were promoted, by how supplies were packaged, by what new lab tests were made available, by which company sponsored a professional presentation, and by which salespersons they saw.

Finally, by the 1960s only medical care itself had not been corporatized. Yet in creating a protected domain where physicians could order what they wanted and have someone pay the bill, the profession created an ideal environment in which corporations could flourish. With the passage of Medicare and Medicaid, which had special provisions that made the corporate practice of medicine very profitable and made it almost impossible to lose money, for-profit hospital and nursing home chains flourished. Soon all kinds of other medical service corporations sprang up. This greatly disturbed the medical profession. Leading physicians saw these corporations as alien invaders who threatened everything they stood for (Relman, 1980), and indeed many observers still do not realize that the rise of corporate *providers* was an integral part of the system that the profession put in place. The irony of professional dominance was corporate dominance.

THE BUYERS' REVOLT

During the 1960s and 1970s, the movement toward a professionally driven health care system increased. Finally, corporate buyers, other employers, and legislators became alarmed at the sharp rise in medical expenses and a number of related problems. The 1970s opened with a burst of criticisms against unnecessary surgery, excessive drug prescriptions, inefficient hospitals, too many specialists who did not care about the patient as a person, the lack of primary care, and the neglect of the poor despite Medicaid. From every sector of society cries arose for national health insurance and a total revamping of what was seen as a chaotic, wasteful system (*Fortune*, 1970; Greenberg, 1971; Ehrenreich & Ehrenreich, 1971; Bodenheimer et al., 1972; Kennedy, 1972; Ribicoff, 1972). Numerous proposals for national health insurance, combined with reforms to contain costs, were made. In response, President Nixon proposed a national network of health maintenance organizations (HMOs). Following the advice of Paul Ellwood, Nixon took these long-despised, anti-American hotbeds of "socialist medicine," and presented them as the ideal business system that integrated all levels of care under one management and managed all aspects of health care in a cost-effective manner. This may be the greatest rhetorical reversal in the history of American health care.

The struggle for national health insurance and reform brought to the surface how deeply entrenched the American system was in a commercial, profit-making industry. Hospital supply companies, medical technology companies, pharmaceutical companies, health insurance companies, hospitals, physicians, and the nursing home industry all mounted intensive campaigns against any bill that would slow down their growth or profits. Of course, universal health insurance would increase their markets, but it came with government regulations if not government administration that were ideologically offensive. Various groups of politicians dug in their heels over different measures. For example, a tax-based system was simply unacceptable to a significant block of legislators, regardless of its fairness to the working class and its much lower administrative costs. Endless politicking over amendments made the choices even more tortured. In the end, nothing passed (Davis, 1975).

In the meantime, during the 1970s, Congress, as the buyer behind Medicare, passed several bills to control costs through regulation. They focused on planning (health service agencies [HSAs]), regionalizing expensive facilities and equipment (certificates of need [CONs]), and reviewing physicians' orders (professional services review organizations [PSROs]). These and similar measures, however, lacked the powers of enforcement, and they had loopholes that health care administrators and consultants quickly learned to exploit. By the end of the 1970s, policymakers concluded that regulation does not work. It would have been more accurate to conclude that weak and partial regulation does not work. The 1970s ended with health care from the medical-industrial complex costing about three times what it had in 1970 and consuming 9.5 percent of GNP (up from 7.5 percent in 1970). Compared to people in other countries who faced similar budgetary crises and brought health care expenditures under control, Americans were not really serious about cost containment. For those costs were the revenues to the medical-industrial complex, one of the strong growth areas in the American economy.

The legal basis of provider dominance and suppressed competition that the medical profession had so carefully built up faced new challenges. In a landmark case involving the issuance of a fee schedule by the Virginia Bar Association, the U.S. Supreme Court ruled for the first time that "learned professions" were exempt from anti-trust laws (*Goldfarb*, 1975). The Court even dismissed the fact that the fee schedule had been approved by the Supreme Court of Virginia and was therefore exempt as a state action. It was judged to be price fixing, plain and simple.

The Federal Trade Commission realized that the *Goldfarb* ruling applied to the practice of medicine, and within months began gathering evidence against medical societies and several specialty societies for restricting advertisement by members and restraining price competition (Pollard, 1981). Soon the dominance of physicians and hospital administrators on Blue Cross and Blue Shield boards came under scrutiny. Laws that the medical profession had put through against the corporate practice of medicine and prepaid health care plans came under attack. In short, the entire structure of legal protections against competitors began to crumble (Havighurst, 1980; Weller, 1983; Gee, 1989). Moreover, many states began to pass new laws to facilitate the creation of HMOs and preferred provider organizations (PPOs).

If one believes that shifts in the law usually reflect shifts in the body politic, and especially in priorities of major interest groups, then the *Goldfarb* case and several other key cases reviewed by the Supreme Court and other senior courts must be seen as part of the profession's fall from grace and the rise of institutional buyers (Havighurst, 1980). It also reflects the almost sacred status that competition holds in American culture. Competition is assumed in most textbooks and conversations to foster high quality at the lowest price, efficiency, productivity, democracy, and liberty. One does not hear about the cases of competition producing dislocation, waste, higher prices, inefficiency, deception, or inferior quality. The Supreme Court captured the competition ethos when it wrote:

> The Sherman act was designed to be a comprehensive charter of economic liberty aimed at preserving free and unfettered competition as the rule of trade. It rests on the premise that the unrestrained interaction of competitive

forces will yield the best allocation of our economic resources, the lowest prices, the highest quality and the greatest material progress, while at the same time providing an environment conducive to the preservation of our democratic political and social institutions (356 U.S. 4 1958).

Evidence for competition doing all these things in health care is scant, except under quite specific circumstances (Light, 1993).

During the 1980s, institutional buyers went into open revolt against the professionally driven system under the banner of competition. Increasingly, they insured themselves and as a consequence managed the health care services for their employees or enrollees more actively. They soon discovered facts about health care that shaped their thinking and have changed the course of medicine. First, evidence had been mounting for years that health care did not improve people's longevity much; the major factors were genetics, social class, environmental hazards and pollutants, and people's health habits. While this interpretation of the evidence can be challenged, doubts about the value of medicine raised the question of what we were getting for our money.

Second, evidence had been mounting that doctors vary greatly in how much they hospitalize or operate on patients with the same kinds of problems, after controlling for many variables that might explain the differences. This further discredited the medical profession and raised the question of whether the high users were wasting other people's money and profiting from it. Given numerous studies indicating that 20 percent to 40 percent of many tests and procedures were unnecessary, buyers suspected that doctors and hospitals were running up bills for overtreatment.

Third, when employers and other buyers brought in specialists to ask them which of several treatments they should be paying for to relieve lower back pain (a common occupational disorder) or to treat breast cancer, they got a roomful of conflicting answers. The implication was that physicians, even board-certified specialists, did not know what worked and what did not. When employers asked their health insurance carriers the same questions, they found that insurance companies did not have any answers either. The issues about the relative efficacy of alternative interventions are in fact subtle, but the message that buyers took away was not.

As a consequence of these rude awakenings, and the goals, values, and policies of institutional buyers (summarized in Figure 2-2), the buyers' revolt led to several new actions. Congress, as the largest buyer of all, got so frustrated that it inaugurated large-scale studies on the outcomes of alternative treatments. Employers were ready to accept any set of criteria by utilization review firms that seemed reasonable for identifying unnecessary tests and procedures. In both responsible and irresponsible ways, these initiatives meant that buyers were taking over the core clinical function of medicine: that of deciding what tests and procedures were clinically useful and which patients needed which ones.

Buyers also campaigned to dismantle and reshape the laws, customs, and institutions so that buyer choice and competition could take place. No longer was there the sacred trust in physicians that had prevailed through the mid-1960s. Doctors were seen as ordering too many tests, prescribing too many drugs, performing too much surgery, and bouncing too many patients from specialist to specialist.

Buyers demanded detailed accounts of what services were being rendered at what cost. To most people's surprise, providers did not know what their services actually cost (only what they *charged*) and did not have good data on the services they gave. Detailed clinical data systems are inherently intrusive; they lead to buyer control through monitoring systems. The battle over the control of data intensified. Even more significant, the demand for accountability has shifted from measuring *inputs* (supplies, equipment, facilities, and medical procedures) to *outcomes* (whose patients get better faster and cheaper).

Employers also started to restructure their contracts to cover all or large portions of health care services. What they sought were organized provider groups that would bid on a package for a price and then deal with these issues of excessive and unnecessary services. This prompted providers to restructure into forms that offered coordinated care. Large group practices, joint ventures between hospitals and physician groups, managed

From Emphasizing	To Emphasizing
Provider dominance (a system run and shaped by doctors)	Buyer dominance (an effort to dismantle and reshape the laws, customs, and institutions established by organized medicine to allow buyer choice and competition)
A sacred trust in doctors	A distrust of doctors' values, decisions, even competence
Quality assured by medical profession as high (but uneven and unattended)	Quality as something buyers want documented and reviewed
A "nonprofit" guild monopoly	Competition for profit (even among nonprofit organizations)
Cottage industry structure	Corporate industry structure
Specialization and subspecialization	Primary care and prevention, with minimal referrals to specialists
The hospital as the "temple of healing"	The home and office as centers of care, with the hospital as a last resort
Fragmentation of services as a byproduct of preserving physicians' autonomy	Coordination of services to minimize error and reduce unnecessary and inappropriate services and costs
Payment of costs incurred by doctor's decisions	Fixed prepayment, with demand for a detailed account of decisions and their efficacy
Cross-subsidization of the poor by the more affluent, of low-tech and service departments by high-tech departments, of medical education by everyone	Cross-subsidization seen as "cost shifting," a suspect maneuver that imposes hidden charges on buyers. An unwillingness to pay for anything but direct services

FIGURE 2-2 The Buyers' Revolt: Dimensions of Change in American Health Care

care systems, and many other kinds of organizational arrangements have grown. The practice of medicine began to change from cost-plus treatment to results-oriented managed care.

Medicare and the Power of Buyer Dominance

In the meantime, as by far the largest institutional buyer, Medicare and its administrators at the Health Care Financing Administration (HCFA) sponsored a wide range of research projects and demonstrations in payment schemes, competitive delivery systems, and methods for monitoring costs. Behind them, as the voice of taxpayers, Congress has steadfastly pressured them to find ways to keep Medicare expenses from rising so fast that they would bankrupt the Medicare Trust Fund. Using its capacity as a dominant buyer to make long-term investments in research and development, HCFA funded a project for over ten years at Yale to design a system for allocating resources within hospitals by diagnostically based utilization rather than by procedure. A bold commissioner of health in New Jersey, Joanne Finlay, proposed using this system to pay hospitals—a radical departure from the way that hospitals had ever been paid, but one that promised to reward hospitals for getting a job done within budget rather than for doing as many procedures as possible. With the support of HCFA, New Jersey imposed this radical payment system by diagnosis-related groups (DRGs) on almost all of its hospitals (Widman & Light, 1988), and in 1983, Congress adopted a stricter version of this system for paying hospitals for Medicare patients. Called the prospective payment system (PPS), the federal version meant that when a patient was admitted, Medicare knew in advance that they would pay only a fixed amount, unless it was a costly outlier. Given Medicare's dominance in the market, almost all hospitals agreed to comply. Subsequently, insurance companies, large employers, and large health care systems adopted it.

PPS had a tremendous impact on the hospital industry and on the health care system in general. Hospital administrators seemed so concerned about PPS that they quickly cut staff, reduced inventory, and had briefing sessions with physicians to encourage shorter stays. They established internal monitoring systems to weed out or reeducate those providers who ran up expenses with too many tests or procedures. Secondary industries arose around maximizing payments and around clinical management systems. Profits (or surpluses) subsequently reached an all-time high, but the era of dehospitalization had begun. Congress responded to the profits by paying less. It did not give the hospitals an increase as large as overall medical inflation until 1989. As a result, profits and surpluses quickly dropped to razor-thin levels, and many hospitals ran deficits. Admissions and length of stay continued to decline.

In addition, Medicare and the administrators of HCFA have developed stronger, more unified programs than the private sector in other areas as well. They restructured and strengthened a national network of peer review organizations and developed specific targets of overuse in each region of the nation. They made another long-term investment in developing a relative value scale based on actual costs of training, time, and resources for paying physicians. The resulting payment system, the resource-based relative value system (RBRVS), is the first nationally used fee schedule in the United States. Finally, HCFA has steadfastly sponsored research on risk factors and how to adjust payments to providers for the risks of their patients.

Each of these tools for cost management is rife with politics and controversy, making it easy to forget from a historical perspective what large advances they were. Although HCFA has been slow to develop and structure Medicare managed care contracts in a sensible way, and in the mid-1990s, was the object of severe criticism, for twenty years it led the private sector in cost controls and developed several tools for controlling costs.

Ironically, although these strong measures were taken in the name of competition under Ronald Reagan, they constituted "the most intrusive government intervention since Medicare . . . by the most conservative President since Herbert Hoover" (Goldfield, 1994, p. 78). One could see the same irony in strong actions taken in the purchase of health insurance coverage by large companies that dominated their local markets. Americans believe deeply in competition, but when they can use their anticompetitive muscle, they will. Likewise, competitive sellers will dominate or control their markets when they can in the name of competition. As Alan Maynard (1993, p. 195), the leading health economist in Britain, where belief in competition is less ideological, has pointed out, the goal of capitalists is to "ensure that they restrict competition, maintain market share and enhance profits: capitalists always and everywhere are the enemies of capitalism!"

The Rise of Managed Care Systems

Besides developing the DRG and RBRVS systems as powerful forms of fiscal management, the federal government strongly supported HMOs. At the time, HMOs were proclaimed to deliver all health care for 10 percent to 40 percent less money than fee-for-service providers and hospitals, and the HMO Act of 1973 *required* employers to offer HMOs as an alternative to regular health insurance (Falkson, 1980). One might call this forced competition, but it did create a national market for cost-effective managed care systems.

The medical and hospital lobbies, however, weighed the HMO Act down with requirements and stipulations that became burdens to growth, and by the early 1980s, the act was considered an obstacle to HMO development—another example of how government regulations keep private markets from developing cost-effective delivery systems. But in fact it was an example of private practitioners using the government to advance their (anticompetitive) goals, for it was the beneficiaries of the cost-plus private market that loaded up the HMO Act with obstructive regulations.

Besides offering HMO options and fostering other forms of managed care, employers increasingly limited their premium contribution for benefits and then let each employee choose from a "cafeteria" of alternative benefit health plans that varied in choice, coverage, and price. That is, employers increasingly went from "defined *benefit*," which guaranteed a certain level of coverage for health care (usually very comprehensive), to "defined *contribution*," which only guaranteed a certain amount of money for health insurance and other benefits. While the cafeteria plan approach gave the employee great choice and fostered intense competition among providers, it protected the company from the relentless increase in health care premiums. Employees

thought the cafeteria plans were giving them more benefits, when over the long run they were getting less. In this context, managed care systems that had few or no charges to patients became increasingly attractive.

During the 1970s, HMOs and employers both pressed for amendments and changes in administrative rules that would make HMOs more competitive. One can see a gradual relaxing of requirements right on through the 1980s to allow HMOs to respond to a wide array of market demands by employers. In addition, preferred provider organizations (PPOs) were invented to provide still more alternatives and flexibility. Essentially, a PPO is any group of providers who agree to discounted fees in return for an employer giving employees incentives to use them. Typically, an employer would cover through health insurance all or most of the treatment provided by a PPO, but if the employee chose another physician outside the plan, he or she would pay anything billed above that discounted level.

Throughout the 1980s, the boundaries between PPOs and HMOs began to blur. On one hand, some PPOs agreed to capitated payments, like HMOs. On the other hand, some HMOs did not provide comprehensive care but were targeted to certain types of medical service, like PPOs. The basic point, however, is that buyers from Medicare on down to mid-sized companies in local markets were hiring managed care companies to tell providers what services they wanted and what prices they thought were reasonable. The buyers' market was greatly aided by a surplus of sellers, that is, by an excess number of hospital beds and an increase in physicians that greatly exceeded population growth.

Paradoxically, these managed care systems, and competition between them and traditional medical services, did not save money. While business leaders proclaimed success at using competition to end professional dominance and spiraling costs, HMOs were attracting healthier employees and shadow-pricing the premiums for traditional plans. This meant healthy profits for the HMOs and rising costs for employers as they paid for their sicker employees (or their dependents) in the open-ended traditional plan. The syndrome feeds on itself: the more sicker employees got left in the traditional plan, the faster its premiums would rise, and thus the faster HMO premiums could rise at a slightly lower shadow price, and the more the employer would pay overall. When the dust settled, the costs of health benefits had risen as fast in the 1980s as in the 1970s, despite the greatest effort in history to use competition in health care.

Crisis and Paradigm Shift in Health Insurance

Several aspects of the buyers' revolt shook the health insurance industry and forced it to rethink its purpose—even what business it was in. After enjoying several decades of an expanding market, the health insurance industry found itself facing a saturated market in the 1970s. Getting new business meant taking it away from a competitor, and the use of risk selection expanded (Light, 1992). When employers started to self-insure, insurance companies not only faced a shrinking market, but were also reduced to being third-party administrators. No longer did they hold huge reserves of funds on which they could earn investment income. Rather they became little more than claims processors.

Certain insurers took the lead in redefining their business and their services by developing managed care services. Initially, some of them served as packagers who would put together a health care network for a large employer. They also developed capacities to do prospective, concurrent, and retrospective utilization review, to do quality assessment, and to assess providers. During the 1980s, these skills and capacities came together to form a paradigm shift: from writing insurance to owning or operating managed care systems. Profits, they discovered, were much greater for them as middlemen who could keep the difference between premiums and the deep discounts they could extract from providers. The surplus of doctors and hospitals has meant that each year they could drive down what they paid providers still farther. Given that contracts in these systems pass nearly all the risk on to the providers, the new business and its sources of profit have little to do with traditional insurance.

National Health Care Reform as a Watershed?

After twenty years of buyers' efforts through competition and direct attempts at regulating medical practices, the United States was the only First World nation that still had not restrained the health care costs of the medical-industrial complex (MIC). Rather, revenues to the MIC (and costs to citizens) had risen from $75 billion or 7.6 percent of GNP in 1970, to $250 billion or 9.2 percent of GNP in 1980, to $666 billion or 12.1 percent of GNP in 1990 (Burner et al., 1992). The costs to employers equaled 100 percent of their post-tax profits. Meanwhile, fewer and fewer working people had health insurance. The "inverse coverage law" of private health insurance (Light, 1992) meant that through exclusion clauses, coverage limits, waiting periods, and reimbursements limited to what the insurance company determines are "reasonable" or "customary" or "prevailing" charges, those with insurance who most needed comprehensive coverage had less coverage.

Dismantling the legal, institutional, and economic features that were built earlier in the century to minimize price competition and cost containment by institutional buyers has been a slow process. Throughout the 1980s and into the 1990s, medical schools still trained largely specialists and provided leadership for the entire profession in state-of-the-art clinical medicine, subspecialization, and new technology—the core values of the professional model and a chief cause of escalating costs (Light, 1989). Licensing and certification rules form a battlement around this core of the professionally driven health care system. The high pay to physicians and great differential in payment between surgeons and primary care physicians remained largely in place. Despite notable savings by some large corporations in some places, the spiraling cost of health care did not slow down, even though politicians proclaimed that it did (Light, 1984, 1994).

Almost twenty years after everyone had demanded national health insurance and reform, everyone demanded it once again. The range of reform proposals was much narrower than twenty years earlier, so that

Clinton's proposal was less comprehensive than Nixon's in 1971 (Garfield, 1994). Nevertheless, 1993 felt like 1973, because the institutional and economic structure of the health care system that had been set during the first half century created entrenched interests against reform. The only difference was that the size of the medical-industrial complex was much greater, and the corporations involved had much more to lose.

The major beneficiaries would be the large insurance companies and the managed care corporations, because all the major reform bills except the single-payer plan of Representative James McDermott (D-WA) and Senator Paul Wellstone (D-MN) would place the nation's health care in their hands. By the end of 1993, however, they realized that the Clinton plan, at least, would close up the loopholes they were so profitably exploiting, and they turned against it. They realized they could do better without it.

Once again, ideological convictions played a major role. Some parties again wanted only a tax-based system; others passionately opposed a tax-based system. Some thought that government intervention was essential to make health care fair and cost-effective; others thought only private markets could do that. The lobbying effort was far larger than in 1973, with far more distorted and erroneous information (Kolbert, 1995; Carlson & McLeod, 1994; Reinhardt, 1995). Most interesting is that employers opposed bills that would relieve them from spiraling costs. Their opposition appeared to be due to three factors. First, employers are wedded to the 50 percent tax break they get on health benefits, even though economists contend that tax-exempt benefits have been a powerful engine driving costs up. Second, national health reform would greatly reduce the size and power of corporate benefits departments, whose directors were the chief advisers to their companies' presidents and board chairs. Third, employers wanted to keep control of benefits as a way to control labor, even though the cost of that control had risen from 50 percent to 100 percent of after-tax profits. Such thinking is oddly American; for employers in no other industrialized country want to add the headaches of health benefits to the complexities of running

their businesses. To put it another way, health benefits is itself a big business inside big business.

A long view leads one to conclude that the Clinton reform effort was not a watershed but rather one more turn in the cycle of spiraling costs and shrinking coverage leading to demands for reform that threaten the institutional, economic, and ideological sources of the spiraling costs and shrinking coverage.

Corporate Medicine in a New Guise

The Clinton reforms seemed to have accelerated efforts by managed care companies and insurance companies, born again as managed care corporations, to buy, build, merge, and otherwise attain market control as oligopolies or monopolies in their principal markets before any die was cast. Thus, in the 1990s, things look different. As the drive for national health reform was collapsing, managed care corporations and insurance companies made a fierce and successful effort to win deep discounts and drive down hospital admissions and bed days per thousand. In areas where they had high market penetration, they succeeded and saved billions of dollars. These savings, however, went largely to executive officers, management teams, and investors' profits, not to the employers and employees who foot the bill.

Employers in a few areas have joined or formed health care coalitions and empowered them to do collective buying. But this is hard to do when each employer has a somewhat different health plan, is structured in a somewhat or very different way, and has a different board of directors. As always, a few large buyers report impressive savings for themselves, but how much these savings are being shifted to others is unknown. One needs to look at declines in real (inflation-adjusted) growth for an entire region, not just for the big buyers.

In short, the principal force behind reducing health care use and cost in the 1990s has been for-profit middlemen and packagers, not employers or Medicare. Many of the major HMO corporations actually provide no health care. These are the new-breed HMOs that are *packagers*, not health service organizations. They take fixed premiums in the front door, pay provider groups under deep-discount contracts out the back door, and keep 18 percent to 30 percent for themselves in the middle. Managerial and marketing costs are high, but there is plenty left for profits. Employers may even save a bit of money. For example, a national survey by A. Foster Higgins found that employers' medical costs declined by 1.1 percent in 1994 (Freudenheim, 1995). However, Harvard health economist Joseph Newhouse sees little evidence of expenditures slowing down (Huskamp & Newhouse, 1994). Rather, most of the 30 percent discounts that the managed care companies negotiate from providers just about matches what they keep. In other words, the managed care revolution of the 1990s has largely been a matter of transferring billions of dollars from doctors, nurses, hospitals, and other providers to executive management teams and investors.

Three-quarters of the new HMOs are for-profit, and consolidation has led to ten firms controlling 70 percent of the HMO market. In mature metropolitan markets like San Francisco, Los Angeles, or Minneapolis, five or fewer firms dominate the market. The larger they are, the deeper the discounts they can negotiate, the more reserves they have to drive out smaller competitors, and the more political clout they have to structure markets to their advantage.

Even more than the early HMOs, which ended up with healthier patients through self-selection, this new breed uses tactics that defy regulation to avoid sicker subscribers. According to two physician-researchers (Woolhandler & Himmelstein, 1994, p. 586), they "place sign-up offices on upper floors of buildings with malfunctioning elevators; refuse contracts to providers in neighborhoods with high rates of HIV infection (an example of medical redlining); structure salary scales to assure a high turnover among physicians (the longer they are in practice, the more sick patients they accumulate); provide luxurious services (even exercise club memberships) for the well, and shabby inconvenience for those with expensive chronic illnesses [so that they will disenroll]."

Given that just 10 percent of the population consumes 72 percent of all medical costs, risk avoidance is the quickest and easiest way to make money. "As a result, society pays twice: once for the high risk people concentrated in high cost plans, and again for the excess profits in plans that succeed in risk selection" (Employee Benefits Research Institute, 1995, p. 586). In the meantime, the number of persons with no health insurance keeps rising, up by about one million in 1993 and another million in 1994 (Employee Benefits Research Institute, 1995).

Soon the discounting will have run its course, and then managed care companies will have to extract profits from direct clinical services. Evidence indicates that this is already happening. A national survey of all managed care enrollees found that they were 2.5 times more likely to rate the quality of services they receive as just fair or poor, and over 4 times more likely to rate their doctors as fair or poor compared to enrollees in traditional plans (The Commonwealth Fund, 1995). Remarkably, people in managed care plans were just as likely to report not having a regular source of care, not getting preventive services, and postponing needed care—the very problems that managed care is supposed to solve. Concerning access, managed care enrollees were much more likely to rate ease of changing doctors, choice of doctors, access to emergency care, and waiting time as only fair or poor. Forty percent had to change their doctors when they joined their current managed care plan. Discontinuity of care was directly related to dissatisfaction. Yet employers and employees are constantly pressured by plans to switch for short-term gains or inducements.

A more telling 1995 survey sponsored by the Robert Wood Johnson Foundation focused only on patients sick enough to be seeing a specialist. Compared to those in traditional unmanaged care, sick patients in managed care were 3.3 times more likely to report that they received inappropriate care, 4.0 times more likely to report that their examination was not thorough, 2.5 times more likely to report they had inadequate time with their physician, and 2.1 times more likely to report that the doctor did not care. Moreover, the out-of-pocket expenses of these sick patients were not zero, as many imagine them to be in managed care systems, but

$1,502. This is only slightly less on average than the out-of-pocket expenses of sick patients in fee-for-service care ($1,735). The picture that emerges is that managed care corporations are already providing worse care for the sick for very little savings to either employers or employees in return for high salaries, large management expenses, and high profits.

Conclusion: The Rhetoric of Competition

American business leaders and politicians continue to believe unquestioningly in the power of competition to make health care efficient and hold down costs. They always prefer the free market though no market is free. Even the market for street vendors is structured by city ordinances, informal but powerful rules about territory, and norms about practices. In fact, health care markets are among the most structured and least free of any on earth. Moreover, competition was widely regarded as impossible in health care until the current period because of the many problems of market failure outlined in Figure 2-3 (Light, 1993, 1995).

There is little evidence that competition can really save money after biased selection, cost shifting, and significantly higher transaction costs are taken into account. It seems like once again the United States is not learning how to contain costs from nations that have done it without sacrificing high-quality care for everyone, but rather has come up with another policy innovation that will not achieve its stated goals. Health care will continue to take money from education, housing, industrial development, and welfare as it consumes an increasing percentage of state and federal budgets.

What makes American health care policy fascinating is that alongside an undying faith in competition, employers and the government impose unilateral changes that are anticompetitive just to be sure competition works! The Reagan administration, for example, talked about PPS being competitive, but it was basically price fixing on a grand scale, and it worked. Just to be sure competition works, employers are cutting benefits. We have already described the continued thinning of coverage for working Americans, and the number with no insurance is rising by about a million per year.

Ideal of Perfect Markets	Actual Hazards of Health Care Markets
Transaction and market costs zero	Large transaction and market costs
Many buyers and sellers	Few buyers and sellers; market capture
Nature, quality, effectiveness, and price of products or service known; no market failure	Nature, quality, effectiveness, and price of products or service incompletely known and variable; some market failure
Power, rules, hierarchy do not exist	Power, rules, hierarchies found everywhere
Manipulations, gaming, cost shifting unknown	Manipulations, gaming, cost shifting prevalent; induced market failure
Losers collapse, disappear	Losers stay around; system carries their inefficiencies
Maximum efficiency	Maximum inefficiencies
Responsive to customers	"Responsive" to customers; induced demand, product or service dilution or substitution, misleading information

FIGURE 2-3 Perfect versus Health Care Markets

Congress is acting out the same ironic syndrome. On one hand, it is seeking to push the elderly and the poor into managed care systems, while on the other hand, it has proposed historically large cuts in the budgets for both Medicare and Medicaid. Put these together and it means that for-profit organizations with a unclear track record of saving money but a good track record of making money are in charge of rationing care to fit within reduced budgets for the elderly and the poor. But even more interesting is the conflict between buyer dominance and competition as two different strategies for keeping costs in line. Strong restraining actions by monopoly buyers are as anticompetitive as restraining actions by sellers, even though the buyers may say they are fostering competition.

Given all the difficulties in creating competitive conditions in health care, competition also fits health care poorly because a competition strategy may destroy professional altruism, commercialize medical care for the sick, and induce providers to play elaborate games in the marketplace without saving much money. Is it buyer dominance we want or competition? If the answer is competition, are we ready for the change from buyer dominance to provider dominance as the baby boom generation grows old and the current surplus of doctors becomes a shortage?

My own analysis is that we are in the middle of a shakedown period in which there is fierce competition between managed care systems for control of large markets in each region. Most of the "savings" will go to the twenty cents to thirty cents they take out of every premium dollar to run their systems. But by the end of the 1990s, there will be only a few major health care corporations in most metropolitan or regional markets, and as oligopolies they will not compete much on price. Overall savings, if any, will occur largely during the shakedown period, and the United States will be stuck with ever-hungrier, multibillion-dollar corporations in control.

On the positive side, the managed care corporations will have cut out (with a hatchet) more fat, faster, than any other approach, and they will have put a large percentage of Americans into capitated delivery systems. They will have restructured the medical profession toward primary care and hospitals toward community care. That is, the excesses of professional dominance over the past sixty years will have been erased.

These changes are very useful for universal health insurance, if Congress decides to do it. In fact, an obvious question may arise: Why pay these corporations 20 percent to 30 percent to run managed care systems when a network of nonprofit institutions like the old Blue Cross network can do it for 10 percent and leave a lot more money for clinical care? In fact, by the year 2000, profits may have thinned out, and the corporations running the managed care systems may be happy to get out of the business and do something else. If something like this happens, then the American health care system will end up having close to an ideal structure for maximizing people's health and dealing with the tidal wave of chronic disease disorders that will roll in with the twenty-first century.

REFERENCES

Anderson, Odin W. (1991). Health services in the United States: A growth enterprise for a hundred years. In Theodor J. Litman and Leonard S. Robins (Eds.), *Health politics and policy* (2nd ed.). Albany, NY: Delmar.

Bodenheimer, Tom, Steve Cummings, & Elizabeth Harding. (Eds.). (1972). *Billions for bandaids*. San Francisco: Medical Committee for Human Rights.

Bulletin of the American Academy of Medicine. (1909). *10* (1), special section, 587–631.

Burner, Sally T., Daniel R. Waldo, & David R. McKusick. (1992). National health expenditures projections through 2030. *Health Care Financing Review, 14* (Fall), 1–29.

Burrow, James G. (1963). *A.M.A: Voice of American medicine*. Baltimore: Johns Hopkins University Press.

Burrow, James G. (1971). *Organized medicine in the Progressive Era: The move toward monopoly*. Baltimore: Johns Hopkins University Press.

Califano, Joseph A., Jr. (1986). *America's health care revolution: Who lives? Who dies? Who pays?* New York: Random House.

Caper, Philip. (1988). Defining quality in medical care. *Health Affairs, 7* (Spring), 49–61.

Caplan, Ronald L. (1981). *Pasturized patients and profits: The changing nature of self-care in American medicine*. Ph.D. diss., Department of Economics, University of Massachusetts (Amherst).

Caplan, Ronald L. (1988). Commodification of American health care: A Marxian reappraisal. *Social Science and Medicine, 28* (11), 1139–1148.

Carlson, E., & D. McLeod. (1994). The "big lie" vs. health reform: Direct-mail firms "raised millions" with scare letters. *AARP Newsletters, 35* (November), 9.

Coburn, David, George M. Torrance, & Joseph Kaufert. (1983). Medical dominance in Canada in historical perspective: Rise and fall of medicine? *International Journal of Health Services, 13* (3), 407–432.

The Commonwealth Fund. (1995). *Managed care: The patient's perspective*. New York: The Commonwealth Fund.

Davis, Karen. (1975). *National health insurance: Benefits, costs, and consequences*. Washington, D.C.: The Brookings Institution.

Employee Benefits Research Institute. (1995). *Sources of health insurance and characteristics of the uninsured*. Washington, D.C.: Employee Benefits Research Institute.

Ehrenreich, Barbara, & John Ehrenreich. (1971). *The American health empire: Power, profits and politics*. New York: Vintage.

Falkson, Joseph L. (1980). *HMOs and the politics of health system reform*. Chicago: American Hospital Association, Robert J. Brady Co.

Ferguson, Charles W. (1937). *Fifty million brothers: A panorama of American lodges and clubs*. New York: Farrar and Rinehart.

Fortune. (1970). Special issue on "Our ailing medical system" (January).

Freudenheim, M. (1995). Health costs paid by employers drop for first time in a decade. *New York Times* (February 14), A1, D9.

Garfield, Norbert. (1994). The looming fight over health care reform: What we can learn from past debates. *Health Care Management Review, 19* (3), 70–80.

Gee, M. Elizabeth. (1989). FTC anti-trust actions in health care services. Washington, D.C.: Federal Trade Commission. (Typescript).

Gist, Noel P. (1940). Secret societies: A cultural study of fraternalism in the United States. *University of Missouri Studies, 15* (4).

Goldberg, Lawrence G., & Warren Greenberg. (1978). The emergence of physician sponsored health insurance: A historical perspective. In Warren Greenberg (Ed.), *Competition in the health care sector: Past, present, and future*. Germantown, MD: Aspen Systems.

Goldfarb v. Virginia State Bar 95 S. S. Ct. 2004 (1975).

Goldfield, Norbert. (1994). The looming fight over health care reform: What we can learn from past decades. *Health Care Management Review, 19* (3), 70–80.

Goldfinger, Stephen E. (1987). A matter of influence. *New England Journal of Medicine, 316* (May 20), 1408–1409.

Greenberg, Selig. (1971). *The quality of mercy: A report on the critical condition of hospital and medical care in America*. New York: Atheneum.

Haley, Edward E., et al. (1911). The evils of the contract system. *New York State Journal of Medicine, 11* (8), 394–396.

Havighurst, Clark C. (1980). Anti-trust enforcement in the medical services industry: What does it all mean? *Milbank Memorial Fund Quarterly, 58* (Winter), 89–123.

Huskamp, Haiden A., & Joseph P. Newhouse. (1994). Is health spending slowing down? *Health Affairs, 13* (Winter), 32–38.

Kennedy, Edward. (1972). *In critical condition*. New York: Simon & Schuster.

Kolbert, E. (1995). Special interests' special weapon: A seeming grass-roots drive is quite often something else. *New York Times, 26* (March), 20.

Langford, T. S., A. S. Kimball, H. B. Garner, E. H. Flynn, & T. E. DeGurse. (1907). Report of the committee on contract practice. *Journal of the Michigan State Medical Society, 6* (7), 377–380.

Larkin, Gerald. (1983). *Occupational monopoly and modern medicine*. London: Tavistock.

Larson, Magali Sarfatti. (1977). *The rise of professionalism: A sociological analysis*. Berkeley: University of California Press.

Leland, Roscoe G. (1932). *Contract practice*. Chicago: American Medical Association.

Leyerle, Betty. (1984). *Moving and shaking American medicine*. Westport, CT: Greenwood Press.

Lexchin, Joel. (1987). Pharmaceutical promotion in Canada: Convince them or confuse them. *International Journal of Health Services, 17* (1), 77–89.

Light, Donald W. (1984). Overstated gains in the war on health costs. *New York Times* (August 6), 30.

Light, Donald W. (1986). Corporate medicine for profit. *Scientific American, 255* (6), 38–45.

Light, Donald W. (1989). Toward a new sociology of medical education. *Journal of Health and Social Behavior, 29* (December), 307–322.

Light, Donald W. (1992). The practice and ethics of risk-rated health insurance. *Journal of the American Medical Association, 267* (May 13), 3503–3508.

Light, Donald W. (1993). Escaping the traps of postwar Western medicine. *European Journal of Public Health, 3*, 223–231.

Light, Donald W. (1994). Medical prices outrun the rate of inflation. *New York Times* (February 18), A23.

Light, Donald W. (1995). *Homo economicus*: Escaping the traps of managed competition. *European Journal of Public Health, 5*, 145–154.

Light, Donald W., & Sol Levine. (1988). The changing character of the medical profession. *Milbank Quarterly, 66* (Suppl. 2), 1–23.

Lytle, Albert T. (1909). Contract medicine—an economic study. *New York State Journal of Medicine, 15* (3),103–106.

Maynard, Alan. (1993). Competition in the UK national health service: Mission impossible? *Health Policy, 23* (January), 193–204.

Medical Benefits. (1986). Payers can be held liable for care limits. *Medical Benefits, 15* (October), 3.

Mintz, M. (1967). *By prescription only* (2nd rev. ed.). Boston: Houghton Mifflin.

Pollard, Michael R. (1981). The essential role of antitrust in a competitive market for health services. *Milbank Memorial Fund Quarterly, 59*, 256–268.

Rayack, Elton. (1967). *Professional power and American medicine: The economics of the American Medical Association*. Cleveland: World Publications Co.

Reed, Louis. (1947). *Blue Cross and medical service plans*. Washington, D.C.: Federal Security Agency.

Reinhardt, Uwe E. (1995). Turning our gaze from bread and circus games. *Health Affairs, 14* (Spring), 33–36.

Relman, Arnold S. (1980). The new medical-industrial complex. *New England Journal of Medicine 303* (17), 963–970.

Ribicoff, Abrahamm, with Paul Danaceau. (1972). *The American medical machine.* New York: Saturday Review Press.

Richardson, J. T. (1945). The origins and development of group hospitalization in the United States, 1890–1940. *University of Missouri Studies, 20* (3).

Robert Wood Johnson Foundation. (1995). Sick people in managed care have difficulty getting services and treatment, new survey reports. *News from the Robert Wood Johnson Foundation.* Princeton, NJ: Robert Wood Johnson Foundation.

Rorem, C. Rufus. (1940). *Non-profit hospital service plans.* Chicago: Commission on Hospital Service.

Rorem, C. Rufus, & Robert P. Fischelis. (1932). *The costs of medicine.* Chicago: University of Chicago Press.

Rosen, George. (1983). *The structure of American medical practice 1875–1941.* Philadelphia: University of Pennsylvania Press.

Rosner, David. (1982). *A once charitable enterprise: Hospitals and health care in Brooklyn and New York, 1885–1915.* New York: Cambridge University Press.

Rosoff, Arnold J. (1984). The "corporate practice of medicine" doctrine: Has its time passed? *Health Law Digest, 12* (12) (Suppl.).

Rothstein, William G. (1972). *American physicians in the 19th century: From sects to science.* Baltimore: Johns Hopkins University Press.

Salmon, J. Warren. (1977). Monopoly capital and the reorganization of health care. *Review of Radical Political Economics, 9* (12), 125–133.

Salmon, J. Warren. (1985). Profit and health care: Trends in corporatization and proprietization. *International Journal of Health Services, 15* (3), 395–418.

Schwartz, Jerome L. (1965). Early history of prepaid medical care plans. *Bulletin of the History of Medicine, 39* (September/October), 450–475.

Selleck, Henry B., & Alfred H. Whittaker. (1962). *Occupational health in America.* Detroit: Wayne State University Press.

Sigmond, Robert M. (1989). Oral history interview (Spring).

Somers, Herman, & Anne Sommers. (1961). *Doctors, patients, and health insurance: The organization and financing of medical care.* Washington, D.C.: The Brookings Institution.

Starr, Paul. (1982). *The social transformation of American medicine.* New York: Basic Books.

Stern, Bernhard J. (1945). *American medical practice in the perspective of a century.* New York: The Commonwealth Fund.

Stevens, Rosemary. (1971). *American medicine and the public interest.* New Haven: Yale University Press.

Vogel, Morris. (1980). *The invention of the modern hospital.* Chicago: University of Chicago Press.

Warner, John Harley. (1986). *Therapeutic perspectives: Medical practice, knowledge and identity in America 1820–1885.* Cambridge, MA: Harvard University Press.

Weber, Max. (1968). *Economy and society: An outline of interpretive sociology.* (Guenther Roth & Claus Wittich, Eds.). New York: Burminster Press.

Weller, Charles D. (1983). The primacy of standard anti-trust analysis in health care. *Toledo Law Review, 14,* 609–637.

Wennberg, John. (1984). Dealing with medical practice variations: A proposal for action. *Health Affairs, 3* (Summer), 6–32.

Widman, Mindy, & Donald W. Light. (1988). *Regulating prospective payment.* Chicago: Health Administration Press.

Williams, Pierce. (1932). *The purchase of medical care through fixed periodic payments.* New York: National Bureau of Economic Research.

Willis, Evans. (1983). *Medical dominance: The division of labour in Australian health care.* Sydney: Allen and Unwin.

Wilsford, D. (1987). The cohesion and fragmentation of organized medicine in France and the United States. *Journal of Health Politics, Policy and Law, 12* (3), 481–504.

Woodruff, John V. (1916). Contract practice. *New York State Journal of Medicine, 16* (10), 507–511.

Woolhandler, Steffie, & David U. Himmelstein. (1994). Clinton's health plan: Prudential's choice. *International Journal of Health Services, 24* (4), 583–592.

CHAPTER

Gridlock and Breakthrough in American Health Politics

James A. Morone

For the past twenty-five years, social scientists recycled the same description of American health policy: health costs rose while access to care shrank. The stubborn problems prompted both liberals and conservatives to dream up all sorts of reforms. Health services researchers added mountains of data to the policy debates. Governments peppered health care professionals with a steady flow of cost-control programs. However, physicians generally found a way to sidestep the controls. The result was a health care politics that featured plenty of activity but few fundamental changes in either health policy or the health care system.

In the 1990s, the "same old story" came to a sudden end. Health reformers got their most promising opportunity to remake the system in three decades—and

were decisively beaten. But defeat did not return us to the old politics of stalemate. For even while Americans debated the Clinton administration's health care reform, a great revolution was taking place. Medicine was rapidly changing from a field dominated by physicians into a corporate enterprise organized and run along business principles. In the process, health care institutions, medical practice, health finance, and the standards of social justice all began to change in fundamental ways.

This chapter considers what happened, what failed to happen, and why. The first part examines the essential political dynamics of the American policy process. The stubborn structural features of the political landscape help explain why some policy innovations succeeded and why others failed. The second part turns to the public sector and examines what may prove to be one of the most important failures in recent American

I am grateful for thoughtful comments from Gary Belkin, Theodor Litman, Leonard Robins, and Deborah Stone.

history: the proposed Clinton health reform. This section examines what went wrong and why it matters. The third part turns to the private sector and the changes now remaking American health care. The emerging American health care regime subordinates physicians, reshapes medicine along unabashedly business principles, and organizes the logic of redistribution right out of the health care system. Ironically, the changes were inadvertently stimulated by the proposed Clinton reforms, which aimed for an entirely different sort of heath care revolution.

POLICY POLITICS IN THE UNITED STATES

On some level, all political systems undergo constant change. The United States has, in the past three decades, turned from Lyndon Johnson's Great Society to Newt Gingrich's "Contract with America." Still, some stable features of the policy process exert a steady and powerful influence on American public policy. Over time, they shape what happens and what does not happen in American health care policy.[1]

Dread of Government

Americans have generally held a profound suspicion of the state—a dread of government. The state occupies an unusually ambiguous place in American society. Right from the start, the Declaration of Independence defined the new nation in a great protest over government intrusion on personal liberty. The Constitution is grounded on precisely the same principle. Citizenship rights, national independence, and the Revolutionary era American state governments were all articulated in a distinctly anti-statist spirit. James Madison contrasted the American Constitution with the development of civil rights in Europe as a "charter of power granted by liberty rather than a charter of liberty granted by power" (Wood, 1969, p. 601). The preoccupation with limiting government has remained a vivid feature of American public life. Alexis de Tocqueville described it

this way in 1832: "the society acts by and for itself . . . so feeble and restricted is the part left to [government] administration" (de Tocqueville, 1966).

One result is that Americans have developed social insurance programs far more reluctantly than most Western democracies. In Europe, benefits were generally proffered from the political center by statesmen bidding for the allegiance of the working classes. Bismarck, Lloyd George, and Napoleon III each tried to coopt labor with social welfare benefits. In the United States, such programs more often provoked debates about the dangers of prompting laziness (and permitting tyranny) rather than the potential for promoting political loyalty. Social policy discussions almost inevitably get tangled up in debates about the legitimacy of state intervention.

To be sure, the symbols evolve. The rhetoric takes new twists. But charges of "tax and spend," "big government," "incompetent bureaucrats," and even "jackbooted state agents" stand in a long and potent American ideological tradition. Naturally, the antigovernment ideology is not always decisive; it can be countered with alternative symbols and rhetorical traditions. However, it is almost always a feature of public policy debates about social welfare programs in the United States. Reformers ignore this ideological tradition at the peril of their plans (Skocpol, 1994).

Civil Service

The United States has never developed a skilled civil service comparable to the ones in Germany, France, Britain, or Japan. Perhaps this is because until the twentieth century, positions were distributed on the basis of political loyalty rather than technical qualifications (Skowronek, 1982). A lingering image of corruption and incompetence still haunts the civil service (often, quite unjustly). Consequently, public service suffers from relatively low prestige, poor resources, and inferior salaries. The low standing of the American civil service was dramatically illustrated by government "shutdowns" during both the Bush and Clinton administrations.

The reluctance to nourish competent public administration is especially debilitating for health policy.

---

[1]For a sustained discussion on the topic of this section, see Morone (1990). For a shorter description, see Morone (1992).

Negotiating with a well-organized, well-financed, and highly skilled profession requires both competence and resources. When civil servants are not up to the job, the American reflex is to curse all government rather than to try and reconstruct a more effective one.

Institutional Fragmentation

Public power in the United States is enormously fragmented. Federal, state, and local governments each pursue their own policies with little coordination of purpose or programs. In Washington, Congress and the presidency have been controlled by different parties for twenty-two of the past twenty-eight years. American legislators are constitutionally forbidden from holding executive offices (as parliamentary leaders hold portfolios to the major ministries). Consequently, conflicts between the branches often develop, even when they are in the same party hands (Steinmo & Watts, 1995).

President Clinton's health reform effort offered an especially vivid case of institutional fragmentation. Thirty-one different congressional committees and subcommittees tried to claim some sliver of jurisdiction over the legislation. Seven actually won a place in the process (Clymer, 1994). Each felt free to substitute its own proposal for the one the president had submitted. As a result, entirely different legislation emerged from different committees. In one case, a subcommittee reported a bill that the full committee (House Ways and Means) then ignored; another committee (Senate Education and Welfare) reported multiple plans. The jumble of reform proposals that emerged from committees faced a daunting political gamut: separate consideration in each chamber, passage, negotiations in a joint committee in order to reconcile the bills passed by the two houses, then back to each chamber for approval. In the Senate, forty-one members could have thwarted the whole process at any point.

Even if the bill had passed, the next steps would have been just as chaotic. First, the president signs the bill (President Clinton unwittingly illustrated the complexity of the process by threatening to veto the legislation if it failed to meet his own priorities). Next, a bureau-

cracy only loosely controlled by either the president or Congress writes (publishes, gathers comments about, and rewrites) regulations. Then the program goes on to the fifty states for enabling legislation. There, organized interests hire local lawyers and lobbyists and a whole new political cycle begins. Finally, all parties adjourn to the courts, where long rounds of litigation shape the final outcome (Morone, 1995, pp. 394–396).

The essential point is simple: the anarchic process makes reform extremely difficult. The American political system has few institutions capable of centralizing political authority over domestic issues. Rather, it is an extraordinarily Byzantine process that has grown increasingly difficult to manage over time. The consequence is a state that makes large-scale reform excruciatingly difficult to win, especially social welfare reform.[2] Ideology and the organization of government reinforce the tendency toward stalemate. It takes a great political event—a landmark election, a mass popular upheaval, a war, a domestic crisis—to temporarily shake off the normal tilt toward timidity and inaction.

GOVERNMENT HEALTH REFORM: THE DEMOCRATS' GREAT CHANCE

The Clinton administration's health reform effort may have been a great political watershed, both for health policy and, more generally, for American politics. What made it so important? And if it was so important, why did it fail?

The Stakes

Even after its electoral victory in 1992, the Democratic Party found itself in a difficult position. American politics still operated in the shadow of President Ronald Reagan. A shrewdly constructed budget deficit blocked progressive reforms. Shrewdly negotiated budget rules required a 60 percent majority in Congress for

---

[2]It is a myth that this is precisely what the founders intended. They were as concerned about "energy in the executive" as they were that "ambition counteract ambition." See Morone (1990).

new spending. A potent anti-tax ideology fed on economic disquiet over job security, the American dread of government, and a middle class angry about stagnant incomes. The rhetoric of aggressive individualism, racial suspicion, and unfettered economic markets ran through American popular culture. The Republican Party mantra against "tax and spend" liberals sent all but the most hardy Democrats scrambling to embrace such Republican themes as crime and free trade.[3]

To reverse such a powerful antigovernment legacy, the political science wisdom calls for a great, popular program that rebuilds old constituencies, reconstructs loyalty to the party that championed the reform, and restores some public faith in government's ability. The obvious candidate for such political reconstruction seemed to be national health care reform. It was a popular idea. It was associated with the Democrats' past— Medicare, after all, was the most popular Great Society effort. In short, health reform offered the great opportunity for the Democrats and, in strictly political terms, a great peril for the Republicans.

In retrospect, this may have been a final possibility for traditional national health insurance. As we shall see in the next section, the American health care system began to evolve in the late 1980s. And what it is evolving into is a classic business enterprise. As health care corporations grow and flourish, large-scale government intervention designed to social welfare specifications becomes increasingly less likely.

However, as the Clinton administration took office in January 1993, health care reform seemed a good bet. It had been dramatically placed on the public agenda by Harrison Wofford's unexpected election to the Senate in a special election in 1991. At the start of that campaign, Wofford had trailed far behind in the polls. He seized health care and skillfully parlayed it (along with the growing dissatisfaction with then President George Bush) into election victory (Rockman, 1995). Long-simmering public dissatisfaction with rising costs and gaps in coverage propelled the issue forward. On both sides of the aisle, congressmen began to propose health

legislation. The Bush administration sponsored a modest bill. Even conservative Republican stalwarts like Senators Phil Gramm (R-TX) and Bob Dole (R-KS) put health proposals forward. However, it was candidate Bill Clinton (now using Harrison Wofford's campaign manager) who seized the issue and made it a major part of his 1992 election campaign. When he won, many observers concluded that, finally, the time for health reform was "ripe."

Why did such an apparently promising reform fail? Future discussions about the government's role in health care are likely to keep returning to the Clinton effort and the question of what went wrong. Consider two levels of analysis: strategic blunders and structural biases.

Strategic Errors

Begin with the simplest explanation: the votes were not there. Even if the administration had enrolled every one of the fifty-six Democratic senators (an almost impossible job), it was still four votes short of breaking a filibuster. The Democrats would have to win over liberal Republicans like John Chafee (R-RI)—but Chafee was waiting for them with his own bill, which was far more modest than the administration's proposal (Brady & Buckley, 1995). This simple explanation, however, is too limited. There would be enormous flux in the positions taken by different members of Congress as they caucused, bargained, and read the polls. After all, at the start of the process, Senate minority leader Robert Dole was a co-sponsor of Chafee's bill; by the end, many Democrats were willing to settle for far less than Senator Chafee had originally proposed.

The reform's prospects were complicated by bald political gaffes. For example, one task force director reportedly kept Congressman Pete Stark (D-CA), chairman of the health subcommittee of the House Committee on Ways and Means, waiting in an outer office for over an hour. In the Washington world of political protocol, this was a serious affront, one that allegedly doomed the Clinton health plan in an important subcommittee. But the failure to bring along congressional allies was just the tip of the political iceberg.

---

[3]For an elaboration of the themes in this section, see Morone (1995).

The deeper blunder was classic Progressive myopia.[4] The original Progressives pursued such elusive muses as scientific management and technical expertise. "Getting it right" mattered more to them than the unsavory rough and tumble of politics. Their intellectual heirs on the Clinton health team repeated the Progressive error—they underestimated the politics. The health reformers gathered sprawling expert task forces that worked so hard on the details that they lost track of political time, causing fatal delays. And, in the end, they produced a proposal that was complex, unfamiliar, and impossible to explain to the public. As a result the reform was easy to caricature and attack. The basic idea in the proposal, managed competition, actually followed from what was happening in the private sector (as we shall see below). But because it was so difficult to explain to the public, it was poorly designed for the rough and tumble of Washington politics.

In true Neo-Progressive fashion, task force leaders like Ira Magaziner would complain long and loud about the harsh political campaign that destroyed their efforts. As Bathhouse John Coughlin, a Chicago politician, could have told them a century ago, "the politics game is not a branch of the Sunday School business." The health plan's "unfair" critics had a great deal at stake. Great changes come at someone's expense—and in this case the losers would have included Republican politicians. As Bill McInturff, a Republican pollster, told his clients, "one of the most important predicates for Republican success [in the 1994 midterm elections] is not having health care pass" (Toner, 1994).

All politicians know the contemporary recipe for defeating an unfamiliar candidate or legislative proposal:

define them before they define themselves. Critics of the president's proposal easily attached negative symbols to the arcane mysteries of the health plan. The critics intoned the familiar conservative liturgy: Tax and Spend, Big Government, Federal Bureaucracy Run Amok, The Destruction of American Medicine. Later, analysts would show that a large portion of the attacks made on the Clinton plan were demonstrably false (West & Heith, 1994; Marmor & Oberlander, 1994). But the attacks worked. Support for the Clinton health plan melted rapidly away. One poll reported 67 percent support in September, 44 percent by February (West & Heith, 1994).

The great symbolic war was no surprise: political historians gave fair warning even before the election (Skocpol, 1994; Marmor, 1994). So did Republican strategists, who were sounding their themes before the administration took office. And the dread of government gave opponents a powerful ideological tradition to draw on as they framed their attacks. The Clintons gamely struggled to respond. But the convoluted, economistic concoction that they were championing was not designed to stir the public or win symbolic wars.

Moreover, something more than the old skepticism of government was at work. This health reform debate produced an ugly, neo-nativist politics of moral repudiation.

In the past, American health insurance debates featured dire alarms about foreign perils: "the Kaiser's throne," "Lenin's keystone to the arch of socialism," "Sovietization" (Morone, 1990, Chapter 8). This time, a more divisive, coded, racialist rhetoric emerged. As one public official put it, "You can't expect the hard working people in suburban Cook County to go into the same Health Care Alliance as the crackheads in Chicago." The middle class, in his view, should not be forced to join (or cross-subsidize) the undeserving: drug abusers, unwed welfare mothers, foreigners, and the like. A bureaucratic mechanism designed to aggregate health risks got tangled up in stereotypes of responsible and irresponsible behavior.

Traditional political wisdom advises that universal programs (like Social Security) are stronger and more legitimate than those that are targeted or means-tested

---

[4]The original Progressive movement arose around the end of the nineteenth century and flourished between 1900 and 1916. Its proponents fought against social injustice, the newly emerging business corporations, and the corruption of party politics. Among the many different reforms they sought was the introduction of scientific principles into government administration. This goal, they imagined, would get American government beyond political squabbles. After all, insisted the Progressives, "there is no Democratic or Republican way to sweep a street." Instead, they argued, get good people who will do the job right. What the Progressives discovered, however, was that in a democratic society it is not possible to get "beyond" politics. Different perspectives and interests will always make themselves heard. See Marone (1990); McConnell (1966); Wiebe (1967); contrast Filene (1970).

(like Aid to Families with Dependent Children). The former are protected by middle-class beneficiaries. The Clinton health debate may mark a decline of the universal social welfare ideal. Long-standing images of community, solidarity, and cross-subsidizations—the essential ingredients of any health reform—are cracking under the strains of an increasingly divided society. The dread of government is now exacerbated by a suspicion of those who are different.

Whereas these nativist sentiments were just whispers during the health reform debate, they became trumpet blasts in the 1994 midterm election that followed. In California, Proposition 187 would sweep undocumented aliens out of the social welfare system. In the new Republican-controlled Senate, Phil Gramm (R-TX) announced that the 40 million people allegedly getting a free ride on welfare would now "get out of the cart and help the rest of us push." In the House, the newly elected speaker Newt Gingrich (R-GA) suggested that illegitimate birth would be "re-stigmatized." One proposal, only briefly discussed, would remove children from unwed mothers who could not afford to care for them. Everywhere, criminals were in the public's mind. All the political indicators appeared to be pointing in the same direction: the populism that swept health reform onto the political agenda in 1992 had turned wrathfully nativist and buried the prospects for progressive government.

What provoked the recrudescence of American nativism? The answer lies in some of the underlying institutional issues that help explain the reform's defeat.

Institutional Realities

On a more fundamental level, Clinton's failure was scarcely a strategic issue. Rather, the political process itself is organized to produce stalemate. The organization—or, more accurately, the disorganization—of American politics doomed the reform (Steinmo & Watts, 1994).

During the debate, this problem of institutional incoherence got lost in the great interest group watch. As health reform lurched forward, endless analysis handicapped each shift in the pluralist constellation. Lee Iacocca, the chief executive officer of the Chrysler Corporation, had hinted that his company's health costs were unsupportable—now would he support reform? How about the rest of corporate America? The big insurers were splitting from the small companies. Would they cut a profitable health care deal with the Clinton administration? The administration plan itself seemed rooted in the interest group logic, almost self-consciously courting some groups within each sector (Ben-David, 1993).

But in American politics, in contrast to the parliamentary democracies, deals do not stick. In Britain, Prime Minister Margaret Thatcher announced a health reform, designed it behind closed ministerial doors, and passed it on to her successor for implementation. In Germany, Christian Democrats (very roughly equivalent to the Republican Party in the United States) held a retreat with Social Democrats (roughly like the Democrats) and hammered out profound changes in the national health insurance arrangements (Morone & Goggin, 1995). In contrast, every bargain in American politics is open to renegotiation elsewhere in the endless political process.

Pluralist images mislead. Toting up the "groups for" and the "groups against" deflects attention from the institutional terrain that has to be negotiated. Never mind where the interest groups stand at the start of the process. Opponents get multiple opportunities to oppose; losers have plenty of institutional venues in which to recoup their losses; supporters can always renegotiate (or cut and run). The organization of the state, however, is only part of the institutional story. The structure of American business also helped wreck health reform.

There is much speculation about why business failed to rally to health care reform. Some point to dogmatic anti-statism (Brown, 1994); others, to the organization of business advocacy. Business associations—like the Chamber of Commerce or the National Association of Manufacturers—amplify the voice of the nay-sayers. If nothing else, potential losers (companies who do not now pay health benefits) opposed reform far more intensely than potential winners supported it (the latter might benefit, but the gains are uncertain and companies would lose some control over their own benefits process) (Martin, 1994).

Beyond these strategic considerations lies a more fundamental and troubling development. Since the 1920s, American corporations have offered their employees what amounted to a private welfare system. Companies have provided health benefits, old age pensions, job security, and vacations. The public welfare state was constructed around the private system—filling the gaps, regulating benefits. The Clinton plan was a typical example: access to health care would have been secured mainly by mandating that large employers provide health insurance for their employees.

Now, after seven decades, the corporate welfare state is coming to an end. A new international economic order is creating an economy of "hollow corporations" and "contingent workers." Rather than hire full-time employees, companies use temporary workers or consultants or simply contract for services. A part-time workforce can swiftly be adjusted to market conditions; and the company saves roughly a third of its personnel costs by getting out of the employee benefits business. In 1992, over one-quarter of the American workforce worked in the "contingent" labor force (duRivage, 1992). Since then, the number has continued to grow rapidly.

For workers, the new order brings job insecurity and haphazard social welfare benefits. It explains why there is such profound anxiety despite a relatively good economy. It suggests why business is apt to resist mandated health benefits with increasing vigor. And it points to the coming crisis in American health care: if business is not going to pay, who will?

In short, we operate with political institutions designed to subvert broad-gauged reform and a private social welfare system that has begun to come apart. The Clinton administration's failure to lock in health care coverage for full-time employees is more than the latest miss in a long line of health reform failures. This time we face the rapid disintegration of American health security—not just the safety net, but the basic infrastructure.

We will, of course, visit health reform again. However, we are likely to do so under a far harsher and more socially perilous economic regime.

THE PRIVATE SECTOR: A NEW MEDICAL CAPITALISM

While public attention was turned to the great political debate over national health reform, the health sector was rapidly remaking itself. The result was a profound set of changes that fundamentally recast health care and health politics in the United States.[5]

The Roots of Corporate Medicine

The new health care can be traced to a series of studies performed by John Wennberg and his associates in the early 1970s (Wennberg, 1973; Morone & Belkin, 1995). Wennberg discovered that physicians in different communities performed the same clinical procedures at sharply different rates. Each local area appeared to have its own "practice style" or "surgical signature." Crucially, the differences did not seem to have any relationship to the diagnoses or patient conditions.

The policy rub came when observers began to attach cost estimates to the variations. In perhaps the most widely cited study, Wennberg and his associates showed large differences in hospitalization rates—and health care costs—between two cities, Boston and New Haven (Wennberg, 1990, pp. 1203–1204; Fisher et al., 1994).

The findings shifted the focus of health policy analysts searching for cost containment. The traditional view featured an unwelcome message. Cost control would mean hard choices—negotiating tough budgets, squeezing physician payments, rationing health care. Here was a far more palatable alternative. Find the unnecessary medical expenditures and squeeze them from the system. Health care cost control could be won by forcing physicians to practice medicine more efficiently. Implicit in this apparently painless route to cost control lay a profoundly subversive conclusion: physicians were treating patients in a haphazard way. Local practice styles rather than medical science were driving health care. The doctors did not know what was best.

How to capture the potential savings? The answer lay in the same kind of health services research that had

---

[5]For an elaboration of the themes in this section, see Morone and Belkin (1995).

unearthed the variations in the first place. If physicians were practicing in arbitrary and expensive ways, social scientists would infuse the medical enterprise with systematic knowledge. The key would be linking specific treatment regimens to medical outcomes while factoring in the costs. Social scientists would statistically determine what worked; payers would subject the results to cost–benefit calculations. Advocates imagined a day when patients would know the probabilities of all relevant outcomes; payers and physicians would have treatments clearly labeled as "appropriate" and "inappropriate" for specified conditions (Morone & Belkin, 1995, p. 2).

In 1989, Congress created the Agency for Health Care Policy and Research (AHCPR) and over the next six years poured $500 million into the outcomes research. Of course, when political stalemate blocks action, studies are the time-honored way for politicians to demonstrate concern without doing anything risky. In this case, however, the researchers were promising particularly useful results. The health services research community was setting out to create a series of medical protocols—statistically verified standard operating procedures that would identify what worked for specified diagnoses (Gray, 1993).

Before the researchers had gotten very far, the political consequences were being felt.[6] The research effort would lead, quite inadvertently, to radical changes in American doctoring, medical organization, and the prospects for health care equity.

The Consequences for Medicine

Many physicians enthusiastically participated in the outcomes research. Protocols, they reasoned, would enhance their profession's diagnostic capacity. But the search for protocols had a more profound result. What is emerging is nothing less than a new model of medical practice.

---

[6]Indeed, the development of protocols may prove less important than the political consequences of *promising* to develop them. Early reports from the researchers engaged in the work suggest that in many cases health care procedures and technologies were changing too rapidly to even permit the development and testing of robust protocols. See Morone & Belkin (1995).

The traditional concept of medicine is rooted in the classic professional ideal. Physicians draw on their education, experience, and internalized norms to make clinical judgments. In doing so they balance two forms of expertise: systematic understanding of the causal mechanisms of disease and highly individualized information about each patient. As with any professional model, ultimate authority over diagnosis and treatment rests in the doctors' hands. Physicians may discuss medical options with their patients; however, they are ultimately accountable not to patient preferences but to the canons of their profession.

What is emerging from the new health services research is an alternative model of medicine. Ultimate authority rests on the results of systematic, replicable, statistical research. For each diagnosis there is a range of treatment options, each with measurable probabilities of success. Medical authority resides in expert panels reviewing aggregate data rather than individual physicians examining individual patients.

Note the crucial shift. Internalized professional judgment becomes suspect. It is unscientific. It creates the costly variations in medical practice that forced the residents of Boston to spend millions of dollars in unnecessary care. In the new model, health services researchers studying outcomes have seized the mantle of scientific authority away from practicing physicians. Some of the health service researchers even developed a certain measure of contempt for traditional medical knowledge. It is based, they argue, on individual case studies more than properly randomized control trials. It is more art than science (Morone & Belkin, 1995, pp. 3–4; Freund, 1994; Tanenbaum, 1994).

The key point is not that the new model is in any sense more accurate than the old. Rather, its significance lies in the policies that it enabled. It broke the long-honored scientific sanctity of individual physician judgments. Now, organizations seeking to control medicine could control individual physicians without violating the canons of scientific medicine. On the contrary, control over clinicians could be asserted with the claim that it was *improving* medicine, rendering it more reliable while reining in its costs.

Long before the researchers could claim "scientifically" robust protocols, however, private insurers had seized on the concept. Crude guidelines were roughed out and pressed into service. In theory, treatment protocols were to be diagnostic guides; in practice, health payers used them to fix reimbursement levels. To the consternation of the medical profession, payers have increasingly required physicians to seek approval before undertaking procedures.

Note the key change. Lay mangers oversee medicine. They approve or disapprove treatments and act as gatekeepers to medical services. The fundamental authority over medical treatment—over who gets what services—shifts from the individual physicians to administrative personnel working for payers touting managed care. The new authority is won with two promises: it will save costs and it will improve medicine by insuring that care is appropriate.

The Consequences for Health Care Business

At the heart of the managed care revolution that is rapidly remaking American medicine is the lay oversight of physicians. An estimated 60 percent of American workers are already in managed care plans (Toner, 1995). And that figure understates the numbers, for payers and hospitals everywhere are instituting controls. Although there are important differences among different kinds of plans, the general trend is clear and powerful.

If lay management of physicians is possible, then physicians become like other workers. The result is a stunning innovation with few parallels in other industrialized nations: the rise of new corporate forms of health care delivery.

In traditional medical settings professional norms and power constituted a formidable barrier to this kind of change. American managers were routinely frustrated in their efforts to discipline the free-spending physicians. Now, managed care rearranges the institutional mechanisms. Concrete management controls reach from health payers into the most micro medical details in American hospitals, clinics, and physician offices. With funding at stake, payers can oversee clinicians, case by case. What the new managerial techniques make

possible is the rise of classic corporate enterprise. With the subordination of physicians, medicine is reconstructing itself into America's largest business.

Of course, the coming of the medical corporation has been predicted before, most famously in the 1980s when for-profit hospital chains appeared poised to transform American medicine. By the mid-1980s, their rapid growth stalled after they had acquired many of the hospitals treating relatively better-off patients in relatively unregulated portions of the United States (Starr, 1982; Gray, 1983). This time, the trend is broader, more fundamental, more powerful. Across the country, corporate enterprise is remaking health care.

There is no systematic analysis, yet, of the new American medicine. But through a frenzy of activity (reported most faithfully in the business press) one can make out the usual signs of corporate capitalism: horizontal or vertical integration as traditional insurers, managed care plans, hospitals, and primary care practices frenetically combine, merge, acquire one another, and sell one another off (Morone & Belkin, 1995, p. 9); the accumulation of enormous pools of capital as health care corporations are traded on the major stock exchanges. For example, in 1995, the nine largest traded health maintenance organizations, taken together, held $9.5 billion in cash (*Medical Benefits*, 1995).

At the same time, health care institutions are accumulating a growing (and for many health care managers, an unprecedented) debt burden. There has also been the development of a powerful managerial class. On the level of health care delivery, physicians often testify that there are managers managing every aspect of medicine. Chief executive officers enjoy salaries typical of Fortune 500 firms (Finkel, 1993).

With the shift in organizational form comes a shift in purpose. The logic of corporate enterprise is no secret. It is designed to make money for investors.

The Consequences for Social Justice

As E. E. Schattschneider (1970) famously observed, "all organization is the mobilization of bias." American health care is rapidly and decisively biasing itself against social redistribution or any sort of "right" to health care.

The right to health care does not easily fit into the rising corporate model.

Of course, the concept of health care as a universal right has been highly contested and only partially won in the United States. Physicians have always operated with a distinctly entrepreneurial spirit (Rothman, 1994). Still, in the past, professional codes proscribed turning away the sick without any care. And loosely overseen funding enabled many physicians to redistribute resources at the point of service—the famous medical "sliding fee." Indeed, physicians once pointed to their sliding fee scales to argue that liberal programs were unnecessary, that no one who needed care was being turned away.

Business logic is different. Managed care is organized precisely to avoid cross-subsidizing other patients. Payers compete to pay as little as possible (so they can offer lower premiums for clients and higher returns for investors). As medicine becomes a product sold to clients by competing corporations, the ethos of health care rights falls outside the logic governing the system.

The Clinton plan was such a complicated contraption in part because its designers tried to embrace both the emerging corporate medicine and universalistic entitlement. Ironically, the process itself stimulated the new market forces as health institutions jockeyed for position under what appeared to be an imminent federal intervention. The plan's ultimate defeat further liberated the entrepreneurs.

Whereas Clinton faced the standard American institutional biases against big reforms, such efforts in the future will find the bias against them even steeper. This time, reform came onto the agenda before business medicine had fully articulated itself as a political interest. Next time, the state will be meddling in America's largest business sector, likely organized and running on unabashedly market principles.

The occasional public outcry only marks the velocity of change. For instance, when health maintenance organizations (HMOs) began to pay for just twenty-four hours of hospital care after normal births, New Jersey and Maryland passed laws requiring insurers to provide mothers with a second hospital day. The critical point lies in the parties that got engaged in the fight: state legislatures, the insurance industry, and HMOs wrangled over what was until very recently a simple matter of clinical discretion.

The conflicts over the length of hospital stays also hint at the future contours of American health politics. Whenever corporations rise up in American industries, politicians tend to respond to public complaints by introducing regulatory controls. Such regulations do not generally alter the new shape of the industry but aim to alleviate the harshest (or least popular) consequences of the emerging corporate regime.

Future American health politics are likely to revisit such traditional issues as cost control and gaps in health insurance. But the old issues will likely be played out in a radically new political context of corporate medical power, constrained (but not fundamentally challenged) by government regulation and occasional public outcries.

Friedrich Hayek, the great Austrian proponent of market capitalism, warned famously about the slippery slope from social welfare to socialism (Hayek, 1946). The slope from social welfare universalism to predatory corporate capitalism may prove to be even more slippery.

REFERENCES

BenDavid, Naftali. (1993). Clinton health plan splits old alliances. *Legal Times, 11* (October), 523–527.

Brady, David, & Kara Buckley. (1995). Health care reform in the 103rd Congress: A predictable failure. *Journal of Health Politics, Policy and Law, 20* (2), 448–454.

Brown, Lawrence. (1994). Dogmatic slumbers: American business and health policy. In James Morone & Gary Belkin (Eds.), *The politics of health care reform: Lessons from the past, prospects for the future.* Durham, NC: Duke University Press.

Clymer, Adam, (1994). Long legislative route for Clinton health plan. *New York Times, 27* (February), A20.

de Tocqueville, Alexis. (1966). *Democracy in America* (J. P. Mayer & Max Lerner, Eds.; George B. Lawrence, Trans.). New York: Harper & Row.

duRivage, Virginia. (1992). Flexibility trap: The proliferation of marginal jobs. *American Prospect, 9,* 85–93.

Filene, Peter. (1970). An obituary for "the progressive movement." *American Quarterly, 22* (1970), 20–34.

Finkel, Marion L. (1993). Managed care is not the answer. *Journal of Health Politics, Policy and Law, 18* (1), 105–112.

Fisher, Elliot, John Wennberg, Therese Stukel, & Sandra Sharp. (1994). Hospital readmission rates for cohorts of Medicare beneficiaries in Boston and New Haven. *New England Journal of Medicine, 331* (15), 989–995.

Freund, Deborah. (1994). Outcomes assessment: Market incentives or regulatory fiat? In Richard Arnould, Robert Rich, & William White (Eds.), *Competitive approaches to health care reform*. Washington, D.C.: Urban Institute Press.

Gray, Bradford. (1993). The legislative battle over health services research. *Health Affairs, 11* (4), 38–66.

Gray, Bradford. (Ed.). (1983). *The new health care for profit*. Washington, D.C.: National Academy Press.

Hayek, Friedrich. (1946). *The road to serfdom*. Chicago: University of Chicago Press.

Marmor, Theodore. (1994). *Understanding health care reform*. New Haven, CT: Yale University Press.

Marmor, Theodore, & Jon Oberlander. (1994). *A citizen's guide to the health care reform debate*. Paper delivered at the 90th annual meeting of the American Political Science Association, New York, September 1–4.

Martin, Cathy Jo. (1994). *Business and the politics of social innovation*. (Working Paper). New York: The Russell Sage Foundation.

McConnell, Grant. (1966). *Private power and American democracy*. New York: Alfred Knopf.

Medical Benefits. (1995). The HMO picture: More consolidation, more growth, more government business. *Medical Benefits, 12* (May 15), A5.

Morone, James A. (1990). *The democratic wish: Popular participation and the limits of American government*. New York: Basic Books.

Morone, James A. (1992). The bias of American politics: Rationing health care in a weak state. *University of Pennsylvania Law Review, 140* (5), 1923–1938.

Morone, James A. (1995). Nativism, hollow corporations and managed competition: Why the Clinton health reform failed. *Journal of Health Politics, Policy and Law, 20* (2), 391–398.

Morone, James A., & Gary Belkin. (1995). *The science illusion and the triumph of medical capitalism*. Paper prepared for delivery at the 1995 annual meetings of the American Political Science Association, Chicago, IL, August 31–September 3.

Morone, James A., & Jan Goggin. (1995). Health politics in Europe: Welfare states in a market era. *Journal of Health Politics, Policy and Law, 20* (3), 557–570.

Rockman, Bert. (1995). The Clinton presidency and health care reform. *Journal of Health Politics, Policy and Law, 20* (2), 399–402.

Rothman, David. (1994). A century of failure: Class barriers to reform. In James Morone & Gary Belkin (Eds.), *The politics of health care reform: Lessons from the past, prospects for the future*. Durham, NC: Duke University Press.

Scattshneider, E. E. (1970). *The semisovereign people*. Hinsdale, IL: Dryden Press.

Skocpol, Theda. (1994). Is the time finally right? Health insurance reforms in the 1990s. In James Morone & Gary Belkin (Eds.), *The politics of health care reform: Lessons from the past, prospects for the future*. Durham, NC: Duke University Press.

Skowronek, Steven. (1982). *Building a new American state*. New York: Cambridge University Press.

Starr, Paul. (1982). *The social transformation of American medicine*. New York: Basic Books.

Steinmo, Sven, & Jon Watts. (1995). It's the institutions, stupid! Why comprehensive national health insurance always fails in the United States. *Journal of Health Politics, Policy and Law, 20* (2), 330–372.

Tanenbaum, Sandra. (1994). Knowing and acting in medical practice. *Journal of Health Politics, Policy and Law, 19* (Spring), Part 1, 27–44.

Toner, Robin. (1994). Pollsters see a silent storm that swept away Democrats. *New York Times* (November 16), A14.

Toner, Robin. (1995). Washington memo: Now it's Republicans who see a health care crisis looming. *New York Times, 23* (April), A1.

Wennberg, John. (1973). Small area variations in health care delivery. *Science, 182*, 1102–1108.

Wennberg, John. (1990). Sounding board: Outcomes research, cost containment and the fear of health care rationing. *New England Journal of Medicine, 323* (17), 1202–1204.

West, Darrell, & Diane Heith. (1994). *Harry and Louise go to Washington: Political advertising and health care reform*. Paper delivered at the 90th annual meeting of the American Political Science Association, New York, September 1–4.

Wiebe, Robert. (1967). *The search for order*. New York: Hill and Wang.

Wood, Gordon. (1969). *The creation of the American Republic*. New York: W. W. Norton.

CHAPTER

The Political Economy
of Health Services:
A Review and Assessment of Major
Ideological Influences and the Impact
of New Economic Realities

Roger M. Battistella
with the assistance of
John B. Ostrick

The attention now commanded by health policy in national political affairs is an indication of the enormously strategic position that the health sector occupies in the general economy. It also reflects a sharp escalation in the clash of interests associated with the difficulty of resolving ostensibly competing and contradictory objectives for efficiency and equity in the production and consumption of health services. Much of this conflict is the manifestation of tensions stemming from a major transition in economic and demographic factors that assault the continuing viability of public and private arrangements for financing health care established under earlier, more favorable circumstances.

Due to developments such as the aging of the population, the growing importance of diseases requiring lengthier and costlier forms of treatment, and rising demands for social and economic justice in the distribution and quality of health services, government and private employers are under constant pressure to increase the size of health outlays. This pressure is occurring, however, at a time of severe macroeconomic disturbances stemming from the financial burden of servicing massive accumulations of public debt, the difficulty of maintaining economic superiority in an increasingly global economy, and the gradual decline in living standards due to disincentives for savings and economically productive long-term investments. Additional disturbances stem from the ascendancy of political ideology wary of growth in the size of central government and spending for social programs. The future of the health sector is further clouded by the decay of confidence in propositions about the relationship between health and medicine and by the waning status and power of the medical profession. Contrary to what was long accepted as true, health spending is now seen as inimical to economic growth, and the medical profession is widely regarded as an obstacle to cost-effective, high-quality patient care.

Since resource scarcity first attracted serious national attention in the early 1970s, following a lengthy post–World War II prosperity in which affluence was popularly assumed to have become a permanent condition of American life, efficiency has emerged as the solution of choice to the dilemma of how to do more without spending more. Disagreement over means, however, has produced a welter of confusing and contradictory initiatives, running the gamut from command planning and regulation to market competition, in which failure is the single constant.

The dissatisfaction and skepticism accompanying the succession of failures to control expenditures obscure recognition of some remarkable health policy achievements beginning in the 1960s. These include the virtual elimination of the hospital and physicians' services utilization gap between upper- and low-income people; the modernization and technological upgrading of the nation's hospitals; the return to the commu-

nity of many physically and mentally disabled persons previously destined to spend their lives in oppressive institutional settings; the correction of aggregate deficiencies in the supply of health personnel; and the improved protection of the aged and low-income groups against the high cost of medical services (Anderson, 1985). Whether attributable to health services or other causes, a notable increase in life expectancy also has benefited U.S. citizens. Another largely unrecognized achievement has been the progress made in converting the organizational and managerial profile of health services from turn-of-the-century handcraft to modern industrial-corporate lines (Battistella & Weil, 1986).

These mixed impressions and events comprise the backdrop for this political-economic review of U.S. health services. Political-economic inquiry involves the study of changes in the economic relationships and the composition of political power within a framework of superordinate values regarding what is fair and just. In the ensuing analysis, health policy is presented largely as the outcome of the interplay of political and economic orientations whose influence has varied over time. For convenience, these orientations have been organized under four principal headings: the normative approach, the rationalist approach, the neoconservative approach, and the Neo-Marxist approach. Following a description of each of these four intellectual influences and a discussion of their significance in the evolution of postwar national health policy, the prospects for continuing equity gains are assessed in the context of more recent developments.

THE NORMATIVE APPROACH

The predominant approach to health services in the United States until recently has been normative in character. That is to say, individuals and groups have sought to influence the role of government in the health services field mainly on the basis of strong convictions about what is or ought to be highly valued.

The normative approach to health services emerges clearly in the uncompleted saga of national health insurance in the United States. Armed with the knowledge of precedents of government intervention in Germany and England, under conditions of widespread unemployment and medical needs similar to those then prevailing in the United States, reformers at the turn of the century unsuccessfully sought to humanize many of the demeaning aspects of charity and welfare medicine institutionalized in practices derived from the Elizabethan poor laws. In doing so, they endeavored to establish the principle that health services ought to be provided as a right on the basis of medical need, regardless of ability to pay (Davis, 1975).

After nearly fifty years of ceaseless but unfulfilled striving, these efforts were partially rewarded with the passage of Medicare in 1965, which established a compulsory program of hospital benefits for retired and disabled workers along with a voluntary program of physicians' benefits for the aged. Treatment of end-stage renal disease for all age groups was included in 1972. At the same time, reformers succeeded in vastly enlarging the influence of the federal government in the operation of state and local public assistance programs, in eliminating some of the harsher features of eligibility tests, and in broadening the reach of welfare medical programs beyond the indigent to include the working poor. Most of these gains were incorporated in the Medicaid program (Fein, 1986).

Marked by sharp ideological divisions, the battle for national health insurance swirled around the issue of whether access to health care was a privilege or a right. Arrayed on the side of privilege were the professional interest groups, the American Medical Association (AMA), the American Hospital Association (AHA), and the American Dental Association (ADA). They feared restrictions on their freedom to pursue unrestricted economic rewards, their autonomy in clinical decision making, and their powers for self-regulation and governance. Their cause was championed by political, commercial, and manufacturing organizations, such as the National Association of Manufacturers, the Chamber of Commerce, and the Young Americans for Freedom, which tended to regard themselves as custodians of competitive market values (Bowler et al., 1978).

Both sides of the national health insurance issue received considerable support from academic economists.

Competitive market economists, led by Milton Friedman (1962), insisted that medical care is a private good in that most benefits accrue to the individual rather than society. The implications for groups outside the labor force through no fault of their own, retirees and the permanently and totally disabled, were frequently obscured in the abstract polemics exalting the competitive market as an instrument for maximizing individual freedom and economic efficiency (Lindsay, 1980).

Because competitive market proponents consider medical care to be much like economic goods and services in general, they, to the consternation of allies in the medical profession, assert that restricting the practice of medicine to licensed doctors of medicine is an abridgment of market efficiency and an enticement to abuse. This is the logical result of their belief that human nature is incorrigibly acquisitive and selfish. Conservative economists are prepared to make only the slightest allowance for negative health care externalities endangering the welfare of others connected to environmental pollution, and such lifestyle hazards as smoking and alcohol and drug abuse. To the fullest extent feasible, they prefer market incentives (taxes and fines) rather than publicly administered programs to safeguard community well-being (Fein, 1980).

On the other hand, economists immersed in the sociopolitical history of medicine stress the vulnerability of the sick to exploitation in the marketplace due to the special dimension of anguish in illness and other constraints on consumer rationality. The professional status of medicine is seen as an instrument for community integration as well as the enrichment of individual welfare. Economists holding that health care is a right typically argue that spending for maternal and child health services and the working-age population is a good investment in economic growth.

Perhaps the best recognized defense of the special character of health service is that prepared by Kenneth Arrow (1963), who concluded that a wide disparity in required and actual relationships severely limits the relevance of competition theory. Sociologists opposed to using the market to ration health services instinctively underscore the moral and utilitarian aspects. The late Talcott Parsons (1951), for example, was foremost among his colleagues in the scholarly defense of the idea that health care is a social good.

Shortcomings of the Normative Approach

The normative approach to health policy prevailed up until the mid-1960s. Since then it has fallen into disfavor. Critics deride the normative approach for being "value-laden," for being overly disputatious and rhetorical, and for using data to buttress policy preferences rather than scientific aims (Battistella, 1972b).

The accusation in brief is that normative analysis tends to simplify the issues and portrays antagonists in hues of good and evil. For example, organized medicine, led by the AMA, often was pictured by reformers as a reactionary monolith, whereas groups favoring reforms in the organization and financing of solo fee-for-service medicine were stereotyped by status quo adherents as disciples of subversive socialist and communist teachings. Likewise, progress in the implementation of welfare-state principles was characterized as well-intentioned but impractical foolishness or, conversely, as tangible proof of the innately noble affinity of human nature for altruism and justice (Battistella & Wheeler, 1978). Amidst such ideological sparring, impulses to enlist government campaigns against poverty invited denunciation of such involvement as disguised paternalism that does more to perpetuate dependency on public programs than to advance responsibility and independence among the disadvantaged.

Criticism of the normative approach, however, is not above reproof. It is seldom dispassionate, since it originates from interests advocating a purportedly superior alternative. Also, the handicaps under which the normative approach functioned were rarely acknowledged. One such handicap that invited appeals to emotion rather than reason was the shortage of reliable data to guide decision making. For example, nationwide registration of births did not occur until 1933. Reliable information on the population's need for health services was not available until passage of the National Health Survey Act of 1956, which provided for a continuing survey and special studies of sickness and disability in the nation (Jonas, 1981). Subsequent improvements have produced an explosion in the amount of informa-

tion on the cost-effectiveness of new technologies and the quality and economy of services given by providers so that facts, assisted by computerized data processing, are more easily obtainable to temper passion in the elucidation of objectives and evaluation of program results. Nevertheless the influence of ideology remains strong. That proponents of social justice in the availability of health services continue to be ridiculed as misguided idealists or worse mirrors a powerful attachment to competitive market doctrine in U.S. culture. The emotional power of this belief system constricts impartial study and discussion of the role of government in national affairs.

In contrast to the experience of most other industrialized free market countries, American free enterprise values successfully withstood the postwar advance of welfare state services. Notwithstanding a substantial increase in public spending following passage of Medicare and Medicaid in the mid-1960s, the nation's health sector remains predominantly private. Public outlays, for example, represent only about two-fifths of total health spending, compared to an average of around three-fourths in Western Europe (Aaron, 1991). The United States, moreover, remains the only major industrial power without a comprehensive national health insurance program. Finally, the situation in the health sector closely resembles that of the economy as a whole, where government spending accounts for only about 37 percent of the gross national product (GNP). In many other highly developed western and northern European countries, on the other hand, the amount of national wealth commanded by government runs between 48 percent and 63 percent (Organization for Economic Cooperation and Development, 1987).

THE RATIONALIST APPROACH[1]

In the midst of sharp controversy throughout the 1970s over the appropriateness of a larger federal presence in the health sector, the simultaneous escalation of

---

[1]Use of the label "rationalist" to identify this school of thought is not meant to imply that the approach is more "rational" than the normative approach (or, for that matter, the Neo-Marxist and neoconservative perspectives introduced later in this chapter). Both approaches are rational since they make

formerly modest and unconnected rates of inflation and unemployment spurred broad agreement on the need to constrain health spending. A pervasive sense of urgency was amplified by annual rates of increase in health spending that were two or more times higher than those for other goods and services. Economic and financial anxieties fostered expectations that the imposition of financial discipline through some form of national health insurance and global budgeting was inevitable (U.S. Department of Health, Education, and Welfare, 1976).

Higher unemployment compounded the strains on government budgets. Loss of wages and private health insurance among the unemployed expanded the size of the population eligible to receive Medicaid coverage and public assistance. Less apparent were the social costs of prolonged unemployment. Subject to different lead times, the combination of physical deprivation and emotional-mental stress was documented to be highly correlated with higher rates of individual pathology and community disorganization (U.S. Congress, Joint Economic Committee, 1980b). Another unanticipated consequence of recession was the stimulus for financially squeezed states to shift welfare costs to the federal government. Creative accounting practices and program restructuring were commonly used to maximize the federal contribution in shared financial responsibility services (Bulgaro & Webb, 1980).

Other financial concerns stemmed from the growth in spending for social welfare services, which together with health spending accounted for roughly one-half of the federal budget. While some observers celebrated this as an irrefutable signal of the triumph of welfare-

state principles, others fretted about the demise of conservative economic and political values. Still others became apprehensive about the potentially negative implications of changes in the composition of the federal budget for the general economy (Janowitz, 1976).

The political and economic tensions accumulating during this period from the activation of government and the ascendancy of welfare-state principles helped provoke a reaction against the normative approach to policy decision making. Although conflict among competing values helped define issues and solutions, there often was a steep price to pay in terms of legislative paralysis. Negotiation and compromise are difficult in a climate of unconstrained ideological fervor. These shortcomings prompted interest in alternatives for expediting decision making. The sheer magnitude of health outlays, moreover, stirred curiosity about the returns to society. In combination with mounting discomfort over the share of national wealth consumed by government, these concerns legitimized efforts to quantify the costs and benefits of government programs (Battistella & Smith, 1974).

Increased political conflict emanating from the slowing of economic growth on the one hand and rising demands for more and better services on the other propelled the emergence of quantitative techniques for depoliticizing decision making. Confronted with a zero-sum environment, elected officials, harried by constituents' complaints and worried about reelection prospects, were predisposed to welcome the introduction of purportedly objective and value-free decision-making methods that diffused responsibility for unpopular decisions. Because these methods characteristically involve an economic or technical means–end orientation in which the calculation of self-interest is synonymous with rational behavior, this form of decision making is described in the policy analysis literature as the rationalist approach (Smith, 1978).

Unlike the image of clarity and conciseness associated with decision making in the private sector, the term "scientific management" is somewhat vague. Among believers in competition, scientific management achieves cost control and efficiency from market discipline and the application of quantitative methods in cost accounting, finance, marketing, and production. Among

---

the same use of reason, are subject to the same rules of logic, and are ultimately subject to the same test of how closely they match reality. The distinction is that one approach (the normative) starts with certain overt beliefs about what should be based on philosophical convictions. In purporting to deal solely with what can be measured, the other approach (rationalist) conceals from view the behavioral assumptions underlying quantitative methods. In point of fact, both are value-laden, since both are based on beliefs about how people should behave. The term "rationalist" is used because of its prominence in the field of policy analysis and to highlight the political implications of allegedly objective-quantitative methods. Another choice would have been to substitute the word "empirical" for "rationalist." The author is indebted to Edmund D. Pellegrino for his suggestion to clarify the reason for choosing the "rationalist" label.

nonbelievers, however, the purpose of these methods is to escape market discipline through the substitution of corporate power and planning for idealized laws of supply and demand. The confusion is multiplied by the contradiction whereby those actually engaged in planning retain ideological loyalty to the sanctity of economic and political relationships derived from the theory of perfect competition (Battistella & Chester, 1972).

Ascension of the rationalist approach coincided with a period of increased activity in the restructuring of health services. The attainment of an organizational pattern of hospital and physicians' services, with fewer but larger vertically integrated units containing vastly improved capabilities for addressing chronic production and quality control deficiencies, was an aspiration that transcended political differences in the health politics of the 1970s. The commonly agreed upon goal was to reconstruct health services delivery from a "cottage industry" to a modern corporate structure (Battistella, 1972b). Since then, the influence of this orientation has grown considerably and it now constitutes one of the main parameters of health reform (Battistella & Buchanan, 1987). The goal of productivity enhancement finds expression in such concerns as surplus capacity in facilities and personnel due to construction and personnel decisions unsupported by sound economic and financial principles because of the lack of discipline associated with open-ended, retrospective, fee-for-service reimbursement. Another important focus is on the diagnostic and treatment advances that are dramatically lowering the demand for costly hospital services and raising the demand for less expensive ambulatory and community services. Technological innovation has sharply reduced dependence on hospitals to the point where two-fifths or more of all acute beds have become redundant. The surplus is destined to grow higher due to new technological breakthroughs and the spread of reimbursement methods that penalize medically questionable and unnecessary admissions and lengths of stay.

Problems of quality management are widespread. Albeit one of the biggest components of the national economy, the health sector ranks among the most backward in matters of quality control. Since systematic inquiry of what happens to patients following the completion of treatment is rare, knowledge about the value of medical and surgical procedures is too limited to enable the formulation of reliable efficacy and cost-effectiveness standards. Scientifically unsupportable claims and anecdotal evidence prevail in the absence of randomized clinical trials and rigorous technology assessment studies. Therefore, an inexact but large amount of what is done to patients is medically questionable or inappropriate.

The language and values of the rationalist approach have a broad appeal that transcends ideological divisions. They capture a rich cultural folklore extolling the innate superiority of market forces over those of government. Their allure extends to persons believing in the efficacy of scientific management, whether in the planning of health services or in the running of complex corporate enterprises.

The popularity of the rationalist approach facilitated the establishment of a consensus for change forceful enough to overcome the status quo in the organization of health services. The merger and consolidation movement among nongovernment community hospitals is but one significant example. Roughly one-half of all hospitals and one-half of all hospital beds in the United States can now be counted as components of multihospital systems, defined as corporations that own, lease, or manage two or more acute care hospitals. This development emulates private-sector managerial principles and is closely patterned after investor-owned health care systems, which comprise over two-fifths of all system hospitals and approximately one-third of all system beds (Haglund & Dowling, 1993). Possibly more significant, given the strong tradition of solo fee-for-service medicine in the United States, is the growth of bureaucratic-contractual modes of medical practice. The percentage of nonfederal physicians working in a group setting has grown from just under 10 percent in 1965 to over 33 percent currently, most of whom are affiliated with a multispecialty group organized as a professional corporation (Williams, 1993; Rodwin, 1993). Physicians also are becoming more dependent for their livelihood on organizations under nonmedical control. About 70 percent of physicians now contract with one or more managed care entities for some portion or all of their income (Gillis & Emmons, 1993). These arrangements, moreover, foretell a major assault on traditional clinical autonomy values inasmuch as their financial performance is a function of monitoring physician practice styles and use of resources.

The ramifications of the rationalist approach for the restructuring of health services are manifold. Rationalist logic and values are imbedded in a number of diverse developments of the 1970s, such as health planning, health maintenance organizations, professional standards review organizations (since revised and renamed professional review organizations), and the imposition of quotas on the supply of medical graduates by specialty. It is unlikely that change of such magnitude could have occurred in such a brief period of time if the policy issues had remained as highly politicized as they were during the peak influence of the normative approach.

Shortcomings of the Rationalist Approach

In retrospect, much of the optimism accompanying the introduction of rationalist methods was misguided. Far more was promised than could be delivered (Battistella & Smith, 1974), and many innate weaknesses have been disclosed.

First, claims that decisions should be based on facts alone and that facts speak for themselves are vacuous. They suggest that irrefutably valid data are readily obtainable and that analytic methods for the accumulation of facts are value-free. Policy decisions about Medicaid reimbursement for abortions, for example, are predominantly valuative ones. The same applies to national health insurance.

Second, the assumptions contained in rationalist models inadequately penetrate the complex environment in which decisions are made. There is nothing indisputably objective in the assignment of interest rates for establishing the relationship between values at different points in time or the assignment of the opportunity cost of capital diverted from more productive alternative expenditures. They involve assumptions about the future that are speculative, and they reflect the values of the analyst. The assignment of high interest and discount rates discriminates against taking actions that produce long-run benefits in preference for the short run. The bias is compounded whenever the economy is beset by high inflation. When all is said and done, these decisions are a matter of judgment.

Third, many aspects of good medical care are difficult to quantify. For example, how is the increased quality of life experience after kidney transplantation measured and compared to the quality of life of a kidney patient surviving on dialysis? Overall, the purpose of medical intervention has become more ambiguous. The concept of cure has no application to the vast number of problems constituting the bulk of health needs today, such as chronic and mental diseases and disabilities. Given the low likelihood of achieving a cure for disorders of this sort, the total effect of medical intervention is more important to assess, and this, too, is highly subjective. Whether people are satisfied with the caliber of medical services they receive and whether they view themselves to be in good or poor health are hard-to-measure social-psychological phenomena that have important effects on utilization of services and treatment outcomes.

For the most part, quantification in cost–benefit forms of analysis works best when what is being studied is accurately reflected in conventional market activities and prices. Oftentimes, the pressures for quantification so disregard common sense that equating health program benefits with market values sanctions socially corrosive consequences. For instance, when discounted future earnings are used to quantify the value of saving lives, investments in white male infants, because of differences in expected lifetime earnings, are easier to justify than are investments in black male infants. Women are similarly disadvantaged by this methodology, as are the elderly.

Fourth, rationality frequently is used as a guise for action based on the philosophical precepts of competitive market theory in which selfishness and greed have been elevated to the status of a moral system. The philosophical case of rational analysis does not accept that medical acts are an important aspect of the human relationship of giving and receiving, constituting the moral experience of mutual help (Campbell, 1978).

Fifth, the mounting realization that many health policy issues are highly subjective and qualitative suggests that allegedly objective techniques may be less important in the future. One such issue involves medical technology and human rights to treatment and dignified death. Another centers on entitlements to publicly supported health services. Limiting illness treatment for the poor to services meeting tests of efficacy and cost-effectiveness from which other socioeconomic groups are exempted is widely repudiated among persons viewing access to care as a form of social validation and caring. The trade-off between economic productivity and the quality of the environment is another example of the saliency of issues that cannot be resolved independently of political and social values. The controversy engendered by the medicalization of abortion and court-countenanced physician-assisted death sentences underscores the moral dimensions of contemporary health policy.

Generally speaking, the application of the rational approach has not succeeded in meeting its economic and efficiency objectives because the delivery of health care ultimately is judged not only in efficiency terms but also in terms of fairness. If anything, there is reason to believe that the calculus of self-interest may have exacerbated government efforts to contain health care expenditures. Indeed, the "rational" models behind the government's cost-containment strategy helped create situations in which health care providers were given "perverse" economic incentives to defeat controls. Assessing performance with commercial accounting principles that measure success by profit and loss encouraged providers to circumnavigate cost controls by artificially inflating the number of procedures performed or by underproviding medically appropriate services, depending on the method of reimbursement. Due to the inability of the rational models to capture the complexities of the health field, government found itself in the bizarre position of reimbursing hospitals for the services of financial experts whose jobs entail devising ways to manipulate or subvert cost-cutting policies (Battistella & Eastaugh, 1980a, 1980b).

Additional unintended consequences may arise in the future from the application of the scientific management paradigm to services that are intrinsically labor-intensive and highly personalized in nature. The scientific management outlook not only contains a bias for technological expansion capable of undermining priorities for cost containment, but it has a bureaucratic proclivity at variance with the essentially human dimensions of the doctor–patient relationship.

It is shortsighted to assume that most health policy problems can be solved by subjecting the medical profession to textbook-style management discipline and control, especially with respect to primary care (Battistella & Rundall, 1978a, 1978b). Such an assumption understates the value to society of the doctor–patient relationship, in which the bond of mutual confidence and respect is the key for minimizing disruptions in social and economic activities, many of which are associated with anxieties and symptoms for which no clinical cause can be established. Given the limitations on the life span and the aging of the population, good health increasingly is the result "of physician and patient working together, often in the face of uncertainty and fear" (Fuchs, 1974) rather than simple, one-time interventions ordered by the physician.

THE NEOCONSERVATIVE APPROACH[2]

Interest groups that have successfully advocated increased health spending certainly merit recognition for corresponding improvements both in medical technology and in social and territorial equity. These successes, however, have compounded economic concerns. Much opposition to future spending increases originates in the contention that present-day totals are too large. Health spending is perceived variously as having reached the stage of diminishing marginal social benefit, or as a drag on economic growth. Since 1950, annual health expenditures have been growing 3 percent

[2]In the policy literature the term "neoconservative" is commonly used as a designation for politically influential and intellectually stimulating left-of-center individuals who agree on the need for a more eclectic and pragmatic approach to social change. This conclusion results from their reexamination of many liberal precepts behind the social and political reforms of the past several decades (Steinfels, 1979). Confusion arises whenever the term "neo-liberal" is used as an expedient for concealing the acquisition of conservative values for tactical political purposes, such as retaining the support of liberal constituencies. Practically speaking, however, the differences are more cosmetic than substantive.

faster than expenditures for all other goods and services. Unless something is done to reduce the gap, health care will consume roughly one-third of the gross domestic product by the year 2030 (Fuchs, 1993). Considering the lackluster state of the national economy, a continuation of high rates of annual increases in health spending is unlikely.

Upwardly spiraling prices for health services attract inquiries about waste and inefficiency that reinforce worries about throwing good money after bad. Inflation also feeds skepticism about whether a positive relationship continues to exist between health status and aggregate health outlays. Indeed, it is now generally accepted that non-health services, such as housing, nutrition, lifestyle, and environmental safety—all highly correlated with income and socioeconomic status—are far more important to the quality of life and that the benefits of early diagnosis and treatment have been greatly overstated (McKinlay & McKinlay, 1977; Ratcliffe et al., 1984; Wilkinson, 1992). Counterevidence that a 10 percent increase in per capita medical care use is associated with a 1.5 percent decrease in mortality rates (Hadley, 1982) is either lost in the mass of criticism or interpreted as confirmation of the diminishing returns from health spending (Altman & Morgan, 1982).

New economic circumstances foreshadow a readjustment of the liberal agenda for health services' reform. Although not always explicit in health policy polemics, the liberal platform traditionally rested on a number of well-reasoned assumptions. Most important of all was the belief that economic growth would produce the resources needed to create a more just society without anyone suffering along the way. Prosperity would be sustained, moreover, by a sufficiently high birth rate for maintaining demand and by a large enough supply of gainfully employed workers to generate the funds to pay for health and social services allocated to the aged and the disabled (Donnison, 1979). The favorable economic and political conditions prevailing at the time of the introduction of Medicare and Medicaid were expected to continue, thereby lessening the chances of a financially driven backlash against an expanding government role. The crowning aspiration of reform was a system of universal health insurance in which comprehensive services were provided free at the time of use on the basis of medical need. These expectations, however, have been shaken by unforeseen economic and social developments.

It is naive for present-day liberals to expect that government will take on a bigger share of health spending along the lines of the British National Health Service or the Canadian example. Since 1983, the economy has enjoyed the longest peacetime expansion in the postwar era, yet the government's ability to absorb costly new social programs remains severely limited. The problem in brief is that relative to previous historical experience, the economy entered a period of slower growth beginning in the early 1970s from which it has not recovered. Measured in the value of lost production, the inflation-adjusted cost to the economy in the two decades following 1973 amounted to roughly $12 trillion, or more than $40,000 per capita (Madrick, 1995). Instead of adjusting to this decline in available resources, government health spending for the most part has continued along its earlier optimistic trajectory.

Paradoxically, the decline in economic growth has also provoked a reconsideration and revision of conservative doctrine. Despite numerous signs of a repudiation of planning and regulation and a preference for free market solutions, current national health policy initiatives do not signify a triumph of competitive market orthodoxy. Although competition and privatization evoke broad support in current political discourse, the words, as elaborated later, have acquired new meaning. Rather than a separation from government, competition now signifies a union of the two and a more complicated approach to regulation. Similarly, privatization does not indicate an end to government intervention in expanding access to health care so much as a change in financing and a more innovative use of public power in pursuit of health care for all. Turn-of-the-century notions of the marketplace are too discordant with contemporary exigencies for tighter controls over health services spending and delivery.

The invocation of absolutes from the political left or right belies the complexities of contemporary policy. Higher requisites for social cohesion point to an innovative search for balance and moderation in the pursuit of interdependent goals of equity and efficiency. Acknowledgment of the necessity for a trade-off between these two goals constitutes the basis for a new political approach: neoconservatism, joining pragmatically minded persons from left and right of center of the health policy spectrum.

Neoconservatives may differ on important issues such as defense spending, affirmative action, and abortion, but they remain supportive of the basic contours of the welfare state. Neoconservatives also concur that the partnership between government and the private sector should be redefined to better accommodate the changing complexities of a mature economy in which low-productivity service industries are the principal source of employment. The challenge of fulfilling political aspirations for equity in an era of economic limits is an overarching preoccupation.

What constitutes grounds for a distinct school of thought is an outlook emphasizing the constraints on political power to effect change and the virtues of public restraint in dealing with complex social problems. In addition to focusing on the difficulties of establishing and sustaining the necessary consensus for effective action in today's social and political environment, neoconservatives are alert to the lengthening administrative and technical lead times required for the solution of many problems. This perspective prompts them to conclude that far more harm than good results from the sharp and erratic short-term actions typical of current government policies. Neoconservatives also share a deep faith in individual opportunity and achievement, rather than parity among social groups through affirmative action quotas, as the best pathway to human progress. Improved balance between self-reliance and government assistance is another hallmark feature, together with the coupling of self-responsibility with social and environmental contributions to behavioral problems (Steinfels, 1979).

Since the onset of macroeconomic malaise in the early 1970s, a heightened regard for what is affordable and attainable has diminished and blurred differences in how all but extreme conservatives and liberals approach health policy issues. This convergence is apparent, for instance, in the broad-based congressional support for free enterprise incentives as practical instruments for overcoming the strong resistance to restructuring and managerial reforms within the health sector (Battistella & Buchanan, 1987). More so than any other single word, pragmatism best conveys the dominant mental attitude within the health-policymaking mainstream today.

The ability of the health sector to enlarge its share of the gross domestic product since 1950 from a modest 4.5 percent to today's disconcertingly high double-digit level was in large part due to the prevalence and depth of trust in some key assumptions and beliefs, which collectively constituted a compelling conventional wisdom. Among these were the following. First, concentrated, large-scale spending for biomedical research and development will significantly improve the population's life expectancy and health levels. Second, the best place to care for patients is in the hospital, since that is where the best technology and medical services are concentrated. Third, medical specialization is both necessary and desirable. In an era of rapid proliferation of knowledge and rising public expectations for technical competence, general practice and family medicine are outmoded. Fourth, spending for health services is finite because of the eventual satiation of unmet medical needs and the benefits of preventive medicine and health education. Fifth, the role of government in health services should be confined to restoring and buttressing the capital requirements of high-technology services and the purchasing power of consumers (Battistella, 1972a).

Dissatisfaction among policymakers with the unintended consequences and failures of actions taken in accordance with these convictions contributed to many of the present uncertainties about the future of public intervention in the health sector. Contrary to a scenario of uninterrupted progress, it became increasingly evident during the 1970s that: (1) spending opportunities for health services were limitless; (2) development of high-technology medical services was reaching the stage of diminishing marginal social benefit; (3) neglect of generalist, first-contact medical services was very costly in economic and human terms; (4) modern medical diagnosis and treatment inadvertently contributed to a surprisingly large amount of illness and disability; (5) there was an oversupply of hospital beds; (6) increasing the supply of physicians was not the solution to problems of maldistribution by location and type of practice; (7) it was perilous to rely on professional self-regulation alone for the attainment of goals of economy and quality; (8) unrealistically high public confidence in the benefits of medical treatment was resulting in the medicalization of many social problems that could be better dealt with through other means; and (9) the magnitude of health spending was a hindrance to economic growth. Skepticism and disillusionment about the value of health services were fostered by a succession of highly critical publications beginning early in the 1970s, both in the United States and abroad (Carlson, 1975; Cochrane, 1972; Fuchs, 1974; Illich, 1976; Lalonde, 1974; Maxwell, 1974; McKeown, 1976; Pocincki et al., 1973; Powles, 1973; Torrey, 1974; U.S. House of Representatives, 1976; U.S. Department of Health, Education, and Welfare, 1976).

The disassociation of many prominent health liberals from the conventional wisdom is possibly best exemplified in the specially prepared 1977 edition of *Daedalus*, "Doing Better and Feeling Worse: Health in the United States," edited by Dr. John H. Knowles. The issue contained a number of far-ranging revisionist interpretations by politically and intellectually influential authors such as David E. Rogers, Donald S. Frederickson, Lewis Thomas, and Renee Fox. Contributions to the publication were linked by a common concern that despite the accomplishments of the U.S. health care system things had recently gone badly and new solutions were required.

While harboring many dissimilar views, health policy neoconservatives have a common orientation regarding some of the more important choices affecting the future of health policy. Given the recency of conversion to this viewpoint, however, the neoconservative movement is less established in experience than in the extrapolation of logical consequences and probabilities.[3] For the most part, health neoconservatives remain committed to the basic goals of the welfare state and retain a preference for equity over efficiency. On the other hand, they accept the reality of resource scarcity and concede the shortcomings of orthodox liberal doctrine geared to the continuing growth of health services and government intervention. As in other applications, practicality is a distinguishing feature.

Health neoconservatives remain open to the possibility that pricing may be acceptable, but only under carefully specified conditions. In an age of limits, what purpose is served by encumbering public financing with services that are of questionable medical value? Assuming that appropriate technology assessment capabilities exist, it is both practical and desirable from a health-promotion and cost-savings standpoint to restrict public financing to services determined to meet safety and efficacy standards (U.S. Congress, Office of Technology Assessment, 1980). Surely services of unproven safety have no commercial place in a society obligated to protect the health of its citizens, although nonharmful services of questionable efficacy might well be left to the market. Nor is it defensible to continue payments for medically questionable and inappropriate diagnostic and treatment services when low-income groups are being deprived of essential services because of constraints on federal and state government spending. The amount of money now spent on medically valueless or questionable procedures is generally conceded to equal 20 percent or more of all outlays (Mitchell & Virtz, 1986; Wolfe, 1988; *Consumer Reports*, 1992). For many frequently performed hospital procedures, research consistently concludes a rate of inappropriate use for surgery, admissions, and testing that ranges from 20 percent to 70 percent (Berwick, 1994).

The shortcomings of quantitative models and techniques aside, neoconservatives generally support efforts to better establish the effectiveness and costs of health services in comparison with alternative expenditures. In the interest of informed decision making they prefer that the hidden values of putatively objective methods be made explicit and that the analyses not be skewed in

---

[3]The writings of Wildavsky (1979) and Glazer (1971) provide some insight into the application of the neoconservative philosophy to health care, as they are members of the broader neoconservative establishment who have commented specifically on health policy.

ways that fail to capture the highly subjective contributions of health services (Wildavsky, 1979).

Pricing may also be acceptable to pragmatists looking for ways to supplement revenues for health services, provided that it does not deter early diagnosis and treatment of efficacious services. In this respect, aggressive cost recovery through the assignment of patient charges based on income and ability to pay is increasingly advocated as a method for husbanding scarce public resources targeted for truly needy persons.

The experience of the 1970s suggests that even among liberals uncomfortable with neoconservatism the practical uses of the market have become widely recognized. In the case of health maintenance organization policy, for example, liberal legislators and union allies sought to accelerate the growth of prepaid group practice by turning competitive market rhetoric against forces of organized medicine, which in the past had successfully used the same tactic in defense of solo fee-for-service practice. Thus confronted, organized medicine no longer was able to condemn the transfiguration of solo fee-for-service practice as socialist-inspired malice (Ehrbar, 1977). Nor did liberals hesitate to support the aggressive anti-trust measures used by the Federal Trade Commission (FTC) to weaken the monopoly powers of the health profession—a move dramatically counter to long-standing historical justifications for the insulation of health services from unbridled competition and for the bestowal of professional privilege (Iglehart, 1978).

Neoconservatives are inclined, furthermore, to believe that the principle of universalism at the core of liberal health policy is politically and financially untenable in a poorly performing economy, and that the interests of the disadvantaged can better be protected by the principle of selectivity. The concept of a totally publicly financed and government-operated service is dismissed as economically and politically unrealistic.

Shortcomings of the Neoconservative Approach

The shortcomings of the neoconservative approach to health policy approximate those of the generic neoconservative movement itself. Proponents of this approach often are viewed as having abandoned their commitment to justice and equity for political expediency. Neoconservativism lacks a clear and simple vision of a "just" society, promulgating instead an eclectic mix of applied principles fraught with ambiguity and inconsistency. Rather than proceeding along a single line, neoconservatives prefer multipronged strategies incorporating elements of regulation and competition more closely resembling actual decision-making conditions. In the world of realpolitik to which they are attuned, the normal rules of mathematics are suspended and the shortest distance between two points is seldom a straight line. While brilliantly inspired, it is doubtful whether the blurring of ideological divisions is conducive to generating and sustaining disciplined political energy for the long-term commitments necessitated by the complexity of many contemporary policy issues.

Putting an end to ideology implies, moreover, a narrow conceptualization of efficiency incompatible with democratic aspirations. In a democracy, ideological exchange serves a valuable function by educating people and alerting them to visions of what is right and just rather than what is workable.

Another hazard is the suppression of equity to economic priorities. With the tide of politics running in a fiscally conservative direction, the pressures for containing costs and government outlays are very strong. Eligibility and benefit reductions in government programs are unquestionably useful for budget-balancing purposes, but unless care is taken to minimize invidious comparisons the social problems created can far outweigh any economic savings. The trade-off between efficiency and equity raises some divisive issues, especially with respect to restricting publicly financed services solely to persons in need. If it makes good economic sense not to give services free to persons who can afford to pay for them privately, what are the longer-run political and moral consequences of a system of health services segmented by differences in employment status, income, and age? Are programs for the poor destined to provide poor services whenever competition for scarce resources occurs between social groups? Even if conducted in strict accord with unambiguous efficacy and cost-effectiveness criteria, rationing introduces the risk of unknown but large costs from the inflamation of class and intergenerational tensions and the disintegration of community solidarity.

THE NEO-MARXIST APPROACH

To what extent recent Marxist writing qualifies for the "neo" appellation is questionable. Much of it is steeped in classical themes of social class oppression springing from capitalists' ownership of the modes of production and their resolute pursuit of profits above all else, including environmental protection, the safety and efficacy of foods and drugs, and the health of workers. The apotheosis of the working class as uncorrupted by materialism also persists, as does belief in the remedial effects of nationalization (Elling, 1977; Krause, 1977; McKinlay, 1979; Sidel & Sidel, 1977).

The chief difference today is in the focus. Rather than proceeding within the framework of entrepreneurial capitalism, contemporary Marxist analysis deals with the effects of new concentrations of power in advanced industrial societies. Hence inquiry is directed at managerial capitalism (the power of national and multinational corporations) and science and technology. Industrialism is regarded as an ideology, independent of private or state ownership, in which health and health services are subordinated to productivity and capital accumulation goals.

From this perspective, power gravitates one-sidedly to the managers of capital (not the owners), to technocrats possessing the necessary skills and knowledge, and to bureaucracies administering and regulating economic activity. One of the consequences is that traditional class conflict is replaced by tension between those at the top responsible for running industrialized society and those at the bottom—the consumers of goods and services. Thus, class has largely lost its importance as a category of social analysis. Due to welfare state policies, the working class in developed capitalist societies has been absorbed as part of the larger consumer mass and is subject to the manipulation of a corporate elite (Waitzkin, 1978).

Applied to the health sector, the conflict pits the medical bureaucracy (notably the medical profession) and the health services delivery system against consumers and patients. The result is manifested in an increase in illness attributable to physicians and health care institutions. In order to perpetuate its power, the medical profession finds it advantageous to medically addict the population (Navarro, 1977). Credence for this line of thinking is derived from widespread concerns among health reform advocates over the pervasive amount of medically questionable and unnecessary procedures perpetuated on unsuspecting consumers.

Despite a proclivity for utopianism and romanticism, the Neo-Marxist school has made some important contributions, particularly the debunking of a number of myths prevalent during the normative period and the steering of public attention to some new realizations. First, belief in the power of morality as an engine for justice has waned. Neo-Marxist writers have argued, with some success, that past reforms are not solely due to the intrinsic altruism of human nature. Change, in their view, is unlikely without the manipulation of events by powerful, self-serving interests in the private sector, such as insurance companies and hospital supply and pharmaceutical corporations. Medicare and Medicaid have been accordingly analyzed, as have the Flexner-inspired reforms of medical education (Berliner, 1973, 1975; Bodenheimer et al., 1977).

As seen by Navarro (1976), the Neo-Marxist emphasis on economic structure and class relations contrasts sharply with the importance given by power-elite theorists to the role of personalities in struggles for reform. Besides acclaiming the contribution of individuals, power-elite writers tend to see change in terms of conflict resolution among different groups and actors in which control of knowledge, technology, money, and the legal right to perform specified services determine the outcome (Alford, 1975: Feldstein, 1977; Marmor, 1973).

Second, belief in the benevolence of the medical profession has diminished, and even middle-of-the-road observers have become alert to the potential use of professionalism as a cover for group aggrandizement (Begun, 1981; Wohl, 1984). Marxist-spirited critics form part of a circle of skeptics divided in ideology but united in their distrust of the profession. It is not unusual, however, to find that traditional left- and right-wing differences intersect and lose much of their clarity when pushed to the outer edges of the political spectrum.

Left-of-center critics are inclined to curtail professional freedom and to demythologize medicine in order to free patients from medical exploitation (Ehrenreich & Ehrenreich, 1974). Bureaucratic discipline in publicly accountable organizations, together with opportunities for citizen participation in the planning, monitoring, and evaluation of services, is the preferred alternative. For the sake of individual freedom and economic efficiency, right-of-center critics recommend going further—the weakening of restrictions on entry to medical practice, on the employment of physicians in bureaucratic organizations, and on competition among medical providers (Freidson, 1970).

From a far-left position, Illich (1976, 1977) has called for yet more extreme measures: (1) the total de-bureaucratization of society; (2) the breaking down of professional and other monopolies; (3) the return to classical market competition, in which enlightened self-interest prevails; and (4) the maximum restoration of individual self-reliance and autonomy in all matters, including self-responsibility for health. In an advanced industrial society, bureaucracy and professionalism, rather than capitalist or class exploitation, according to this perception, are an omnipresent danger to individual freedom and the exercise of free will.

Dissolution of belief in the monolithic structure of organized medicine is a third contribution of Neo-Marxism. Until the mid-1960s, the stereotype of an all-powerful, reactionary American Medical Association entered into most policy deliberations. The medical schools and teaching hospitals, in contrast, seemed to be virtuous exceptions. This image was terribly simplistic and sidetracked awareness of the implications of a shift in real power to scientific and technological interests.

Neo-Marxist observers were among the first to report that the major teaching hospitals and medical centers had become big obstacles to cost containment and better health care access for the poor. Few recognized at the time that the enormous capital requirements of high-technology, superspecialty medicine were being served without proper consideration for cost-effectiveness or the availability of primary health care to underserved populations (Ehrenreich & Ehrenreich, 1970).

Not only were Neo-Marxists among the first to understand the powerful forces in biomedical science and technology causing medical centers to take on many of the features of private corporations, but they also pointed the way for an analysis of the implications of this trend for the provision of medically questionable procedures and the availability of first-contact services attuned to everyday health needs (Kotelchuck, 1976).

Finally, belief that medicine possesses little in common with big business has declined. The corporatization of U.S. medicine and the attractiveness of investments in the health economy to major financial and industrial corporations are subjects developed by Neo-Marxist analysts (Salmon, 1977) and popularized by others in terms of a medical-industrial complex (Relman, 1980; Starr, 1982; Wohl, 1984).

Shortcomings of the Neo-Marxist Approach

Conceptualization of health services as an instrument in the service of a ruling establishment certainly is insightful. The drawing of connections between medicine and the structural features of society opens the mind to the realization that reforms are not always conducted purely for noble reasons. The manner in which Marxist-oriented analysts examine industrialization as a process cutting across national differences in ideology allows the identification of factors more fruitful than those bound to individual personalities or highly localized circumstances. On the other hand, as noted by Higgins (1980), this approach has a number of weaknesses.

First, the presumption of selfish intent is one-sided. In taking a pessimistic view of the motives of the powerful, Neo-Marxism suffers the same limitations ascribed to conservative believers in the doctrine of market competition, the only difference being that the latter see selfishness as universal to human nature.

Second, Neo-Marxist analyses are frustrating to follow. They tend to rely heavily on assertion instead of data. The theory often suggests a conspiratorial group design to keep and expand controls. The proclivity is to generalize on the basis of a series of policy decisions that may not be representative.

Finally, there is a disturbing disregard for precision in the use of concepts and categories. Neo-Marxist writing is encased in confrontational-pugnacious rhetoric that deters serious reflection and thoughtful analysis, by appealing more to prejudice than intellect. It seldom is clear just what is meant by "the ruling class," "the state," or "the system." Vagueness is a major impediment to good analysis.

PREVAILING POLICY IMPERATIVES AND NEW ECONOMIC REALITIES

Although ideology unquestionably does and will continue to influence health and welfare policy, its significance has been superseded by large-scale structural movements in the economic and social spheres mentioned earlier—notably, the decline of productivity and the aging of the population. Following a prolonged period during which government engaged in extensive borrowing to compensate for revenue shortfalls in the vain hope that slow economic growth was a short-term phenomenon, it is now widely accepted that the affluent post–World War II decades marking the expansion of generous social programs were an exception rather than a permanent fixture of economic life. Compared to the prosperous decades between 1950 and 1969, when annual growth averaged almost 4 percent, the economy has been mired in a much slower phase hovering in the vicinity of 2.5 percent, which translates into slightly less than a 40 percent decrease in annual output.[4]

Much of today's pressure to cut government spending and the financial stresses affecting family stability are attributable to the cumulative effects of this shortfall. Over the twenty-year period prior to 1994, the federal government would have received around $2.4 trillion in additional revenues at present rates of taxation, if the economy had grown but one percent faster a year. Had this amount been used to reduce debt, the government, according to Madrick (1995), would have saved more than $1.2 trillion in interest payments, the deficit would have been eliminated by the late 1980s, and current budgets would be running a significant surplus—thereby making the cost of government more affordable and possibly permitting modest tax relief as well. In an ensuing salubrious spiral, demand for labor would have gone up along with wages and salaries, and income for the typical family would have been $5,500 or more higher in 1993. Over the entire two-decade span, total income gain for a typical family would have amounted to approximately $50,000—a sum sufficient to enable many uninsured low-income persons to purchase private health insurance, to broaden home ownership among young couples, and to permit higher family savings and living standards in general. Regrettably, there is no basis, as indicated by the Congressional Budget Office (1995), for anticipating a return to higher growth any time soon, given the failure of past attempts and the worry now driving fiscal and monetary policy that faster growth carries the risk of unwanted higher inflation because of capacity shortages in the economy.

As described by the World Bank (1994) and the Organization for Economic Cooperation and Development (1994), the tensions caused by an aging population and slower economic growth are not a peculiarly American phenomenon. Many other countries are similarly affected. In the United States and other highly developed countries the adaptation of public opinion to the consequences of these developments comprises a principal test of leadership ingenuity and integrity.

Awareness of international similarities underscores and solidifies the dominant view in domestic policy today that government can no longer afford the costly health and welfare programs enacted in earlier times of a rapidly expanding economy and fewer older people. As the gravity of the situation receives broader dissemination and the public becomes better educated, politicians who know what must be done but are reluctant to do so for fear of invoking voter displeasure will become more emboldened. Progress in this direction is evident

---

[4]Compiled from tables contained in *Statistical Abstracts of the United States,* published by the Census Bureau in Washington, D.C., in the years 1984 (Table 720), 1993 (Table 931), and 1994 (Table 1367).

in the recent narrowing of formerly large Republican and Democratic differences in Washington, as indicated by the proceedings of the Bipartisan Commission on Entitlement and Tax Reform (1994), and the agreement in principle between the president and Congress on the need to balance the budget within seven years through cuts in government spending (Calmes, 1995).

Politicians no doubt will continue to loudly trumpet their differences for partisan advantage, but the similarities now far outweigh the differences. In addition to agreeing on a timetable for balancing the budget, there is strong bipartisan support for economies in Medicare and Medicaid through the replacement of fee-for-service with managed care delivery systems (Prospective Payment Assessment Commission, 1996). This coalescence represents an accommodation to the inescapable conclusion that American living standards are endangered by a decline in productivity for the reasons that the nation spends too much, saves and invests too little, and borrows indiscriminately to satisfy immediate gratification instead of providing for future needs. In borrowing to compensate for spending more than it takes in, the federal government has been depleting the supply of savings available for private investment and contributing to a decline in both workforce productivity and workers' real hourly wages (Bipartisan Commission, 1994; Peterson, 1994; Concord Coalition, 1992; Rivlin, 1992).

Unlike the situation between 1950 and 1970, when real average income doubled, the income of most Americans has since stagnated or declined, except among the wealthy who have continued to do well. After peaking in 1973, real earnings have dropped by close to one-fourth among persons in the bottom 20 percent of the income distribution, while it increased by 10 percent for persons in the top 20 percent. Young males have been especially hard hit. Male workers with only a high school education experienced a 30 percent decline in real income between 1973 and 1993. Incomes have gone down in correspondence with productivity. Between 1947 and 1973, productivity and income both rose by 3 percent a year. However, between 1973 and 1991, productivity slowed to 0.7 percent a year and worker compensation grew by a paltry 0.3 percent (Rattner, 1995).

Regardless of any short-term improvement in economic conditions that may benefit the private sector, the long-term forecast for government is grim because of the effects of past overspending and unrelenting pressures for growth in hard-to-control entitlement programs. In addition to comprising a major proportion of federal outlays, entitlements contain contractual provisions for expansion outside the scope of yearly spending limits. More than half of the current federal budget goes to entitlement programs, among which Social Security, Medicare, and Medicaid represent the largest share. In contrast, that share was only 30 percent in the late 1960s. Entitlement spending is growing so much faster than other forms of spending that by the year 2004 it will absorb nearly two-thirds of federal outlays. The aging of the baby boom generation will continue to drive the share higher yet, to the detriment of other government programs. Barring major reforms, the government will consist of only four programs by the year 2029: Medicare, Medicaid, Social Security, and federal pensions. Nothing else! No education assistance, no research and development, no low-income housing, no conservation programs, no public works—all these and more will be squeezed out of the budget. Consequently, no political claim to spending or deficit control, according to the Congressional Budget Office (1994), can be taken seriously in the absence of a plan for reining-in entitlement spending. The challenge of doing so is complicated by the massive accumulation of debt.

Now hovering in the range of 15 percent, debt service is the largest component of the federal budget (Concord Coalition, 1992). Clever financing may give some temporary relief, but at great danger to future economic stability. Recently completed financial maneuvers to lower debt service through the substitution of lower-cost short-term borrowing for costlier long-term loans has, for instance, created substantial savings in interest payments, approximately $50 billion, but at the risk of increased exposure to interest rate hikes that may outpace the government's ability to compensate through commensurate cuts in spending. Nearly three-fourths of the national debt now is funded at five years or less, with about one-third in obligations of one year or less. The significance of this is that for every percentage-point rise in short-term rates, another $200 billion will be added to the debt service load (Armstrong, 1995). The actual situation is even more precarious. Were it not for the questionable accounting practice of adding loans from the surplus in Social Security trust funds to general revenue calculations, the actual size of annual deficits would run some $50 billion higher (Concord Coalition, 1992).

The fixed nature of debt service obligations and broad-based congressional belief that additional deep cuts in defense will dangerously compromise national security and foreign policy heightens the significance of entitlement programs in deficit reduction. Arguments that entitlements ought to be exempt from the normal rules of budgetary management because they are a form of payroll savings fully paid for by beneficiaries during their working years are only partially valid. In point of fact, most retirees receive far more than they contribute—in the case of Medicare, for example, about $100,000 more (Posner, 1996). Everyone also comes out comfortably ahead in the Social Security program, particularly moderate- and low-income workers, due to the redistributive element whereby they are subsidized by high-income earners. Most currently retired Americans, according to Peterson (1994), receive benefits that are two to five times more than what they and their employer paid in.

Because of recently introduced taxes on benefits received by higher-income retirees and a scheduled rise in the eligibility age, future retirees will not be as fortunate. Posner (1996) calculates that people who retired in the mid-1980s will get about two-thirds more in Social Security than what they contributed. Soon-to-retire workers who paid the maximum payroll tax over their careers possibly may find themselves roughly breaking even, and by 2030 they, along with some average-income workers, actually may receive less than their full contribution, but most beneficiaries will continue to do well (American Association of Retired Persons, 1995).

The elderly are a highly privileged group in federal budgetary politics. Excluding interest on the national debt and military spending, about half of the budget goes to people over sixty-five. The same applies to entitlement spending, which is disproportionately focused on the elderly. They receive roughly three-fifths of all outlays. While this special attention has done much to improve the living conditions of older Americans, it is questionable whether such a disproportionate concentration of limited resources on 12 percent of the population is in the national interest, especially if it hinders the ability of future generations to compete successfully in the new economy. Per capita federal spending on the elderly exceeds federal spending on children by a ratio of eleven to one. As pointed out by Peterson (1994), poor children outnumber poor elderly Americans by five to one and in no other major industrial country is the poverty rate for children so high.

Underlying the age discrepancy in federal resource distribution are two opposing stereotypes—despondent helplesness and raw political power—both of which give the elderly a substantial advantage. A perception of the elderly as impecunious and financially vulnerable persists despite vast improvements in income security derived from inflation and adjusted Social Security payments, together with Medicare and other government programs that insulate the elderly from economic insecurities encountered by younger population groups. When combined with the tendency of politicians to pander to the vaunted political organization and electoral strength of the elderly, this outdated vision of impoverishment constitutes a compelling formula for preferential treatment.

Insofar as Social Security and health programs are designed to meet the daily living needs of recipients they represent a form of consumption that detracts from savings and investment. This applies especially to health services. Whatever the investment value in health spending, it paradoxically diminishes with socioeconomic progress, mainly because of the effects of population aging and larger numbers of pensioners. Even in more auspicious demographic circumstances, the value of health spending is dubious because of the paucity of hard evidence concerning the benefits of treatment. Much of what is done has not been subjected to rigorous evaluation. Instead of quantifying treatment outcomes, medical practice standards focus disproportionately on inputs and processes, the effects of which are assumed to be relevant. Therefore, there is little real knowledge of which treatments work best in comparison with the cost-effectiveness of alternatives (Eddy & Billings, 1988; Ellwood, 1988).

Presumably, government can raise investment funds and lower the deficit through tax increases instead of cutting entitlements, but this risks introducing disincentives that would further weaken the economy. Ultimately, the economy can only grow stronger if workers become more productive. This necessitates spending more on elementary and secondary education and worker training; on industrial modernization, better production methods, and new technologies through research and development; and on essential infrastructure, such as transportation, communications, and energy. Otherwise, the prospects for breaking out of the existing slow-growth, low-investment cycle are remote.

Following a review of government and private saving rates in thirty-six industrial and developing countries, Edwards (1995) concluded that the two best ways to increase the supply of savings for investment purposes are through public thrift and entitlement reform. Government saving is a stimulus for private saving. For every one percent increase in government savings, overall savings go up 0.45 percent. Entitlements produce an opposite result. Lower private savings are clearly related to the generosity of pension schemes and associated entitlement programs.

The magnitude of investment required to revitalize the economy far surpasses the capacity of the public sector. Since the private sector accounts for a close to 70 percent share of the national economy, its cooperation is indispensable. For the private sector to do its part, however, it has to have access to affordable capital, of which there is, as mentioned above, an insufficient supply due to the decline in domestic savings and government borrowing to finance activities that contribute little to long-range economic improvements and national wealth.

Since the 1960s, aggregate national savings has fallen by one-third to roughly 3 percent of GDP whereas the size of annual deficit has tripled to 3 percent of GDP. The combined effect on investment has been drastic. Less than 3 percent of national income is now invested annually in comparison with 9 percent between the end of World War II and the early 1970s. An astounding 97 percent of net national product is spent on consumption. Of what little is invested, roughly a third of the net

is funded by foreign creditors. This dependence on external sources introduces two dilemmas. Coincidentally with the possible loss of flexibility in domestic economic policy arising from the need to satisfy the demands of international creditors, on the one hand, there is the equally alarming prospect, on the other hand, that inflows may slow or disappear if confidence in the U.S. economy diminishes or more attractive investment opportunities develop elsewhere, including the possibility that capital-exporting countries may acquire a need to consume more of their national income and savings at home (Peterson, 1996). The dangers to the economy from overconsumption will intensify as the economy becomes more global in reach, inasmuch as trade rivals that save and invest more acquire a competitive advantage that inevitably magnifies domestic unemployment and balance-of-payment difficulties.

Whether viewed from a public- or private-sector perspective, control of entitlement spending is pivotal to raising the level of investment. Social Security is now in surplus, but shortly after the baby boom generation begins to retire outlays will exceed revenues at an accelerating rate and cause annual deficits to mushroom. The surplus is predicted to run out sometime between 2013 and 2019. By 2030, the trust fund will go broke, at which time the government will have to raise taxes substantially on workers to somewhere between 29 percent and 37 percent of payroll in order to fulfill its obligations and thereby run the risk of creating work disincentives or otherwise compromise the economy (Concord Coalition, 1992).

In the short run, the elderly share of the population will not change much beyond today's 12.5 percent. But after 2010, it will climb to over 16 percent and when it peaks between 2030 and 2040, at roughly 20 percent, one in five Americans will be over sixty-five years of age. Not only will there be more older people but they will be living longer as well. The strains on the economy will be enormous. In company with more and longer pension payments, more will be spent on health care, since health services utilization and expenditures rise sharply with age. The elderly use four times as much health care as the general population. Per capita expenditures among persons over eighty years of age run about two and one half times higher than those for persons in the sixty-five to sixty-nine age group and seven times higher than those for the under-sixty-five population (Garber, 1996; Schmid, 1991).

In future years the working-age populations will not grow correspondingly so that the number of elderly supported by each worker will rise. Contrasted with today's situation, where there are five workers for each retiree, the ratio will diminish by 2040 to two or fewer workers, excluding any unforeseen changes in birth rates and immigration (Committee on Ways and Means, 1993; Peterson, 1996). Unless productivity and economic growth improve markedly, an aging population ultimately will exhaust the capacity of entitlement programs and strain the ability of government to provide for the health and income security needs of retired and disabled populations, along with the welfare of children and other important functions. It boggles the mind to realize that spending for Medicare, Medicaid, and Social Security will double by the year 2030, even assuming the improbable elimination of all sources of inflation in these programs so that per capita outlays grow in tandem with the economy (Bipartisan Commission, 1994). This unfortuitous juxtaposition of unkind economic and demographic forces emits unrelenting pressure on policymakers to become more aggressive in altering the scope and composition of health and other entitlement programs.

The government's ability to meet Social Security obligations depends more on the future strength of the economy than on the solvency of Social Security trust funds per se. This is because the money collected is not set aside in interest-bearing accounts but lent to the federal government to finance day-to-day operations. Thus, benefits due in any given time must be paid for either by government revenues collected in that year or by borrowing. The only way to make either measure easier is to raise the resource base by assisting economic growth and the accumulation of national wealth as much as possible through higher government savings (Congressional Budget Office, 1991; Woods, 1994). While the case for higher growth is strong, the issue of whether it should proceed in tandem with deficit reduction is less clear. Rohatyn (1996), for example, believes that it is economically imprudent and probably too socially disruptive within the existing slow-growth environment to commit to balancing the budget within a short timeframe. Reliance solely on economic growth, according to this traditionally liberal view, offers a less disruptive means than spending cuts for achieving a balanced budget. Among those believing in the necessity of spending reductions in conjunction with faster growth, however, the value of an abbreviated deadline is that it forces coming to grips with difficult choices that are better made sooner rather than postponed until the actual onset of a predictable crisis.

How the deficit is brought under control will greatly affect the size of the economy in future years when the size of the retired population soars upward. If higher taxes are counterproductive, then the issue centers on what to cut. Social Security has been spared for the time being, but something will have to be done soon. Delay will only exacerbate matters. Any accompanying social and economic dislocations will be far less severe if phased-in over a longer time period. Considering the risks of a political backlash from cuts in such a popular program, politicians will be inclined to proceed cautiously. Natural instincts for self-preservation predispose a preference for minimizing conflict through indirection and concealment—for example, low-key adjustments to incomprehensibly complicated cost-of-living allowance and benefit formulas. More direct measures, such as the following, are sure to arouse greater controversy: raise the eligibility age in correspondence with life expectancy gains occurring since the program's inception; increase payroll contributions; lower benefits; tax all benefits as regular income, except among lower-income recipients whose liability would be limited to benefits that exceed their contributions; and invest all or part of future revenues in private stock and bond funds that generate higher yields than trust-fund government securities (Poortvliet & Lane, 1995; Wyatt, 1996).

Privatization attracts considerable favorable interest because of the anticipated stimulative effects for investment capital and economic growth together with higher returns for Social Security beneficiaries, but it also contains some significant hazards. The temptations for political interference in free markets will increase and the security of retirement income will be jeopardized by unpredictable market movements and bad investment choices on the part of individuals too poorly informed to manage their money wisely.

Similar pressures to cut spending apply to private-sector retirement and health programs, where the old "social contract" between large employers and their employees is no longer valid (Conte, 1996). Regarding pensions, there is a pronounced movement within business and industry to replace fixed benefit plans, in which employers assume complete financial responsibility for monthly payments based on length of service and earnings, with defined contribution plans, in which workers take responsibility for investing tax-free monthly payroll contributions that may or may not be matched by employers. The rapid increase in this type of coverage is disclosed in the fact that it now pertains to 27 percent of full-time private-sector workers, in contrast to 17 percent in 1988 and 3 percent in 1983 (Woods, 1994; Silverman & Yakoboski, 1994).

The employment-based health insurance system that provides most of the nation's health care financing is also acquiring a new appearance. Like entitlements in the federal budget, the cost of fringe benefits has become an obstacle to investment and economic prosperity. Consequently, many employers who provide insurance to workers and their dependents at little or no cost are reconsidering and revising this arrangement. Along with having workers assume a bigger share of the cost of insurance, many employers are cutting benefits. When the cost of fringe benefits becomes a noticeable drag on profits, firms tend to react by doing everything possible to get out of the business of providing health benefits. This applies particularly to firms having an older workforce and a large number of retirees, where the cost of health insurance can reach 20 percent or more of payroll in comparison with an average 6 percent for business and industry in general (Morrison et al., 1991; Edwards et al., 1992; Battagliola, 1994).

For most firms the concern is not so much the level of health spending but the steep rate at which it is growing as seen in the following data. Health spending represented 7.6 percent of employee compensation in 1991, compared with 1.8 percent in 1965. Relative to fringe benefits it jumped from 21 percent in 1965 to 49 percent in 1991. In magnitude it now equals the size of after-tax profits, whereas it accounted for only 36 percent in 1970 and 43 percent in 1980 (Center for Health Economics Research, 1994).

The emerging global marketplace greatly intensifies the disadvantages of high health insurance and other fringe benefits expenditures to business and industry. Within the confines of a domestic economy firms usually have opportunities to pass costs off to others—to workers in the form of lower wages, to consumers in the form of higher prices, or to shareholders by way of smaller dividends. But in an international free trade economy, low-wage, low-cost rivals gain markets and profits at the expense of corporations that raise consumer prices or undermine investor confidence. Even in the absence of other constraints, the lead times required to adjust wages downward, because of contractual restrictions, employee resistance, or tight labor markets, is a big handicap to high-cost producers. In fast-moving contests for market share and economic survival there is little solace in the economists' standard assurance that wages invariably adjust in the long run (Fuchs, 1996). By then it may be too late. Short-run wage adjustments are difficult (U.S. Department of Labor, 1992).

Narrow-minded insistence among economists on the compensation equilibrium achieved through fringe benefit and wage trade-offs fails to comprehend that employers may be under pressure to reduce rather than simply hold the line on unit labor costs. Whether due to a decline in profits measured as a return on assets resulting from inadequate capital spending on productivity improvements or to tougher competition from lower-cost nonunion and foreign producers, high-labor cost manufacturers in order to survive in today's economy are cutting labor costs.

The effects of global competition clearly are manifest in the changing composition of the labor force. Job insecurity and unemployment are common occurrences. High fringe benefit costs induce corporations to shift production to low-wage, low-tax locations, cut costs by eliminating positions, and replace full-time employees with part-time workers and independent contractors for whom they are not obliged to provide health insurance. Thus, over half of all new jobs today are part-time (Oravec, 1993) and one-fourth of all workers fall in the contingent category (Pierce, 1991). Fortune 500 companies, which accounted for about one-fifth of all full-time workers in 1970, now employ only around one-tenth of the full-time workforce (*The Economist*, 1992).

Small firms are especially limited in how they can cope with fringe benefit burdens even when insulated from the competitive stresses of global trade. Insurance companies typically charge them 10 percent to 40 percent higher premiums for a given amount of health insurance (U.S. Department of Labor, 1992). Lacking the financial resources and market power of big corporations, they have fewer opportunities to shift costs to consumers. Consequently, the offering of health insurance to employees is related to firm size. The lower wage levels common to small firms allows less flexibility for wage and fringe benefit trade-offs. Marginal-income workers understandably resist any decline in take-home pay and there is no room whatsoever to maneuver among minimum-wage earners.

Close to one-fifth of all workers are employed by firms that do not offer health benefits. Over half are in firms employing fewer than ten workers and nearly three-quarters are in firms with fewer than twenty-five workers (U.S. Department of Labor, 1992). Small companies, on the other hand, are a principal source of new jobs. Under existing economic conditions, this presents a dilemma for society—whether in a zero-sum business climate the public interest is better served by opting for low-wage, meager fringe benefit jobs conducive to employment growth or for higher wages and better fringe benefits that multiply unemployment and punish unskilled workers and add to welfare dependency among low-wage earners. According to the Employee Benefits Research Institute (1996), firms with fewer than one hundred employees create roughly three-fourths of new jobs. The predicament is highlighted in the reaction of minimum-wage employers to the subsequently failed Clinton administration's health reform provision to make work-based health insurance compulsory. Be-

cause of an inability to lower wages to compensate for the requirement that they pay 80 percent of each worker's health insurance premium, employers believed they would have had to cut employment and that up to one hundred thousand jobs would have been lost (Klerman & Goldman, 1994).

Squeeze on Equity

The numerous efforts to slow and control health costs to date have been only partially successful. Instead of despair and resignation, however, failure has led to more intensive endeavors and a preoccupation with efficiency and savings that dulls attention to equity. Following the arrest of robust economic growth beginning in the early 1970s, access to health care has diminished for many Americans, especially the uninsured, who number 40.9 million and represent 18.1 percent of the nonelderly population (Employee Benefits Research Institute, 1995b).

On the public-sector side, budgetary constraints have eroded the accomplishments and aspirations of programs instituted in the mid-1960s to extend health care across price and income barriers. Medicaid was designed originally to eliminate gaps in access among both the indigent and the medically indigent, but following some initial successes it has failed to fulfill its mandate. Savings have been achieved mainly by curtailing coverage of the poor and low-income workers to the effect, ironically, that government has become a major contributor to the problem of the uninsured. From a previous high of 70 percent, achieved shortly after the program's implementation, only about 40 percent of the federally defined poor currently have Medicaid coverage. What care they do receive is provided in sparsely available and underfunded public facilities, or through means of charity and uncompensated services. On the assumption they are less needy, the medically indigent have suffered greater reductions and together with the poor they account for most of the uninsured (Fuchs, 1993).

Measures to save money through the underpayment of health providers, in both Medicaid and Medicare, also adds to the ranks of the uninsured, albeit in a less direct manner. Hospitals and physicians pressed to meet their financial objectives compensate for money-losing public-financed services by charging private payers more, a practice popularly referred to as cost shifting. This is equivalent to a hidden tax on business, inasmuch as most private health insurance is provided by employers. The effect is that employers end up subsidizing public programs and the uninsured by a substantial amount, estimated at $17 billion or more (Center for Health Economics Research, 1994). In an ensuing negative spiral, many employers react by cutting coverage of workers' dependents and retirees. Yet more damaging to the economic security of full-time workers is the growth in part-time employees and independent contractors, who command fewer and less costly fringe benefits. Loss of employment-based health insurance further expands the ranks of the uninsured.

Downsizing of employment in manufacturing firms that commonly provide good fringe benefits, coupled with increased employment in the services sector where fringe benefits are less plentiful, is responsible for much of the drop in employment-based health insurance coverage. The corollary social dislocations are amplified by the corrosive effect steep health cost increases have on the willingness of employers to provide health insurance and by declines in real wages, prompting workers to opt for higher take-home pay in exchange for reduced fringe benefits. In 1988, 62 percent of workers had health insurance through their jobs. Today only 58 percent do and, unless macroeconomic circumstances improve, this downward trend will continue. Manufacturing employment is becoming less significant. It is projected that 96 percent of the 25 million net increase in nonfarm jobs between 1992 and 2005 will occur in the services sector, and that stiffer international competition, along with technological change, will further depress wages among less-educated, less-skilled workers while adding to the amount of part-time and temporary employment (Shactman & Altman, 1995). In 1993, over 16 million workers did not participate in their employers' sponsored health plan. Over 50 percent elected not to be covered, another 36 percent were ineligible or denied coverage, 11 percent did not participate for some other reason, and the remaining 2 percent were not ascertainable. Among the ineligible workers, two-thirds did not

participate because they were part-time, contract, or temporary workers (Employee Benefits Research Institute, 1994). Confidence in the future security of their financial protection has coincidentally declined among workers and nearly half of them openly worry about their ability to retain the health benefits they have (Edwards et al., 1992). These developments cast considerable doubt on the future reliability of employment-based health insurance coverage.

Payroll financing clearly is more applicable to situations of a youthful labor force and when, moreover, domestic firms are insulated from low-cost foreign competition. These structural impediments to employment-linked health and social programs are magnified by the current spread of underwriting practices which assign premiums to employers based on their labor force's specific risk profile, in contrast to social insurance principles where premiums are less variable due to the subsidization of high-risk groups by low-risk groups. All these factors feed the escalation of fringe benefit costs relative to profits and real wages and further support the rationale for decoupling health insurance from employment. The fringe benefit disincentives encountered by employers have substantially increased in the wake of recently imposed accounting rules compelling the financial disclosure of previously unreported future health insurance obligations and to fully fund retirement programs formerly conducted on a pay-as-you-go basis (Employee Benefits Research Institute, 1994).

As presently constituted, employment-based insurance has the additional disadvantage of distorting labor market efficiency. It does this by influencing workers' choice of job, decisions on whether to change jobs, and the timing of retirement. Employer decisions in the areas of hiring, training, promotions, and labor force cutbacks also are affected (Fuchs, 1993; Pauly & Goodman, 1995).

What is happening in government and business are the surface indications of the fundamental predicament distressing policymakers: the country is spending far more on health care than it can afford. A bizarre effect of socioeconomic advancement is that medical progress has complicated the problem of resource scarcity inasmuch as it enables people to live who otherwise would have succumbed to illness and disability. Although modern medicine successfully treats symptoms and prolongs life, it seldom cures, thereby enlarging the population for whom the cost of appropriate health and social support services is high, such as the aged and low birth weight infants.

As discussed earlier, one of the big issues confronting political leadership centers on expenditure management and the redirection of spending from consumption to investment. Furthermore, government needs to become more supportive of business and industry by ending practices that add to the cost of production, hamper competitiveness in global markets, and contribute to higher unemployment. Toward this end, a restructuring of the relationship between health insurance and employment is unavoidable. The major problem with rising health care costs is the historical accident whereby health benefits were linked to employment to get around wage controls during World War II. This has encouraged employees to think that health care is free to them and that somebody else is paying for it. This mindset has been augmented by Medicare and Medicaid coverage. Today, only one-fifth of health costs are paid out of pocket compared to 60 percent in 1960 (Levit et al., 1994; Center for Health Economic Research, 1994). The only way to contain spending is to reverse the trend and have individuals take greater control over their own spending. Making the consumer the purchaser of health care also would cause health plans to become more directly accountable for the price and quality of their services, insofar as individuals are free to chose among plans competing for market share and survival.

Convincing the public of the need to accept redirections in programs that have assumed the status of rights to which everyone is entitled is admittedly difficult. It entails a radical reformulation of government philosophy and practice deeply ingrained in post–World War II orthodox thinking whereby in return for higher taxes individuals and families are relieved of the need to make provision for many of life's vicissitudes.

Union of Political and Market Forces

Expectations that health reform can be successfully accomplished from within the health sector are im-

plausible. More significant than the inertia and delay natural to large-sized organizational entities, health providers are subject to the same human impulses that predispose individuals to put their self-interest ahead of others'. Health providers differ principally from other occupations in the greater freedom they have in controlling their working conditions, due to the historical deference granted to physicians and the many practical justifications for clinical autonomy. In the best of circumstances, the service ethic and self-restraint provide only a partial check on self-interest. This is why health services everywhere around the world exhibit signs of being run more for the convenience of providers than for patients (Timely Surgery, 1991).

The circumvention of powerful self-interest groups through the use of market mechanisms is, as said previously, a concession to the limitations of political power and planning in the conduct of complex and controversial changes. A strong attraction of market strategies is that they depersonalize responsibility for hardship while allowing individuals and interest groups an opportunity to control their own futures during periods of economic difficulty. The invisible hand and inexorable laws of supply and demand, moreover, provide a means for avoiding the due process delays and polarization hindering managerial efficiency in public administration. Whether mythical or not, what counts most is that people believe in and accept the power of markets for resolving resource allocation issues. The process and results unquestionably are imperfect, but among pragmatists partial deliverance from otherwise insuperable health care problems of surplus capacity, backward productivity, and quality controls is preferable to the inaction and procrastination associated with political methods and paralysis by coordination occasioned by orthodox planning and regulation. In their eschewal of government solutions, policymakers subscribing to the practical applications of market principles have much in common with the neoconservative movement discussed earlier and this outlook is now ascendant both in the United States and abroad (Battistella, 1993).

Two related but nonetheless distinct objectives mark the direction taken by the competitive market strategy—price discipline and managed care. Greater awareness of the true cost of health resources among both consumers and providers is basic to curtailing the profligacy perpetrated when services are provided free in an open-ended manner. By merging price consciousness and self-interest, market incentives lead individuals to weigh the financial consequences of wants and demands in ways that spur economy and efficiency. The federal government's prospective payment system for hospitals (DRGs), introduced in the mid-1980s, is an illustration of how market incentives can be used successfully to advance public objectives inasmuch as it has stimulated rapid and lasting reductions in both patient lengths of stay and occupancy rates. Despite frequently expressed concerns about possible perverse effects, there is no strong evidence to date to support fears that quicker discharges and the substitution of ambulatory care are detrimental to quality of patient care. But this conclusion may not necessarily apply equally to other health delivery settings (Fuchs, 1993).

Perhaps because the out-of-pocket requirements are not high enough relative to disposable income, documentation of the effects of higher consumer co-payments on utilization of physician and hospital services is ambiguous. Studies conducted by the Rand Corporation indicate that utilization is not much affected until co-payments reach around 25 percent. At this level consumers begin to differentiate between necessary and unnecessary care. The drawback of such a flat payment method, however, is that it is regressive and less selective in the case of low-income persons, who Rand researchers found may put off or avoid beneficial preventive services (Newhouse, 1994).

Price clearly achieves the intended effects in consumer choice of health plan. Within the workplace, the imposition by employers of higher premium and co-payment charges is inducing workers to move from traditional fee-for-service indemnity insurance to managed care plans, where the appeal of lower out-of-pocket charges and more extensive benefits overrides any distaste for restrictions on physician choice. About 70 percent of employees are presently enrolled in managed care compared to only 29 percent in 1988 (Davis et al., 1995; Myerson, 1996). Comparable efforts by the government to get the elderly to shift from fee-for-service indemnity plans to managed care plans has been less

successful because of the ease with which they can obtain affordable private insurance to supplement and expand Medicare fee-for-service coverage. This will change quickly, however, once the government becomes more aggressive in increasing the price and benefits differential between conventional indemnity Medicare coverage and managed care options.

Ten percent of Medicare recipients are now enrolled in some form of managed care, about two-thirds of whom are in HMOs. Because of comparable financial pressures Medicaid also is in the process of moving away from retrospective, open-ended provider reimbursement. Nearly all of the states have introduced some form of managed care, which presently covers approximately one-fourth of the Medicaid population; and this percentage, given present trends, is expected to climb to four-fifths or more by the year 2000 (Standard & Poor's, 1995; Anders & McGinley, 1995; Winslow, 1995).

As described by Iglehart (1992), the term "managed care" is used permissively to encompass any restriction on the clinical autonomy of physicians and consumer freedom of choice, but has as its main defining feature the integration, in varying degrees, of the financing and delivery of health care through contracting with selective providers for the delivery of comprehensive health care services to enrolled members for a predetermined monthly premium. HMOs, whose origins go back more than a half century, set the standard in managed care. Anchored in principles of prepaid health insurance, they contract with health providers for the care of enrolled members who, in return for a fixed fee, are entitled to a range of benefits rendered by affiliated hospitals and physicians. Other kinds of managed care include preferred provider organizations (PPOs), in which employers and insurers contract with providers for services at a reduced rate; and point-of-service plans (POSs), which are hybrid HMOs that permit members to use services outside the plan in return for sharing part of the cost.

All forms of managed care seek to control costs by modifying physician practice styles and dissuading patients from the inappropriate use of medical specialists and nonparticipating physicians. Unlike unmanaged care, where they occupy a secondary role, primary care practitioners are the main source of patient care services and regulate access to costly specialty services on the basis of medical need. The quintessential aim of managed care is to have providers compete against one another on the basis of price and quality within a framework where there are clear-cut winners and losers. The need to declare prices in advance causes providers to become more cost-conscious and the dynamics of competition promote the rationalization of previously fragmented and uncoordinated services. Competition is strengthened by accompanying management information system requirements permitting the public disclosure of provider performance data for informing purchasers and enabling them to become more discriminating buyers.

Managed care incentives are geared to saving money through fewer hospital admissions, shorter lengths of stay, use of less expensive procedures and tests, and greater use of preventive services. The degree of discipline applied to providers varies considerably, but HMOs generally exercise more vigorous and sophisticated controls than other forms of managed care. In areas where HMOs have a strong presence, inpatient utilization rates are from one-third to one-half less than the national average (Standard & Poor's, 1995), and savings of 10 percent to 13 percent are customary, without any discernible reduction in quality of care (Miller & Luft, 1994).

Influence over the entire system generally becomes felt when 20 percent of a population is enrolled and increases steadily thereafter. Because this plateau has already been reached in most parts of the nation, the positive spillovers from additional HMO growth on hospital and physician utilization will become rapidly more pronounced in future years. Concentration of purchasing power inevitably will result in stronger pressures on providers to merge into fewer but larger-sized entities for the delivery of better-coordinated health services. As competition stiffens, the instinct for survival will stimulate providers to become more responsive to the price and quality concerns of purchasers through measures that tighten controls over utilization; trim unnecessary managerial and staff positions; stan-

dardize treatment plans for a wide variety of conditions and diagnoses; develop better quantitative indicators of quality; speed the development of integrated delivery system capabilities over a wider range of services enveloping acute, chronic, rehabilitative, and preventive services, as well as community and inpatient care.

Managed care leverage over the organization and delivery of health services actually is much higher than indicated by HMO penetration alone. Enrollment in all forms of managed care presently accounts for about three-fifths of the private insurance market, and more than one-half of all hospitals and about three-fourths of all physicians now are subjected to its direction by way of some sort of contractual relationship. This signifies a continuing marginalization of retrospectively reimbursed fee-for-service medical practice (Standard & Poor's, 1995).

Although often criticized for diffidence in the imposition of productivity and quality controls, whether because of insecurities characteristic of immature industries or the numerous opportunities to make profits through easier means (like selective enrollment practices and curtailment of unnecessary hospital utilization), managed care has evolved to the stage where cost-effectiveness will be pursued more vigorously, if for no other reason than the stronger insistence of big business, government, and other major purchasers of health care for better price and quality improvement results.

Whether consolidation ultimately will enable hospitals and physicians to reassert their former ability to control price is problematic. Trends favor a continuing shift of economic power from providers to purchasers and the growth of a buyer's market. If managed care organizations attain oligopolistic and monopoly status within a medical service area they can easily be undercut by self-insured buyer coalitions that either bypass intermediate organizations by relating directly to individual providers on a competitive contract basis, or by dealing with growth-oriented external managed care entities anxious to expand into new geographic areas (Weissenstein, 1995). Should restructuring culminate in too few remaining providers for meaningful competition to occur, then other ways will have to be found to harness the power of private interest for social good that are compatible with the macroeconomic exigencies propelling health policy, among which the public utility model is a good example. For most of the nation, however, this contingency appears far off due to the vast amount of surplus capacity remaining to be eliminated from the health sector.

Whatever the oscillations in the pendulum swing affecting the provider–purchaser relationship, managed care has become an irreversible juggernaut. Nearly all forms of health care already are subjected to some form of managerial control, including traditional fee-for-service medicine, where clinical decisions routinely are screened by insurers for compliance with medical treatment norms. Although often highly rudimentary and diffuse in nature, managerial controls steadily are becoming more refined and systematically applied (American Medical Association, 1994).

The possibility that medical savings accounts (MSAs) may emerge as an alternative mechanism for health reform will not endanger the future of managed care. Contrary to managed care industry fears noted by Friedman (1996) of an MSA-sparked revival of waning freedom-of-choice, fee-for-service medicine, managed care firms that provide superior quality at a good price will do well in a value-conscious environment.

Where MSAs are more apt to make a difference is hastening the withdrawal of business and industry from the provision of insurance to workers for whom discretionary control over a health spending account and the opportunity to convert health dollars into general purpose funds is a more attractive alternative than a fringe benefit provided in lieu of wages, particularly among low- and moderate-income employees. Opposition to granting workers this choice on the grounds that it gives them an incentive to forgo needed health care is overreactive. The deductible and co-insurance features routinely found in insurance plans today are a bigger deterrent to primary care access for low-income persons, considering that such out-of-pocket payments consist of after-tax money.

Because MSA money is tax-free, there is less of an out-of-pocket penalty for using it. Briefly stated, MSAs allow workers to spend their employer's tax-sheltered health insurance at their discretion and retain whatever they save by being prudent buyers. To protect themselves and society against large-sized out-of-pocket expenditures, participants are required to purchase catastrophic insurance (Jensen & Morlock, 1994; Goodman & Musgrave, 1994).

MSAs also are applicable to the disengagement of government from open-ended Medicare spending. The presently favored process of increasing out-of-pocket and benefit differentials between unmanaged and managed care in order to motivate the elderly to relinquish traditional indemnity fee-for-service coverage is fraught with political divisiveness. The difficulty of getting individuals to surrender freedom of choice of provider, as discussed by Ferrara (1995), likely will pale in comparison to the backlash of resentment and polarization inevitably aroused when the government subsequently moves as expected to ration care more severely by squeezing payments to managed care firms in the vain hope of obfuscating responsibility for cuts in services. In contrast to the difficulty of getting the elderly to acquiesce to government-enjoined rationing, freedom to choose is less unsettling. It provides a more harmonious path for transforming Medicare from a defined benefit into a defined contribution plan, analogous to the private-sector initiative for disengaging from costly retirement programs. In addition to their share of Medicare contributions to a tax-sheltered account, the elderly might be permitted to include some part of their average out-of-pocket expenditures, including possibly premium payments for private supplemental Medicare coverage, in the interest of expediting acceptance of an MSA option paralleling that available to the gainfully employed. To the extent that MSAs put older and sicker retirees at a disadvantage, Medicare payments could be adjusted to assure that they have enough money to purchase adequate insurance protection.

Future Equity Prospects

Market competition unquestionably is a powerful stimulus for efficiency and cost-effectiveness, but in matters concerning access to care among low-income and geographically isolated populations there are serious problems. Because of the unacceptably high social costs of practices that disadvantage the poor and other high-risk groups, some degree of regulation is inevitable regardless of the level of disagreement about what constitutes the right mix of centralized controls and free market elements.

Controversy over managed competition spans a broad continuum. Ideological purists are averse to the juxtaposition of ostensibly antithetical regulatory controls with entrepreneurial incentives, whereas proponents of entitlements and the right of all persons to care regardless of ability to pay are predisposed to view managed competition as a subterfuge for the advancement of efficiency and savings at the expense of the disadvantaged. True believers in competition, on the other hand, regard managed competition as a backdoor approach to socialized medicine. Among pragmatists, however, the eclectic composition of managed competition commands approval for symbolizing a results-oriented, open-minded commitment to what works instead of a mindless dedication to ideological dogma and unattainable ideals (Battistella, 1993).

Present political and economic conditions seem unfavorable to the furtherance of equity, but appearances are misleading. Economy and efficiency are not the inescapable enemies of equity. Albeit difficult, it is possible to pursue ostensibly discordant objectives in complementary and mutually beneficial ways. Consistent with this possibility, a continuation of congressional interest in health reform is predictable, ranging from such low-controversy health care proposals as slowing benefit growth, raising the age for full benefit eligibility, and higher out-of-pocket charges based on ability to pay to more radical system-wide changes in which individuals and households are required to purchase private coverage in return for lower payroll taxes. The politics of deficit reduction also augur greater congressional focus on ways to capture an estimated $90 billion in unlimited tax deductions granted annually for company-paid health care insurance that disproportionately benefits upper-income workers more than low-income workers in terms of the imputed after-tax values to individuals and families (Butler, 1991; Peterson, 1996).

At a more abstract and philosophical level, one should not misconstrue as reactionary movements to spend more on investments essential to the health of the economy and the accumulation of wealth for raising living standards and advancing the well-being of future generations. Similarly, the reformulation of entitlement philosophy and practice away from traditional principles of universality toward a greater acceptance of selectivity is not antagonistic to values of fairness and social justice. The same applies to mounting congressional interest in the partial privatization of entitlement programs and increased price consciousness among consumers as mechanisms for slowing disturbingly high rates of spending growth and for conditioning voter psychology to accept greater self-reliance and individual responsibility.

In assessing future prospects for equity it is useful to note that most of what the government spends on health care today goes to the non-needy; only one-fifth of current outlays go to the poor. Nearly 90 percent of Medicare outlays and virtually all of the tax subsidies granted to employment-based health insurance benefit individuals who are not poor (Darman, 1991). Contrary to popular belief, the poor are not the sole beneficiaries of Medicaid. Although originally designed for the poor, around half of all expenditures support people with incomes above the federal poverty line (Darman, 1991); this is largely due to the financial legerdemain practiced by middle- and upper-class elderly who insulate their assets from the high cost of nursing home care through the exploitation of financial loopholes in Medicaid eligibility. Needy children consequently are deprived. These children account for roughly half of the Medicaid population, but only 15 percent of the program's budget is spent on them. Nearly one-third of payments go to the 11.9 percent who are elderly (Committee on Ways and Means, 1993). With respect to Social Security and Medicare, the elderly collect far more than what they contribute, mainly in the form of health benefits. Most currently retired persons receive benefits that are two to five times greater than the value of their contributions. In the case of Medicare, the return is five to twenty times more (Peterson, 1994).

Limiting federal assistance to needy persons would free close to $200 billion annually—a sum sufficient to allow for substantial deficit reduction and add to savings for financing economic growth while also providing for the health and social service needs of the truly needy.

Moreover, a properly guided government disengagement strategy could actually renew and strengthen values of social justice. But fairness in the distribution of sacrifice is essential. Within the framework of managed competition, public policy must do the following in any shifting of responsibility to individuals and families: eliminate the problem of the uninsured by compelling households to purchase health insurance; affirm social equity by capping individual and family responsibility as a reasonable percentage of disposable income, possibly somewhere in the range of 8 percent to 10 percent with a somewhat higher figure for the elderly, given the decline in living expenses following retirement and the completion of child-raising expenses; subsidize on a sliding scale the cost of health insurance for low-income and poor households, whether through tax credits, vouchers, or other means; develop a basic package of services that all insurance companies must provide; establish uniform rules for all insurers concerning enrollment practices that do not discriminate against high-risk individuals or groups; facilitate the formation of purchasing groups to lower enrollment cost and adverse risk-selection problems; and assist the power of self-interest to accelerate the growth of managed care through means of lower subsidies to persons opting for traditional fee-for-service insurance (Battistella & Kuder, 1993).

Competition for market share and survival within a properly regulated environment is a powerful inducement for insurers to monitor and evaluate health services more closely with respect to efficiency and quality performance that inevitably stimulates the growth of coordinated care networks among physicians and hospitals and the expansion of managed care principles throughout the health care industry. Collateral benefits derive from better-informed consumer decision making and more prudent use of health services. Since any savings in health expenditures go directly into their pockets, consumers acquire an incentive to become better informed and more assertive in dealing with health providers. Financial incentives also are conducive to enhancing self-responsibility for health, complementing the idea that individuals have a responsibility to apply good judgment in choice of lifestyle.

Conclusion

Radical modifications in the financing of public and private health programs are unavoidable if the country is to successfully resolve the multifaceted dilemmas imposed by demographic forces and a decline in economic growth and living standards. Philosophical disagreement undoubtedly will continue to produce strong dialogue over how to proceed, but what is most important to recognize in the midst of acrimony is that parties of different political outlook are now coming to some of the same general conclusions about fundamental ideas defining the future of health and social programs. This applies particularly to the concept of fairness. Rather than the conventional redistributionist philosophy of wealth, interest is shifting to the creation of wealth geared, as noted by Rohatyn (1996), to an economy where everyone willing and able to work can find employment and the opportunity for a higher living standard. Toward this end, a thriving private sector driven by high levels of investment and supportive public services is increasingly regarded as the best hope for minimizing the dislocations associated with technological change and globalization.

Among knowledgeable observers, the cost of inaction—higher taxes on the most productive members of society and a further weakening of the economy—is unacceptable. Informed measures to bring federal spending under control inevitably include substantial changes in the structure of Medicare and Medicaid because, except for Social Security, that is where the biggest potential savings are. Together they account for nearly one-fifth of the budget. Flurries of activity involving modest changes in the health insurance market to extend private coverage to more individuals are but sideshows to the main event—balancing the budget and dealing with Medicare and Medicaid. The realities driving health policy indicate that national health insurance based on a vast increase in public spending or imposition of higher taxes on business and industry is not in the national interest. A substantial withdrawal of government entitlements and the decline or even elimination of employment-based health insurance implies neither an improvement nor a deterioration in health care so much as that health care will be different.

The vagaries of politics and future events being what they are, public policy is not foreordained to adhere tightly to detailed prescriptions for health reform; many variations are possible from those described here. Implacable economic and demographic realities nonetheless indicate a pattern of movement whereby principles of selectivity will acquire greater significance in the composition of entitlement programs and the pressures to disengage government and employers from the financing of health services will intensify. Continuity of progress in this direction is problematic, however, unless public policy initiatives are accompanied by a commitment to personal responsibility that extends beyond narrow self-interest to encompass those most vulnerable and least able to provide for themselves unassisted.

The tensions described in this inquiry into the political economy of health services did not occur overnight, nor can they be attributed mainly to the policies of competing political parties. They were observable in the early 1970s, and the implications were evident in broad outline (Battistella, 1972b). Indeed, one could have seen as early as then that comprehensive universal health insurance paid entirely by the government was impractical (Battistella, 1973). The only subsequent major changes that have occurred involve matters of degree more than of kind and a broadening awareness within the health community that things will not improve soon regardless of the outcome of national political elections. Evidence from many other highly industrialized nations of widely differing political and economic backgrounds suggests that the causes of the reformulation of postwar health policies are structural in nature. They are the manifestation of a process of adjustment to large-scale institutional changes resulting from the transition from industrialization to a service economy and an aging population (Battistella, 1978; deKervasdoue et al., 1984; World Bank, 1994).

The complexities of the changes now occurring in social, political, and economic institutions are a reminder that establishing the right balance in health policies between equity and efficiency will not be easy. The enormous challenges of accommodating public policy to an unfamiliar decision-making environment, in which selectivity rather than universality is becoming the rule, deserves the attention of all groups committed to the preservation of equity in an era of limits.

REFERENCES

Aaron, Henry J. (1991). *Serious and unstable condition: Financing America's health care.* Washington, D.C.: The Brookings Institution.

Alford, Robert R. (1975). *Health care politics: Ideological and interest group barriers to reform.* Chicago: University of Chicago Press.

Altman, Drew E., & Douglas H. Morgan. (1982). The role of state and local government in health. *Health Affairs, 2* (Winter), 7–31.

Amara, Roy, J. Ian Morrison, & Gregory Schmid. (1988). *Looking ahead at American health care.* Washington, D.C.: McGraw-Hill Book Co.

American Association of Retired Persons. (1995). Social Security: Your questions answered. *AARP Bulletin* (July/August), 10–11.

American Medical Association. (1994). *The future of medical practice* (Order No. OP211594). American Medical Association.

Anders, George, & Laurie McGinley. (1995). Managed elder care, HMO's are signing up new class members: The group in Medicare. *Wall Street Journal* (April 27), A1, A8.

Anderson, Odin W. (1985). *Health services in the United States: A growth enterprise since 1875.* Ann Arbor, MI: Health Administration Press.

Armstrong, Martin A. (1995). The Clinton debt crisis [op-ed]. *Wall Street Journal* (April 19), A14.

Arrow, Kenneth J. (1963). Uncertainty and welfare economics of medical care. *American Economic Review, 53,* 941–969.

Battagliola, Monica. (1994). Workers shoulder more health care costs. *Business and Health, 12* (11), 31–36.

Battistella, Roger M. (1972a). Post-industrial Europe: Implications for health services structure. *International Journal of Health Services, 2* (November), 465–476.

Battistella, Roger M. (1972b). Rationalization of health services: Political and social assumptions. *International Journal of Health Services, 2* (August), 331–348.

Battistella, Roger M. (1973). Towards national health insurance in the USA: An examination of leading proposals. *Acta Hospitalis, 13,* 3–22.

Battistella, Roger M. (1978). Health policy development in other highly industrialized nations. In Roger M. Battistella and Thomas G. Rundall (Eds.), *Health care policy in a changing environment* (pp. 23–51). San Francisco, CA: McCutchan Publishing Co.

Battistella, Roger M. (1993). Health services reform: Political and managerial aims—An international perspective. *International Journal of Health Planning and Management, 8* (October–December), 265–274.

Battistella, Roger M., & Robert J. Buchanan. (1987). National health policy: Efficiency–equity syncretism. *Social Justice Review, 1*, 329–360.

Battistella, Roger M., & Theodore E. Chester. (1972). Role of management in health services in Britain and in the United States. *The Lancet, 1* (March 18), 626–630.

Battistella, Roger M., & Steven R. Eastaugh. (1980a). Hospital cost containment. In Arthur Levin (Ed.), *Regulating health care: The struggle for control* (pp. 192–205). New York: Proceedings of the Academy of Political Science.

Battistella, Roger M., & Steven R. Eastaugh. (1980b). Hospital cost containment: The hidden perils of regulation. *Bulletin of the New York Academy of Medicine, 56*, 62–82.

Battistella, Roger M., & John M. Kuder. (1993). Making health reform work without employer mandates. *Journal of American Health Policy, 3* (3), 18–22.

Battistella, Roger M., & Thomas G. Rundall. (1978a). The future of primary health services in the U.S.: Issues and opinions. In Roger M. Battistella & Thomas G. Rundall (Eds.), *Health care policy in a changing environment*. San Francisco, CA: McCutchan Publishing Co.

Battistella, Roger M., & Thomas G. Rundall. (Eds.). (1978b). *Health care policy in a changing environment*. San Francisco, CA: McCutchan Publishing Co.

Battistella, Roger M., & David B. Smith. (1974). Towards a definition of human services management: A humanist orientation. *International Journal of Health Services, 4* (Fall), 701–721.

Battistella, Roger M., & Thomas P. Weil. (1986). Pro-competitive health policy: Benefits and perils. *Frontiers of Health Services Management, 2* (May), 3–27.

Battistella, Roger M., & John R. C. Wheeler. (1978). Ideology, economics, and the future of national health insurance. In Roger M. Battistella and Thomas G. Rundall (Eds.), *Health care policy in a changing environment*. San Francisco, CA: McCutchan Publishing Co.

Begun, James W. (1981). *Professionalism and the public interest: Price and quality in optometry*. Cambridge, MA: MIT Press.

Berliner, Howard. (1973). The origins of health insurance for the aged. *International Journal of Health Service, 3*, 465–474.

Berliner, Howard. (1975). A larger perspective on the Flexner Report. *International Journal of Health Services, 5* (4), 573–592.

Berwick, Donald M. (1994). Eleven worthy aims for clinical leadership of health system reform. *Journal of the American Medical Association, 272* (September 14), 797–802.

Bipartisan Commission on Entitlement Reform. (1994). *Interim report to the president* (Stock No. 040-000-0064305). Washington, D.C.: Bipartisan Commission.

Bodenheimer, Thomas, Steven Cummings, & Elizabeth E. Harding. (1977). Capitalizing on illness: The health insurance industry. In V. Navarro (Ed.), *Health and medical care in the U.S.: A critical analysis* (pp. 69–84). Farmingdale, NY: Baywood Publications.

Bowler, Kenneth M., Robert T. Kuderie, & Theodore R. Marmor. (1978). The political economy of national health insurance: Policy analysis and political evaluation. In Kenneth M. Friedman & Stuart H. Rakoff (Eds.), *Toward a national health policy*. Lexington, MA: Lexington Books.

Bowsher, Charles A. (1991). *Canadian health insurance: Some lessons for the United States*. Testimony of the comptroller general before the House Committee on Government Operations (GAO-HRD-91-35). Washington, D.C.: U.S. Government Printing Office.

Bulgaro, Patrick J., & Arthur Y. Webb. (1980). Federal–state conflicts in cost control. In Arthur Levin (Ed.), *Regulating health care: The struggle for control* (pp. 92–110). New York: Proceedings of the Academy of Political Science.

Butler, Stuart M. (1991). A tax reform strategy to deal with the uninsured. *Journal of the American Medical Association, 265* (May 15), 2541–2544.

Calmes, Jackie. (1995). Clinton plan on budget gets wary welcome. *Wall Street Journal* (June 15), A3, A16.

Campbell, Alastair V. (1978). *Medicine, health and justice: The problem of priorities*. New York: Churchill Livingstone.

Carlson, Rick. (1975). *The end of medicine*. New York: John Wiley & Sons.

Center for Health Economics Research. (1994). *The nation's health care bill: Who bears the burden?* Waltham, MA: Center for Health Economics Research.

Cochrane, A. L. (1972). *Effectiveness and efficiency: Random reflections on health services*. London, UK: Nuffield Provincial Hospitals Trust.

Committee on Ways and Means, U.S. House of Representatives. (1993). *Green book: Overview of entitlement programs* (WMCP No. 103–18). Washington, D.C.: U.S. Government Printing Office.

Concord Coalition. (1992). *Citizens for America's future*. Washington, D.C.: Concord Coalition.

Concord Coalition. (1994). *The zero deficit plan*. Washington, D.C.: Concord Coalition.

Congressional Budget Office. (1991). *The economic effects of uncompensated changes in the funding of Social Security*. Washington, D.C.: Congressional Budget Office.

Congressional Budget Office. (1994). *Reducing entitlement spending*. Washington, D.C.: U.S. Government Printing Office.

Congressional Budget Office. (1995). *The economic and budget outlook*. Washington, D.C.: Congressional Budget Office.

Consumer Reports. (1992). *How to resolve the health care crisis: Affordable protection for all Americans*. New York: Consumer Reports Books.

Conte, Chris. (1996). The changing world of work and employee benefits. *Employee Benefit Research Institute Notes, 17* (3), 1–4.

Cooper, Richard. (1992). Seeking a balanced physician workforce for the 21st century. *Journal of the American Medical Association, 272* (September 7), 680–687.

Darman, Richard. (1991). *Introductory statement: The problem of rising costs*. Testimony before the Senate Finance Committee. Washington, D.C.: Executive Office of the President.

Davis, Karen, Kathy Scott Collins, Cathy Schoen, & Cynthia Morris. (1995). Choice matters for consumers. *Health Affairs, 14* (2), 99–112.

Davis, Michael M. (1975). *Medical care for tomorrow*. New York: Harper.

deKervasdoue, Jean, John R. Kimberly, & Victor G. Rodwin. (Eds.). (1984). *The end of an illusion*. Berkeley: University of California Press.

Donnison, David. (1979). Social policy since Titmuss. *Journal of Social Policy, 8*, 145–156.

The Economist. (1992). The economy: Small business, small beer. 31 (July 25).

Eddy, David M., & John Billings. (1988). The quality of medical evidence. *Health Affairs, 7* (Spring), 19–32.

Edwards, Jennifer N., Robert J. Blendon, & Robert Leitman. (1992). In Robert J. Blendon & Tracey S. Hyams (Eds.), *The future of American health care:* Vol. 2, *Reforming the system: Containing health care costs in an era of universal coverage* (pp. 61–82). New York: Faulkner and Gray.

Edwards, Jennifer N., Robert J. Blendon, Robert Leitman, Ellen M. Morrison, J. Ian Morrison, & Humphrey Taylor. (1992). In Robert J. Blendon & Tracey S. Hyams (Eds.), *The future of American health care:* Vol. 2, *Reforming the system: Containing health care costs in an era of universal coverage* (pp. 125–139). New York: Faulkner and Gray.

Edwards, Sebastian. (1995). *Why are savings rates so different across countries? An international comparative analysis* (Working Paper No. 5097). New York: National Bureau of Economic Research.

Ehrbar, A. F. (1997). A radical prescription for medical care. *Fortune, 95*, 164ff.

Ehrenreich, Barbara, & John Ehrenreich. (Eds.). (1970). *The American health empire*. New York: Vintage Books.

Ehrenreich, Barbara, & John Ehrenreich. (1974). Health care and social control. *Social Policy, 5*, 26–40.

Elling, Ray H. (1977). Industrialization and occupational health in underdeveloped countries. *International Journal of Health Services, 7* (2), 209–235.

Ellwood, Paul M. (1988). A technology of patient experience. *New England Journal of Medicine, 318* (June 9), 1549–1556.

Employee Benefits Research Institute. (1994). *Questions and answers on employee benefit issues* (Issue Brief No. 150). Washington, D.C.: Employee Benefits Research Institute.

Employee Benefits Research Institute. (1995a). *Databook on employee benefits* (3rd ed.). Washington, D.C.: Employee Benefits Research Institute.

Employee Benefits Research Institute. (1995b). *Sources of health insurance and characteristics of the uninsured: Analysis of the March 1994 current population survey* (Issue Brief No. 158). Washington, D.C.: Employee Benefits Research Institute.

Employee Benefits Research Institute. (1996). *The changing world of work and employee benefits* (Issue Brief No. 172). Washington, D.C.: Employee Benefits Research Institute.

Fein, Rashi. (1980). Social and economic attitudes shaping American health policy. *Health and Society, 58*, 350–385.

Fein, Rashi. (1986). *Medical care, medical costs: The search for a health insurance policy*. Cambridge, MA: Harvard University Press.

Feldstein, Paul J. (1977). *Health associations and the demand for legislation: The political economy of health*. Cambridge, MA: Ballinger Publishing Co.

Ferrara, Peter J. (1995). Gingrich can avert GOP disaster over Medicare. *Wall Street Journal* (May 1995), A20.

Freidson, Elliot. (1970). *Professional dominance: The social structure of medical care*. New York: Atherton.

Friedman, Milton. (1962). *Capitalism and freedom*. Chicago, IL: Phoenix Books.

Friedman, Milton. (1996). A way out of Soviet-style health care [op-ed]. *Wall Street Journal* (April 17), A20.

Fuchs, Victor. (1974). *Who shall live?* New York: Basic Books.

Fuchs, Victor. (1993). *The future of health policy*. Cambridge, MA: Harvard University Press.

Fuchs, Victor. (1996). Introduction. In Victor R. Fuchs (Ed.), *Individual and social responsibility: Child care, education, medical care, and long-term care in America* (pp. 3–12). Chicago: University of Chicago Press.

Garber, Alan M. (1996). To comfort always: The prospects of expanded social responsibility for long-term care. In Victor R. Fuchs (Ed.), *Individual and social responsibility: Child care, education, medical care, and long-term care in America* (pp. 143–169). Chicago: University of Chicago Press.

Gillis, Kurt D., & David W. Emmons. (1993). Physician involvement with alternative delivery systems. *Socioeconomic characteristics of medical practice 1993* (pp. 15–19). Chicago, IL: American Medical Association, Center for Health Policy Research.

Glazer, Nathan. (1971). Paradoxes of health care. *The Public Interest, 22,* 67–77.

Goodman, John C., & Gerald L. Musgrave. (1994). *Patient power: The free-enterprise alternative to Clinton's health plan.* Washington, D.C.: Cato Institute.

Hadley, Jack. (1982). *More medical care, better health?* Washington, D.C.: Urban Institute.

Haglund, Claudia L., & William L. Dowling. (1993). The hospital. In Stephen J. Williams & Paul R. Torrens (Eds.), *Introduction to health services* (4th ed. pp. 135–176). Albany, NY: Delmar Publishers, Inc.

Higgins, Jan. (1980). Social control theories of social policy. *Journal of Social Policy, 9,* 15–21.

Iglehart, John K. (1978). Adding a dose of competition to the health care industry. *National Journal, 10,* 1602–1606.

Iglehart, John K. (1992). Health policy report: The American health care system. *New England Journal of Medicine, 327* (September 3), 742–747.

Illich, Ivan. (1976). *Medical nemesis: The expropriation of health.* New York: Pantheon Books.

Illich, Ivan. (1977). *Disabling professions.* London, UK: Boyars.

Janowitz, Morris. (1976) *Social control of the welfare state* (pp. 41–71). New York: Elsevier.

Jensen, Gail A., & Robert J. Morlock. (1994). Why medical savings accounts deserve a closer look. *Journal of American Health Policy, 4* (3), 14–27.

Jonas, Steven. (1981). Population data for health and health care. In Stephen Jonas (Ed.), *Health care delivery in the United States* (pp. 37–60). New York: Springer Publishing Co.

Klerman, Jacob A., & Dana P. Goldman. (1994). Job loss due to health insurance mandates. *Journal of the American Medical Association, 272* (August 17), 552–556.

Knowles, John K. (Ed.). (1977). *Doing better, feeling worse: Health in the United States.* New York: W. W. Norton.

Kotelchuck, David. (1976). *Prognosis negative: Crisis in the health care system.* New York: Vintage.

Krause, Elliot A. (1977). *Power and illness: The political sociology of health and medical care.* New York: Elsevier.

Lalonde, Marc. (1974). *A new perspective on the health care of Canadians.* Ottawa, Canada: Ministry of National Health and Welfare.

Lindsay, Cotton L. (1980). *New directions in public health care.* San Francisco, CA: Institute for Contemporary Studies.

Luce, Bryan R. (1994). Medical technology and its assessment. In Stephen J. Williams & Paul R. Torrens (Eds.), *Introduction to health services* (4th ed., pp. 245–268). Albany, NY: Delmar Publishers, Inc.

Madrick, Jeffrey. (1995). *The end of affluence.* New York: Random House.

Marmor, Theodore R. (1973). *The politics of medicine.* Chicago, IL: Aldine.

Maxwell, Robert J. (1974). *Health care: The growing dilemma.* New York: McKinsey.

McKeown, Thomas. (1976). *The role of medicine: Dream, mirage or nemesis?* London, UK: Nuffield Provincial Hospitals Trust.

McKinlay, John B. (1979). A case for refocusing upstream: The economy in illness. In E. Gartly Jaco (Ed.), *Patient, physicians, and illness* (3rd ed., pp. 9–25). New York: The Free Press.

McKinlay, John B., & Sonja A. McKinlay. (1977). The questionable contribution of medical measures to the decline of mortality in the United States in the 20th century. *Milbank Memorial Fund Quarterly, 55* (Summer), 405–426.

Middleton, Timothy. (1996). Can retirees' safety net be saved? *New York Times* (Feburary 18), F1, F4.

Miller, Robert M., & Harold S. Luft. (1994). Managed care performance since 1980. *Journal of the American Medical Association, 271* (May 18), 1512–1518.

Mitchell, Samuel A., & John R. Virtz. (1986). Health care cost containment: What is too much? *Health Affairs, 5* (Winter), 112–120.

Morrison, J. Ian, Ellen M. Morrison, & Jennifer N. Edwards. (1991). Large employers and employee benefits: Priorities for the 1990's. In Robert J. Blendon & Jennifer N. Edwards (Eds.), *The future of American health care: Vol. 1, System in crisis: The case for health care reform* (pp. 103–124). New York: Faulkner and Gray.

Myerson, Allen R. (1996). A double standard in health coverage. *Wall Street Journal* (March 17), F1–F13.

Navarro, Vicente. (1976). *Medicine under capitalism.* New York: Prodist.

Navarro, Vicente. (Ed.). (1977). *Health and medical care in the U.S.: A critical analysis.* Farmingdale, NY: Baywood Publications.

Newhouse, Joseph P. (1994). Economic analysis of the Clinton plan. *Health Affairs, 13* (1), 132–146.

Oravec, John R. (1993). Economy: Part-time, temporary jobs fuel jobless recovery. *AFL-CIO News, 38* (September 20), 10.

Organization for Economic Cooperation and Development. (1987). *The control and management of government expenditure.* Paris, France: Organization for Eeconomic Cooperation and Development.

Organization for Economic Cooperation and Development. (1994). *New orientations for social policy* (Special Policy Studies No. 12). Paris, France: Organization for Economic Coooperation and Development.

Parsons, Talcott. (1951). *The social system.* New York: The Free Press.

Pauly, Mark V., & John C. Goodman. (1995). Tax credits for health insurance and medical savings accounts. *Health Affairs, 14* (1), 125–140.

Peterson, Peter G. (1994). *Facing up: Paying our nation's debt and saving our country's future.* New York: Simon & Schuster.

Peterson, Peter G. (1996). Will America grow up before it grows old? *Atlantic Monthly, 277* (5), 55–86.

Pierce, Wayne. (1991). *Exploiting workers by misclassifying them as independent contractors.* Testimony before the U.S. House Committee on Government Operations. Washington, D.C.: U.S. Government Printing Office.

Pocincki, Leon S., Stuart J. Dogger, & Barbara P. Schwartz. (1973). The incidence of iatrogenic illness. In *Report of the Secretary's Commission on Medical Malpractice* (Pub. No. OS, 73–89). Washington, D.C.: Department of Health, Education, and Welfare.

Poortvliet, William G., & Thomas P. Laine. (1995). A global trend: Privatization and reform of Social Security pension plans. *Benefits Quarterly, 11,* 63–84.

Posner, Richard. (1996). *Aging and old age.* Chicago: University of Chicago Press.

Powles, John. (1973). On the limitations of modern medicine. *Medicine and Man, 1,* 1–28.

Prospective Payment Assessment Commission. (1996). *Report and recommendations to the Congress: Medicare reform.* Washington, D.C.: Prospective Payment Assessment Commission.

Ratcliffe, John, Lawrence Wallack, Francis Fagnani, & Victor Rodwin. (1984). Perspectives on prevention: Health promotion vs. health protection. In Jean deKervasdoue, John R. Kimberly, & Victor G. Rodwin (Eds.), *The end of an illusion: The future of health policy in Western industrialized nations* (pp. 56–84). Berkeley: University of California Press.

Rattner, Steven. (1995). GOP ignores income inequality [op-ed]. *Wall Street Journal* (May 23), A22.

Relman, Arnold S. (1980). The new medical-industrial complex. *New England Journal of Medicine, 303* (October 23), 963–970.

Rice, Dorothy P. (1989). *Caring for the elderly.* Baltimore, MD: Johns Hopkins University Press.

Rivlin, Alice M. (1992). *Reviving the American dream: The economy, the states, and the federal government.* Washington, D.C.: The Brookings Institution.

Rodwin, Marc A. (1993). *Medicine, money and morals.* New York: Oxford University Press.

Rohatyn, Felix G. (1996). Recipe for growth [op-ed]. *Wall Street Journal* (April 11), A18.

Salmon, J. W. (1977). Monopoly capital and reorganization of the health sector. *Review of Radical Political Economics, 8,* 125–133.

Schmid, Gregory. (1991). Demographic, social and economic changes in the 1990's. In Robert J. Blendon & J. N. Edwards (Eds.), *The future of American health care:* Vol. 1, *System in crisis: The case for health care reform* (pp. 31–52). New York: Faulkner and Gray.

Shactman, David, & Stuart H. Altman. (1995). *A study of the decline in employment-based health insurance.* Washington, D.C.: Council on the Impact of Health Care Reform.

Sidel, Victor W., & Ruth Sidel. (1997). *A health state.* New York: Pantheon Books.

Silverman, Celin, & Paul Yakoboski. (1994). Public and private pensions today: An overview of the system. In D. L. Salisbury & N. S. Jones (Eds.), *Pension funding and taxation: Implications for tomorrow* (pp. 7–42). Washington, D.C.: Employee Benefits Research Institute.

Small Business Administration. (1988). *The state of small business: A report to the president.* Washington, D.C.: U.S. Government Printing Office.

Smith, David G. (1978). Policy analysis and liberal arts. In William D. Coplin (Ed.), *Teaching policy studies* (pp. 37–44). Lexington, MA: Lexington Books.

Standard & Poor's Health Care Industry survey. (1995). *Health care products and services basic analysis.* New York: Standard & Poor's.

Stano, Miron. (1994). Outcomes research: High hopes, low yield? *Journal of American Health Policy, 4* (2), 50–52.

Starr, Paul. (1982). *The social transformation of American medicine.* New York: Basic Books.

Steinfels, Peter. (1979). *The neoconservatives: The men who are changing America's politics.* New York: Simon & Schuster.

Timely Surgery. (1991). *The Economist* (May 4), 57–58.

Torrey, Fuller. (1974). *The death of psychiatry.* Radnor, PA: Chilton.

U.S. Congress, The Joint Economic Committee. (1980). *The social costs of unemployment.* Ninety-sixth Congress, 1st Session. Washington, D.C.: U.S. Government Printing Office.

U. S. Congress, Office of Technology Assessment. (1980). *The implications of cost effectiveness analysis of medical technologies.* Washington, D.C.: U.S. Government Printing Office.

U.S. Department of Health, Education, and Welfare. (1976). *Theme: Preparing for national health insurance, forward plan for health FY 1977–1981* (Pub. No. 0826-50046). Washington, D.C.: U.S. Department of Health, Education, and Welfare.

U.S. Department of Labor. (1992). *Health benefits and the work force.* Pension and Benefits Administration. Washington, D.C.: U.S. Government Printing Office.

U.S. House of Representatives, Subcommittee on Oversight and Investigations of the Committee on Interstate and Foreign Commerce. (1976). *Report of the cost and quality of health care: Unnecessary surgery.* Ninety-fourth Congress, 2nd Session. Washington, D.C.: U.S. Government Printing Office.

Waitzkin, Howard. (1978). A Marxist view of medical care. *Annals of Internal Medicine, 89* (August), 264–278.

Weissenstein, Eric. (1995). Cut out the middleman: Coalition seeks big savings by taking the direct approach. *Modern Health Care, 25* (July 3), 28–29.

Wildavsky, Aaron. (1979). *Speaking truth to power: The art and craft of policy analysis.* Boston, MA: Little, Brown.

Wilkinson, Richard G. (1992). National mortality rates: The impact of inequality. *American Journal of Public Health, 82* (August), 1082–1084.

Williams, Stephen J. (1993). Ambulatory health care services. In Stephen J. Williams & Paul R. Torrens (Eds.), *Introduction to health services* (4th ed., pp. 108–134). Albany, NY: Delmar Publishers, Inc.

Winslow, Ron. (1995). Medical upheaval, welfare recipients are a hot commodity in managed care now. *Wall Street Journal* (April 12), A1, A8.

Wohl, Stanley. (1984). *The medical industrial complex.* New York: Harmony Books.

Wolfe, Sydney. (1988). Waste not, want not. *Wall Street Journal, Special Report on Medicine and Health* (April 22). R30–R31.

Woods, John R. (1994). Pension coverage among the baby boomers: Initial findings from a 1993 survey. *Social Security Bulletin, 57,* 12–25.

World Bank. (1994). *Averting the old age crisis: Policies to protect the old and promote growth.* New York: Oxford University Press.

Wyatt, Edward. (1996). A windfall for Wall Street? *New York Times* (February 18), F4.

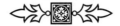

PART TWO

HEALTH POLICY AND THE POLITICAL STRUCTURE

The chapters in this section have two objectives: the first is to describe the role of various government institutions in health policymaking; the second is to evaluate the effects of institutional changes on health policy outcomes.

William Lammers in his discussion of the presidency makes it clear that the president has a powerful, but by no means all-powerful, role in health policymaking. One can also presume that if military spending continues to slowly decline and no foreign crisis equivalent to the Cold War arises, the power of the presidency will decline, for it is the inevitable predominance of the president in foreign affairs that has been the main engine for the expansion of presidential power.

Lammers, as do many of the other authors, also forcefully addresses one of the main recent controversies in health politics: the reasons for the failure of the Clinton health reform proposals. While fully discussing the Clinton administration's tactical errors, he places primary emphasis on the inherent difficulty of enacting comprehensive legislative reform.

David Falcone and Lynn Hartwig also address the failure of the Clinton health reform proposals, but from the perspective of whether the structure of Congress made their defeat inevitable. While recognizing the serious obstacles congressional procedures and norms place in the way of major health reform, they conclude that major health reform is not inevitably doomed to failure.

They also examine the effects of recent changes in congressional procedure on health policy outcomes. Their general belief is that changes that emphasize increased "openness" have had little effect. However, changes that view health issues from the perspective of their impact on the budget have been more important. Moreover, the changes made by House Republicans in 1995—increasing the power of the Speaker and limiting the use of seniority—may be even more important.

Frank Thompson's chapter on policy implementation is a careful examination of what the bureaucracy can reasonably be expected to do well and, conversely, when one should not be very much surprised to discover policy implementation failures. Thompson's perspective is that of "contingency theory," that is, under what set of circumstances is implementation likely to be successful and under what set of circumstances is it likely to fail. This nuanced perspective is particularly useful in analyzing health care delivery programs, for they are rarely either total successes or unmitigated disasters.

Thompson also insightfully assesses one unique perspective on the American bureaucracy: the public's total loathing of it. While not making a case for loving your local bureaucrat, he shows how dysfunctional this is and paradoxically how it often results in the cautious, by-the-rules behavior that the public so dislikes.

Debra Lipson concludes this section by examining the role of the states in health policy. She generally maintains that their role has increased in inverse proportion to the distrust of the federal government, that a major and increasing state role is probable in the foreseeable future, and that this increased role constitutes, on balance, good public policy.

In her description of empirical reality, Lipson is clearly correct. Whether this is desirable is more debatable. Even here, however, Lipson has shown that earlier arguments stressing the states' administrative shortcomings are much less true today and that the real issue is whether comprehensive health reform is inherently a function of the national government.

Overall, the authors in this section take the view that the structure of American government makes comprehensive health reform, as well as the enactment and implementation of other major social reforms, uniquely difficult, but by no means impossible. Their useful lesson is that health reformers should not be advocating proposals that seem ideal in the abstract, but rather the best possible reforms consistent with probable enactment and effective implementation by the institutions of American government.

CHAPTER

Presidential Leadership and Health Policy

William W. Lammers

Americans frequently look to the possibility of strong presidential leadership in the search for possible sources of major change in health policies. President Lyndon Johnson's role in the passage of Medicare is frequently cited as a prime example. Often, the hope for presidential leadership emphasizes the importance of making a fast start, as occurred in Roosevelt's first hundred days and with Reagan's passage of his economic program in the first months of 1981.

In the wake of the stunning congressional rejection of President Clinton's proposed health reform package in 1994, it is essential to reconsider the potential for presidential leadership. After an introduction to the concepts being used, this chapter examines the successes and failures of presidents in the pursuit of changes in health policy. Implications of previous experiences are then considered in an assessment of possible future presidential roles.

THE PRESIDENT'S ROLE AND THE POLICYMAKING CYCLE

To effectively examine presidential actions in the development of health policy, it is necessary to consider two sets of relationships. First, leadership roles and strategies need to be assessed across the policymaking cycle. Second, as a basis for evaluating a president's performance, it is essential to consider the factors that have shaped his level of opportunity for achieving changes in health policy.

The formation and implementation of health policy occurs in a policy cycle comprised of five components: issue raising, policy design, public support building, legislative decision making, and policy implementation. These activities are likely to be shared with Congress and interest groups in varying degrees. As a result, it is essential to consider interest group and legislative actions as well as presidential roles when examining cases of major policy change. Presidents nonetheless have a wide variety of possibilities for effective action in each aspect of the policy cycle.

Issue-Raising Activities

Issue-raising activities are clearly essential in the policy formation cycle. The enactment of a new policy is generally preceded by a variety of actions that first create a widespread sense that a problem exists that needs to be addressed. Social conditions, in other words, do not automatically produce the attitude that there is a problem that requires solution (Kingdon, 1995). Specific actions are necessary to produce a perception that a problem requiring solution does exist. In the issue-raising process, presidents have multiple opportunities. Periodically, presidents have chosen to emphasize major health policy issues in their campaigns. The list of presidents who have made major efforts to expand interest in health policy changes during their campaigns includes not only Clinton, but also Truman, Kennedy, Johnson, and Carter.

Once elected, presidents possess a number of potential issue-raising opportunities. These actions may signal to members of Congress as well as the public that a health policy issue is going to take on considerable importance. Presidents may encourage others to act by underscoring the importance of an issue in their State of the Union Address. In seeking to increase general public interest in health policy issues, presidents on occasion have included health policy issues in major addresses. In 1993, President Clinton took a unique step in elevating the importance of health policy issues by appointing his wife, Hillary Rodham Clinton, to head his task force on health care reform. Once that step had been taken, it became clear to those interested in health policy that a major effort would be undertaken.

Design of Specific Proposals

The second component of presidential policymaking activity involves the development of specific proposals. This has been a particularly difficult undertaking in health care because there are many different ways of changing its organization and financing. As a result, one has frequently seen, as in 1993–94, major conflicts involving different policy approaches among members of Congress and interest group leaders who agree that "something needs to be done."

Presidents have substantial resources at their disposal for developing new policy proposals. They may call upon segments of the executive branch of government, such as the Health Care Financing Administration and policy staffs within the Department of Health and Human Services. In some instances, interagency task forces have also been employed. Some presidents, however, including Kennedy and Johnson, viewed policy design processes oriented around cabinet members and their staffs as too likely to be tied to narrow and existing policy ideas.

The alternative preferred by both Kennedy and Johnson was the use of outside task forces. Kennedy used task forces that included a health group dealing with health care in 1961, and Johnson used that process quite extensively in 1964–65. Clinton, on the other hand, took an unusual approach to health policy development in that he involved both a uniquely large outside task force and a group of cabinet members to participate in the development of a set of final recommendations. While outside task forces can be highly effective, there are potential difficulties surrounding the lack of practicality in the resulting proposals (Wolanin, 1975).

Along with the structure that is used to develop policy proposals, a variety of strategic issues are involved. One question concerns the level of specificity that will be contained in the materials submitted to Congress. In 1992, President Bush submitted a health proposal that was quite general and did not directly address financing issues. The prospect of presenting only the general outlines of a legislative proposal and "leaving things up to Congress" may facilitate a bargaining process, but is often resented in Congress. The present congressional requirement that the Congressional Budget Office "cost out" legislative proposals also reduces the extent to which that strategy can be employed.

A second issue surrounds the extent to which previously developed proposals will be absorbed into the materials the president ultimately submits to Congress. Presidents often like to stress the extent to which they will be presenting new policies once they arrive in Washington. Nonetheless, analyses that are sometimes touted during a campaign are no substitute for an actual legislative proposal. Often, presidents promoting major changes in the first year have actually been working with existing policy designs. This was substantially the case for both Roosevelt in 1933 (Freidel, 1973) and Reagan in 1981 (Stockman, 1986). The use of existing policy proposals is particularly important when a president is emphasizing speed, since the effort to sift through options and develop new approaches is likely to be time-consuming. Such use also has the potential advantage of generating proposals that are familiar to policymakers and the public. But if few changes have occurred in the partisan and ideological composition of Congress, there is the danger that they may quickly reproduce earlier partisan and ideological divisions in Congress.

The final question a president faces in developing policy design involves issues of potential support. Presidents and their policy designers in varying degrees may: (1) shape their proposal in relationship to assessments of public opinion, (2) negotiate with interest group leaders, or (3) seek the guidance and support of key members of Congress. Presubmission negotiations can be a difficult process, but are usually an important key to success.

Support-Building Roles

Presidents can also choose from a variety of support-building roles. This includes not only major addresses to the nation, but efforts to mobilize their administration to make public appeals and organized attempts to increase support among interest groups. As emphasized by Kernell (1986), presidents on occasion have been able to expand public support with major addresses. A example of this is President Reagan's successful effort in building public support for his economic policies in 1981. The initial favorable response to Clinton's September 1993 health policy address is another important example of this strategy.

The mobilization of members of the administration involves not only public addresses, but television appearances on various interview programs. It is now quite common for a key member of the president's staff to develop a systematic plan for those appearances. Presidents now also operate with an Office of Public Liaison, which seeks to maintain continuous contact with interest groups that are important to a president's legislative program.

Legislative Roles and Strategies

Presidents and key staff and department officials interact with Congress in several different ways. Presidents generally meet with legislative leaders several mornings each month in an effort to shape the coming legislative agenda and to identify possible problems as bills move through various committees. Beginning in particular with the Kennedy administration, presidents have developed fairly large liaison offices for dealing with Congress (Walcott & Hult, 1995). Actions taken by those staff members seek to develop support among members of Congress by helping with issues relating to their districts and addressing patronage concerns, while also gaining information presidents can use regarding individuals whose voting decision may be modified by various presidential actions. Presidents have also quite frequently had their chiefs of staff engage in direct contact with important members of Congress as well as those whose favorable vote is being pursued. In addition, presidents can mobilize officials within key departments and agencies to promote their legislation at congressional hearings.

One of the president's most important roles is to focus congressional energies on a particular issue. Although this may overlap issue-raising activities to some extent, such presidential actions may include stressing a specific issue in the State of the Union Address, sending messages and specific proposals to Congress, and arranging to have a proposal entered as the number one bill in the House and Senate.

In their agenda-setting role, presidents face important questions surrounding the extent to which they attempt to use a "fast-start" approach in their first year.

Presidents are encouraged to seek a fast start for several reasons. Their popularity is likely to be higher at the outset of their administration, and there may be an initial sense of a honeymoon with Congress. If they have made a major case for a policy change in the campaign and won convincingly, they may also be able to claim a mandate. In addition, the second year is likely to see increased congressional concern with reelection politics and the president's party usually loses votes in the midterm elections.

Data presented by Light (1982) clearly support the fast-start strategy. In his study of presidential requests to Congress in the first year, he found that between 1960 and 1977, the success rate of legislative items submitted between January and the end of March was 72 percent, but only 39 percent in the next three months and 25 percent by the third quarter of the year. Presidents may nonetheless confront difficulties in pursuing a fast-start strategy if they seek to develop a new policy design at the outset of their administration. It is for this reason that Light recommends policy design strategies that utilize existing proposals rather than seeking to develop an optimum new policy design.

Presidents may pay a price for a fast start by enacting legislative proposals that have been hastily developed and require subsequent modification. This was dramatically the case for Roosevelt in the wake of his first hundred days (Freidel, 1990). On the other hand, in some instances they may find that changing circumstances facilitate success later in their first term. This was also the case for Roosevelt, who actually passed his most important programs in his third year in office. Nonetheless, the fast-start approach in the first year can give presidents advantages in their degree of influence in Congress.

In their efforts to persuade members of Congress to support their preferred positions, presidents often confront serious limitations. Interpretations of legislative voting by Bond and Fleisher (1990) and Edwards (1989) have emphasized the extent to which legislative votes are shaped by partisan affiliation and ideology. While this pattern clearly holds for a large number of the votes being cast each session, presidents do have some potential for influencing a few important individual votes. Patronage considerations and aid for a legislator's district may be helpful. A president may also become involved in cross-policy area trades, such as agreeing to support a legislator's favored program in another area. Tobacco state legislators, for example, have periodically used presidential support for government programs aiding tobacco growers as a basis for granting their support for a president's health policy proposal. Appeals to partisan considerations and efforts to persuade by advocating a policy on its own merits may also be successful.

While their ability to influence legislative voting decisions is quite limited, presidents can also influence legislative outcomes in several ways. Often, the key decision-making roles occur in a particular committee. Chairmen are often highly independent, as was the case on Medicare with Wilbur Mills (D-AR). Nonetheless, at least occasionally they may be able to encourage desired action by committee chairs or individual committee members.

Presidents also have important opportunities for influencing congressional outcomes through their efforts to develop compromises that allow bills with at least some of their preferred outcomes to be passed. On some occasions, that battle involves efforts to prevent legislative stalemates over divisions between those who want to do more than is being proposed and those who want to do less.

Beginning in the 1980s, legislative decision making has also found presidents and their key aides involved with a few congressional leaders in efforts to develop widespread compromises in bills that include many major provisions (Davidson, 1992). This form of top-level negotiation has grown in part because of the desire for broad deficit reduction packages. The decision process in 1990 in which President Bush abandoned his "no new taxes" pledge was one important example of top-level negotiation in an effort to achieve deficit reduction. Such a strategy, however, is more likely to operate successfully if there is strong pressure to reach an immediate decision. On the difficult issue of reform in the Social Security system, top-level negotiation was used to achieve the "shared pain" compromises that produced a broad package of changes in the Social Security system in 1983 (Light, 1985). In this case, there was a very real threat that the absence of some decision would leave the Social Security Administration without the funds needed to operate in the coming year. Therefore, a president who is well prepared with measures he wants to promote in top-level negotiations and adopts effective bargaining strategies can have an important influence.

Policy Implementation

Presidents also have important roles in the shaping and implementation of health policies. In some instances, this comes as a result of somewhat vague legislation written to facilitate compromise among interest groups. In other instances, important issues of timing will be involved regarding the implementation of a policy Congress has enacted. In some instances, presidents will be able to act in their administrative role even while Congress is debating a possible change in policy. This occurred in 1995, when President Clinton used his administrative role to have waivers quickly granted to states wanting to experiment with new variations in their AFDC and Medicaid programs while Congress was still debating possible steps to broadly shift greater responsibility for those programs to state governments.

Opportunity Level

Studies of presidential leadership in recent years have given increasing attention to the factors that shape opportunities for presidential successes in achieving major policy change (Light, 1988; Jones, 1995). The first set of factors involves election results. These include: (1) the size of the president's winning margin, (2) the president's share of the total vote cast, and (3) the size of the president's party in Congress.

A second line of analysis has been developed by Kingdon (1995), who conceptualized the existence of a "window of opportunity" if a combination of three basic factors occurs. These are: (1) a widespread view within the electorate and among key policymakers that a given problem needs to be addressed; (2) a substantial amount of agreement regarding a possible choice of a specific policy design; and (3) a set of political relation-

ships that are conducive to change. A somewhat similar approach has been utilized by Starr (1982) in his assessment of changes in health policy from the Progressive Era to 1980.

In addition, several other factors also are seen as important dimensions of a president's opportunity level. As reviewed in an assessment of recent studies by Michaelson (1994), presidential popularity may have an impact on a president's level of success with Congress. Such influence, for instance, is most apt to occur when a president's popularity is tied to his position on major issues before Congress. Public confidence in government can also shape a president's opportunity level. The general level of activism in the electorate, as existed between about 1964 and 1974, has been found by Mayhew (1991) to be a factor contributing to the passage of an extensive amount of major legislation during that period. Finally, economic and budgetary conditions often shape a president's level of opportunity for addressing major health policy issues.

CASE STUDIES OF PRESIDENTIAL LEADERSHIP

The following discussion examines major cases of health policy change and attempted change during each presidency beginning with that of Franklin Roosevelt. The case studies were selected from a review of major works on each president and the enumeration of major policy enactments between 1947 and 1990 developed by David Mayhew (1991).[1] By considering each president's opportunity level and leadership roles, it is possible to assess the extent to which each president was successful in using his opportunities for achieving changes in health policy.

---

[1]The materials reported are drawn from a study of presidential leadership on major cases of domestic policy change during the first term of each president, beginning with Franklin Roosevelt. Along with published sources, research materials for Kennedy, Johnson, Nixon, Carter, and Reagan were gathered by the author at their presidential libraries. The Clinton case study is based on books and newspaper accounts, plus Washington interviews with and an examination of the papers of the Health Care Task Force. For the larger study, see William W. Lammers, *Comparing presidents: Leadership and domestic policy* (Washington, D.C.: CQ Press, forthcoming).

President Roosevelt (1933–45)

The absence of any significant health care legislation during the Roosevelt years raises an important question regarding possible lost opportunities. During his first term Roosevelt enjoyed large Democratic majorities, which reached 319 in the House and 69 in the Senate after the 1934 midterm elections. In addition to being elected decisively in 1932, he was reelected by a landslide majority in 1936.

In the context of those advantages, Roosevelt nonetheless made it clear to his Committee on Economic Security that he did not want to include a battle over health insurance with the American Medical Association (AMA) as part of his proposed Social Security program in 1935. As a result, the Social Security Act excluded a health component while including an insurance-based pension system for the elderly, unemployment insurance, some benefits for impoverished individuals, and benefits for widows and children that would later evolve into today's Aid to Families with Dependent Children program.

As one considers a wider range of factors involved in shaping Roosevelt's level of opportunity in 1935, it is quite clear that no obvious opportunity was missed (Starr, 1982). In part, the primary public concern at the time was with economic assistance for the elderly and the unemployed rather than health insurance. Also, the pressing concern in many quarters with the size of the deficit reduced potential support for an expensive new program.

The difficulties Roosevelt encountered in Congress with a program that did not include health care also suggest the likelihood of even greater difficulty with a broader proposal. While there was considerable sentiment in Congress for creating some form of assistance for the elderly, Roosevelt confronted resistances from southern Democrats that required compromises such as the elimination of coverage for agricultural workers (Quadagno, 1994). In addition, considerable presidential lobbying was still required to push the bill through the House Ways and Means Committee, which was stacked with southerners. At the same time, Roosevelt also had to prevent supporters of broader pension plans such as the Townsend Plan (which would have given $200 a month to persons over sixty) from acting in ways that would make it more difficult for his far more limited plan to pass. While Roosevelt had a high opportunity level in 1935, considerable skill was required to pass the Social Security Act even without a health care component.

During Roosevelt's final eight years in office, the promotion of health insurance came primarily within Congress (Poen, 1979). Roosevelt indicated that he would push for a major health program after the war, but no action had been taken at the time of his death. Roosevelt may have missed an opportunity for the federal government to take some initial steps on health policy during the 1937–45 period. Nonetheless, this opportunity for achieving major policy change was seriously reduced in this period despite his reelection landslide. Beginning in 1937, a conservative coalition of Republicans and southern Democrats who constituted more than one hundred members of the party's strength in the House came together to effectively oppose many of Roosevelt's domestic policy initiatives. Interestingly, it is this same coalition that would continue to reduce the prospects for new health policy initiatives for succeeding Democratic presidents.

President Truman (1945–53)

Despite Truman's repeated advocacy of a system of national health insurance, the only major piece of health legislation that passed was the Hill–Burton Hospital Construction Act. Although interest in a hospital construction program was promoted to a very limited extent by Truman's emphasis on the issue in his initial broad statement of health policy objectives in September 1945, actions taken by the American Hospital Association had far greater importance.

During both his first term and again in 1949, Congress rejected Truman's proposals for national health insurance. In 1945, former Roosevelt aide Samuel Rosenman was the key figure in developing the message Truman submitted to Congress, as he drew upon ideas contained in a plan first introduced in 1943 by Senators Robert Wagner (D-NY) and James Murray (D-MT) and Representative John Dingell (D-MI). Truman's plan was broader, however, as he proposed a single system that would include all segments of American society rather than one that included the needy in a separate category.

In his first three years in office, Truman did little more with his proposal than make his annual message to Congress. His inaction accurately reflected the constraints facing a president who (1) had not been elected in his own right, (2) was seeking to lead a country through extensive adjustments to a peacetime economy, and (3) faced a Congress controlled by the Republicans in the wake of their fifty-five seat gain in the 1946 midterm election.

The 1948 election produced renewed interest in health care issues. Truman stressed national health insurance, partly in an effort to attract potential supporters of Progressive Party presidential candidate Henry Wallace and partly as a basis for attacking the "do nothing" Republican Congress. Despite a measure of newfound energy that emerged as a result of his surprising election victory, he was nonetheless still in a relatively weak position. He had won by a margin of only 2 million votes and was not a particularly popular president. Although the Democrats won control of Congress with 263 members in the House and 54 in the Senate, those figures did not accurately reflect Truman's potential level of support because of the conservative views held by many southern Democrats.

The manner in which Truman's proposal failed was markedly similar to that observed with the Clinton administration virtually a half century later. In this instance, the American Medical Association (AMA) mounted an intense campaign against what they called "socialized medicine" and spent the then unprecedented sum of $2.5 million to defeat it. Truman on the other hand was not particularly effective with his own limited appeals, which further reduced potential public support. A level of support that stood at 58 percent at the beginning of 1949 dropped to only 38 percent by the end of that year (Poen, 1975).

In his attempt to move his health insurance proposal through Congress, Truman lacked the public support-building skills of a Franklin Roosevelt or the skill in dealing directly with Congress of a Lyndon Johnson. Given the circumstances Truman confronted, however, it is likely that either of those more highly skilled presidents would also have experienced enormous difficulties in trying to push a system of national health insurance through Congress in 1949. The one significant action that did occur in the wake of the defeat of Truman's initiative was a shift toward a program focused upon the elderly. This occurred with the efforts initially undertaken by Oscar Ewing (head of the Federal Security Agency) to develop a proposal for initial coverage of the elderly. That proposal would ultimately contribute to the development of interest in Medicare at the end of the 1950s. In the meantime, a rapid expansion of employer-based health benefits for union members and a growth of private insurance for the middle class reduced pressure for national health insurance during the 1950s.

President Eisenhower (1953–61)

In electing Eisenhower in 1952, the voters placed in the White House a popular general with good skills in leading "behind the scenes" but not a strong advocate of new health care programs. Moreover, except for the 1953–54 period, control of the House and Senate rested in the hands of the Democrats. Interestingly, Eisenhower did develop one extremely limited reinsurance proposal in his first term, which he thought would be a useful step toward precluding future interest in "socialized medicine." When the AMA moved to block his proposal, however, he concluded that it was led by "a little group of reactionary men dead set against change" (Ambrose, 1984).

The politics of health care basically shifted to Congress, with an increased amount of activity on issues involving health care for the elderly at the end of the decade. The latter was fueled by the problems the elderly were facing as the group in society with the largest health costs and yet virtually lacking the private coverage that had been growing for younger segments of the population in the 1950s. In this context, the Eisenhower administration in 1960 presented a limited proposal that would have provided a federal subsidy for the purchase of private health insurance for the elderly.

The resulting passage of the Kerr–Mills Act in 1960 was nonetheless primarily a result of political forces within Congress and the desire of Senator Robert Kerr (D-OK) and Congressman Wilbur Mills (D-AR) to achieve some legislation prior to the fall elections. The system they promoted "rocked no boats" in terms of established interests. Instead, it promised to build upon existing means-tested programs for which the states were already receiving some assistance. The new act provided for larger federal matching grants to the states and also established a new category of "medically indigent" individuals who were poor but were not receiving cash assistance from other assistance programs. Its structure, which was a forerunner to Medicaid, entailed open-ended federal cost sharing, without limits on individual payments or total state expenditures, and with cost control left to the states. This could hardly be viewed as a complete answer to the health insurance problems of the elderly, however, because it only began payments when individuals had already become poor. Despite the fanfare that surrounded the passage of Kerr–Mills during the 1960 elections, state responses were generally quite limited (Stevens & Stevens, 1974).

President Kennedy (1961–63)

The 1960 election brought to the White House a president who had been a strong promoter of federal health insurance for the elderly during his final two years in the Senate (David, 1985). His level of opportunity, however, was fairly limited. He emerged as a popular president and there were Democratic majorities in both houses. Nonetheless, he had won by a razor-thin margin of only 113,000 votes and was confronted by the strong opposition of key committee chairmen in both the House and Senate along with the familiar resistance from southern Democrats.

Interest group support showed growing activity on the part of the elderly, first as the labor-backed group initially organized as Seniors for Kennedy and later reorganized as the National Council of Senior Citizens. There were also important indications of support from such groups as nurses and labor unions. At the same time, the AMA remained adamantly opposed, as did major business groups such as the Chamber of Commerce (Marmor, 1973).

In the quest for specific approaches to his health policy initiatives, Kennedy turned to Wilbur Cohen. As chairman of the president's health task force, Cohen brought to that responsibility an extensive understanding of health policy issues, derived from extensive roles in both promoting Social Security legislation in Congress and studying those issues as a professor at the University of Michigan. The proposal that his task force produced was quickly endorsed by Kennedy, with its call for an expansion in the hospital insurance proposal that had been previously developed in Congress.

As he sized up the Congress he would have to deal with, Kennedy decided it was important to seek an expansion in the House Rules Committee since that twelve-person committee presented a difficult hurdle for liberal legislation with the tendency of southern Democrats to vote with Republicans to prevent programs they disliked from reaching the floor for deliberation and a vote. Even with a strong effort by Speaker Sam Rayburn (D-TX), success in expanding the committee to fifteen members required an extensive effort and passed by only five votes. The resulting expansion helped on some domestic measures, but did not resolve the problems being created by chairmen such as Wilbur Mills (D-AR) who were reluctant to have their committees pass new proposals.

The primary action on Medicare occurred in 1962 rather than 1961. During Kennedy's initial year in office, possible action was slowed in part because of resistance toward Medicare on the part of the extremely influential chairman of the House Ways and Means Committee, Wilbur Mills. In 1962, the Kennedy administration considered the Senate to be a more likely source of an initial victory and made a major outside "going public" effort to achieve passage of its Medicare bill. The outside strategy included speeches by some twenty-one members of the administration along with an address by the president to an audience of senior citizens at Madison Square Garden. While Kennedy's address was well received by his immediate audience, it was judged to have been one of his poorest efforts for the wider listening audience. As an important indication of the tensions that can occur between strategies of "going public" and efforts to achieve compromise within the legislative arena, Wilbur Cohen was critical of the emphasis on the public strategy being promoted by Ivan Nestingen, another top Kennedy appointee in the Department of Health, Education, and Welfare (David, 1985).

Prior to the floor vote on the Medicare bill in the Senate, Kennedy made a number of personal appeals. Nonetheless, in the midst of skillful maneuvering by legislative opponents, the measure was defeated by a vote of 48 to 52. The majority that formed to defeat that measure was comprised of thirty-one Republicans and twenty-one southern Democrats. In the wake of that defeat, Kennedy retreated from any further major effort in 1963. Progress, however, was made in dealing with Wilbur Mills, who had agreed to hold hearings just before Kennedy's death.

In the more limited area of medical education, President Kennedy played a fairly significant role in producing new legislation. He promoted a broad plan of assistance in 1961, and in 1962 his message on education included a ten-year program of matching grants for a variety of medical and other health-related professional schools. In 1963, his health message again called for construction grants, while his financial assistance proposal changed to loans rather than his previously recommended scholarships. At a key point as the bill was being delayed in the House Rules Committee, he appears to have successfully used very pointed press conference remarks to put additional pressure on two southern Democrats, including the chairman, to avoid delaying the bill. A somewhat modified form of Kennedy's initial proposal subsequently passed handily in each house of Congress (*Congressional Quarterly Almanac*, 1963).

Despite his ability to achieve passage of a medical education bill, Kennedy's failure to pass his Medicare proposal understandably constitutes the major issue in evaluating his performance. For revisionists such as Parmet (1983), Kennedy is portrayed as a president with limited interests in many domestic policy issues and a reluctance to act in an assertive manner in his relationships with Congress.

Kennedy clearly did not pursue legislative relations with the aggressiveness displayed by Johnson. At the same time, Kennedy did undertake leadership roles on several aspects of the policy cycle. On Medicare he contributed to issue raising during the campaign, promoted a modified policy design in 1961, and undertook a public support-building and legislative bargaining effort in 1962. When considered in light of the forthcoming discussion of the different opportunity levels Johnson enjoyed, the Kennedy case underscores the need for not only leadership skill but also a high level of opportunity if a president is going to be successful in achieving major changes in health policy.

President Johnson (1963–69)

President Johnson clearly enjoyed a uniquely high level of political opportunity as he addressed Medicare and several other health policy issues. In 1964, efforts to reach a compromise on Medicare made substantial legislative progress, but ultimately produced a deadlock at the conference committee stage. As the bargaining process evolved, Johnson concluded that he would be in a stronger position in 1965 and was reluctant to give away too much in 1964 (David, 1965).

Johnson achieved the passage of Medicare in 1965 in the context of an unusually favorable level of political opportunity and an effective use of leadership skills on some aspects of the policy formation cycle. He had been elected by a landslide vote of over 60 percent in 1964 and enjoyed fairly high levels of popularity. That election not only produced a landslide victory for Johnson, but also impressive gains of 37 Democrats in the House to give him a total of 295 Democrats in the House along with 68 in the Senate. As one indication of the shift in opportunity, a memorandum by legislative aide Mike Manatos (1964) indicated that in his best judgment the Medicare bill had gained a likely increase of ten additional supporters in the Senate as a result of the fall election. In addition, Medicare enjoyed substantial support by the general public, and the program's most vocal opponent—the American Medical Association—suffered a serious loss as many of the candidates it had backed in the 1964 election were defeated. In terms of budgetary prospects, the substantial economic growth experienced in 1964 made the prospects of new expenditures more plausible than in 1961. As seen by Mayhew (1991), a rise in general activism on domestic policy issues was also affecting the potential for substantial new domestic policy actions.

In the context of his high level of opportunity, Johnson took several important leadership roles. As he planned for a new initiative on Medicare in 1965, Johnson used a combination of an advisory panel and staff work by Wilbur Cohen along with contributions from Nelson Cruikshank representing the AFL-CIO to produce some expansion in the previous legislation. Along with producing some changes in the new bill, that process had the positive consequence of furthering consensus in support of the bill among key constituencies. Fortunately for a president who was never able to develop a particularly effective speaking role in promoting his legislative agenda, public roles beyond his strong endorsement of Medicare in the 1964 presidential race were not crucial to legislative success.

The key changes in Medicare in 1965 came about in an unexpected way. They were not initiated by the president but by Chairman Wilbur Mills of the House Ways and Means Committee. Johnson was initially concerned that Mills was trying to change the legislative package in a way that might contribute to its defeat. But after receiving assurances that the chairman was acting in good faith to expand the bill, the president quickly threw his support behind Mills' efforts.

The maneuver Mills undertook was to add proposals that proponents had seen as alternatives to Johnson's proposal as additional components of that proposal. This included both coverage for visits to physicians and an expanded needs-based system to build upon the 1960 Kerr–Mills legislation. Thus, the program that would emerge as Medicaid was in fact the plan that the AMA had been promoting as an alternative to Medicare.

Johnson was nonetheless an important player in the passage of the new combined legislative package in several ways. In an effort to prompt swift legislative action, Johnson arranged to have Medicare given the symbolic designation as the number one bill in each house. As a classic display of Johnson's skills in dealing with potential problems in Congress, he also put pressure on Senator Robert Byrd (D-WV) to report the bill out of committee in a timely manner. This occurred as Byrd was invited to a meeting at the White House and discovered to his surprise as the meeting ended that television cameras were present. In that setting, Johnson asked if the bill would soon be reported out, and Byrd somewhat reluctantly gave an affirmative response. Johnson also played an important role in thwarting an attempt by Senator Russell Long (D-LA) to shift the emphasis of the program toward catastrophic health insurance when the measure reached the Senate Finance Committee. The central legislative role Johnson performed was thus not seeking to change the votes of a significant number of legislators, but rather one of helping steer the legislation away from possible roadblocks or unwanted detours. While these skills were important, the situation had changed dramatically from the one Kennedy had confronted in 1961. For, as one legislator noted, anyone introducing both Medicare and Medicaid in 1960 would have had his sanity questioned (David, 1985).

In the implementation of Medicare, Johnson also had an extremely important role. Some members of the AMA had been publicly discussing the prospect of boycotting the new program, and the question of how the program was to be implemented took on considerable importance. In this context, Johnson gave a pep talk to a group of eleven AMA leaders the day before the bill was to be signed. This talk found Johnson dealing from one of his strengths—the ability to be persuasive with small groups. Although relationships between the federal government and the AMA remained cool, the implementation of Medicare was carried out quite smoothly.

One final issue needs to be considered regarding Johnson's role regarding Medicare. In neither the process of legislative enactment nor the implementation phase was there extensive consideration of having a direct government role in controlling the prices that would be charged by hospitals and doctors. As a concession to the medical profession, congressional leaders worded the reimbursement procedure so that doctors could claim their "usual and customary fees." Doctors quickly raised their fees at the beginning of the program, in part because of a fear of future regulations. Later, in the 1980s, this issue would be revisited with forms of price regulation for both doctors and hospitals.

On another health care measure, Johnson's leadership also had an important impact. In July 1964, Johnson instigated the establishment of a number of task forces that were used with considerable effectiveness throughout his entire presidency. One result of this process was the passage of a measure authorizing the construction of a system of regional heart, cancer, and stroke programs. The commission initially had recommended the establishment of 450 "stations" across the country to provide such services as screening, diagnosis, outpatient care, and training of physicians (*Congressional Quarterly Almanac*, 1965). The legislation Johnson subsequently developed dropped the call for stations, and focused on grants for the establishment of unspecified number of medical "complexes" affiliated with medical schools and hospitals.

Johnson sought to build congressional interest in the latter proposal through the use of a special message to Congress in early 1965. The measure quickly encountered opposition, however, as the AMA voiced strong objections at its June 20, 1965 national convention. After the Senate had passed a somewhat modified bill, the AMA requested that Johnson defer action until 1966, with a rather clear threat that its passage would likely jeopardize the AMA's cooperation with the Department of Health, Education, and Welfare in regulating Medicare. Johnson refused to delay, but asked his new HEW secretary, John Gardner, to work with an AMA committee to find ways to make the bill less objectionable. Despite substantial changes, the AMA representatives said that they still could not support the bill although it was clearly less objectionable than the original pro-

posal. Johnson, too, was not pleased with some of those changes, nor with additional changes made in congressional committees, but decided that they were the price one had to pay for passage of the bill.

The final measure called for a total expenditure of $340 million over fiscal years 1966–68 for grants to develop medical centers and established a thirteen-member National Advisory Council on Regional Medical Programs to advise and assist the surgeon general in the implementation of the new program. As part of the effort to at least soften AMA resistance, the act stipulated that no patient would be furnished care unless he or she had been referred to the facility by a practicing physician.

In sum, Johnson was obviously skilled in his dealings with Congress and had a strong commitment to an expanded federal health policy effort. He was also aided in having uniquely favorable opportunities in 1965. Because of those unique opportunities, it is conceivable that Johnson yielded too readily on aspects of Medicare's final program design (Marmor, 1973). The primary lesson that emerges from the Johnson case, however, is that major policy change requires both presidential skill and favorable opportunities.

President Nixon (1969–74)

In assessing President Nixon's level of opportunity, the situation in his first term was in some respects quite limited. He had received only 43 percent of the total vote, and his margin over Hubert Humphrey had narrowed to approximately a half million votes. In an election that had focused on foreign policy issues, he could not realistically claim voter support for any health policy initiatives. He also faced the rare situation of being the first newly elected president in over a century to face opposition party control of both houses of Congress. Public approval ratings during his first term were also no more than average.

Despite such obvious limitations, two major factors were operating in Nixon's favor. Most centrally, the high level of public-sector activism that had begun in 1964 continued to a substantial degree until 1974. In addition, in terms of issue agendas, a growing concern with both access questions and cost control was producing substantial interest in major and potentially fundamental changes in the nation's health care system.

The passage of three major pieces of health legislation during Nixon's presidency came with varying degrees of presidential leadership. In the development of an expanded federal government commitment to combatting cancer in 1971, there was issue-raising activity both in Congress and in Nixon's 1971 State of the Union Address. In the midst of legislative conflict that centered primarily on organizational issues, however, Nixon took the position that he did not have a preference when the issue reached the conference committee stage.

The actions leading to federal support of health maintenance organizations (HMOs) in 1973 represent a particularly controversial aspect of health policy development during the Nixon presidency. The proposal for government encouragement of prepaid health efforts found the Nixon presidency performing unusually active issue-raising and policy design roles, with the president paradoxically also engaged in interest group and legislative bargaining efforts that reduced the scope of the final legislation. As the final compromise emerged, Congress got the broad goals desired by liberally oriented reformers, and the Nixon administration won in the desire to promote limited funding.

The emergence of HMOs as a new approach for controlling health costs is a fascinating story of presidential health policy leadership. In the desire to find some strategy that would assist in the control of health costs, top officials in Nixon's Department of Health, Education, and Welfare turned to the ideas being advanced by Paul Ellwood Jr., a physician and head of a Minneapolis-based policy study group (Brown, 1983). There was an initial receptiveness based on a sense of urgency in light of the president's promise of new strategies for cost control, combined with a desire to do something different. Nixon was initially enthusiastic about the concept of federal HMO encouragement, and included that approach as a centerpiece in his major health policy statement to Congress in early 1971. To an unusually high degree, Nixon and his top health

advisers were responsible for choosing a particular policy approach as the preferred strategy for fighting the rapid increases in health care costs in the private sector. Quite strikingly, as they took that step they were promoting a strategy that initially had the support of only a third of the public (Brown, 1983). Although the concept of prepaid health plans had been in existence for several decades, it is doubtful that HMOs could have emerged as a major focus for changes in health care organization without the strong actions taken by the Nixon administration.

The unusual aspect of HMO politics during the Nixon presidency surrounded his subsequent retreat from a support-building role. The stage for Nixon's shift was set as the Democratic majority in Congress (and in particular Senator Edward Kennedy) became increasingly interested in using HMOs to advance a variety of their policy objectives, while the American Medical Association expressed increasing alarm over the prospect of federal support for a significant shift away from independent physician and fee-for-service forms of organization (Falkson, 1980). By 1973, as a modified bill was passed, legislative bargaining occurred in which the Nixon administration expressed substantial concern regarding the size of the future HMO effort. Thus the Nixon administration's role was significant in somewhat contradictory ways—in raising an issue and promoting interest in a new policy approach, while also working to restrict the scope of the new initiatives when Congress began to promote a major expansion. In the implementation phase, the Nixon administration was left with a difficult law to administer, and through the 1970s the level of HMO development fell substantially below the original optimistic projections.

On an even more far-reaching second-term initiative, the results were quite different as a major health insurance proposal ended in complete defeat. The proposal that Nixon presented included a continuation of private policies, with the government providing insurance for those not covered by private plans. Administration of the plan was to be carried out by existing insurance companies, and the government's financial contribution was to be 75 percent of an individual's medical costs up to an annual maximum of $1,500.

In addition to the Nixon proposal, two other approaches were also debated in Congress. Senator Edward Kennedy (D-MA) along with a labor-promoted Committee of One Hundred for National Health Insurance advocated the most sweeping change. Their proposal included federal funding, comprehensive coverage, and the use of the federal government (rather than private insurance companies) in the administration of the new plan. For proponents, this step represented a logical extension of Medicare with its coverage of the elderly. A third alternative involved a variety of approaches to catastrophic insurance. This option had been periodically considered in earlier debates, and was advanced by Senator Russell Long (D-LA). The basic thrust of this approach was for individuals to be assisted with medical costs when they reached variously defined maximum expenditure levels in a given year.

In a pattern that would be repeated in 1993–94, the existence of three options all having some support made coalition building difficult. By the spring of 1974, two additional factors complicated the development of a compromise. The increasing preoccupation with Watergate drew attention away from health care reform on the part of not only the Nixon administration itself, but also Congress and the public. In addition, in a situation that reversed party positions two decades later, the Democrats began to sense that they would experience major congressional gains in the 1974 elections and became increasingly reluctant to compromise. These forces, along with the persistent difficulty of trying to get reform-minded legislators and interest groups to agree on one specific approach prevented possible action at a time in which concern for health care reform was high and the nation had not yet experienced the dual impacts of inflation and spiraling budget deficits that would reduce the prospect for fundamental change in the nation's health care system for a substantial time.

While Nixon was not in a position to decisively push his own health policy preferences during his first term, the 1973–74 period as seen by Starr (1982) did present an opportunity for a major step toward an ex-

panded federal health care role. This was an activist period, the public was generally supportive of an expanded federal role, and there was substantial interest in reform proposals on Capitol Hill. Although one cannot know if more decisive presidential leadership might have forced a compromise, it is clear that a beleaguered Nixon presidency by 1974 reduced chances for major new legislation.

Congress, on the other hand, did take one significant step in this direction, just as Nixon was leaving office. The enactment of the National Health Planning and Resources Development Act of 1974 represented an additional effort to restrain rapidly rising health care costs, and included a fairly elaborate system of required approvals for new equipment and new hospital construction. In this case, the ideas for policy design were drawn in part from early state-level efforts. Rather than being a catalyst for the program, however, the Nixon administration worked to reduce the scope of the new federal and state regulatory process.

This episode then demonstrates another important example in which major legislation has emerged with a president seeking to reduce the size of the program rather than using his political resources to build support for a larger federal effort.

President Ford (1974–77)

During his brief interlude in office, President Ford displayed quite dramatically the problems that can confront a president who is weak on virtually all of the components of political opportunity. In addition to the absence of the legitimation that comes from winning an election, Ford's popularity fell by some 17 percentage points in the wake of his pardon of Richard Nixon. His position was further weakened following the 1974 congressional elections, which saw the size of the Republican delegation fall to only 144 seats in the House and 37 seats in the Senate.

To make matters worse, there was a rapid increase in the costs of Medicare and Medicaid in the 1975–76 period, intensifying budgetary concerns. Economic conditions in general also deteriorated, as the country began in 1974 a period of heightened concern over an economy that was generating relatively high levels of both unemployment and inflation. In this context, President Ford withdrew references to national health insurance in his State of the Union Address in 1976.

President Carter (1977–81)

The Carter years also witnessed a lack of success in presidential efforts to achieve fundamental changes in major health policies. On the two related and highly visible issues of hospital cost control and expanded access through the adoption of one of the competing proposals for national health insurance, the Carter administration was unable to achieve congressional action.

Carter's lack of success occurred in the context of political opportunities that were quite limited. He had been elected by a 2 million vote majority, but he had not provided a sufficient focus on health policy to claim any sort of a mandate. While Democratic margins in Congress were high (292 House seats and 61 Senate seats), these figures were inflated by both conservative southern Democrats and those Democrats who had won on the basis of voter repudiation of Republicans after Watergate. Support for policy changes within the electorate was more uncertain in the face of economic uncertainties.

In the health field itself, spiraling costs were judged by some to be creating a problem of increasing magnitude. After the removal in 1974 of the hospital cost controls that Nixon had established three years earlier as part of an attempt to combat inflation, annual increases in hospital costs soared past 15 percent in the following two years. Yet at the same time, as viewed by Kingdon (1995), the policy area was still characterized by substantial disagreement on specific alternatives for reform. Public perceptions also reflected uncertainty. Although a slim majority favored some help for those without any health insurance, 62 percent favored keeping the existing system (Braverman, 1978).

Carter decided to resist making health care a top first-year issue as he placed his highest priority on a year-long but unsuccessful effort to enact a comprehensive new energy policy (Jones, 1988). Regarding health care policies, he took the position that enactment of effective cost controls must precede the enactment of a new federal program addressing the problems of those who lacked health insurance. In addition, he wanted to develop his own proposal.

Carter's fight for cost-control legislation was undertaken as a second-year strategy and with actions that included policy design, support building, and legislative-bargaining efforts. His secretary of health, education, and welfare, Joseph Califano, was instrumental in developing a proposal for controlling hospital costs. Carter, Califano, and Carter's legislative liaison team were quite extensively involved in the quest for legislative support. In addition, Carter also undertook an active effort to build public support, including speeches to special groups, talk show sessions, and references to this issue in major addresses. His skills in this effort were no more than average, and his public liaison efforts were somewhat below average. For Jones (1988), Carter's difficulties in generating public support stemmed in part from the extent to which large segments of the public were shielded by their health insurance from the direct costs of hospital price increases. In a more forceful manner than he had used with his major legislative initiative in 1977, Carter also made a number of direct appeals to key legislators in efforts to gain needed support for this legislation.

The net result, however, was that Congress rejected hospital cost control plans in both 1978 and 1979. These defeats included an original proposal that would have provided a cap on hospital costs in relationship to the consumer price index and a 1979 proposal that excluded nonprofessional wages from a more flexible cap (in an effort to win union support) and provisions designed to protect areas experiencing rapid population growth. The only immediate development was a hospital industry pledge to voluntarily constrain the annual rate of increase, which had been running at approximately 15 percent.

Carter was equally unsuccessful in the pursuit of a program of national health insurance. After delaying action in 1977, in his second year Carter only went as far as stating a set of guidelines rather than designing a specific proposal (Califano, 1981). As a result, Senator

Kennedy and his supporters then chose to go their own way, and developed a proposal that was in some respects a forerunner of the managed competition ideas found in President Clinton's proposal fifteen years later. This plan called for private health plans and HMOs to compete for subscribers, who would receive a health insurance card entitling them to hospital and physicians' care and a variety of other basic health services.

In retrospect, it seems unlikely that Carter missed a significant opportunity for fundamental change in health policy. Some were disappointed that he did not take a fast-start approach. To take that route, however, he would have had to either proceed with existing policy designs or work very quickly to develop an alternative approach. His lack of success with his energy policy initiative, which he did make a centerpiece of his first year (after rapidly seeking a new policy design), suggests that substantial difficulty would have occurred had he used a similar strategy in search of a fundamental change in the nation's health care system.

President Reagan (1981–89)

President Reagan came to office in 1981 with a ten-point victory margin over Carter and a surprising increase in Republican strength in Congress, which produced control of the Senate and an increase to 192 seats in the House. He had emphasized his economic policies of cutting taxes and domestic spending during the campaign, and was thus able to assert the existence of a voter mandate. He then moved quickly to implement a fast-start strategy with a combination of effective public appeals and a legislative effort that included extensive efforts to gain support from southern Democrats. The result was a presidency with "one big year" followed by markedly fewer efforts to develop new program initiatives (Peterson, 1990).

Although Reagan and his White House staff devoted far less attention to health policy issues than occurred with the passage of his economic program, a general concern over mounting health care costs among business leaders along with key members of Congress generated several significant efforts to modify health policies. These included the establishment of new Medicare cost control approaches for hospitals and physicians along with the establishment of additional Medicare coverage for the elderly.

The first of these, the change in hospital reimbursement within Medicare in 1983, produced another case of shared policymaking roles. In early 1982, Secretary of Health and Human Services Richard Schweiker indicated that a procompetition proposal would be forthcoming, but by the end of the year he was supporting a prospective payment plan.

The prospective payment approach that did emerge provided for hospital reimbursement on the basis of established reimbursement rates for 467 diagnosis-related groups (DRGs). This included an element of competition, since hospitals that were more efficient would be able to realize a greater profit. Rather than being paid on the basis of their charges for services rendered, hospitals would be paid a fixed amount for treating individuals in various DRG categories. By 1982, prospective payment systems had been used in a number of states, and in a few instances there were efforts to apply this system to private hospital charges as well as those being reimbursed through government programs. In Washington, the Health Care Financing Administration (HCFA) had developed an interest in this approach and had encouraged experiments using this system. This interest had been spawned in part by the difficulties policymakers had faced in the effort to develop effective cost controls after the defeat of Carter's efforts in 1978 and 1979. There was also interest in this approach in Congress, as manifested by a requirement that HCFA report to Congress on their analyses of prospective payment systems.

The shift to DRGs for Medicare came with several roles being carried out by the Reagan administration, but also included major legislative action. The policy design itself borrowed heavily from state experiences as well as analyses undertaken by HCFA. The most important role, however, was undertaken by Secretary Schweiker (Green, 1992). There were no presidential addresses on hospital cost containment or significant references to it in any of Reagan's major speeches. As the measure moved to Congress, the Reagan administration played a more important role. For instance, their willingness to confront the opposition of the American Medical Association (AMA) and its (well-founded) fear that the system would subsequently be expanded to include physicians was a supporting influence with some members of Congress. At the same time, the president's adamant opposition to proposals that would expand the same system beyond Medicare reduced possible development of a broader system. In addition, the emphasis on the importance of the need for quick action to address rising Medicare costs contributed to the congressional desire to act quickly (Demkovich, 1983).

In the implementation stage the Reagan administration also resisted efforts by the hospital industry to achieve a delay in the implementation of the new program. Public and legislative support building was essentially unnecessary in this situation, since Democratic legislators were inclined to be supportive and the word went out to Republicans that this was an important measure to support. As a result, a program that was characterized by Demkovich (1983) as "the most significant change in Medicare in seventeen years" fundamentally altered the manner in which hospitals were reimbursed by Medicare.

In contrast to Reagan's public silence on the hospital reimbursement issue, the establishment of the Medicare Catastrophic Coverage Act (MCCA) did include an initial public role. Beginning in 1983, catastrophic insurance received a brief but recurrent inclusion in each of the president's State of the Union Addresses. Rather than promoting a system of catastrophic insurance for all Americans as had periodically been advocated, however, Reagan chose to focus only on some of the limitations in hospital coverage for the elderly under Medicare. Nonetheless, with his periodic references to catastrophic health care costs, Reagan helped create a political environment that was conducive to some form of legislative action.

Whether intentional or not, Reagan's selection of Otis Bowen as his secretary of health and human services in 1985 constituted a crucial step in the ultimate development of MCCA. Bowen was an Indiana physician and former governor who was strongly committed to catastrophic insurance in part because of personal experiences. Bowen affirmed a strong interest in catastrophic insurance at his confirmation hearings and began to develop a proposal once he assumed office.

As the Reagan administration was debating its final proposal in late 1986, Republican as well as Democratic members of the House Energy and Commerce Committee were sending word to the president that they were about ready to act whether the White House submitted the Bowen proposal or not. Reagan's subsequent endorsement was an important step in its signaling of presidential support, but it did not represent the seizing of an initiative that would otherwise have remained dormant in Congress as of early 1987.

In the development of the design for catastrophic insurance that finally emerged, significant roles were performed within both the Reagan administration and Congress. In the effort to build support for this bill, Reagan used a radio address on February 14, 1988, to express his support. Congressional action in turn broadened the bill beyond Reagan's initial proposal. Yet at the same time, his adamant opposition to and threatened veto of a final bill that would have included a major long-term care benefit or financing that was not based upon higher premium payments by those enrolled in Medicare served to dampen legislative support for a broader piece of legislation. In the actual process of negotiation that occurred to produce the final bill, the key interaction took place between committee chairs in the House and Senate. Congressman Henry Waxman (D-CA) played a particularly important role in the process. Intense conflict emerged, for example, as the Pharmaceutical Manufacturers Association fought tentative provisions in a prescription drug benefit that would have increased Medicare funding for generic drugs rather than the more expensive brand-name products. Representatives of the elderly, led by the American Association of Retired Persons, also provided a strong lobbying role in supporting a program that went beyond the president's original proposal.

Although the final bill did go beyond the administration's original proposal by including provisions for prescription drug reimbursement and a minor amount of nursing home assistance, Reagan was successful in his insistence that the program be self-financing. In sum, congressional as well as presidential actions were clearly important in shaping this Medicare expansion.

In 1988, Congress also took the action that AMA leaders had feared in the debate over Medicare hospital reimbursement and established a system of reimbursement for physicians. The impetus for this plan was also from Congress rather than the Reagan administration. The new approach was based on complex formulas, with the general objective of increasing reimbursement for general practitioners and reducing reimbursement for specialists.

Health policy development in the Reagan years did not produce instances of health policy leadership comparable to his bold actions on economic policy in 1981. Both the dominant public concerns in 1981 and Reagan's campaign emphasis largely dictated a focus on economic policy rather than major health policy changes. It seems likely that Reagan would have confronted major difficulties had he attempted to promote a more radical change toward market-oriented reforms. Political resistance to such approaches as vouchers for Medicare would in all likelihood have doomed such an effort. At most, an effort to address health reform issues more broadly from a conservative perspective would have generated some additional interest in those options. Overall, this was a period in which Congress as well as the presidency were involved in shaping policies with motivations that were driven in considerable part by the constant rise in federal health care spending.

President Bush (1989–93)

In contrast to Reagan's situation in 1981, Bush entered the presidency in 1989 with a lengthy list of limitations. He had raised few domestic issues in the campaign, and he faced Democratic majorities in both houses of Congress. While he enjoyed relatively high popularity, this was not tied to specific domestic policy goals. In addition, he was constrained by the size of the deficit and his "no new taxes" pledge.

Perhaps the most unusual development during the Bush presidency was Congress's unprecedented repeal of the Catastrophic Coverage Act only one year after its adoption. This occurred in response to a protest in 1989 primarily on the part of higher-income elderly recipients of Medicare, who concluded that the combination of premiums and benefits in the modified program was inferior to what they could obtain through private "medigap" policies. The only position taken by President Bush was on the question of how changes in the law would affect deficit calculations in relationship to the Gramm–Rudman requirements, which mandated significant reductions in the deficit each year. The ultimate result of that conflict was that Congress did respond to the lobbying effort on the part of segments of the elderly population and rescinded MCCA.

Interest in health policy reform increased dramatically in 1991 and 1992 due to continuing increases in health costs coupled with increases in the portion of the electorate lacking health insurance. The dramatic triggering event was Democrat Harris Wofford's stunning upset of former governor Richard Thornburgh in a special U.S. Senate election in Pennsylvania to fill the seat of Republican Senator John Heinz, who had been killed in an airplane crash. The relatively unknown Wofford focused on the need for health care reform to defeat Thornburgh,who had resigned his position as attorney general,in the Bush administration to seek the Senate seat.

In the House, efforts were unsuccessfully undertaken by Democratic Party leaders to develop consensus around a specific approach to reform. The Bush administration also sought to at least show that the president was addressing health care concerns by submitting the broad outlines of a plan in 1992. Richard Darman, the head of the Office of Management and Budget, was the primary author of that proposal, and acted so hastily that initial copies of the proposed budget had to be withheld so that revisions sought by key Republican members of Congress could be included. The final proposal left numerous specifics to be resolved, and received scant attention from a Democratically controlled Congress in which many preferred a larger effort; moreover, electoral concerns mitigated against any effort to rally behind the initial Bush proposal.

Given his limited opportunity level, Bush was in a poor position to promote major changes in health policy. At the same time, his reluctance to become involved with public roles and hesitancy in carrying out some of his relationships with Congress increased the extent to which Congress shaped health policy developments while he occupied the White House.

President Clinton (1993–)

During his first two years in office, Clinton was able to generate a national focus on health care reform that was at least as extensive as any domestic policy debate the nation has experienced in several decades. While clearly warranting high marks as an issue raiser, Clinton nonetheless came away empty-handed after a two-year effort. As with the earlier case studies, it is helpful to examine this outcome in the context of opportunity levels and leadership roles.

Opportunity Level

Clinton's opportunity level during his first two years was higher than that for a number of his predecessors, but nonetheless contained major weaknesses. Clinton had won by a 5 percentage point margin over Bush, but had received only 43 percent of the total vote; Democratic gains in Congress were very minimal. While these numbers included fewer conservative southern Democrats than in earlier decades, the size of the party's legislative majorities was substantially lower than that enjoyed by either Johnson or Carter and somewhat below that of Kennedy.

Several other legislative factors were also involved. Clinton faced a Congress that had become increasingly partisan. After being out of power for twelve years, Democrats in 1993 had a fairly strong sense of importance attached to their being able to show that the Democratic Party could successfully address major issues. While this had the potential for creating a high level of Democratic support, it also intensified the question of how much support might be forthcoming from Republicans (Pfiffner, 1994).

Several other factors also limited Clinton's opportunities. In terms of popularity during his first two years

in office, his average ratings were the lowest of any president since Truman, and his figure after three months in office was the lowest on record for a newly elected president. At the same time, voter lack of trust in government was unusually high. Whereas responses to the question "Do you trust the government in Washington to do the right thing most of the time?" found over 70 percent agreeing in 1964, only 22 percent gave that response in 1993 (Phillips, 1994).

Clinton was also handicapped by the size of the deficit he had inherited. In 1992, the recession had swollen the deficit to over 21 percent of total spending, the largest fiscal burden any newly elected postwar president has had to confront. The magnitude of the deficit and the promotion of deficit concern by various political figures, including independent candidate Ross Perot, created an opportunity for deficit reduction that Clinton seized as a major first-year commitment (Woodward, 1994; Drew, 1994). That deficit reduction commitment nonetheless had two major constraining impacts on Clinton's opportunity for achieving health care reform. The allocation of time and political resources to deficit reduction limited the effort that could be devoted to health reform. Moreover, the inclusion of new taxes in the deficit reduction package virtually eliminated prospects for including additional taxes to support health care reform. For example, legislative leaders such as House Ways and Means Chairman Daniel Rostenkowski (D-IL) had made congressional opposition to additional taxes very clear by July 1993.

Clinton's opportunity level was also influenced by two other factors. A clear majority of Americans indicated to pollsters in the spring of 1993 that the health care system needed to be substantially rebuilt. As subsequent polling and events would indicate, however, that preference for rebuilding in many instances only went as far as reducing costs and insuring portability of insurance coverage (Skocpol, 1995). In addition, as emphasized by Kingdon (1995), there was still widespread disagreement among both policymakers and the general public regarding the specific reforms that should be undertaken. As the policy struggles from at least the early 1970s have revealed, an inability to coalesce those who desire change around one specific proposal has proven to be a crucial stumbling block in the efforts to achieve fundamental reform of the nation's health care system.

Policy Design

In the face of this situation, the strategy Clinton pursued was that of an attempted fast start coupled with a major effort to produce a new policy design. The decision to develop a new policy design stemmed from several sources. In part, public opinion polls were judged to be highly encouraging. There were also forceful arguments being made to the effect that because of the interrelatedness of the health care system, incremental change would not be sufficient. Such an argument was being made, for example, as a reason for not proceeding with an expansion of Medicare to cover additional groups (Starr, 1993).

Clinton, in turn, rejected at the outset an effort to proceed with a Canadian-style single-payer system. He concluded that the public would not be willing to accept the large increase in taxes necessary for a federally financed health care system even though their payments for private insurance coverage would be eliminated. As viewed by Marmor (1994), one of the consequences of that decision was that the policy design process was oriented toward the development of new institutional arrangements that were more complex than those that a direct switch to federal financing would have entailed.

At the outset of his planning process, Clinton was favorably inclined toward the concept of managed competition as that plan had emerged from a series of discussions held over a period of several years among health policy experts, practitioners, and health insurance company leaders under the leadership of Paul Ellwood in Jackson Hole, Wyoming. There was also interest in the ideas that had been developed by California's commissioner of insurance, John Garamendi.

The specific process Clinton used in developing his proposal was to have First Lady Hillary Rodham Clinton undertake the leadership of a Health Care Task Force and Ira Magaziner, a business consultant and long-time friend, direct its planning process. The task force was expected to produce a report within three months to enable Clinton to meet his campaign promise of submitting a health reform proposal within one hundred days of his inauguration.

The task force was comprised of some five hundred individuals drawn primarily from congressional staffs and federal agencies, along with consultants from the private sector. These individuals were organized into thirty-four working groups and were asked to work their way through an elaborate series of some 840 decision points (called "gates") in a process Magaziner had utilized in the private sector when elaborate plans were to be developed in a short period of time. These groups would work at a frenetic pace. Their meetings would run well into the evening in their effort to complete their deliberations by early May.

Along with the efforts to weigh the merits of specific components to be included in a revised system, political feasibility considerations were given significant attention. This included, first of all, polling conducted by Clinton's primary pollster, Stanley Greenberg (Woodward, 1994). Political considerations were also involved in the effort to structure components of the plan in ways that would make it politically attractive. This was a period in which the strategy as viewed by Starr (1995) was one of attempting to make the proposal as attractive as possible to those groups and legislators who would have preferred a presidential commitment to a single-payer system. Various components of the plan that sought to attract the support of particular groups included the scope of benefits for the elderly, assistance for corporations in the financing of health benefits for their early retirees, subsidies for small businesses to reduce the size of their mandated benefits, and opportunities for individual states to experiment with a single-payer system.

There was also a variety of interactions with interest groups, including by both mail and fax. Moreover, with the inevitable Washington process of news leaks (both intended as well as inadvertent), additional communication of preferences was achieved. Although there was no formal representation of interest groups on the task force working groups, there were a substantial number of meetings with them. A memoranda prepared for Ira

Magaziner by Barbara Woolley et al. (1993), for instance, lists over five hundred meetings with various health and consumer groups. As assessed by Skocpol (1995), these tended to involve opportunities for expressing concerns and preferences rather than actual bargaining sessions.

The final aspect of concern with political feasibility involved interactions with members of Congress. With the inclusion of a large number of legislative staff members in the planning process, one level of information flow was established. This tended, however, to be quite compartmentalized. During the spring and in subsequent months, both Magaziner and the First Lady also engaged in an extensive series of meetings with key health policy leaders in Congress. As summarized by Woolley et al. (1993), this included visits with 65 senators, and 156 members of the House. The most extensive interaction occurred in meetings with Representative Henry Waxman (D-CA), who had four visits from the First Lady, three visits from Magaziner, and two visits from other staff members. While consultation was clearly extensive, many of these visits were primarily designed to convey information.

Approximately five months elapsed between the time the working groups concluded their deliberations in May and the full 1,346-page proposal was delivered to Capitol Hill on October 27, 1993. During that time, deliberations were undertaken that included cabinet and staff members who were concerned about the size and complexity of the proposal. As a result, substantial modifications were made to the original proposal (Starr, 1995). Steps were also taken to have additional reviews of the proposal by outside experts, and to have the revenue aspects of the plan subjected to additional analysis.

In addition to the time spent in directly debating and modifying the proposal, the lapse of time was also a result of other factors, including the primary focus of Clinton and top aides on the deficit reduction package, a desire not to have two major initiatives competing for attention, and (in October) the president's primary focus on American policies for Somalia in the wake of the killing of eighteen American soldiers (Woodward, 1994).

The plan that emerged called for a standard benefit package as well as the formation of health purchasing alliances to control future costs by creating additional competition and provisions for the possible use of price controls if target figures for cost control were not being achieved. The financing component relied primarily on future savings in federal health programs (particularly Medicare) along with employer mandates to expand private-sector spending.

Public Support Building

The effort to build support for the Health Security Act began with a major and quite successful presidential address to Congress and the nation in September 1993. In his speech the president laid out his major themes while stressing universal coverage as the most crucial requirement. Press commentary was quite favorable, and opinion polls showed an increase in support from 43 percent to 55 percent (Keen, 1993). Clinton's knowledge of his proposal (which allowed some necessary ad libbing due to a TelePrompTer error) and ability to empathize with the problems people were having with the present health care system were clearly assets.

Despite the president's successful initial speech, the Clinton administration clearly lost the ensuing battle for public opinion. The resulting decline in public support for the Clinton plan as the debate continued was dramatic. According to one major poll, support for his proposal dropped from 58 percent in September 1993 to only 37 percent by July 1994 (Yankelvich, 1995). Another clear indication of the unsuccessful promotion of the plan is the finding that the number of people who told pollsters that they felt they understood the Clinton plan was never more than 20 percent. That figure went down rather than up as the public debate continued (Yankelvich, 1995).

A number of accounts of Clinton's handling of his campaign for public support have been quite critical (Yankelvich, 1995; Peterson, 1995). He has been criticized for: (1) trying to proceed with slogans rather than a serious educational campaign; (2) being unable to mount a televised campaign that compared with the highly effective "Harry and Louise" commercials aired by the Health Insurance Association of America;[2] and (3) not having a sufficient focus on the extent to which middle-class Americans were looking in very personal ways for indications that the president's proposals would improve their specific situation. As viewed by Skocpol (1995), the crucial loss occurred during the final three months of 1993.

Critics in this instance may be imposing overly high standards regarding the extent to which an effective dialogue could have been created. Nonetheless, two points are relevant in interpreting Clinton's situation. First, his proposal was difficult to explain in simple terms and invited attack because of its complexity. Second, he was attempting to promote a major and complex new plan at a time when many voters regarded him with suspicion.

Legislative Relations

The most immediate cause for the defeat of health reform in 1994 was the inability of the major committees to report out compromise legislation that had a chance of carrying majority support in each house. Among the powerful committee chairmen who were unable to steer the legislation through their committees was Congressman John Dingell (D-MI), who had hoped that he would be able to finally achieve the goal his father had sought starting in 1943 with his House sponsorship of a system of national health insurance.

The deadlocks that occurred at the committee stage stemmed from several sources. Declining public support was obviously one key dimension, and may well have been decisive. A second factor, however, was that in the various compromise plans that did not include an employer mandate, the analyses of cost projections by the Congressional Budget Office were extremely sobering to would-be promoters (Starr, 1995). A third influence was the emergence among some Republicans of the (ultimately very correct) view that they could at once defeat health care reform and also profit as a party in the midterm elections.

An Opportunity Lost?

In the end, Clinton proved unable to gain approval of even a limited new policy step. To evaluate Clinton's record, it is important to consider both his opportunity level and his leadership approach.

President Clinton was obviously in a far less promising position to pass landmark social legislation than Roosevelt in 1935 and Johnson in 1965. The case studies have also repeatedly shown that presidents with moderate or lower opportunity levels have not been able to achieve success with landmark new health policy initiatives that involve high stakes for major interests. Limitations in Clinton's electoral and congressional support can certainly be used to argue that he did not miss an opportunity to create the single-payer system some have long supported. In retrospect, the plan Clinton sought to enact was simply too ambitious for a president in his position.

While it is always easier to see problems in presidential strategies after they have been tried, it is useful to compare Clinton's approach in 1993 to the actions of several other presidents. In considering the proposal itself, a frequent criticism has focused on the proposal's complexity and length (Drew, 1994). Although it is startling to recall that the Social Security Act required thirty-two pages in comparison to the proposed Health Security Act's 1,342 pages, the issue of length needs to be put into perspective. In the 1990s, lengthy legislative proposals are not that uncommon. Rival health proposals were also in excess of one thousand pages. Moreover, both the North American Free Trade Agreement and the crime bills, which were successfully passed, were of comparable length (Pfiffner, 1994).

The sense of complexity in the Health Security Act was not simply a reflection of its length, but rather the number of new institutional arrangements that were being proposed. Comparisons with two other efforts at landmark change in social policy illustrate the difficult challenge the Clinton health policy design created.

---

[2]These television commercials featured a husband and wife discussing Clinton's health plan in ways that cast doubt on its merits for average Americans.

When Roosevelt chose the insurance model as part of the Social Security design in 1935, one of his important concerns was that he wanted to be able to explain his new system by using examples that were part of the experiences of many Americans (Perkins, 1946). When Medicare was created in 1965, it built upon the existing and popular Social Security system for financing while avoiding changes in doctor–patient relationships and maintaining existing insurance company roles as intermediaries. Although there were substantial cost-control limitations with the Medicare program when it was adopted, that approach did enhance prospects for legislative success. By proposing new institutional arrangements without obvious parallels with which the public and members of Congress were familiar, the task force produced a plan that would prove highly vulnerable to attack by its opponents.

To put Clinton's early planning process in perspective, it was clearly undertaken with greater attention to political feasibility than occurred with Carter's planning process on energy policy in early 1977 (Kerbel, 1991). At the same time, it did not reach the level of negotiation and support building among key groups that occurred in the formation of successful new proposals such as Roosevelt's interaction with a wide variety of groups and legislators in 1933 (Freidel, 1973) or Johnson's actions on several of the programs that were adopted as part of his Great Society in 1964–65.

The design process President Clinton employed worked in combination with his own uncertainty in shaping his first-year agenda to produce a damaging delay in his ability to engage Congress in deliberations over his proposal. In a major *New York Times* summary article, Clymer et al. (1994) viewed the loss of time as a serious handicap. Similarly, Starr (1995) also stressed the issue of timing, arguing that there was a window of opportunity in 1993 that closed quite quickly.

One can obviously not know for sure whether other strategies and levels of skill would have been successful in achieving at least some degree of policy change. The strategy that President Clinton pursued was a difficult one, however, in that he undertook the development of a new policy design and chose a proposal that was sweeping in scope and difficult to explain to the American public. For multiple reasons, he was then unable to deliver a specific proposal to Congress until October 27, 1993. Proceeding in this manner, Clinton did not lose an opportunity to profoundly transform the health care system, but he did reduce his chances for achieving some degree of change. By completely retreating from health care reform issues after September 1994, he contributed to a marginalizing of his own role in the 104th Congress.

LESSONS AND IMPLICATIONS

Presidential actions surrounding major health policy changes suggest important lessons and conclusions regarding both past performances and future leadership prospects. Despite the sobering impact of Clinton's experiences, there are also indications of numerous ways in which future presidents may contribute to the evolution of the nation's health policies.

One major lesson from these cases is that successful presidential leadership in achieving landmark changes in health policies can occur only when a convergence of political opportunity, political skill, and commitment occurs. Opportunities were uniquely abundant for Johnson in 1965, and he effectively handled his legislative role. Presidents Truman, Kennedy, and Carter might have promoted their proposals with greater skill, but were fundamentally thwarted by their level of opportunity. During Nixon's second term there may have been an opportunity for major change, but his faltering presidency and limited skill in dealing with Congress ended reform prospects. Clinton enjoyed a uniquely high level of public interest in health care reform, but failed in part because of other weaknesses in his level of opportunity.

The second lesson from the case studies is that instances of major policy adoption have occurred with a sharing of roles and influence between presidents and Congress. The passage of the Hill–Burton Act was the clearest case in which issue raising, policy design efforts, and negotiations with interest groups occurred with very peripheral presidential involvement. In some instances, however, presidents have made efforts to reduce the scope of final legislation an important part of their effort to shape new legislation. As illustrated by Nixon's role with HMO legislation and Reagan's role with the expansion of Medicare to include catastrophic care, however, the effort to constrain the size of the final legislation came after some initial policy design and issue-raising activity.

From a presidential perspective, none of the cases shows a dominance of all aspects of the policy cycle or an ability to simply force a president's program on Congress. Johnson was in the strongest position to deal with health policy issues in 1965, and yet it was unexpected steps by Wilbur Mills that expanded the president's Medicare proposal while also adding the Medicaid component. Conversely, in his effort to establish regional health care centers Johnson played a strong role in generating initial interest and in developing a specific proposal, but nonetheless found it necessary to make major concessions in order to have the proposal enacted.

The results of the case studies also have important implications for future efforts to modify health policies. Presidents clearly have a wide variety of policymaking roles they can choose from, including their capacity to raise issues and to focus congressional attention on a particular policy issue by submitting an initial proposal. Implementation roles, as in the past, are also likely to have major significance. Support-building efforts will continue to find presidents facing stiff competition from interest groups, but they also have significant resources for promoting public support. In bargaining processes, top-level negotiation between presidential aides and legislative leaders is also likely to be an important option.

In the not too distant future, another president may well seek to implement a fast-start strategy. On the basis of Clinton's experience and the actions by presidents who have been successful with this approach, a president is likely to increase his chances of success if he: (1) tries to build on existing policy designs rather than attempting to quickly develop an entirely new approach, and (2) engages in a substantial amount of early negotiation with interest group leaders. The results of a hasty effort may well require major subsequent modifications and leave important decisions to be made as policies are implemented. Nonetheless, in a political system in which

major changes are difficult to achieve, an effective fast-start strategy can increase a president's level of influence.

The skills presidents possess and the strategies they pursue can clearly make a difference in the evolution of health policy. At the same time, the emphasis on shared roles suggests that a wide variety of actions will affect future policy developments. Along with congressional actions, that list of important influences includes such factors as: (1) the quality of the public debate that takes place on various issues such as the appropriate allocation of resources among various age groups and disease categories; (2) the extent and effectiveness of various innovations that are attempted by federal and state governments as well as private-sector organizations; and (3) the extent to which interest group activities and electoral politics create potential support for new policy commitments. Future presidents will differ in the skill with which they maximize their opportunities, but a broad range of factors will shape their potential for providing effective leadership.

REFERENCES

Ambrose, Stephen E. (1984). *Eisenhower the president.* New York: Simon & Schuster.

Bond, Jon R., & Richard Fleisher. (1990). *The president in the legislative arena.* Chicago: University of Chicago Press.

Braverman, Jordan. (1978). *Crisis in health care.* Washington, D.C.: Acropolis Books, Ltd.

Brown, Lawrence D. (1983). *Politics and health care organizations: HMOs as federal policy.* Washington, D.C.: The Brookings Institution.

Califano, Joseph A., Jr. (1981). *Governing America.* New York: Simon & Schuster.

Clymer, Adam, et al. (1994). For health care, time was a killer. *New York Times* (August 29), A1.

Congressional Quarterly Almanac. (Select years). Washington, D.C.: Congressional Quarterly.

David, Sheri I. (1995). *With dignity: The search for Medicare and Medicaid.* Westport, CT: Greenwood Press.

Davidson, Roger H. (1992). *The post-reform Congress.* New York: St. Martin's Press.

Demkovich, Linda. (1983). Who says Congress can't move fast? Just ask hospitals about Medicare. *National Journal* (April 2), 704–707.

Drew, Elizabeth. (1994). *On the edge: The Clinton presidency.* New York: Simon & Schuster.

Edwards, George C. (1989). *At the margins: Presidential leadership of Congress.* New Haven: Yale University Press.

Falkson, Joseph L. (1980). *HMOs and the politics of health system reform.* Chicago: American Hospital Association and Robert J. Brady Co.

Freidel, Frank. (1973). *Franklin D. Roosevelt: The launching of the New Deal.* Boston: Little, Brown.

Freidel, Frank. (1990). *Franklin D. Roosevelt: A rendevouz with destiny.* Boston: Little, Brown.

Green, David S. (1992). *Paying for Medicare: The politics of reform.* New York: Aldine de Gruyter.

Jones, Charles O. (1988). *The trusteeship presidency: Jimmy Carter and the U.S. Congress.* Baton Rouge: Louisiana State University Press.

Jones, Charles O. (1995). *Separate but equal branches: Congress and the presidency.* Chatham, NJ: Chatham House Publishers, Inc.

Keen, Judy. (1993). Health plan gets thumbs-up. *USA Today* (September 27), A1.

Kerbel, Matthew R. (1991). *Beyond persuasion: Organizational efficiency and presidential power.* Albany: State University of New York Press.

Kernell, Samuel. (1986). *Going public: New strategies of presidential leadership.* Washington, D.C.: CQ Press.

Kingdon, John. W. (1995). *Agendas, alternatives, and public policies.* New York: HarperCollins.

Light, Paul C. (1982). *The president's agenda: Domestic policy choice from Kennedy to Carter.* Baltimore: Johns Hopkins University Press.

Light, Paul C. (1985). *Artful work: The politics of Social Security reform.* New York: Random House.

Light, Paul C. (1988). The focusing skill and presidential influence in Congress. In Christopher Deering (Ed.), *Congressional politics* (pp. 239–261). Chicago: The Dorsey Press.

Manatos, Michael. (1964). Memo to Lyndon Johnson, dated November 17, 1994. Manatos papers, November 1994 folder. Johnson Presidential Library.

Marmor, Theodore R. (1973). *The politics of Medicare.* New York: Aldine Publishing Co.

Marmor, Theodore R. (1994). *A citizen's guide to the health reform debate.* Paper prepared for delivery at the 1994 annual meeting of the American Political Science Association, New York, September 1–4.

Mayhew, David R. (1991). *Divided we govern: Party control, lawmaking, and investigations, 1946–1990.* New Haven: Yale University Press.

Michaelson, Melissa R. (1994). *The effect of public approval on presidential power.* Paper prepared for delivery at the 1994 annual meeting of the American Political Science Association, New York, September 1–4.

Parmet, Herbert S. (1983). *J.F.K.: The presidency of John F. Kennedy.* New York: Dial Press.

Perkins, Frances. (1946). *The Roosevelt I knew.* New York: The Viking Press.

Peterson, Mark A. (1990). *Legislating together: The White House and Capitol Hill from Eisenhower to Reagan.* Cambridge: Harvard University Press.

Peterson, Mark A. (1995). The health care debate: All heat and no light. *Journal of Health Politics, Policy and Law, 20* (2), 425–430.

Pfiffner, James P. (1994). *President Clinton and the 103rd Congress: Winning battles and losing wars.* Fairfax, VA: The Institute of Public Policy, George Mason University.

Phillips, Kevin. (1993). *Boiling point: Republicans, Democrats, and the decline of middle-class prosperity.* New York: Random House.

Poen, Monte E. (1979). *Harry S. Truman versus the medical lobby: The genesis of Medicare.* Columbia: University of Missouri Press.

Quadagno, Jill. (1994). *The color of welfare.* New York: Oxford University Press.

Skocpol, Theda. (1995). The rise and demise of the Clinton plan. *Health Affairs, 14* (Spring), 66–85.

Starr, Paul. (1982). *The social transformation of American medicine.* New York: Basic Books.

Starr, Paul. (1993). Why not Medicare for all? Here's why. Advisory memo dated March 25, 1993. Starr file, Box 2180, Clinton White House Interdepartmental Working Group. College Park, MD: U.S. Archives.

Starr, Paul. (1995). What happened to health care reform? *American Prospect, 20,* 21–31.

Stevens, Robert, & Rosemary Stevens. (1974). *Welfare medicine in America: A case study of Medicaid.* New York: The Free Press.

Stockman, David A. (1986). *The triumph of politics: Why the Reagan revolution failed.* New York: Harper & Row.

Walcott, Charles E., & Karen M. Hult. (1995). *Governing the White House from Hoover through LBJ.* Lawrence: University of Kansas Press.

Witte, Edwin. (1963). *The development of the Social Security Act.* Madison: University of Wisconsin Press.

Wolanin, Thomas F. (1975). *Presidential advisory commissions: Truman to Nixon.* Madison: University of Wisconsin Press.

Woodward, Bob. (1994). *The agenda: Inside the Clinton White House.* New York: Simon & Schuster.

Woolley, Barbara, et al. (1993). Memo to Ira Magaziner, April 21. List of Interest Groups/Consumer Meetings. Richard Brown file, Box 1792.

Yankelvich, Daniel. (1995). The debate that wasn't: the public and the Clinton plan. *Health Affairs, 14* (Spring), 7–23.

CHAPTER

Congress and Health Policy: "Dynamics without Change?"

David Falcone and Lynn Hartwig

In 1976, Robert Alford coined the phrase "dynamics without change" to describe action in U.S. health policy. It is fitting that the book in which he expressed this view won the Woodrow Wilson Award. The political scientist Wilson would not have been at all surprised by Alford's observation. In *Congressional Government* (1956), Wilson described a legislative process designed to maintain a nightwatchman state. In the early 1950s, E. E. Schattschneider (1956) and others (Dahl, 1966) revitalized Wilson's call for a reformation of the legislative process.

From the perspective of health policy, recent sentiment for congressional reform—at least intensified disgruntlement with the status quo—has been one by-product of the failure of health care reform in the 103rd Congress (1993–94). But, dissatisfaction with Congress's role in health policy had been building for some time; in fact, the Renewing Congress Project, a joint undertaking of The Brookings Institution and the American Enterprise Institute, was begun in 1992 to "respond constructively" to critiques of Congress (Mann & Ornstein, 1995). Of course, Congress is only one

This chapter was completed shortly before the senior author's untimely death at the age of fifty-one. David Falcone was a major figure in the field of health politics, having served as book review editor of the *Journal of Health Politics, Policy and Law* for many years while he was at Duke University, where he was instrumental in persuading the university to become the journal's official sponsor. His contributions to the field were many, the

least of which was his agreeing to prepare a chapter on the role of Congress in health policy for each of the three editions of this book. That he did so this final time in spite of his illness is a reflection of his dedication and commitment to the field. He will be deeply missed. So, too, will his long-time collaborator, Lynn Hartwig, who also passed away a few months later. We mourn both of their untimely losses.

135

component of the institutional nexus of health policy-making, but it is the focal point for translation of what is perceived to be public demand into public policy.

This chapter examines the relationship between the congressional process and health policy in the post–Medicare and Medicaid era. In so doing, we show that changes in congressional procedures and structures in the 1970s did little to further progress begun by Medicare and Medicaid toward national health insurance (NHI). In fact, variations in congressional structure and process may have been less consequential than other factors affecting the pace and direction of health policy. The same observation can be made about the 1980s. And, despite a spate of "Congress bashing" over the past few years, the failure of health care reform in 1993–94 may not be directly attributable to congressional variables. There is no doubt that "congressional government" frustrates architectonic, that is, nonincremental health policy reforms. However, other causes of policy stasis have to be taken seriously and should quell enthusiasm for fundamental, constitutional change as a recipe for health policy reform (or, for that matter, reform in any other policy area). Furthermore, the productivity of the 104th Congress may dispel, at least for a time, cynicism about the role of congressional change in policy change.

Before addressing the issues of procedural change and policy change, some definitional underbrush should be cleared. First, when we talk about congressional health policy, we mean legislative decisions directly affecting principal actors and institutions in their roles in the health field. Several identifiable legislative structures that deal with bills that directly affect the organization, delivery, and financing of health services can be identified. There is, however, little to distinguish the politics of health legislation other than this structural differentiation in Congress, whereby responsibilities are assigned for health issues, and the particular "concentration of interests" that characterizes pressure group demands in the health policy arena (Falcone et al., 1994).

Second, we contend that the legislative process with regard to health issues is not immune to the factors that have affected all policy areas over the past thirty years. In her book, *Stability and Change in Congress*, Barbara Hinckley (1983) asked "what is the effect, if any, of congressional variations on environmental policy, or education or any other policy area?" She is not the only observer of legislative behavior who has asked this type of question. A highly controversial body of literature has challenged the traditional political science view that places significance on procedural reform (Dye, 1980). The studies making up this literature—referred to, among other labels, as "determinants analyses"—have at least forced people to consider, in qualitative as well as quantitative terms, whether the variations in structure and process that have been the foci of reform efforts, such as the professionalization and institutionalization of state legislatures, have been merely coincidental with, rather than causes of, policy change.

In this chapter, after discussing what we mean by health policy, we delineate the major modern reforms in congressional procedures, most of which occurred in the 1970s, assess their impact on legislative decision making in health, and examine the question of whether these changes have made any significant difference in health policy. Procedurally, we note that the influence of the general budgetary policy process has grown in importance relative to the specific health policy process. We hypothesize that disjointed incrementalism (which we use interchangeably with the term "decrementalism")[1] remains an appropriate description of the health policy process even if more rationalistic "models" now may better fit the budgetary process. The disjointed

---

[1]"Disjointed incrementalism" refers to the tendency for policy changes to be marginal from year to year for a variety of reasons, among which are the necessity for compromise built into the structures of decision making in a modern polity; the attractiveness of a relatively certain past in an environment where predications are unreliable; and the fact that ideological constraint among decision makers is low and "satisficing" outputs are acceptable (Simon, 1955). This modern notion popularized by Lindblom (1969, 1992) has its roots at least as far back as Adolf Wagoner's law of expanding state expenditure (Wagoner, 1964), where government expenditure as a function of gross domestic expenditure was viewed as a linear function of gross domestic product per capita. The direction of government expenditure was incremental as long as GDP was expanding. When it is not, or not at a pace sufficient to cover increasing government expenditures, then "decrementalism" is a more appropriate description of what Dahl, Lindblom, et al. initially envisioned.

incrementalism description is reinforced by the failure of health reform in 1993–94.

Substantively, the general conclusion reached is that it is nearly impossible to ascribe policy developments, or the lack of them, in the health field to variations in the structure and process of congressional decision making. This is not to say that congressional reforms have been insignificant, only that changes in both policy and procedure may also spring from, among other sources, economic and, perhaps consequently, ideological variables, from the substance and style of the presidency, from "rational" evaluations of the efficacy, efficiency, and effectiveness of past policies, and from a residual category of situational factors that have characterized reform efforts.

HEALTH POLICY

Several types of policy directly affect or seek to affect health. Those that come readily to mind are primarily legislative, but they also include judicial and executive decisions. Specific subjects include the rates of production, geographic and specialty distribution of health personnel, health care financing, assurance of the quality of health personnel, institutions, and services, occupational safety and environmental protection, and attempts to limit consumption of destructive substances such as alcohol, tobacco, and synthetic carcinogens. In some instances, the indirect effects on health of housing, income maintenance, or other welfare policies may be even more consequential than the direct effects of policies that patently deal with health (Falcone et al., 1994; Feldstein, 1993). Nevertheless, it is useful to limit the conception of health policy to the conventional notion of public decisions that seek primarily to affect health or principal actors, both professional and institutional, in their roles in the health arena. Using this restriction allows statements to be made, such as the one posited above, that some other policies may ultimately have a more telling impact on health than more strictly health ones, or that there is a need for integrating different policy areas (health and welfare are perhaps those most frequently cited).

Health Legislation, Johnson to Bush: Surge and Decline

This section reviews legislative developments in the health arena prior to the health reform debate of the 1990s in an attempt to depict the forward thrust in policy activity, particularly from 1965 through 1975, followed by a diminution of government intervention from the late 1970s through the late 1980s. The 1970s was a period of major congressional reform, and an issue addressed here is the influence of this reform on congressional decision making in explaining policy shifts.

Before 1960, health care policy in the United States focused on improving the quality of care through activities of the health professions and state governments. After the Flexner Report in 1910, for example, a number of medical schools in this country were closed as the educational process for physicians was standardized and the basis for scientific and specialty medicine was created in the basic science departments of educational institutions. At the same time, states passed licensing laws restricting entry into practice to graduates of accredited schools (Stevens, 1971).

Federal public health activities were limited to hospitals for special populations, communicable disease control, and some maternal and child health programs. These functions were overshadowed after World War II by the passage of the Hill–Burton Hospital Construction legislation and the buildup in the 1950s and early 1960s of the research programs of the National Institutes of Health (NIH). The first major federal social policy thrust, on the other hand, the Social Security Act (SSA) of 1935, purposefully omitted health proposals. Framers of the act feared medical profession opposition would subvert the entire program. While some of the above policies, such as the reduction in medical school openings, negatively affected access, others, such as Hill–Burton, increased access and improved the quality of the facilities in small communities.

In 1960, a new emphasis on access as a goal, and the shift to greater federal involvement in policy decisions generally, resulted in a fifteen-year period of legislation designed to reduce financial, geographical, organizational, and other barriers to care. The decision makers placed their faith in input and process policies, assuming that the outcome would be beneficial; that is, if people were provided resources, they would get the health care they needed and improved health status would result. Within a very short period, federal health policies laid the foundation for increases in facilities, personnel, and money. Amendments to the Hill–Burton legislation (PL 87-395, PL 88-442, and PL 91-296) provided support for outpatient facilities, nursing homes, and the modernization of hospital and health care facilities in urban areas.

In 1963, health manpower legislation (PL 88-129) authorized support to medical schools for the first time. Later, legislation encouraged existing schools to expand enrollment, funded new schools, supported programs to train new health practitioners and primary care physicians, and created area health education center (AHEC) programs. Federal policies were directed at preventing an impending physician shortage that was predicted in numerous studies in the 1940s, 1950s, and early 1960s (Sorkin, 1977).

The legislative debates over Hill–Burton, health manpower, and research funding were mild compared to the debates that raged over national health insurance. Several factors limited controversy. For one thing, it was difficult to argue with the need for physicians, hospitals, and research. In addition, the policies were perceived as essentially distributive in nature, benefiting the professional and academic interest group constituencies without directly depriving anyone else of support.

Far more controversial was legislation that finally passed creating government-funded health insurance coverage for those over sixty-five and some of the poor. Marmor (1973) charts Medicare's progress from impossible in the 1950s to enactment in 1965 and notes that the House Ways and Means Committee had a central role, first in preventing passage and then, after the 1964 election made the legislation virtually inevitable, in greatly expanding the Johnson administration's proposals.

While policymakers from 1961 to 1964 focused public attention on the battles between the American Medical Association (AMA) and the AFL-CIO, the most crucial negotiations took place between then Assistant Secretary of Health, Education, and Welfare Wilbur Cohen and Ways and Means Committee chairman, Wilbur Mills (D-AR). According to Marmor's analysis, Mills had the political sensitivity, power, and technical expertise to block legislation before 1964 and then to steer his own version of Medicare through the Ways and Means Committee and the House. Many of the legislative reforms in the 1970s were aimed directly at breaking Mills' power on Ways and Means, and it is doubtful whether by 1980 any member of Congress could exercise the control Mills did through "persuasion, entreaty, authoritative expertise and control of the agenda" (Marmor, 1973).

Other key elements of President Johnson's health policy were regional medical programs (RMPs) designed to help move the latest medical knowledge into communities through a cooperative arrangement between academic institutions and community physicians, and comprehensive health planning (CHP). As with many federal programs, CHP began as a permissive program and later became mandatory.

Health legislative activity continued under the Nixon administration, and in 1970 eleven major acts of legislation were passed, including such new areas as occupational health and safety, alcohol abuse, and the National Health Service Corps. In 1971, the president's declared war on cancer resulted in substantially increased support for comprehensive programs targeting this disease.

The major features of legislation passed between 1961 and 1971 were improved access through increased numbers of physicians and other health professionals, construction of facilities, and payment for care. Policymakers before 1972 showed little concern for either actual or future cost as legislation was passed creating program after program. At the end of this period, health policy, as other policy areas, changed in three ways: (1) the magnitude of government spending at all levels in health rose both in absolute terms (from $6.6 billion in 1960 to $104.2 billion in 1980) and as a percent of total health expenditures (from 24.7 percent to 42.2 percent) (Gibson & Waldo, 1981); (2) policymaking and decision making shifted to the federal level; and (3) the goals of the policy process became more redistributive and explicitly aimed at improving access to health care.

By 1972, the costs of these programs had become visible, whereas their effectiveness, measured in terms of improved health status, had not. The prospect of some form of national health insurance seemed imminent, and the consequent effect on inflation was viewed with alarm by federal policymakers (Russell, 1977). A significant change in the rhetoric of the health policy debate was evident in Congress by 1972 during consideration of professional standards review organization (PSRO) legislation and discussion of the National Health Planning and Resources Development Act (PL 93-641). Cost containment was the prevailing justification for peer review. Policymakers believed that if unnecessary hospitalization and surgery could be averted, Medicare and Medicaid costs could be reduced. The containment of costs was also the justification for a stronger health planning law. As time for the legislative authority of Hill–Burton, regional medical programs, and comprehensive health planning began to run out, Congress recognized that government programs had proliferated in an uncoordinated fashion and that inflation in the health system was significantly greater than general inflation. For those in health policy circles desiring to expand health insurance in the United States, regulation was one method of centralizing control of the system. On January 4, 1975, a few days after the National Health Planning and Resources Development Act was signed into law, a staff member of the Subcommittee on Health of the Senate Labor and Public Welfare Committee told an audience of health planners that "you are providing the foundation of an effective, efficient national health insurance program" (Biles, 1975).

Ironically, the same year that PL 93-641 was passed, the health manpower legislation was allowed to expire. For two years Congress was unable to pass renewal authorization. While the new health planning system was given authority to determine the need for health professionals, it had no control over the training or distribution of physicians. After ten years of federal funding of health professionals' education, Congress realized that, while the medical schools had responded to federal policy by increasing the output of physicians—nearly doubling the number of student spaces by 1974—the increased numbers had not altered geographical and specialty maldistributions. Suggested solutions that would be less costly were to direct physicians into primary care, use nonphysician health personnel, and increase the number of areas receiving members of the National Health Service Corps. Differences between proposals supported by Senator Edward Kennedy (D-MA) and Congressman Paul Rogers (D-FL) prevented final congressional action (LeRoy & Lee, 1977). Rogers' philosophy ultimately was reflected in the Health Professions Assistance Act of 1976. Medical students were not required to enter primary care specialties or practice in underserved areas, but medical schools were required to have 50 percent of their graduates enter primary care, and Congress chose the least controversial but also less meaningful definition—graduates entering internal medicine, family medicine, pediatrics, and obstetrics-gynecology.

Cost containment was also used as justification for the health maintenance organization legislation passed during the Nixon presidency, although with an entirely different rationale than PSROs and HSAs. The purpose of federal support of HMOs was to instill competition in the health care system and to encourage effective preventive medical care. Senator Kennedy's attempt to turn the administration's bill into a much stronger initiative to reform the health system resulted in a bill that contained proposals (such as open enrollment) making it difficult for federal HMOs to compete. AMA pressure resulted in a bill that provided limited funds for feasibility studies and development grants (Price, 1975). Subsequent revisions of the act created a more economically realistic set of criteria for HMO development, but far fewer applicants than had been expected qualified for federal status.

Between 1970 and 1975, Congress created a host of new programs. The prevailing ideology still expected government to provide solutions to the problems identified in the health system. But instead of the open-ended financing of the 1960s, such programs needed to be justified in terms of cost-effectiveness. New program costs had to be offset by savings to the system. This belief, and the presence of two subcommittee chairs

(Rogers and Kennedy) intent on establishing reputations in the health arena, made this period a particularly productive one.

As health care costs continued to escalate at rates above general inflation during the Carter presidency, the Democrats were divided over how to proceed. Senator Kennedy argued that costs could be controlled only by centralizing the insurance system. The president and more fiscally conservative senators and representatives feared that until a mechanism was in place to control at least hospital costs, expansion of the insurance system could strain the federal budget to the breaking point. National health insurance took a back seat to proposals to control fraud and abuse in the system and change hospital reimbursement to a formula reflecting historical costs and growth in the GNP. Carter was successful in the former, but not in the latter effort. The Hospital Cost Containment Act failed to pass in the Ninety-fifth and Ninety-sixth Congresses, largely due to lobbying efforts on the part of the hospital industry and the initial success of its "voluntary effort" cost-containment program. In addition, the difference between general inflation and that in the hospital sector briefly decreased, thereby temporarily quelling the desire for reform.

With the election of Ronald Reagan, the terms of the health policy debate were significantly altered. After twenty years of government expansion, Reagan promised to balance the budget and to reduce the size and scope of federal activity. Congressional policymaking was caught between a popular president and growing concern in both the public and private sectors over the federal deficit. Initially, Reagan's proposals spared Medicare, but when Congress showed a willingness to include this program in serious budget cuts, the administration "soon came around" (Iglehart, 1985). The president's initial budget proposed replacing the categorical health grant structure with two block grants for health and preventive services. Responsibility for allocating resources among the programs would be shifted to the states. The amount of funds transferred to the states for the programs would be reduced by 15 percent on the argument that states would have lower administrative costs and duplication of effort could be reduced. For other programs, such as the health planning system,

PSROs, and HMOs, the Reagan administration proposed they be defunded entirely. For Medicaid, Reagan proposed a cap on the federal contribution. Within a year of taking office, he proposed a swap calling for, among other things, federalizing Medicaid and turning the food stamp program over to the states.

Congress was forced to respond to Reagan's agenda. Substantial changes were made in the block grant proposal (four block grants were created with restrictions on funding and ten programs were left out of the block grants); many of the other Reagan proposals were incorporated in the Omnibus Reconciliation Budget Act of 1981. Federal contributions for Medicaid were reduced by 3 percent in fiscal year 1982 and 4 percent in fiscal year 1983, and the out-of-pocket costs borne by beneficiaries increased by 25 percent. Congressman Henry Waxman (D-CA), chair of the House Energy and Commerce Subcommittee on Health and the Environment, was more successful than any other legislator in countering the administration's proposals, and the continued authorization of many health programs was the result of his efforts, efforts that were often in vain when the programs went unfunded (Iglehart, 1983).

By 1985, the health planning system had been dismantled and funding for HMOs and the new scholarships for the National Health Service Corps had ceased, but the competitive deregulated health system Reagan envisioned never materialized. No coherent competitive strategy ever emerged from the Reagan administration. What became obvious during the budget debates of 1981 and 1982 was that Reagan's focus would be on controlling the cost of federal programs, particularly Medicare and Medicaid, not attempting to restructure the private sector, as Carter's hospital cost-containment legislation had sought. Congress preferred to reduce spending for all programs rather than discontinue them. And by the end of Reagan's first term, spending cuts were beginning to be restored, including a major expansion of the Medicaid program to include poor women and children in households not previously eligible, a proposal originating in Waxman's subcommittee.

Since discretionary health spending (i.e., all programs other than Medicare and Medicaid) accounted for only 14 percent of the total health outlays and Medicare alone accounted for 60 percent (Davis, 1987), it was obvious that Medicare and Medicaid costs had to be contained to effect significant budget reductions. During the 1980–87 period, Congress enacted more than thirty laws that affected the Medicare and Medicaid programs. An analysis by the General Accounting Office (U.S., 1988b) of the five laws[2] having the most telling effects on program and beneficiary costs concluded that had prior cost growth trends continued, actual inflation-adjusted Medicare expenditures would have been about $17.3 billion more than they actually were.

Congressional health policymaking in the Reagan years was characterized by changes in both process and content. Decision making shifted from the authorizing and appropriating processes to the budget reconciliation process. Health subcommittees came to play a much smaller role than they had previously. Traditional interest groups found they were much less able to follow policy proposals as they emerged in consolidated budget acts, let alone influence the process (Lawton, 1981).

The policy process within Congress in the 1980s was conditioned by two environmental factors—the election of Reagan and the budget deficit. By 1981, even the most committed government interventionist had to bow before the reality of the costs of social programs put in place in the 1960s and 1970s. Policymaking became a zero-sum game. Explicit redistribution was necessary between government policy areas (e.g., defense and domestic policy) as well as between groups and classes of citizens (e.g., young and old). As Price (1985) observed, Congress is not only better at distributing benefits than redistributing them but generating ideas and representing particular interests than enacting policies that are integrative and broadly representative of the national interest. Congress in the 1980s found itself in the dilemma of having to enact policies it was least equipped structurally and least comfortable politically to address. It reacted by avoiding making decisions un-

til the last possible moment, which resulted in a government run by continuing resolution for days to months after the start of fiscal years, and making policy through the budget reconciliation process, largely invisible to outsiders, and for which accountability largely disappeared.

HEALTH POLICY AND THE LEGISLATIVE PROCESS

Twenty years ago we would have described the U.S. Congress by noting that it was distinctive among Western democratic legislative assemblies with respect to the power it has retained vis-à-vis the executive, despite the fact that the complexities of policy formation have increasingly placed the responsibility for policy initiation, priority determination, and formulation with the executive branch of government.[3] Whereas legislatures in most countries have had as their principal function the refinement of executive proposals, Congress has remained comparatively capable both of generating policy and of posing the threat of thwarting executive initiatives so that, at least, the calculus of anticipated legislative reaction has been a significant factor in influencing the shape of major policies.

Key Structures in the Health Policy Legislative Process

Congressional decision making is so fluid and complex (e.g., each session of the House and Senate establishes its own procedures although some are eminently predictable) that it is an oversimplification to single out the components of the legislative process responsible for health policy. Nevertheless, it is fairly clear that certain standing committees are central, most notably Ways and Means and Commerce in the House, Finance and Labor and Human Resources in the Senate. Their respective turfs are not so readily identifiable since committees are regularly engaged in jurisdictional disputes and because some proponents of legislation used the

---

[2]They were the Omnibus Budget Reconciliation Act of 1981, the Tax Equity and Fiscal Responsibility Act of 1982, the Deficit Reduction Act of 1984, the Consolidated Omnibus Budget Reconciliation Act of 1985, and the Omnibus Budget Reconciliation Act of 1986.

[3]We borrow this "staging" of the policy process from Van Loon and Whittington (1987).

machine gun approach in advancing their causes; that is, they targeted several committees in the hope that one would be a hit. The House elected in 1994 banned such multiple submissions.

Given norms of subspecialization partly owing to the complexity of modern legislation, particularly health legislation, subcommittees are key working units in the congressional process. An exception is the absence since 1981 of a Senate Subcommittee on Health within the Committee on Labor and Human Resources (formerly the Committee on Labor and Public Welfare).

In addition, there periodically are select committees (i.e., those assigned responsibility for issues of emerging importance) that consider health issues. Moreover, all legislation must undergo the scrutiny of the House Rules Committee and the Senate and House Budget Committees. Finally, the Appropriations Committees of both houses are divided into subcommittees with functional responsibilities, one of which is health. Their support is crucial, since many authorizations are beefed up or, more likely (White, 1995a), watered down at this stage. Authorizations usually cover a period of several years, whereas appropriations are voted on yearly.

Other committees occasionally assume prominence in dealing with health issues when their central concerns intersect with this policy area. For example, the Banking and Currency Committees were especially important during the early to mid-1970s because of the impact of the Economic Stabilization Program (wage and price controls) on health care institutions.

The potential confusion in the legislative process surrounding the health arena mirrors the difficulty in labeling health policies: most not only seek to affect quality of care, access, and financing but also, explicitly or implicitly, call for regulation and redistribution of resources. For example, consideration of National Health Insurance (NHI) schemes could require decisions about revenue (House Ways and Means Committee and the Senate Finance Committee), health services delivery (Interstate and Foreign Commerce Committee in the House and the Labor and Human Resources Committee in the Senate), federal–state relations (Judiciary in each house), and the organization of government to administer the plan (Government Operations in the House and Senate).

The effects of fragmentation of responsibilities in the congressional process traditionally have been mitigated to varying degrees by an agile and vigorous leadership, norms of reciprocity and specialization, as well as presidential direction. The 1970s reforms, however, may have undercut the informal structures and processes that "greased the skids" of this very frictional mechanism. The irony in this turn of events is that the intention of the reformers was to smooth the way for "liberal" legislation.

Congressional Reforms of the 1970s

Between 1970 and 1975, Congress, particularly the House of Representatives, passed a series of primarily procedural reforms (*Congressional Quarterly*, 1976). These reforms sought to dismantle a pattern of legislative decision making that evolved from 1911 until the late 1960s whereby Congress was dominated by powerful committee chairmen who rose to their positions by virtue of their ability to be reelected. Many of these posts, especially the critical positions on the House Rules and Ways and Means Committees, were held by conservative southern Democrats who were adept at delaying or defeating liberal legislation.

The 1964 election dramatically changed the context of policymaking and the characteristics of Congress. The reforms of the 1970s date to this election. From the Johnson landslide of 1964 to that of the congressional Democrats in 1974, the composition of Congress reflected the effects of the proportional increase in the number of young voters and the growing demand of minorities and women for influence and power. Murphy (1974) has characterized the results of these movements as a "new politics" involving three major effects on Congress. The first was a significant decline in the power of the conservative coalition. Southern Democrats in both houses of Congress were being challenged by Republicans in general elections; primary competition was greater; and the constituency in the suburbs, traditionally Republican strongholds, became less conservative. The second and related change was that the composition of the House became more diverse. Black membership increased from five in 1960 to sixteen in 1974. Although their numbers did not increase, women began to play a more important role. Finally, public interest lobbying forces, such as that of Ralph Nader and the Sierra Club, emerged as a counterbalance to the traditional interest groups.

Reforms were so numerous during the 1970s and affected so many areas of congressional activity that the particular problems to which they were directed are difficult to discern (Jones, 1977). The problems appear, however, to fall into the following five categories:

1. an unequal and ineffective relationship with the executive
2. the concentration of power in senior committee chairmen
3. too many barriers in congressional procedure, which allowed a minority of legislators to block programs
4. the inability of junior members, particularly freshmen, to play an active role in the legislative process
5. a weak party structure and inability to effect party platform commitments

The reform movement began with the formation of the Democratic Study Group, an unofficial alliance of liberals concerned about social policy legislation. In 1968, they pushed to revive the Democratic caucus, and in 1973, they were instrumental in creating the Democratic Steering and Policy Committee. Through procedural reforms, power and authority were transferred to these structures and away from the House Ways and Means and Rules Committees, which were viewed as major stumbling blocks for liberal legislation.

Initially, the reforms worked to the benefit of the liberals who proposed them. The rejuvenated caucus and Steering and Policy Committee provided a forum for discussion. The majority of the Democrats were relatively liberal and therefore could control votes taken within the party caucus. The freshman and junior members had been guaranteed seats on major committees and subcommittees hitherto impossible to achieve and, at the height of the reformists' power, three senior committee chairmen (all conservative southern Democrats) were removed from their posts. The visibility

of the legislative process was enhanced when teller votes were recorded, committee sessions were opened to the public, and the budget acts required explicit priority setting in the appropriations process. With this increased visibility, coalition building and compromises became more difficult to negotiate. Members found their interest group constituencies paying closer attention to their voting record and uninterested in the necessity to sometimes "make deals."

The intended outcomes of the reforms were to strengthen the party leadership, remove barriers in the legislative process, and democratize (i.e., give more power to more members) the decision-making structure. Observers of the reforms (Rieselback, 1977; Ornstein & Rhode 1977; Oleszek, 1977) maintain that the cumulative effect was to decentralize power so severely that committee chairs could no longer manage their committees. The sharing of authority and expertise (e.g., staff) with subcommittee chairmen led to the characterization of the 1970s as an era of "subcommittee government" (Davidson, 1977).[4]

The effect of the reforms on the health subcommittees proved less crucial than in other areas. Rogers and Kennedy, though very different in style, were able to get their bills skillfully to conference. Rogers' subcommittee was known as one of the most productive in the House. During the Ninety-second Congress more than one-third (twenty) of the total bills reported by the Commerce Committee were in the area of health, and all cleared the House (Price, 1978).

Health care issues, especially research, personnel training, and hospital building, remained popular. The lower level of AMA opposition and the emergence of interest groups representing numerous other health constituencies meant considerable demand for legislation viewed as distributive or self-regulatory (Feldstein, 1977). By the late 1970s, when legislation was increasingly viewed as redistributive, the presence of all these groups, their ability to focus almost exclusively on a small number of subcommittee members, and the

---

[4]Somewhat ironically, perhaps, the percentage of partisan votes has increased since the 1970s (Schick, 1995). The irony is dispelled when one views party voting as a sign of inability to forge bipartisan agreements.

addition, at least in the House Subcommittee, of more conservative members, prevented Chairman Rogers from mobilizing a moderate, centrist consensus.

The Impact of the Budget Containment Movement of the 1980s[5]

The policy impact of major procedural reforms of the 1970s has been partially obscured by the effects of the budget containment movement of the 1980s. The 1970s reforms did produce results (Sinclair, 1985; Hinckley, 1983; Dodd & Openheimer, 1985): the committee chairs no longer wielded the power they once did; the process of their selection remained more open; subcommittees assumed more ability to initiate, refine, and obstruct. However, assessing the impact of these changes on the politics of congressional decision making and on the shape and pace of policy in general, and health policy in particular, is confounded somewhat by the recognition in the late 1970s and early 1980s that fiscal responsibility would have to guide congressional behavior more visibly than ever before. Policies previously regarded as distributive began to be seen as patently redistributive (Ellwood, 1985; Schick, 1994).

Much attention has been focused on the Gramm–Rudman–Hollings legislation as an enforcer of fiscal responsibility. In fact, the budget reconciliation movement began with the Congressional Budget and Impoundment Control Act of 1974, which created the House and Senate Budget Committees and contained provisions that made members go on record for higher spending, or taxes, or deficits, if Congress could not live within its own budget guidelines.

Describing the subsequent transfer of power from the appropriations to the budget committees, John Ellwood (1985, pp. 328–329) noted:

> During the first stage of the development of the new procedures (1975 through 1979), both budget committees and especially the House Budget Committee, acted as brokers for the claimants within each chamber. Their budget resolutions frequently reflected a balance among the wants of the various committees, the party leaders, and the president. In this role the committees were traffic cops of a bottom-up (that is, from the subcommittees and committees) budgetary process. Over time, however, the budget committees became budget guardians because they alone were in a position to add up the effects of the incremental requests and actions of the other committees. The appropriations committees had abandoned their role as guardians of the purse and had become claimants for federal money. The budget committees were able to build their power to the extent that they could work their will on the budget process.

The budget consciousness movement is manifest in the titles of the major bills that affected health policy in the 1980s: the Omnibus Reconciliation Act of 1981; the Tax Equity and Fiscal Responsibility Act of 1982; the Deficit Reduction Act of 1984; the Consolidated Omnibus Reconciliation Act of 1986. The shift of power and responsibility from authorization and appropriations committees by centralizing costs as well as benefits made partisan and ideological rifts more pronounced relative to clientele and interest group bargaining. It thereby gave the congressional leadership more power relative to committee and subcommittee chairs.

This development is related to a centralizing tendency in the bureaucracy, with budget requests aggregated at the Office of Management and Budget and interagency allocations then made on a top-down basis. Ellwood (1985) has contended that this dynamic lessened the validity of disjointed incrementalism and made more descriptive a "rational" synoptic model that envisions economic reasoning exerting increasing influence on policy.

His observation is apt if one examines general trends in U.S. policy, which have been the result of compromises struck between supporters of presidential and congressional leadership budget proposals. The proposals of Presidents Reagan and Bush tended to be geared to deficit reduction targets that reflected a commitment to maintenance (at least) of expenditure levels, downscaling of domestic programs, and a related ideological (or economic) commitment to reduction in the tax burden on those regarded as most prone to pro-

---

[5]For a rounded description of the reconciliation process, see Schick (1994).

duce and consume in accordance with supply-side economics. "Alternative budgets" proposed by congressional leaders, on the other hand, took a decidedly different tack: they proposed transfers from defense to domestic programs. But within the health policy arena, disjointed incrementalism in the 1980s was perhaps more evident than ever in the two largest health programs: Medicare and Medicaid (Hinckley & Hill, 1988).

Until recently, Medicare and Medicaid have been regarded as "uncontrollable" categories of expenditure, although their growth in fact has been marked by a decrease in the rate of acceleration of government spending. This "negative growth" has occurred largely through almost arbitrary marginal program cuts: per visit reimbursement levels to physicians were frozen and they were forced to bill at a rate in effect when services were rendered rather than in the next year; the nursing care differential, whereby hospitals were reimbursed more for extra costs incurred in nursing care for the elderly, was eliminated and indirect medical education allowances were reduced; hospitals now are prospectively reimbursed; Medicare enrollees' deductibles and Part B premiums have been raised to the extent that, as a proportion of their incomes, out-of-pocket health expenditures by the elderly now are higher than before Medicare.

This "decrementalism" thus has been disjointed: within reduced expenditure outlay ceilings and revenue enhancement targets, hospitals, physicians, and program enrollees have borne, to varying extents at different times, the brunt of efforts to keep federal budgets under control. The federal budget cuts, in either coverage under entitlements or net expenditures on entitlements, have occurred in seemingly uncoordinated fashion; they have been guided by expectations about where there was the most fat or where they would be least politically painful to impose, rather than by systematic cost–benefit analysis. This microview seemingly contrasts with Ellwood's (1985) more macroscopic view, in which OMB-aggregated budgets, tempered by presidential preferences, are pitted against Congressional Budget Office-shaped budgets pushed by congressional leaders. These views, however, are reconcilable. Within

major health programs, the chess pieces in this titanic game are still maneuvered under the gaze of special interests who have high stakes in the size and location of the expenditure decrements.

Further, Ellwood focuses his attention on manifestly redistributive policy. Increasingly, redistribution is being effected (albeit perhaps implicitly and haphazardly) via regulation. (Regulative policy eludes many of the generalizations Ellwood [1985] makes about overall revenue and expenditure policies.) In fact, the reform that has had the most profound impact on the health system was the quiet adoption of the prospective payment system (PPS) for Medicare, which replaced cost-based hospital reimbursement with prospective rates for diagnosis-related groups (DRGs) (Mann & Ornstein, 1995). Variants of this payment system were adopted by several Medicaid programs and other payers. The relationship between the congressional process and regulative policy within the context of the new shape of legislative–executive interaction clearly needs new research in light of old typologies.

Assessing the Impact of the 1970s Congressional Reform

Whatever the comparative utility of frameworks for viewing the legislative process, and whether that utility varies by policy scope, function, or area, we must confront the question posed by Hinckley (1983): What difference does the congressional process make on policy? What impacts on policy, not just process, are attributable to congressional reforms of the early 1970s and the heightened budget consciousness of the late 1970s and 1980s?

At the outset of this discussion it should be pointed out that it is assumed that the procedural reforms of the 1970s represented a significant alteration in the power structure of Congress, and that the reconciliation process did heighten Congress's sense of fiscal responsibility. If this seems to be a banal proposition, consider another view: that the reforms were merely cosmetic, simply exchanging subcommittees for full committees as the principal fiefdoms in the feudal domain of congressional decision making; reconciliation could simply have replaced appropriations committees with budget committees. (In this view, what we have regarded as a set of independent variables affecting policy change really amounts to a constant and, for this reason alone, cannot be expected to have explanatory power.)

However, even eschewing such procedural nihilism, as most observers of congressional behavior have done, and assuming that the legislative changes noted were more than chimerical, there are still difficulties in attributing health policy trends to legislative developments. Other potential causes of policy retrenchment have to be considered.

Economic Circumstances

Perhaps the most obvious of the coincidental and interrelated causal factors that compete with legislative reform is the economic downturn that began in the 1970s, followed by the rapid accumulation of the national debt in the next decade. This trend illuminates the fact that many health policies are reallocative and that they, therefore, rest on the presumption that there will be resources to allocate. Theories of public finance (Bird, 1971; Dye, 1980) that view government expenditures as led by "luxury" categories such as health and welfare and that posit the existence of a ratchet effect that underlies an irreversible incrementalism have to be reconsidered. In short, the law of expanding state activity, which envisions almost inexorable "progress," should be called into question for reasons quite apart from changes in congressional behavior patterns. As noted previously, the dynamics of the law (and its variants) also could be used to explain decrementalism.

During the past twenty years, we have accumulated a sizable national debt, one whose service now requires more than 14 percent of the federal government's annual expenditures. There are strongly conflicting views on whether the deficit really should be a preoccupation of public policy (e.g., GAO, 1988; Morris, 1989; Friedman, 1988). Nevertheless, unless one assumes very persuasive and pervasive disingenuity on the part of the leadership of both parties, the deficit has been perceived as critical and perception is reality in viewing constraints on government expenditure programs.

Experience of Government Health Programs

Another factor coinciding with congressional change as an explanation of policy change has been the experience of government programs. By way of illustration, Medicare and Medicaid have been far more expensive than predicted and have been accompanied by numerous regulations not unanticipated by watchful observers. Mechanic (1981) has observed that the hesitant and, therefore, perhaps awkward approach to government-sponsored health insurance programs has disaffected both the right and left sides of the ideological spectrum. Medicaid, in particular, has not resulted in easily available and accessible services for those citizens it targets (e.g., it covers only 58 percent of the poor nationally). Moreover, it has become extremely costly, particularly in recent years as it has grown from 10 percent (1987) to 20 percent of the typical state's budget.

There is also a less cynical interpretation of the impact that experience with government health programs has had; that is, such programs have actually achieved a measure of success and, therefore, have quieted demands for policy change (Mann & Ornstein, 1995). Most obviously, Medicare has helped make a wide (if not totally comprehensive) range of services accessible to the heaviest users of health care. Medicaid does cover most of the designated poor, although in a less than ideally humanitarian fashion. And what perhaps largely escapes public attention is that government tax expenditures in effect subsidize the private health insurance industry. This has had more than a trivial effect on the numbers of people covered and is somewhat analogous to the more explicit government subsidization of sickness funds in the Federal Republic of Germany and Sweden, for example. The fact that the income tax exemption accorded employer-paid health insurance premiums constitutes a form of government expenditure, in terms of foregone revenues to the Treasury (Surrey & McDaniel, 1985), did not go unnoticed by the Reagan administration and Republican Senate. As a result consideration was given to the termination of such indirect government support as a means of curtailing government expenditures by putting potential consumers at greater risk and, at the same time, generating revenues.

In addition, health care tax expenditures have not escaped the attention of the House Ways and Means Subcommittee (Falcone & Warren, 1988). In this policy posture, the government is perhaps further mending the patchwork quilt of programs that has forestalled a more comprehensive health policy.

Another impact of government programs has been the increasing trend toward oligopsony (or bilateral oligopoly) that they have furthered. As Marmor et al. (1976) and others pointed out some time ago, concentrated interests result in decision makers becoming more cost-conscious purchasers of health services. This historical observation is corroborated by cross-national comparison (Falcone et al., 1994).

The United States still falls in the mixed, pluralistic source of funding classification, but, over time, expenditures have become increasingly centralized. Medicare has had a more profound effect than Medicaid in this regard (Marmor et al., 1976), but the sheer amounts of money required to underwrite the Medicaid program have also piqued the fiscal sensitivity of federal, state, and county governments. Of course, governments are not alone in the trend toward oligopsony. Managed care plans are forcing deep discounts where market penetration is extensive, which is occurring in an ever-increasing number of areas in the United States. Now with devolution of Medicaid on the near horizon, the impact of this program's expenditures will be concentrated at the state level.

Ideological Orientation

In addition to the cynicism and cost consciousness engendered by government health programs and the resource limitations faced by recent Congresses, there has also been a political and ideological shift to the right. This has not been a distinctively U.S. phenomenon, as it seems that in every one of the Big Seven nations (i.e., those with the largest gross domestic products), the basic role of the state is being questioned. In light of this attitudinal movement in favor of reprivatization (or, at least, a climate of opinion not conducive to intensified government activity), health policy retrenchment is as explainable, by conventional, civics text notions about the responsiveness of legislators to their constituents' preferences, as it is on the basis of economic, pragmatic, or procedural considerations. This is an issue we discuss below in attempting to explain the recent failure of health care reform.

Again, however, the impact of ideology on policy is questionable. First, it is nearly impossible to separate the rhetoric that underlies policy change from that which merely is convenient to justify it. Second, whatever the casual mechanism involved, the media seem to have adjudged that there has been an ideological shift, and that may amount to a self-fulfilling prophecy in that the assessment is as important as the phenomenon being analyzed. Third, ideological constraint, even among the elite (i.e., political leaders), is limited. Support for process reform is rarely divorced from substantial policy implications (e.g., those who favor limitations on debate typically oppose the positions of those who likely will be using the filibuster or other tactics to obstruct legislation). Finally, to summarize the effects of ideology, this classification is simply too convenient. Political language is often couched in ideological terms, and post factum analyses of political events tempt people to exchange ideas in the coin of the realm. Historians and journalists perhaps are especially prone to succumb to this fallacy, but other social scientists are not immune to such entrapment.

THE FAILURE OF HEALTH REFORM— THE 103RD CONGRESS

The debate over health care reform that virtually preoccupied the 1993–94 congressional session will be difficult to rival as the legislative spectacle of the 1990s. Explanations of the resultant "Failure of Health Care Reform" (*Journal of Health Politics, Policy and Law*, 1995) have employed various perspectives on Congress's internal decision-making mechanisms, susceptibility to influence by powerful interest groups, faithfulness as a mediator/translator of public opinion into public policy, and other roles and responsibilities.

Conditions seemingly were as ripe as possible for the enactment of comprehensive national health reform legislation by the 103rd Congress. Bowler, Kuderle, and

Marmor (1977), writing in a similarly propitious climate, posited two conditions that were necessary, albeit insufficient, for adoption of a social model of national health insurance: (1) a president who sets a high priority on health care reform and (2) whose party has a majority in both houses of Congress.

There was no doubt about the Clinton administration's commitment to substantial health care reform. And the administration's proposal initially was supported by the House and Senate leadership. The Guaranteed Health Insurance Act of Congressmen Richard Gephart (D-MO) and Thomas Foley (D-WA) and Senator George Mitchell's (D-ME) Health Security Act differed only slightly from Clinton's Health Security Act with respect to universal mandated (employer and individual) insurance coverage with a comprehensive benefits package (Kaiser Commission, 1994). The result, according to Mark Peterson (1995b), was that the debate progressed further than ever before, and he cites the reportage of bills by committees in support of his optimism. Schick (1995), on the other hand, argues that the reported bills were not passable. Still, we wound up with, in Alford's (1976) memorable phrase, "dynamics without change," and, according to Theda Skocpol, "an enormously costly lost opportunity" (1995a, p. 485).

Why did reform fail? Most answers to this question feature congressional structures, processes, and behavior. These answers can be categorized with respect to their emphasis on Congress's role as a shaper and articulator of public opinion; an arena for the accommodation of elite interests; and an institution designed for inaction, particularly in the case of complex, systemic health reform. Another answer focuses on distinctive features of the Clinton plan and the congressional debate it engendered. None of these categories of answers is entirely satisfying, but they shed light on how the congressional process deals with health policy issues.

Congress and Public Opinion

Years ago V. O. Key, echoing Walter Lippman, noted that decision-mandating opinion clusters were an extreme rarity in American politics; rather, policies typically have required the mobilization of "supportive" consensuses by elite cue givers. In the case of health care reform, there initially was an amorphous but potentially resonant climate of supporting opinion, if not demanding change (Brodie & Blendon, 1995; Jacobs & Shapiro, 1995; Brady & Buckley, 1995), which members of Congress failed to mobilize (Navarro, 1995; Yankelovich, 1995). Their failure in this regard was compounded by media coverage devoted to sound and sight bytes (Marmor, 1995; Yankelovich, 1995). Marmor (1995), with grim humor, has compared the media's obfuscation of the health policy debate with the relatively informative coverage of the highly publicized 1994–95 O. J. Simpson murder trial.

As for the tenor of congressional debate on health reform, Marmor (1995, p. 499) termed it a "debate without deliberation" while Peterson (1995b) characterized it as "all heat and no light." Part of the reason for this cynical view was the attempt of middle-range reform advocates (i.e., those favoring "play or pay" "managed competition" plans versus a single-payer approach) to obviate addressing ideological issues in the interest of political feasibility. As Theda Skocpol (1993) observed early on in the debate, these reformers thought that gridlock could be overcome through bargaining, that ideological battles did not have to be fought openly as such. As a result, she argues, the opponents of reform were able to create ideological metaphors while reform advocates were not. And, the reformers may have missed a golden opportunity. For instance, Blendon, Brodie, and Benson's (1995) survey research indicates that Hawaii's employer mandate plan would have had more public appeal than did the Clinton proposal.

On the other hand, some authors hold that the 103rd Congress accurately reflected public opinion, at least so far as the latter can be characterized as a generalized distrust of government (Smith, 1995; White, 1995b; Blendon et al., 1995). And, as White (1995b) notes, the fact that a majority of the public supports the goal of universal health insurance is irrelevant; what is crucial is support for plausible means of achieving universal coverage.

According to this line of reasoning, there sometimes can be majorities who believe that a problem exists and that it should be corrected. However, agreement breaks down when the posited solutions call for *government* (particularly federal government) intervention, at which point American skepticism about government overrides substantive concerns (Smith, 1995). This logic borders on the "American exceptionalism" argument that several authors (Falcone et al., 1994; Broyles & Falcone, forthcoming; Marmor & Bynum, 1992; Steinmo & Watts, 1995) have sought to discredit. One way the exceptionalism argument can be laid to rest is simply to juxtapose the Canadians' acceptance of national health insurance and their attitudes toward government(s), which make putative American antipathy look tame (Kornberg & Clarke, 1992). Americans may be "ambivalent" in their desire for reform and distrust of government, but this alone clearly cannot explain the repeated failure of reform in this country (see also Fukuyama, 1995).

Congress and Elite Interests

The argument that elite interests stalled congressional action has been put succinctly by Cathie Jo Martin (1995), who wrote that "compounded by a Republican leadership refusal to entertain serious bipartisan compromise and by full-scale mobilization against the bill by vested interests, healthcare reform once again floundered on the shoals of divided government and interest group liberalism, the age-old villains in the story of American governance" (p. 431). Navarro (1995), on the other hand, although claiming that most of the blame for the failure of health reform could be placed on the Democrats' abandonment of "class politics," also recognized the important role played by the linkage between Congress and the "medical-industrial complex." In a more expansive view, Schick (1995) partially attributes the failure of reform to "hyperpluralism" (i.e., the fracturing of interest group coalitions).

The elite accommodation argument for the failure of reform can be overstated. As will be seen in the case of the institutional argument that follows, the influence of vested interests hardly determined the failure of reform. If, in fact, vested interests were very influential in defeating reform, this can be partially attributed to situational factors rather than the existential supervening

power of such interests. History shows the influence of health groups can be forestalled, as in the case of the establishment of the prospective payment system (Smith, 1995; White, 1995a), or overcome, as in the case of Medicare. Also, in comparative perspective, vested interests are everywhere powerful (Glaser, 1993; Saltman, 1992); therefore, their role cannot explain U.S. health policy uniqueness among Western developed nations. Constants do not explain variables.

Congress and American Politics: "It's the Institutions, Stupid!"

The quotation above is part of the title of an article by Steinmo and Watts (1995) in which the authors contend that America's most recent failure to pass comprehensive national health care reform is attributable to the same cause of failure as it was in 1948, 1965, 1974, and 1978: American political institutions are structurally biased against this kind of comprehensive reform (p. 330). James Morone, who has advanced a similar argument in several places (1990, 1995), has vividly described the obstacle course confronting any executive proposal as "an extraordinarily byzantine process that has grown increasingly difficult to manage" (1995, p. 395). He noted that when the Clinton plan reached Congress, thirty-one committees tried to claim jurisdiction, seven won claims, and each was free to substitute its own bill for the president's. Further, committee jurisdiction is more divided on health care than on any other issue (Baumgartner & Talbert, 1995). Morone also reminds us of the imposing role the bureaucracy would have faced in designing regulations in the unlikely event a legislative proposal as ambitious as NHI would have been successful (1995).

It is difficult to deny the constraints placed on policymaking by the United States' distinctive, if not unique, political structures and processes. Still, American politics are not necessarily *determining* in this regard. As White (1995b, p. 375) points out, very few nations that have national health insurance have a British model of responsible party government and "[t]he multiparty coalitional politics in most other nations seems an unpromising basis for decisive government action."

Further, White points out, as does Smith (1995), that the passage of the prospective payment system was not a trivial stage in the regulation of the health industry. This leads White to suggest that the real culprit in health care reform was the nature of the debate which, in turn, was largely prefigured by the package being debated.

The Clinton Plan and the Nature of the Debate

In an admirably parsimonious argument, Brady and Buckley (1995) hold that the Clinton administration's plan was unsuccessful because it departed too radically from the "median congressional voter" with regard to the crucial issues of who pays, the scope of coverage, and the quality of care. They note that, with never more than thirty votes, the Clinton plan failed to mollify the concerns of the conservative Democratic members at the median and represented a far too costly alternative to the status quo. And, even gainsaying the ideologically unappealing aspects of the plan, it simply called for too much change (Skocpol, 1995b). As White (1995b, p. 374) dramatically pointed out, "[n]o other democratic state has ever reformed anything that big, whatever the political system, barring revolution." Further, it must be recalled that Clinton did not win a majority campaigning on health care reform (Blendon et al., 1995). Finally, technical aspects of the bill, such as its very consequential uncertainty about the fiscal impact of the tax treatment of employer mandates (Nichols, 1995), did not inspire confidence.

That the failure of health reform in the 103rd Congress may be plausibly attributed to distinctive features of the reform proposal and the issue orientations of members of Congress is grounds for optimism. Whatever one thinks health reform should look like, the inherent pessimism of the institutional structure and American exceptionalism arguments are not reassuring. Institutional and cultural determinists ultimately have to answer the perennial question of "What is to be done?" "Situationalists/contextualists," those who attribute the failure of health care reform to the features of the major proposals and their appeal, or lack thereof, to various contituencies in 1993–94, can answer that question at the next round of the confirming debate on

health care reform. The plan advanced should be simpler, more marketable, and advocated with less ideological trepidation. The experience of the 104th Congress thus far underscores the validity of this recommendation, although many would not argue with the substance of the reforms that are being enacted.

THE 104TH CONGRESS: THE REPUBLICAN REVOLUTION?

We have noted that, following the 1974 elections, there were substantial changes in congressional structures and processes that may have contributed to stasis in health policy. The 1970s legislative changes had no counterpart in the 1980s. There was a temporary aberration of sorts when the Republicans took control of the Senate after the 1982 elections, but the change in partisanship did not occasion any major procedural change (other than Orrin Hatch dissolving the Health Subcommittee of the Labor and Public Welfare Committee), certainly not any that could be linked to health policy change. The major policy changes in the 1980s, the advent of prospective payment, and the passage and repeal of Medicare's catastrophic coverage cannot be readily traced to procedural variables.

The 1990s are a radical departure from the previous decade with regard to the pace of change in health policy and the congressional process. It would be difficult to overestimate the suddenness and force of the changes. Both are driven by a new conservative ideology (Ornstein & Schenkenberg, 1995) that embraces, among other things, a smaller federal role in health care financing and a level of deficit reduction thought achievable only through severe fiscal restraints on Medicare and Medicare. Because each set of changes, legislative and policy, is so enmeshed in the same ideological movement, it is virtually impossible to view one set as causing the other.

This ideological drive gives rise to some apparent anomalies. For example, in the House, Newt Gingrich (R-GA) has exercised a near unilateral discretion over the selection of committee chairs unmatched by any Speaker since the early part of this century. On the other hand, freshmen have been appointed to key committees and their views have been accommodated when they diverged from those of the leadership. Both leaders and followers have seen procedural change as clearly linked to fulfillment of the substance of the "Contract with America." Perhaps this cohesion is what most differentiates the 104th Congress from its look-alike twenty years earlier: the firebrands in the 1970s saw leadership standing in the way of reform; their 1990s counterparts see vigorous leadership as an instrument of needed change.

While the Senate's modus operandi was not very much affected by the Republican sweep in 1994, the changes in the House were many and swift. The only "failures" that Gingrich and his cohorts registered were owing to the fact that the very slim Republican majority (230 seats) was insufficient to pass constitutional measures such as term limits or a balanced budget amendment. A sampling of the changes enacted in the first (very long) day: the elimination of three committees; cutting professional staff by one-third; prohibiting the Speaker from referring a bill to more than one committee; a ban on proxy voting in committee; limiting the Speaker's tenure to four consecutive terms; more minor party representation on committees; and giving the minority party the right to move to recommit a bill (Ornstein & Schenkenberg, 1995).

More important, perhaps, than these rule changes has been the transformation of the Speaker's role. Although Gingrich delegated the management of legislation and administration of the House and Capitol to Majority Leader Dick Armey (R-TX), he monitors the delegated operations with sophisticated software and a regularly consulted staff of whips. In turning his immediate attention away from day-to-day concerns, Gingrich effectively postured as a legislative leader, at least on a par with the president. For example, he became the first Speaker to request an opportunity to address the nation on television, other than to respond to a president, and the request was granted (Ornstein & Schenkenberg, 1995). Former presidential candidate Eugene McCarthy describes Gingrich's demeanor as prime ministerial and, indeed, Ornstein and Schenkenberg (1995) depict the legislative behavior of the 104th Congress as more parliamentary than congressional.

With regard to substantive policy, after having vented their spleen over Public Broadcasting, the National Endowments for the Arts and Humanities, the Republicans turned to their two main themes: government dismantling and budget balancing. These imperatives moved Medicare and Medicaid to center stage (Ornstein & Schenkenberg, 1995). Proposed changes in Medicaid would give states very broad latitude in making decisions about spending on health care services for the poor. In the case of Medicare, expenditure growth would be slowed significantly with greater cost sharing by beneficiaries indexed by income.

Conclusion

This chapter has examined developments in the legislative process and health policy. We have shown that the first emphasis of health policy during that period was on access enhancement. One major barrier to demand for health services, price, had been eliminated for a substantial proportion of the population. The next major barrier to access was seen as availability, which was targeted through regional planning and human resources policies. Except for a window of opportunity for national health insurance in the early to mid-1970s, which reopened wide during the 103rd Congress, the primary target of policy has shifted from access enhancement to expenditure control, albeit efforts to improve access have often also been touted as cost-effective. The concern with cost is understandable in view of the fact that the levels of federal expenditure on Medicare and Medicaid are exceeded only by those on defense and interest on the national debt. Therefore, control of health care expenditures is likely to remain a policy preoccupation.

It is difficult to lay the blame for this shift in policy emphasis—from access to cost—on the structures and processes of congressional decision making in the health arena, although some pundits were moved to do so after the failure of health reform in the 103rd Congress. Perhaps that is because congressional behavior, with its visibly complex patterns, is such an easy target. So it seemed in the 1970s, when zealous Democratic newcomers dismantled congressional structures and wound up with little (actually perhaps nothing) to show for their efforts in terms of health policy. We have argued that this is evidence that there is not a clear link between changes in congressional structures and processes and health policy.

This argument gains weight from the experience of the 104th Congress, where there have been changes in both congressional decision-making patterns and health policy, but both have been part and parcel of an ideological movement. The recent Republican "revolution" leaves little doubt that Congress can churn out health policy initiatives, and the fact that the Republican policies are truly initiatives is undeniable. And, even though watered down in the legislative process and bargaining with the administration, they still represent significant departures from trend lines, that is, aberrations to disjointed incrementalism or "decrementalism." "It's the institutions, stupid!" has lost resonance, even if the current congressional enactments fail to survive political developments in the coming years with their ideological integrity intact.

REFERENCES

Alford, Robert. (1976). *Health politics: Dynamics without change.* Chicago: University of Chicago Press.

Barber, James D. (1972). *Presidential character.* Englewood Cliffs, NJ: Prentice-Hall.

Baumgartner, Frank, & Jeffrey Talbert. (1995). From setting a national agenda on health care to making decisions in Congress. *Journal of Health Politics, Policy and Law, 20* (Summer), 437–446.

Biles, Bryan. (1975). Regional orientation session health resources planning. Unedited transcript of remarks, Atlanta, GA, January 13–14.

Bird, Richard. (1970). *The growth of government spending in Canada.* Toronto: Canadian Tax Foundation.

Blendon, Robert, Mollyann Brodie, & Joan Benson. (1995). What happened to America's support of the Clinton plan? *Health Affairs, 14* (Summer), 7–23.

Blumstein, James F. (1977). Inflation and quality: The case of PSRO's. In Michael Zubkoff (Ed.), *Health: A victim or cause of inflation* (pp. 245–295). New York: Prodist.

Bowler, M. Kenneth, R. T. Kuderle, & Theodore Marmor. (1977). The political economy of national health insurance: Policy analysis and political evaluation. *Journal of Health Politics, Policy and Law, 2* (Spring), 100–133.

Brady, David, & Kara Buckley. (1995). Health care reform in the 103rd Congress: A predictable failure. *Journal of Health Politics, Policy and Law, 20* (Summer), 447–454.

Brodie, Mollyann, & Robert Blendon. (1995). The public's contribution to congressional gridlock on health care reform. *Journal of Health Politics, Policy and Law, 20* (Summer), 403–410.

Brown, Lawrence. (1986). Introduction to a decade of transition. *Journal of Health Politics, Policy and Law, 11* (Spring), 569–584.

Brown, Michael K. (1988). The segmented welfare system: Distributive conflict and retrenchments in the United States, 1968–1984. In M. K. Brown (Ed.), *Remaking the welfare states: Retrenchment and social policy in America and Europe* (pp. 182–205). Philadelphia: Temple University Press.

Broyles, R., & D. Falcone. (Forthcoming). Health care reform: An American obsession with prescriptive incrementalism. *Journal of Health and Human Resources.*

Congressional Budget Office. (1981). *The impact of PSRO's on health care costs: Update of EO's 1979 evaluation.* Washington, D.C.: U.S. Library of Congress.

Congressional Quarterly. (1976). *Inside Congress.* Washington, D.C.: Congressional Quarterly Press.

Cooper, Theodore. (1976). Federal health policy. *Journal of Health Politics, Policy and Law, 1* (Spring), 9–12.

Dahl, Robert. (1966). *Pluralist democracy in the United States: Conflict and consensus.* (Chapter 5). Chicago: Rand-McNally.

Davidson, Roger. (1977). Breaking up those cozy triangles: An impossible dream? In Susan Welch & John G. Peters (Eds.), *Legislative reform and public policy* (pp. 30–53). New York: Praeger Publishers.

Davis, Karen. (1987). Reagan administration health policy. *Journal of Public Policy, 2,* 312–331.

Davis, Karen, & Cathy Schoen. (1978). *Health and the war on poverty: A ten year appraisal.* Washington, D.C.: The Brookings Institution.

Department of Health, Education, and Welfare. (1978). *Health 1976–77.* Washington, D.C.: U.S. Government Printing Office.

Dodd, Lawrence C., & Bruce I. Oppenheimer. (1985). The House in transition. In Lawrence C. Dodd & Bruce Oppeheimer (Eds.), *Congress reconsidered* (3rd ed., pp. 380–411). Washington, D.C.: Congressional Quarterly Press.

Dye, Thomas. (1980). *Understanding public policy* (4th ed.). Englewood Cliffs, NJ: Prentice-Hall.

Ellwood, John W. (1985). The great exception: The congressional budget process in an age of decentralization. In Lawrence C. Dodd & Bruce I. Oppenheimer (Eds.), *Congress reconsidered* (3rd ed., pp. 345–362). Washington D.C.: Congressional Quarterly Press.

Etzioni, Amatai. (1967). Mixed scanning: A "third" approach to decision-making. *Public Administration Review, 27,* 385–442.

Falcone, David, Robert Broyles, & Steven R. Smith. (1994). American health policy in temporal and cross-national perspective. In Stuart Nagel (Ed.), *The encyclopedia of policy studies* (2nd ed.). New York: Marcel Dekker.

Falcone, David, & David Warren. (1988). The shadow price of pluralism: The use of tax expenditures to subsidize hospital care in the United States. *Journal of Health Politics, Policy and Law, 13,* 735–751.

Feldstein, Paul. (1977). *Health associations and the demand for legislation.* Cambridge: Ballinger Publishing Company.

Feldstein, Paul. (1988). Straight talk about deficits. *Wall Street Journal* (December 14).

Feldstein, Paul. (1993). *Health economics.* New York: Delmar.

Friedman, Milton. (1988). Straight talk about deficits. *Wall Street Journal* (December 14).

Fukuyama, Francis. (1995). *Trust: Social virtues and the creation of prosperity.* New York: The Free Press.

Gibson, Robert M., & Daniel R. Waldo. (1981). National health expenditures. *Health Care Financing Review, 4,* 35.

Glaser, William A. (1993). How financing caps and targets really work. *Milbank Quarterly, 7* (1), 97–127.

Hinckley, Barbara. (1983). *Stability and change in Congress* (3rd ed.). New York: Harper & Row.

Hinckley, Kathryn, & Bette Hill. (1988). *Biting the bullet? Post-1980 congressional process and Medicare/Medicaid decisions.* Paper presented at the 1988 annual meeting of the American Political Science Association, Washington, D.C., September 2–4.

Iglehart, John K. (1983). The Reagan record on health policy. *New England Journal of Medicine, 308* (January 27), 232–236.

Iglehart, John K. (1985). The administration's assault on domestic spending and the threat to health care programs. *New England Journal of Medicine, 312* (February 21), 525–528.

Iglehart, John K. (1988). The administration responds to the cost spiral. *New England Journal of Medicine, 305* (November 26), 1359–1364.

Jacobs, Lawrence, & Robert Shapiro. (1995). Don't blame the public for failed health care reform. *Journal of Health Politics, Policy and Law, 20* (Summer), 411–424.

Jones, Charles. (1977). How reform changes Congress. In Susan Welch & John Peters (Eds.), *Legislative reform and public policy* (pp. 11–29). New York: Praeger Publishers.

Journal of Health Politics, Policy and Law. (1995). Special Section: The failure of health care reform. *20* (2), 329–352.

Kornberg, Allan, & Harold Clarke. (1992). *Citizens and community: Political leadership in a representative democracy.* New York: Cambridge University Press.

Lawton, Stephen E. (1981). Budget reconciliation: The new legislative process. *New England Journal of Medicine, 305* (November 19), 1297–1300.

Leroy, Lauren, & Philip Lee. (1977). *Deliberations and compromise.* Cambridge: Ballinger Publishing.

Lindblom, Charles. (1969). The sciences of "muddling through." In Amatai Etzioni (Ed.), *Readings in modern organizations* (pp. 154–165). Englewood Cliffs, NJ: Prentice-Hall.

Lindblom, Charles. (1992). *Inquiry and change.* New Haven: Yale University Press.

Lowenberg, Gerhard. (1971). *Modern parliaments: Change or decline.* New York: Aldine Publishing Company.

Mann, Thomas, & Norman Ornstein. (Eds.). (1995). *Intensive care: How Congress shapes health policy.* Washington, D.C.: American Enterprise Institute and The Brookings Institution.

Marmor, Theodore. (1973). *The politics of Medicare.* New York: Aldine Publishing Company.

Marmor, Theodore. (1995). A summer of discontent: Press coverage of murder and medical care reform. *Journal of Health Politics, Policy and Law, 20* (Summer), 495–502.

Marmor, Theodore, & Daniel Bynum. (1992). American medical reform: Are we doomed to fail? *Daedalus,* 174–194.

Marmor, Theodore, Donald Wittmann, & Thomas Heagy. (1976). The politics of medical inflation. *Journal of Health Politics, Policy and Law, 4,* 69–84.

Martin, Cathie Joe. (1995). Stuck in neutral: Big business and the politics of national health reform. *Journal of Health Politics, Policy and Law, 20* (Summer), 425–430.

Mechanic, David. (1981). Some dilemmas in health policy. *Millbank Memorial Fund Quarterly/Health and Society, 59* (Winter), 1–15.

Morone, James. (1995). Nativism, hollow corporations, and managed competition: Why the Clinton health care reform failed. *Journal of Health Politics, Policy and Law, 20* (Summer), 391–398.

Morris, Charles R. (1989). Deficit figuring doesn't add up. *New York Times Magazine* (February 12).

Murphy, Thomas P. (1974). *The new politics: Congress.* Lexington, MA: Lexington Books.

Navarro, Vicente. (1995). Why Congress did not enact health care reform. *Journal of Health Politics, Policy and Law, 20* (Summer), 455–462.

Nichols, Len M. (1995). Numerical estimates and the policy debate. *Health Affairs, 14* (Spring), 56–59.

Oleszek, Walter J. (1977). A perspective on congressional reform. In Susan Welch & John Peters (Eds.), *Legislative reform and public policy* (pp. 3–10). New York: Praeger Publishing Company.

Ornstein, Norman, & David W. Rhode. (1977). Revolt from within: Congressional change, legislative policy and the House

Commerce Committee. In Susan Welch & John Peters (Eds.), *Legislative reform and public policy* (pp. 247–256). New York: Praeger Publishing Company.

Ornstein, Norman, & Amy L. Schenkenberg. (1995). The 1995 Congress: The first hundred days and beyond. *Political Science Quarterly, 110*, 183–206.

Peterson, Mark. (1995a). Editor's note: Political perspectives on policy defeat. *Journal of Health Politics, Policy and Law, 20* (Summer), 271–274.

Peterson, Mark. (1995b). The health care debate: All heat and no light. *Journal of Health Politics, Policy and Law, 20* (Summer), 425–430.

Price, David. (1975). *The Commerce Committees*. New York: Grossman.

Price, David. (1978). Policymaking in congressional committees: The impact of "environmental" factors. *American Political Science Review, 72*, 548–574.

Price, David. (1985). Congressional committees in the policy process. In Lawrence Dodd & Bruce Oppenheimer (Eds.), *Congress reconsidered* (3rd ed., pp. 220–311). Washington, D.C.: Congressional Quarterly Press.

Rieselback, Leroy N. (1977). *Congressional reform in the 70s*. Morristown, NJ: General Learning Press.

Russell, Louise. (1977). Inflation and the federal role in health. In Michael Zubkoff (Ed.), *Health: A victim or cause of inflation?* (pp. 225–244). New York: Prodist.

Saltman, Richard B. (1992). Single-source financing systems: A solution for the United States? *Journal of the American Medical Association, 268* (August 12), 744–779.

Schattschneider, E. E. (1956). United States: The functional approach to party government. In S. Neumann (Ed.), *Modern political parties* (pp. 194–218). Chicago: University of Chicago Press.

Schick, Allen. (1994). *The federal budget: Politics, policy, process*. Washington, D.C.: The Brookings Institution.

Schick, Allen. (1995). How a bill did not become a law. In Thomas Mann & Norman Ornstein (Eds.), *Intensive care: How Congress shapes health policy* (pp. 227–266). Washington, D.C.: American Enterprise Institution and The Brookings Institution.

Simon, H. (1955). A behavioral model of rational choice. *Quarterly Journal of Economics, 69*, 99–118.

Sinclair, Barbara. (1985). Agenda, policy and alignment change. In Lawrence Dodd & Bruce Oppenheimer (Eds.), *Congress reconsidered* (3rd ed., pp. 300–314). Washington, D.C.: Congressional Quarterly Press.

Skocpol, Theda. (1993). Is the time finally ripe? Health insurance reform in the 1990s. *Journal of Health Politics, Policy and Law, 18* (Fall), 531–550.

Skocpol, Theda. (1995a). The aftermath of defeat. *Journal of Health Politics, Policy and Law, 20* (Summer), 485–490.

Skocpol, Theda. (1995b). The rise and resounding demise of the Clinton plan. *Health Affairs, 14* (Spring), 66–85.

Smith, Steven R. (1995). Commentary—the role of institutions and ideas in health care policy. *Journal of Health Policy, Politics and Law, 20* (Summer), 385–390.

Sorkin, Alan L. (1977). *Health manpower*. Lexington, MA: D. C. Heath.

Steinmo, Sven, and Jon Watts. (1995). It's the institutions, stupid! Why comprehensive national health insurance always fails in America. *Journal of Health Politics, Policy and Law, 20* (Summer), 329–372.

Stevens, Rosemary. (1971). *American medicine and the public interest*. New Haven: Yale University Press.

Surrey, Stanley, & Paul McDaniel. (1985). *Tax expenditure*. Cambridge, MA: Harvard University Press.

U.S. General Accounting Office. (1988a). *The budget deficit*. Washington, D.C.: U.S. Government Printing Office.

U.S. General Accounting Office. (1988b). *Medicare and Medicaid: Updated effects of recent legislation on programs and beneficiary costs*. Washington, D.C.: U.S. Government Printing Office.

U.S. Senate. Committee on the Budget. (1988). The congressional budget process: An explanation. 100th Congress, 2nd Session, *Proceedings*, 100–189.

Van Loon, Richard J., & Michael Whittington. (1987). *The Canadian political system*. Toronto: McGraw-Hill.

Wagoner, A. (1964). Three extracts on public finance. In A. Peacole & R. Musgrve (Eds.), *The theory of public finance* (pp. 1–20). New York: St. Martin's Press.

White, Joseph. (1995a). Budgeting and health policy making. In Thomas Mann & Norman Ornstein (Eds.), *Intensive care: How Congress shapes health policy* (pp. 53–78). Washington, D.C.: American Enterprise Institute and The Brookings Institution.

White, Joseph. (1995b). Commentary—the horses and the jumps: Comments on the health care reform steeplechase. *Journal of Health Politics, Policy and Law, 20* (Summer), 373–384.

Wilson, Florence, & Duncan Neuhauser. (1976). *Health services in the United States*. Cambridge: Ballinger Publishing Company.

Wilson, Woodrow. (1956 [1885]). *Congressional government*. New York: Meridian Books.

Yankelovich, Daniel. (1995). The debate that wasn't: The public and the Clinton plan. *Health Affairs, 14* (Spring), 7–23.

CHAPTER

7

The Evolving Challenge of Health Policy Implementation

Frank J. Thompson

The ground under health care policy implementation has shifted radically in the 1990s. The decade began by testing whether we could adequately fathom the implementation issues that would emerge from the adoption of comprehensive health care reform in the United States. It will end by gauging our capacity to cope with the implementation conundrums posed by efforts to reinvent, shrink, and dismantle health care programs, including the popular and successful Medicare. The constant in all this turmoil is that implementation issues continue to matter enormously. Although they exist in the penumbra and shadow of American political life, the administrative politics and processes that play out after a health bill becomes law are as important a part of the policy process as those in evidence prior to passage.

In some respects, the pessimism of the 1990s about government programs can trace its origins to early studies of policy implementation. These studies focused disproportionate attention on good policy intentions gone awry through underperformance, delay, soaring costs, and other factors (Pressman and Wildavsky, 1973; Bardach, 1977; Foltz, 1975). Their dominant theme was that "the great American weakness . . . lies in implementation" (Heclo & Wildavsky, 1974, p. 12).

Clearly, the political culture and institutions of the United States present major challenges for those committed to efficient, effective, and accountable policy implementation. The country features a distinctive political tradition—one built on suspicion of government in general and of centralized power in particular. This political culture with its emphasis on individualism and mistrust of government combines with such institutional factors as the separation of powers, federalism, and weak political parties to fragment power and provide a perilous context for policy implementation (Morone, 1993).

Although it would be folly to discount the implementation potholes on the road to sensible health care policy, it is probably more damaging to exaggerate their significance—to let them become an excuse for not traveling the road at all. As this chapter shows, federal and state governments have enjoyed considerable success in their efforts to implement health care programs (e.g., Thompson, 1981; Goggin, 1987; Moon, 1993). On balance these programs have improved access to medical care, its quality, and the health of the citizenry.

This chapter assesses several important factors that shape policy implementation in the health care arena, including:

- the design of policy mandates—their precision and plausibility as well as their tools, targets, and chosen participants
- the capacity and commitment of administrative agencies
- the implications of using private agents (partners?) to carry out the government's health programs
- the role of federalism—a topic of utmost importance in a period when the national government seems bent on devolving major health programs to the states with less funding

Prior to discussing these factors, however, certain basic ingredients of the implementation process need to be discussed.

IMPLEMENTATION INGREDIENTS

"Health policy implementation" is a deceptively simple phrase. Its meaning seems obvious until matters of formal definition arise; then consensus vanishes. Where, exactly, in the seamless web of the policy process does implementation begin and end? Is it best viewed as carrying out policy, or as the evolution of that policy in new directions (e.g., Goggin et al., 1990; Ingram, 1990; Majone & Wildavsky, 1979)? While these

and related questions are important, I will for present purposes rest content with defining health policy implementation as the program processes generated by a particular health policy mandate or law. These processes lead to some *output* (such as the delivery of care to a patient in a Veterans Administration hospital), which in turn yields some *outcome* (the veteran's health improves, stays the same, or gets worse).

Outputs and outcomes mingle with costs and norms of democratic accountability to provide at least a partial foundation for assessing the degree to which a program succeeds or fails. Do implementing agents operate within the general bounds set by law and the policy preferences of their political masters (the chief executive, the legislative body, and the courts)? Does the program do well on various measures of accomplishment, such as increasing access to medical services, enhancing the quality of care, constraining medical costs, and, ultimately, improving the health of the populace (effectiveness)? How impressive are the benefits engendered by the program relative to the economic costs of operating it (efficiency)? The criteria embedded in these questions certainly fail to exhaust the list of those that can be used to evaluate policy implementation. They do not, for instance, address important symbolic outcomes of implementation that might be part of a health program's report card.[1] But they comprise a set of core categories that deserve a place on that card.

Implementation combines many ingredients, including the strategic, the routine, and the fortuitous. Bardach (1977, pp. 57–58) captures the strategic aspect of implementation when he defines it as "the playing out of a number of loosely interrelated games whereby . . . elements are withheld from or delivered to the program assembly process on particular terms." For instance, the implementation of Medicare features federal administrators, private insurance companies, medical providers, advocacy groups for the elderly, the White

---

[1] A health policy also has symbolic connotations that may yield significant sociopolitical outcomes regardless of whether officials vigorously move to implement it. Laws that administrative agencies do not or cannot implement may nonetheless reinforce commitment to important values in the health arena. In some cases, these policies buy time for government to develop the means for delivering on these value commitments.

House, congressional committees, and others as critical players. These participants bring diverse goals and preferences to the Medicare game. They mobilize power resources, forge coalitions, and plot strategies designed to influence who gets what, when, where, and how from Medicare. Bargaining and compromise often ensue. The health program assembled and delivered in response to strategic maneuvering in countless implementation games may, of course, differ so greatly from the one envisioned by the founding statute as to undercut any notion of implementation as the "carrying out" of health policy.

The processes that give birth to the administrative rules governing health programs often serve as an important focal point for strategic interaction. The federal bureaucracy does not simply impose major administrative regulations and guidelines as it hands down its official interpretation of the law. Rather, civil servants typically draft and publish them in the *Federal Register* with an eye toward giving various interest groups a chance to respond.

In December 1989, for instance, Congress approved a new approach for paying physicians who treated Medicare patients—resource-based relative value scales (RBRVS). This system sought to establish a nationally recognized value for an array of physician services that would reflect the demands of the professional work involved, practice expenses, the cost of professional liability insurance, and the norms of the geographic area where the physician worked. In implementing RBRVS the federal Health Care Financing Administration eventually proposed to reduce the amount paid for surgeries and other highly specialized procedures and to boost the rate for delivering primary care. This approach triggered skirmishes with various physician groups adversely affected by the new system. Notices of proposed rule making in the *Federal Register* become an invitation to negotiate and bargain over the rates (Moon, 1993).

In addition to the strategic, implementation processes feature behavior that occurs with relatively little of the calculation associated with participating in a competitive game. Some of this behavior occurs almost without thinking. The institutional structures and cultures of administrative agencies breed standard operating procedures and informal decision rules that can markedly shape the performance of government programs. These procedures and rules facilitate the reliable performance of tasks by ordinary people. Intake workers at Veterans Administration hospitals, for instance, adhere to certain decision criteria for processing and admitting veterans who seek care from them.

Beyond the strategic and the routine, chance events shape the implementation mosaic for a health program. Conveying the importance of the fortuitous runs against the grain of social scientists who by training tend to emphasize regular or predictable patterns of interaction. Some of them, however, have taken major strides toward capturing these random factors (e.g., Cohen et al., 1972; Kingdon, 1984). One such perspective sees aspects of policy implementation as a process of organized anarchy. In this view, some implementation processes can best be seen as the product of four streams: problems, solutions, participants, and choice opportunities. Although none of the streams is completely independent of the others, this model holds that implementation decisions often derive from a somewhat fortuitous confluence of the four. For instance, the purchase of new computers and utilization review software (a solution) by the Veterans Administration plus the hiring of a new medical director could give those concerned (participants) with the excessive prescription of certain drugs and services (the problem) a chance (choice opportunity) to correct the excesses.

Whether policy implementation in a health care program finds primary expression as a game, as standard operating procedures, informal decision rules, or professional norms, as a somewhat random intersection of streams, or as some other pattern, certain critical factors shape these processes. In this regard, policy design looms particularly large.

HEALTH POLICY DESIGN

The content and structure of the founding statute and subsequent legislative amendments usually reveal the essence of a policy design. A well-designed policy greatly increases prospects for program success. The smartest and most talented administrators can seldom salvage a poorly constructed mandate. In a perfect world, lawmakers would create statutes based on a plausible theory, or hypothesis, about how the health care arena works—that if the government does a, b, and c, then x, y, and z will result. In fact, however, limits to their knowledge and the political dynamics of policy formulation often impede this development. Many features of a policy design shape program fortunes. These include the precision of the statute, policy tools, targets, and the administrative agents invited to the implementation table.

Precision: A Siren Call?

The precision of a statutory mandate is a function of the degree to which it defines terms, quantifies objectives, specifies timetables for obtaining them, indicates priorities among objectives, and prescribes the administrative structure and procedures to be used in implementing the program (Sabatier & Mazmanian, 1979). Highly precise laws provide clear directions for administrative agents.

Precise policy possesses considerable appeal in a democratic society. It seems consistent with the rule of law and the thwarting of unaccountable bureaucratic power. Aside from keeping elected officials in the driver's seat, some experts (for instance, Sabatier & Mazmanian, 1979) see it as a springboard to efficiency and effectiveness. Precise mandates presumably give an agency a weapon to turn against those who oppose its mission; these mandates also win praise for reducing prospects that administrators will lose their sense of direction or dissipate energy by skirmishing with one another over how to interpret the law. In addition, precise mandates allegedly expedite program evaluation and the detection of noncompliance or program difficulties. Some evidence from the health policy arena points to the value of precision. Analyses of such initiatives as the early and periodic screening, diagnosis and treatment program (Foltz, 1975) and the now defunct National Health Planning and Resources Development Act of 1974 point to statutory ambiguity as one source of implementation problems (Thompson, 1981).

If policy designers are not careful, however, the quest for precision can quickly become a search for fool's gold. In rejecting the New Deal tradition of delegating vast discretion to the executive branch, Congress has tended to pass longer and more detailed laws (Melnick, 1994, p. 32). These detailed statutes can pose as many implementation problems as shorter, more ambiguous mandates.[2] The Health Security Act proposed by President Clinton in 1993 is a case in point.

The Clinton Health Plan: Precision to the Fore

President Clinton's proposal for comprehensive health care reform ran 1,431 pages. It drew on the advice of some of the best policy analysts in the country, went to great lengths to specify goals and means, and achieved a remarkable degree of consistency. Yet the girth of the proposal not only exposed it to much criticism in the ensuing debate in Congress; many of the proposal's details would in fact have created serious implementation problems for program administrators had the bill passed. As Paul Starr, a leading expert involved in drafting the plan, subsequently noted: "we had failed to edit the plan down to its essentials and find familiar ways to convey it" (Starr, 1995, p. 25).

Space does not permit a synoptic review of the implementation issues that the Clinton health plan would have created, but a snapshot of its quality assurance provisions provides a useful illustration. The Health Security Act sought to motivate competing health plans to achieve high levels of performance by requiring them to provide report cards to facilitate informed consumer choice. Under the Clinton proposal regional alliances established to select and monitor participating health plans would "make available to eligible enrollees information in an easily understood and useful form, that allows such enrollees . . . to make valid comparisons among health plans" (Thompson, 1994, p. 90). These report cards on cost, access, and quality were to be made available to consumers in a brochure published at least annually. The act called for a newly created federal qual-

---

[2]Lengthy, detailed laws need not, of course, be precise if they contain many contradictory provisions or fail to establish priorities among goals.

ity management council to control the specifics of these report cards. Working with others the council was to develop performance indicators for the health plans concerning the degree to which these plans provided access to appropriate health care services, achieved suitable health outcomes, and ensured consumer satisfaction with care.

Ultimately, the Clinton proposal was extremely ambitious. It asked plans to produce data for report cards that no one had ever systematically assembled before on this scale (e.g., on the health outcomes of a range of treatments). The plans would inevitably face difficulties obtaining and "scrubbing" the data to ensure their validity. Had the Health Security Act passed, implementing agents would not have been able to produce the required report cards in the time frame envisioned by the law. The same can be said of many other provisions in the Clinton health plan.

Vague Laws as the Fount of Creative Evolution

If precise laws at times undermine effectiveness, vague laws can on occasion lead to program success. In 1970, for example, Congress passed an ambiguous, four-page statute that authorized placement of Public Health Service physicians in medical shortage areas as part of what eventually became known as the National Health Service Corps (NHSC). This foggy mandate made it possible for the program to undergo a metamorphosis in the 1970s. At first, agency officials stressed the objective of retaining NHSC physicians in private practice within shortage areas after they left the corps—an effort that met with little success. By the end of the decade, agency officials had turned their backs on this concern. Instead, they stressed the placement of such physicians in community health centers and other federally supported organizations that provided care to the poor in larger cities. They emphasized reenlistment in the NHSC after a physician's term of duty had expired rather than placement in the private sector. In critical respects, this shift permitted the program to achieve a higher level of effectiveness. The corps served those who otherwise faced difficulty obtaining care. Retention rates rose along with various measures of physi-

cian productivity (Thompson, 1981). Although the Reagan administration radically reduced the flow of funds to the program, it nonetheless remains useful as an example of creative program evolution.

Ultimately, debates about administrative discretion and the importance of statutory precision cannot be settled without understanding context. Under what circumstances will less precise statutes more readily foster positive program results? Several factors, among others, loom large.

First, statutory ambiguity more readily generates creative evolution when lawmakers cannot turn to a good underlying theory in drafting legislation and problems seem so pressing that something must be done (throwing money at the problem may be the only hope). Policymakers may experience uncertainty about the best path to a widely agreed-upon goal. For example, Congress simply does not know how best to allocate funds to specific research projects to guarantee a reduction in the cancer mortality rate. But uncertainty may be even more fundamental. Policymakers may feel compelled to act but uncertain about their preferences. In this regard, March (1978, pp. 595, 603) has argued that when decision makers have confused and contradictory preferences, "precision misrepresents them." Policymaking involves guesses not only about the future consequences of various alternatives but also about preferences for these consequences. At times, policymakers discover their preferences as they see a program evolve—even when it goes in directions they did not originally anticipate. Congress, for instance, was aware of the significant shift in the direction of the NHSC and continued to support the program.

Second, specific health statutes seem less fruitful when rapidly changing social and economic factors promise to threaten the validity of any precisely worded hypothesis. It would, for example, make no sense for policymakers to specify in great detail appropriate care for certain kinds of illnesses in light of rapid advances in medical technology.

Third, creative program evolution in the face of an ambiguous statute occurs more readily when a tempered consensus exists within the implementing agency as to its fundamental mission and this mission is not at odds with the general thrust of the statute. In the case of the NHSC, for example, top officials responsible for the program shared a strong commitment to delivering care to the disadvantaged through group practices such as community health centers. Without internal accord of this kind, vague legislation can fuel internal tensions and dysfunctional delay as civil servants fight with one another over the proper definition of program goals and means.

The wrong kind of consensus can, of course, impair implementation. Tempered commitment exists within an implementation agency when its key personnel strike a reasonable balance between skepticism and dogma. Skepticism or hostility can breed sabotage or lethargic program implementation. The concept of tempered commitment also recognizes that too much commitment (dogma, zealotry) can hurt a program. Implementors who are "true believers" often fail to acknowledge evidence of program shortcomings and tenaciously cling to certain strategies and tactics no matter how dysfunctional. Innovative administrators must be open to admitting their mistakes and learning from them.

Fourth, ambiguous statutes more readily spark creative evolution if the implementing agents face an environment less dense with groups and individuals intensely opposed to the efficient and effective implementation of the program. Where such resistance exists, program officials typically need more precise grants of statutory authority and persistent backing from the courts, the legislative branch, and the chief executive. For example, state agencies charged with regulating payment rates to providers need clearly specified statutory grants of authority to accomplish this.

Finally, precise legislation becomes less appealing when doubts exist about the efficacy of key principals (legislative bodies, the chief executive, and the courts). Efficacy increases to the degree that these actors possess the capacity and commitment to formulate theoretically sound and coherent policies as well as to engage in learning that allows them to repair programs. Efficacious principals effectively exploit the knowledge base available in society to guide policy development.

Efficacy of this sort is often in short supply. Policymakers frequently show little sensitivity to issues of ad-ministrative capacity and implementation feasibility in formulating policy. The fragmentation and fractiousness of the American political system can make coherent policy design very difficult to achieve. Compared to various parliamentary democracies, legislation in the United States tends to be drafted with less care. "Many American statutes lack coherence, fail to resolve key controversies, or even incorporate inconsistent requirements" (Melnick, 1994, pp. 10–11). These conditions bode poorly for efforts to draft precise legislation. It deserves emphasis that statutory ambiguity need not automatically become a recipe for less democratic accountability so long as policymakers possess ample information on the direction and nature of program evolution. As Ingram (1990, p. 473) has observed, "passage of a statute needs to be seen as a benchmark from which to measure, not the achievement of the embodied objectives, but progress toward doable and agreeable policy."

Many Tools

Health policy design also involves choices of tools, or instruments, to accomplish certain ends (Elmore, 1987, p. 175; see also Salamon, 1989). The search for a parsimonious typology of tools represents a small-scale version of the quest for the Holy Grail. Scholars seek a typology that would allow them to predict precisely the implications of employing a particular tool. So far, however, the world of public policy has proven too messy and complicated to permit this quest to succeed fully. Among other things, policies typically draw on a mix of tools to accomplish their ends, which makes it hard to isolate the effects of using a particular instrument. Nonetheless, we can acquire some insight into the challenges of health policy implementation by focusing on two general types of tools: regulatory and allocative.

Regulatory Tools

Certain policies call on government to prescribe and control the behavior of a particular target group by monitoring the group and imposing sanctions if it fails to comply. Examples of regulatory approaches abound in the health care arena. Federally funded peer review organizations (PROs), for instance, develop and enforce standards concerning appropriate care under the Medicare program. State insurance departments across the country regulate health insurance companies in their jurisdictions in an effort to protect the customers of these companies from insurer financial failure, excessive premiums, and other mendacious practices. States regulate the division of labor in the health care sector by insisting that only medical doctors can perform certain functions as opposed, say, to nurses or physician's assistants.

When health policy designers adopt a regulatory approach, at least four basic questions about implementation immediately surface. First, what rules or standards should the agency promulgate to define acceptable and unacceptable behavior? The founding statute seldom spells out the answer, in no small part because it is a very tough question. For instance, government agencies responsible for quality assurance in the medical sector face the perplexing task of defining what quality care means in a given case. Definitions of quality vary and grappling with them plunges one into a dense empirical and ethical thicket. Impenetrable underbrush often obscures the causal relationship between medical care and health outcomes. Norms of "appropriate" care vary from one region of the country to the next (Thompson, 1994).

Second, how should regulators disseminate information about the rules to the target group? For example, regulators need to make sure that providers understand their definition of what constitutes appropriate care—to get the message out.

Third, how should monitoring occur to detect failure to comply with standards? Regulatory agencies typically lack the resources to monitor their environments thoroughly to discover all infractions of the rules. For instance, many state insurance agencies lack the resources to do annual reviews of licensed health insurance companies and to conduct in-depth analysis when they initiate reviews. As a result, they may fail to head off financial debacle. In 1990, for instance, the West Virginia Blue Cross and Blue Shield failed and fifty thousand policy holders were stuck with nearly $40 million in unpaid claims (U.S. General Accounting Office, 1993).

Fourth, what penalties or remedial action should the regulator impose on those discovered to be in violation of the rules? Should, for instance, the government withdraw medical licenses for extended periods from physicians convicted of malpractice? Or, in the interest of not wasting a critical resource and promoting access to medical care, should the government make the penalty milder and permit the doctor to "reform" and practice again in the relatively near future?

Allocative Tools

These tools involve the direct provision of income, services, or goods to groups of individuals who usually see benefit in receiving them. Allocative tools in the health care arena appear in myriad forms. These tools subsidize providers to deliver care to specific groups (e.g., the elderly, the poor, and veterans), the construction of facilities (e.g., hospitals and the Hill–Burton program), the development of personnel (e.g., medical education for those who participate in the National Health Service Corps), the initiation of certain institutional forms (e.g., health maintenance organizations), and the production and dissemination of knowledge (e.g., the basic medical research of the National Institutes of Health, the medical practice guidelines prepared by the Agency for Health Care Policy and Research).

One set of questions faced by those implementing allocative programs involves targeting the benefit. How can they focus distribution of the resource on those who need it most in a manner consistent with law? In this regard, state Medicaid administrators have faced constant pressure from the federal government to reduce their eligibility error rates—especially miscues that allow ineligible individuals to receive benefits.

Administrators also face temptations to spread benefits over many congressional districts even if this shifts program resources from those most in need. During the 1970s, for instance, officials at the Department of Health, Education, and Welfare came under increasing pressure to broaden the definition of primary care shortage areas because such areas were eligible for National Health Service Corps physicians. Having published the criteria and an initial list of shortage areas in

1974, administrators soon moved to expand the roster. The result was that the total number of primary care shortage areas soared from just over 500 in late 1974 to nearly 1,200 by September 1978. To accomplish this expansion, administrators abandoned their initial rule that a shortage area needed to have a population to primary care physician ratio of greater than 4,000 to 1. They instead decided that a ratio of 3,500 to 1 should serve as the cut point, or even 3,000 to 1 if certain other circumstances applied (Thompson, 1981, pp. 80–108).

Although direct payments from the government's coffers represent a pervasive approach, allocative tools also assume such guises as loans, loan guarantees, and tax expenditures. For instance, the Health Maintenance Organization Act of 1973 sought to encourage the development and proliferation of certain kinds of managed care organizations that policymakers hoped would be more efficient than standard fee-for-service practice. Qualified public or private nonprofit organizations could receive loans during their initial thirty-six months of operation to meet deficits encountered in providing services. Other proprietary entities could apply for federal loan guarantees for planning, development, and initial operation if they proposed to serve a "medically underserved" population.

Obviously the appeal of loans or loan guarantees to policymakers is that they can induce behavior without actually appearing in the budget as an expenditure. From the perspective of policy implementation, however, the task is to steer loans and loan guarantees to those who would not otherwise have engaged in the activity desired by the government. At the same time, officials do not wish to channel funds to those who will default on payment and thereby convert the loan or loan guarantee into a failed government grant. In the case of the HMO program, federal officials worked hard to prevent bad loans but at the risk of not having much stimulative impact. As Brown (1983, p. 327) notes:

> The HMO act authorized loans to HMOs to cover their early operating deficits. To obtain the loan, however, the plan had to be qualified as an HMO as defined by law and regulations. One criterion for qualification was that the plan be financially viable. But many plans needed the loan

to attain that condition, and for many, time was of the essence . . . the difference between survival and bankruptcy.

In the case of tax expenditures, another important policy tool, the government uses the tax code to provide an incentive for firms and individuals to engage in certain behavior in the health care arena. The tax system in the United States affords people who obtain health insurance through their place of employment more favorable treatment by excluding from federal taxation the subsidy the employer provides them to obtain health insurance. This policy costs the federal treasury nearly $100 billion per year in taxes that would otherwise be paid (Pauly & Goodman, 1995, p. 131). It provides an incentive for employees to seek compensation from employers in the form of health insurance rather than other taxable benefits. So long as the Internal Revenue Service can achieve reasonable compliance with the tax law, this policy tool poses fewer implementation issues than many others. However, calibrating the tax expenditure to motivate just the "right" amount of certain behavior in the health arena often boils down to guesstimates.

Qualities of the Target Group

Policy design also involves the formal selection of a group to be targeted for benefits or regulation. The resources and other characteristics of this group can markedly shape the implementation challenge. The social construction of the target—the cultural characterization or popular images of it—matters greatly. Other things being equal, the implementation of programs that seek to help favorably viewed groups such as the elderly tends to be easier and more vigorous than programs aimed at groups less popular with the public, such as welfare mothers (Schneider & Ingram, 1993).

In the case of regulatory policies, high-status groups such as physicians and hospitals frequently enjoy more opportunities to engage in self-regulation. In terms of allocative policies, programs that redistribute from the more affluent to serve means-tested target groups usually face more difficulties sustaining important political support. In this sense, "a program for the poor is a poor program."[3] Medicare, which subsidizes health care for nearly all of the elderly regardless of their income, enjoys broader, more supportive constituencies and generally faces fewer implementation problems than Medicaid, which relies heavily on means tests for eligibility and focuses on the poor.

Of course, the social construction of the elderly is not the only factor at work here. The propensity of the elderly to vote and participate politically no doubt figures into the clout the group possesses in implementation processes. More affluent, educated, and politically participative target groups stand a better chance of obtaining administrative deference to their needs than groups without these resources.

The Implementation Lineup

Policy design also involves selecting the official lineup of players who will participate in the implementation game. Other uninvited players may enter the game later, but the founding mandate usually establishes a number of key participants.

In the abstract, of course, there is nothing to stop policymakers from keeping things simple by holding the number of implementation players to a minimum. In the case of the Veterans Administration medical system, for instance, Congress charged a single federal agency (now the Department of Veterans Affairs) with carrying out a program to ensure that veterans have access to medical care for service-related and other health problems. The culture and institutions of the American political system, however, tilt overwhelmingly against such a direct approach. Skepticism (and in these times, an epidemic of cynicism) about government and centralized authority has fueled tendencies to rely on private-sector providers to deliver a vast array of health care programs. The institutions of federalism also open the door to participation by state and local governments as implementing agents.

As in selecting the lineup for a sports team, at least two key questions loom large: Do those selected have

the capacity both individually and as a team to achieve victory—to deliver the program efficiently, effectively, and accountably? Do they have the commitment to do so? The next three sections of this chapter take up some of the issues suggested by these questions.

AGENCY CAPACITY AND COMMITMENT

The commitment and capacity of the agencies formally charged with implementing a program greatly affect its destiny. As suggested earlier, program prospects improve when key personnel sustain tempered commitment—a willingness to work hard to achieve program goals without falling prey to zealotry or dogma. At times concerns about agency commitment enter into policy design. When, in the late 1980s, Congress moved to pass legislation placing greater emphasis on research that would yield practice guidelines for physicians, the American Medical Association and others successfully argued that the program should be placed in a new Agency for Health Care Policy and Research rather than in the Health Care Financing Administration (HCFA). The physicians group believed that HCFA's strong commitment to saving money in Medicare and Medicaid would influence its selection of research and shape the practice parameters it issued. In contrast, they hoped that the Agency for Health Care Policy and Research would be more open to practice guidelines that promised little or no cost savings (Morone, 1993).

Agency capacity depends on the presence of at least three major factors, among others:

- adequate resources, that is, status (or prestige), authority, money, personnel, information or expertise, and physical facilities and equipment
- skilled leadership and management sensitive to the technical core of the agency's mission and the art of administrative politics
- institutional arrangements, especially standard operating procedures, conducive to accomplishing program objectives

---

[3]This was the dictum of program executives in the Social Security Administration (Derthick, 1979, p. 217).

No simple index exists to monitor administrative capacity, but most agencies must contend with powerful forces that can erode their ability to deliver health care programs.

Among the factors that threaten implementation capacity, none ranks higher in importance than the limited status, or prestige, of public administration in the United States. Compared to their counterparts in other industrialized democracies, civil servants in the United States suffer from low public esteem. One observer aptly notes that "the ineffectiveness and inefficiency" of the public sector is a belief "so widely and firmly held that one . . . can regard it as a unifying theme of our creed" (Waldo, 1980, p. 17). Suspicion and mistrust of bureaucracy show up even among liberals who support government action to accomplish health care reform (Jacobs, 1993). Sensing this vulnerability, the media, oversight committees in Congress, and others often caricature the performance of public bureaucracies. They become expert at blaming administrative agencies—at making them "the fall guys of American government"—rather than at helping administrators keep their programs on track (Derthick, 1990, p. 181).

Health agencies with excellent performance records may dodge some of the problems spawned by the limited status of public administration. But even they cannot escape it completely. The Medicare program, for instance, has much lower administrative costs per benefits paid than private insurance companies. Yet various political players sporadically toss brickbats at the program, claiming that it is bureaucratic and wasteful.

Nor is this prestige deficit confined to the federal government. In its assessment of the status of public Health Departments across the country, the Institute of Medicine (1988, p. 85) noted that "Public Health agencies suffered from the generally poor image of bureaucrats." One state legislator interviewed for the institute's study called public health officials "eunuchs" and "consummate bureaucrats." Some members of the medical community described public health workers "as passive survivors, 'also rans' in the world of health."

The limited status of public administration makes it harder for the government to secure the other critical resources it needs to achieve high performance. Attracting and retaining the "best and the brightest" employees becomes more arduous. Low status also opens agencies up to charges that they are fat and can readily be downsized at no cost to program efficiency and effectiveness. It heightens the appeal of cumbersome control systems designed to reduce the potential for administrative abuse, rather than for systems that enhance prospects for innovation and effectiveness. Low status magnifies the risk that policy implementation will become a defensive and nonexperimental exercise where officials spend much time maneuvering to avoid scrutiny, blame, and responsibility (Bardach, 1977, p. 37). It makes administrative agencies more dependent on support from outside groups even though catering to them can deflect these agencies from their mission.

In these and countless other ways, the limited status of government service in the United States assures that capacity problems will be chronic—a persistent, severe, and nagging cold that gets better from time to time but never seems to go away. Although few would prefer a political system where public administration enjoys such high esteem as to breed government complacency or arrogance, the United States has pushed so far in the opposite direction as to make this problem remote.

In spite of this difficult context, the administrative agencies of the government often manage to sustain sufficient capacity to score impressive victories. At times the bureaucracy's mastery of highly technical subject matter allows it to innovate and resist debilitating external pressures. Consider the evolution of Medicare payment approaches for hospitals and physicians. When Medicare started in 1965, it used a cost-based reimbursement formula that provided generous payments to providers and fueled program inefficiencies. In the wake of congressional action, HCFA moved in the early 1980s to develop a hospital payment strategy based on diagnosis-related groups (DRGs). By the early 1990s, the agency introduced payment for physicians based on resource-based relative value scales. In both cases, the mind-numbing complexities of these formulas gave HCFA officials the opportunity to exploit their expertise to exert substantial leverage. The technical nature of this implementation game heightened the entry costs for other players and made it difficult for them to use cultural stereotypes about the "incompetence" of public bureaucracies (Morone, 1993).

PUBLIC MONEY FOR PRIVATE DELIVERY

Policymakers frequently insert private entities into the implementation lineup. The single largest health care program in the nation, Medicare, stands as vivid testimony to this approach. Medicare provides health insurance to over 38 million elderly and disabled people and had projected outlays of nearly $178 billion in fiscal 1996 (about 11 percent of total estimated federal spending). Yet HCFA, the agency charged with implementing it, employs only four thousand personnel to accomplish this mammoth task. The reason for this gaping disparity between budget and personnel is simple. HCFA contracts with seventy-nine insurance companies to ensure payment to the nonfederal hospitals, physicians, and other providers who deliver services to Medicare recipients.

Observers have appropriately touted Medicare as a major implementation success story (e.g., Moon, 1993). Its contracting insurance carriers and intermediaries process huge numbers of claims—roughly 650 million in fiscal 1992—and pay providers with reasonable dispatch (National Performance Review, 1993a). Medicare eligibles have had great freedom to choose their providers and without question the program has improved their access to medical care and contributed to their health and longevity. Moreover, its administrative price tag has been relatively low. Medicare's administrative costs are about 3 percent of its expenditures compared to roughly 10 percent for private health insurance plans (Moon, 1993, p. 209).[4]

---

[4]Technical debates flourish over how precisely to define and measure administrative costs. The U.S. Office of Technology Assessment (1994, p. 14) notes, for instance, that official estimates of Medicare's administrative costs do not include a pro-rated portion of the cost of acquiring the contracting insurer's administrative infrastructure. Private insurance companies have this infrastructure in place to serve their nonfederal customers. But the Office of Technology Assessment makes no effort to estimate the "true" administrative costs of Medicare. Nor is it crystal clear that these infrastructure estimates are not already included in Medicare's administrative costs.

Medicare's accomplishments do not come automatically, of course. Privatized service strategies do not end the need for sophisticated management by the government; to the contrary, they often increase it. Medicare's leaders and managers must daily cope with difficult administrative problems and certainly do not escape all implementation pitfalls.

Advocates of privatization believe that it galvanizes efficiency and effectiveness via a market stimulus. Private agents presumably compete vigorously with one another to become the supplier of some government good or service. They seek to impress purchasers with the amount and quality of the output they deliver relative to its cost. Government officials and (in the case of Medicare) program beneficiaries have access to information about the performance of private agents and readily understand it. If these agents fail to deliver the promised service or product at a reasonable cost, purchasers can fire them and move on to another agent. In fact, of course, this model often bears little resemblance to reality. Limited information, constraints on competition, and a potpourri of political factors often vitiate its logic. Medicare's relationship with its carriers and intermediaries serves as a case in point.

HCFA and Its Contractors

Are the health insurance companies who contract to process Medicare claims the masters or servants of the government? In a world where the government was the master, HCFA officials would have discretion to contract with private companies that would deliver the most bang for the buck. HCFA would inform hospitals and physicians which company would process their claims. These companies would be subject to HCFA direction and terminated if they failed to produce. In fact, however, HCFA's relationship with contracting carriers (which pay physicians) and intermediaries (which reimburse hospitals) departs greatly from this model.

At the time of Medicare's birth in 1965, insurance companies claimed that their close relationships with medical providers would allow them to establish effective payment and utilization review practices. Subsequent events revealed these assertions to be long on promise and short on delivery. Program costs soared. Federal frustration with the performance of these companies grew to the point that, in 1973, the Department of Health, Education, and Welfare established the Perkins Committee to examine Medicare's contracts with the insurance industry. Among other things, the committee recommended development of more systematic means for measuring the performance of insurance companies, defining ways of terminating those contractors that performed poorly, and improving cost reporting and accounting. Subsequently, the federal government inched toward implementing some of these recommendations (U.S. House Committee on Appropriations, 1977).

But problems persisted. Twenty years after the establishment of the Perkins Committee, the Clinton administration's initiative to reinvent government, the National Performance Review (1993b), singled out Medicare's relationships with its insurance contractors as an area in need of reform. The National Performance Review diagnosed two main infirmities in Medicare's contracting provisions (National Performance Review, 1993a, pp. 80–83; see also 1993b).

First, laws handcuffed HCFA in selecting contractors to process claims. Hospitals under Medicare Part A had the right to choose the intermediary that would process and review the bills they submitted. This approach created incentives for insurance companies to appease these hospitals, especially in the initial phases of the program. A contracting company that tried to get tough with hospitals faced the prospect of being "fired" and seeing the hospital shift to a contractor with a reputation for being a softer touch. As for Medicare Part B claims—those submitted primarily by physicians—HCFA by law can only contract with insurance companies to perform this service. Other kinds of firms are excluded.

Second, the multiple business interests of carriers and intermediaries at times conflicted with their Medicare obligations. Insurance companies have often attempted to make the government pay a disproportionate share of their overhead costs. By so doing, they enhance their competitive position when they market their private plans to employers and others. Moreover,

contracting companies at times skirt the Medicare requirement that the federal government pay the bill only if the patient does not have private health insurance. Contractors often fail to catch bills that should be submitted to private insurance companies—perhaps themselves—and instead let the government pick up the tab. To impede federal investigation of the degree to which this problem exists, insurance companies exerted influence in Congress to get laws passed that restrict HCFA from insisting that contractors share insurance information concerning their private businesses with their Medicare claims processing units. One study suggests that less than 10 percent of the contractors routinely perform data matches with their private insurance to identify when Medicare should be the secondary payer (National Performance Review, 1993a, pp. 80–81).

These and related constraints prompted the report of the National Performance Review (1993a, p. 80) to conclude: "No other government agency operates under the same constraints as HCFA in managing its contractors. Legal, regulatory, and local political constraints undermine HCFA's ability to contract competitively with those contractors who can best perform claims processing activities."

HCFA Exerts More Leverage

If aspects of the HCFA's relationship with contractors and providers hardly project the image of a powerful bureaucracy, it would be misleading to portray the federal government as putty in the hands of insurance companies. Over time, HCFA has evolved a more exacting set of performance standards that it expects carriers to meet as it processes claims. Much of contemporary theorizing about reinventing public administration emphasizes the importance of setting performance targets for contractors, giving them wide latitude in how they pursue these targets, and holding them accountable for achieving results. This argument makes considerable sense. But as the case of Medicare indicates, the quest to find the right productivity measures can be complex indeed.

Understandably, HCFA wants its contractors to pay only the valid claims of providers. Invalid provider claims may spring from fraud, clerical errors, and poor judgment about the most efficient and effective care. To avoid these sources of waste, HCFA officials understand that they must provide their insurance contractors with incentive to say "no" to providers when they submit illegitimate claims.

Medicare officials have in fact found a way to get these companies to scrutinize and reject claims. In fiscal year 1993, for instance, Medicare carriers turned down 19 percent of all Part B (physician) claims submitted. The program saved some $17 billion in denied claims for Part B—about 18 percent of all billed charges (U.S. General Accounting Office, 1994, p. 2). Although most claim denials result from routine administrative checks (e.g., rejections of duplicate claims for the same service), many involve more subjective judgments concerning what constitutes appropriate care. In some instances, HCFA has established national standards to guide carriers in dealing with this issue. But in the case of other diseases, the agency has respected the fact that medical treatment norms vary considerably from one area of the country to the next and granted carriers the discretion to develop and apply their own practice protocols for screening claims.

Given this discretion and the incentive carriers have to get along with providers, how does HCFA prod them into denying so many claims? Much of the answer lies in the contractor performance evaluation program, which HCFA established in the late 1970s. This program required each carrier to achieve an overall return of some number of dollars saved ($5 in 1988) for every administrative dollar HCFA gave the carrier for medical review. As a result, carriers have a strong incentive to deny claims if they wish to preserve the profit they receive from Medicare.

Performance indicators, however, often take on a life of their own—creating incentives for behavior of dubious value. Ironically, the performance standards established by HCFA provide carriers with no incentive to educate physicians to reduce the number of erroneous claims. If physicians were to submit only valid claims, the carrier would not be able to show X dollar savings from its review activities unless it denied legitimate submissions (Grogan et al., 1994). At times the system has

encouraged carriers to be aggressive about denying certain claims when a less confrontational and abrasive approach might well be better. For instance, carriers receive significant numbers of claims that cannot be processed because of incomplete information on the form. One way to approach this would be to return the claim for completion or to obtain the needed information in some other way. When HCFA recommended that the denial option be eliminated for handling incomplete claims, however, insurance carriers protested because returned claims would not count in their workload data in the way that denials do (U.S. General Accounting Office, 1994, pp. 16–18).

The conundrums of establishing appropriate performance targets for contractors illustrate the persistent challenges that the program faces. Considerable room for improvement exists. But these trees should not obscure the forest. Medicare has scored impressive achievements. Originally placed in a very weak position, relentless cost pressures have buttressed the ability of the federal bureaucracy to hold contractors and providers more accountable. Although HCFA may not yet be the master in its dealings with contracting carriers and intermediaries, it is at least an implementation partner.

DEVOLUTION TO THE STATES

By the 1990s, the states had firmly established themselves as critical implementing agents in any effort to change the health care system. President Clinton's plan to provide health insurance to all Americans assigned a major role to them. After Republicans seized control of Congress in 1994, their quest to cut taxes and budgets drove them to advocate a block grant for Medicaid and other health programs that would give vast new discretion to the states along with less federal money.

Students of implementation have viewed state involvement with ambivalence. Some see it as a sure-fire way to lower the odds for program success. In this view, states emerge as a very mixed assortment of implementation partners, the worst of which may be marginally competent, dilatory, and feckless when it comes to carrying out the spirit of federal legislation. At a bare minimum, they see states as multiplying the transaction costs of delivering federal programs. Others, however, see the involvement of states as the ticket for ensuring that federal policy sustains its legitimacy and democratic flavor by remaining responsive to preferences found in different areas of the country. They credit state lawmakers and administrators with being closer to the problem and having more insight than the federal government concerning how to deliver a health care program efficiently and effectively. The degree to which the pessimistic or optimistic scenario comes closer to the mark depends largely on whether federal policy design takes into account issues of state commitment and capacity.

Commitment: Race to the Bottom?

As noted elsewhere in this volume, states vary greatly in their political cultures and institutions. This translates into significant differences among them in their commitment to carrying out and maximizing the impact of federal health policy, especially when such policy seeks to help the poor.

When state officials lack interest in implementing a federal policy, Washington usually faces major (although not necessarily insurmountable) problems in persuading them to do so. Efforts to discipline an errant state will typically unleash pressure on the federal agency from that state's congressional delegation and others. Forcing states to comply by taking them to the courts is cumbersome and not always a viable option for federal officials. These officials can exert leverage by threatening to withhold federal funds for state health care programs. But this is a blunt weapon because it threatens most the very beneficiaries (e.g., the poor) that the federal government wants to help.

Most of the time, however, states can realize their preferences without open resistance. Federal policy usually provides room for state governments to express varying degrees of commitment to a program. Nowhere is this variation more patent than in the case of Medicaid—a program that has provided states with wide latitude concerning eligibility, payment, and service decisions. One indicator of state commitment to

implementing the program is the percentage of Medicaid recipients to the persons in poverty in a given state. As of 1991, this indicator ranged from 165 percent in Rhode Island to 42 percent in Nevada. Among the five most populous states (which encompass just over 35 percent of the country's population) Pennsylvania ranked first on this indicator of commitment (95%), followed by New York (90%), California (83%), Florida (60%), and Texas (58%). Thanks in part to the expansion of federal mandates requiring states to expand eligibility to certain categories of pregnant women and children, state variation on this indicator dropped appreciably from 1979 through 1991 (Coughlin et al., 1994, pp. 72–73). However, the move toward enhanced state discretion under Medicaid in the late 1990s could well bring back higher levels of state variation.[5]

In an era when states will acquire increased discretion to implement health programs, the question naturally arises: Will they engage in a race to the bottom, especially in the case of programs that involve taxation of the more affluent to serve the poor? Competition among states for economic development could unleash this bid-down effect. Decisions to provide generous benefit packages could drive up state taxes. At some threshold higher taxes for such purposes tend to discourage firms and affluent individuals from remaining in or moving to the state, thereby eroding its revenue capacity. Simultaneously, generous redistributive programs may become a magnet, attracting needy people to move to the state and thereby placing additional fiscal stress on that government (Peterson & Rom, 1988; Peterson et al., 1995).

The exact degree to which firms and people migrate in response to state tax policies and the generosity of health care programs for the poor remains uncertain. But state officials often perceive that they do. These concerns have, for instance, been among those driving Governor George Pataki in New York to propose major cuts in that state's Medicaid program. Businesses fre-

---

[5]Other indicators of state commitment to Medicaid showed less convergence. For instance, interstate variation in Medicaid expenditures per adult and child recipient remained essentially unchanged between 1984 and 1991. Individual states, however, did change their rankings (Coughlin et al., 1994, p. 76).

quently use the threat of exit to influence state and local policies. Although this is partly an exercise in crying "wolf," state officials cannot safely dismiss this warning, especially in light of factors that have heightened the ability of firms to move in response to uncompetitive tax rates. These factors include (Rivlin, 1992, p. 138):

- improvements in transportation and communication that greatly enhance the geographic mobility of people, goods, and services
- an economy dominated by large companies that operate in multiple locations and can easily shift activities and jobs from one place to the next
- the greater incidence of service industries, many of which can relocate and perform their activities at a substantial geographic distance from their customers

If the dynamics of state competition for economic development in fact spark a race to the bottom, what patterns of behavior would occur in an era when states have increased discretion? Above all, we would expect to see a diminution in the expenditure effort that most states devote to Medicaid—measured, for instance, as the proportion of total state personnel income spent on Medicaid payments to providers minus the federal financial contribution (Barrilleaux and Miller, 1988). States would, under this scenario, also become more comparable in effort as generous states lowered benefits in an attempt to close the gap between themselves and their more parsimonious counterparts. Even if these two developments occur, however, state Medicaid programs could still vary considerably in payment strategies, eligibility standards, and the service packages they provide. States that achieved greater creativity in developing and implementing their programs might purchase more medical care access and quality per dollar spent. Moreover, to the degree that some states enjoyed greater prosperity, they could invest much more heavily than other states in the Medicaid program even though their expenditure effort, as defined above, did not increase.

Whether in fact states will race or drift to the bottom under the new Medicaid remains, of course, an open question. The next decade will in all probability provide a golden opportunity to test whether the pessimists or optimists have more accurately assayed the commitment of the states to Medicaid.

State Capacity: Forward and Backward

Up until the 1960s, most state governments were political and administrative backwaters. Their legislatures and bureaucracies lacked professional staffs; their governors did not have authority over many line agencies; relatively low pay and patronage characterized personnel administration; election processes assured that urban areas lacked proportionate representation in state legislatures; many southern states ruthlessly denied minorities the right to vote and engage in meaningful political participation.

Those days are now gone. Virtually everyone agrees that in the past thirty years, states have surged forward in bolstering their capacity for efficient, effective, democratic governance. As the U.S. Advisory Commission on Intergovernment Relations put it in the mid-1980s, state governments had become "more representative, more responsive, more activist, and more professional in their operations than they ever have been" (1985, p. 365). Hence, those concerned with health care policy can turn to the states with more confidence that they have the wherewithal to be effective implementation partners.

If states have unquestionably become better candidates for implementing federal health policy, it would nonetheless be a big mistake to adopt a sunny outlook on the subject. Patches of drizzle and some destructive storms quickly become apparent when we examine the administrative, political, and ecological capacity of the states.

Clouds on the Horizon for Administrative Capacity

Many states continue to struggle with issues of administrative capacity. As discussed earlier, such capacity refers to institutional features of state implementing agents as well as their ability to obtain and manage such critical resources as personnel and information. Proponents of reinventing government have noted that many of the progressive reforms of the past have come full circle to become systemic obstacles to more efficient and effective performance. For instance, the National Commission on the State and Local Public Service (1993a, pp. 1, 4) observed that states often "hamstring their chief executives by diffusing their power. They operate with antiquated and obsolete personnel, procurement, and budget systems. They fail to invest in the most critical resource they have: their rank and file personnel. . . . In many ways it could be described as a system undergoing death by a thousand paper cuts."

Analyses focused specifically on state health agencies have noted similar problems (e.g., National Commission on the State and Local Public Service, 1993b; Institute of Medicine, 1988). For example, a study of barriers to the effective management of Medicaid agencies in four states—California, Minnesota, Mississippi, and New York—found that staff cutbacks, civil service restrictions, and an "eternal crisis atmosphere" consistently posed problems. Structural fragmentation at times undercuts the program. In New York, for instance, management responsibility for Medicaid is fragmented among several state agencies and county governments—a pattern that can sap managerial coherence and boost the leverage of interest groups. In other instances, rapid turnover of those in top leadership positions in health care agencies undermines prospects for efficient and effective implementation (Sparer & Brown, 1993).

Nor can state administrators necessarily count on enjoying higher public esteem than their federal counterparts. For instance, when asked who would do the best job of managing health care in the United States, 18 percent of a random sample of adults identified the federal government; 19 percent, the states; and 48 percent, the private sector (Fact Finders, 1994). When asked more generally about their confidence in different levels of the federal system, state governments at best enjoy only a marginal advantage over their federal counterpart (Thompson, 1993, pp. 10–11).

Like members of Congress, state lawmakers tend to devote scant attention to issues of organization building, capacity, and implementation. As two seasoned observers of state health care policy observe, "underinvestment in state management and implementation capacities [by policymakers] is penny-wise, pound-foolish, perverse, and predictable" (Tallon & Brown, 1994, p. 58).

State initiatives to introduce managed care plans under Medicaid drive this point home. The number of Medicaid enrollees in these plans increased greatly in the early 1990s. Start-up of these initiatives often bordered on the chaotic, as the experience of the widely heralded TennCare program in Tennessee attests (Holahan et al., 1995). At the program's starting date, January 1, 1994, Tennessee Medicaid officials had not completed contracting with providers to establish the managed care networks. Some Medicaid recipients had to choose a plan without knowing whether the physician who had treated them in the past would be part of it. Nor had the state developed smooth systems for processing provider bills, which resulted in slow payment. Data on patient encounters that the networks were to submit to state officials so that access to and the quality of care could be monitored were not complete one year after the program had begun. A survey of Medicaid recipients found that 45 percent of enrollees who previously received care under Medicaid's fee-for-service program expressed less satisfaction with TennCare (U.S. General Accounting Office, 1995a, p. 41).

Threats to Political Capacity

Questions of administrative capacity are part of a broader set of issues related to the ability of states to govern effectively and responsively. Being an implementation agent in the federal system requires action not just by administrative agencies but by an array of other political players. In this regard, questions loom large as to whether states possess the political institutions to govern democratically and effectively so that, for instance, they can set and maintain priorities, reconcile conflicting objectives, manage societal cleavages, and represent diffuse, unorganized interests in addition to concentrated, well-organized ones (Weaver & Rockman, 1993, p. 6).

Although states have on the whole increased their capacity for democratic governance, several complications have arisen. One of the chief storm clouds has been a movement to hamstring the states fiscally by requiring legislative supermajorities for tax increases. By 1994, ten states had decided to put on these fiscal handcuffs. Eight of the ten adopted these provisions over the past twenty-five years—three in the decade of the 1990s (see Table 7-1). Hence, even if those who support greater commitment to Medicaid or some other health policy can build a majority coalition to increase taxes to support that objective, they may not be able to overcome the power of a concentrated minority to block change. The fiscal arena in the states has increasingly become a breeding ground for minority rule and obstruction.

A possible paradox of reform is also a flashing yellow light for those who see states as steadily building their capacity. Over the past quarter century, the executive, legislative, and judicial branches in the states have boosted their capacity and assertiveness. The problem is that in a system that constitutionally fragments political power, increasing the capacity of the parts may not bolster the capacity of the whole. The sheer number of increasingly sophisticated and interdependent participants taking part in state policymaking may well congest and bog down the process of governance; it may in some states fuel friction, "fragmentation, disarray, confusion, and lack of leadership" (Murphy, 1981, pp. 125, 135). The implementation strategies produced in such contexts may well tend to be farragoes.

Ecological Capacity: Persistent Inequality of Wealth

Critical features of a state's economy, society, and culture also affect its capacity to serve as an effective implementation partner of the federal government. For instance, as states in general have become more affluent, their ability to share the costs of federal health care programs and to afford a more professional and competent administrative apparatus has grown. But substantial inequality in wealth persists among the

TABLE 7-1 States Requiring Supermajorities for Tax Increases, 1994

State	Year Adopted	Legislative Majority Required	Applies to
Arizona	1992	2/3	All taxes
Arkansas	1934	3/4	All taxes except sales and alcohol
California	1979	2/3	All taxes
Colorado	1992	2/3	All taxes[a]
Delaware	1980	3/5	All taxes
Florida	1971	3/5	Corporate income tax[b]
Louisiana	1966	2/3	All taxes
Mississippi	1970	3/5	All taxes
Oklahoma	1992	3/4	All taxes
South Dakota	1978	2/3	Sales and income

[a]Tax increases automatically sunset unless approved by voters at next election.
[b]The constitution limits the corporate income tax rate to 5 percent; 3/5 vote needed to increase beyond 5 percent.

SOURCE: "Revenue and Expenditure Limits," remarks by Scott Mackey to the National Education School Finance Seminar, Atlanta, Georgia, May 19, 1994.

states and one can find little evidence that they will become more equal in per capita income any time soon; in fact, over the past quarter century some movement exists in the opposite direction (Thompson, 1993, p. 18). Hence, federal programs that fail to consider the differential wealth of states in their funding approach can expect great variation in the capacity of states to become aggressive implementing agents.

Overview

From the vantage point of administrative, political, and ecological capacity, developments in the states should not be portrayed as some inexorable march of progress. Backsliding has occurred in some states in terms of their ability to serve as effective implementing agents of federal health policy. Institutional arrangements that boosted state capacity at one point at times have undercut it.

None of these concerns should gainsay the constructive role that states can and do play in the implementation of health policy. But their positive involvement requires sensible policy design by the national government—design that reflects serious assessment of the appropriate division of labor in a federal–state partnership. For instance, building pertinent mandates into federal law about required service packages, eligibility, and funding formulas can reduce state propensities to race to the bottom. Sensible policy design can help ensure that coherent rather than incoherent federalism undergirds the implementation of health policy.

AN ENDURING AND EVOLVING CHALLENGE

Twenty years of studying health policy implementation leave me impressed with the enduring challenges it poses as well as the degree to which these challenges have evolved in new directions. One predicament clearly persists. It involves balancing a desire to diagnose the infirmities of health programs without falling prey to excessive pessimism. As this chapter has shown, numerous potholes can sidetrack implementation—faulty policy design, public agencies lacking in capacity or commitment, the convolutions of trying to get private entities to do the government's work, the frictions of federalism, and more.

Too often, however, a preoccupation with these maladies has crossed the line into administrative hypochondria. Putting deleterious details under the microscope can block out the big picture. A more balanced perspective suggests that by most reasonable standards, officials have implemented the government's health programs in ways that have greatly benefited the citizenry. If, for instance, we focus on the three medical service programs targeted at civilians that consume the most federal dollars—Medicare, Medicaid, and the Veterans Administration medical system—an array of evidence points to substantial success in achieving objectives efficiently, effectively, and accountably.[6] Is the glass full with respect to these programs? Of course not. Each of them has faced major management and implementation problems. Their performance could be improved. But after acknowledging these difficulties, the glasses in these three cases look pretty full—maybe 80 percent or even higher in the case of Medicare.

Not that the successful implementation of these policies can cure all that ails the U.S. health care system. In fact, as administrators progress in improving the performance of their particular programs, they may exacerbate problems outside their domains. As the Medicare program became more efficient through such strategies as using prospective payment, hospitals found it harder to shift the costs of treating the uninsured to Medicare. Hospitals therefore faced new incentives to either cut services to the uninsured or find alternative subsidies to pay for such care. Important as it is, successful implementation is no elixir. Achieving a better balance among quality, access, and cost in the U.S. health care system will require new policies.

A second enduring problem is that, after years of exhortation about their importance, implementation and public management continue to be afterthoughts in the policy formulation process (DiIulio & Nathan, 1994). The proposal to enhance state discretion over Medicaid by converting it to a block grant is only the most recent example. The approach taken by proponents of block grants can best be termed "fire, ready, aim."[7] Toss the program into the laps of the states and worry about the consequences later, if at all. Amorphous assurances by a number of Republican governors that states are up to the task constitute the only form of implementation analysis that figures prominently in the debate. More serious assessments of whether states have the commitment and capacity to use their new discretion to provide critical health services efficiently and effectively play little, if any, role in policy deliberations.

A fragmented and fractious political system means that taking time to consider implementation will often

---

[6]My claim concerning the Veterans Administration medical system may seem the most debatable. No doubt various reforms would heighten its efficiency and effectiveness (U.S. General Accounting Office, 1995b). But this observation should not cause us to overlook the substantial achievements of the system (Thompson, 1981; Wolcott & Smith, 1991).

[7]I am indebted to Thomas Anton for drawing this point to my attention.

be unappealing to policymakers. Lawmakers may increasingly sense the need to move aggressively in those fleeting moments when policy windows are open. As proponents of President Clinton's Health Security Act learned to their dismay, too much detail about implementation can fuel opposition. In such a climate, the sensible strategy may be: strike while you can and zero in on implementation later. Worry less about avoiding mistakes than fixing them later. This repair phase may provide more fertile soil for implementation analysis; if the program can sustain itself politically through initial implementation breakdowns, policy fixers stand a better chance of adopting the approach embedded in "ready, aim, fire!"

If these and other issues have persistently appeared on the radar screen of policy implementation, new blips have also shown up. The 1990s have ushered in and reinforced dramatic developments that could markedly alter the implementation of health policy. Four trends deserve particular note.

First, critical implementation issues will increasingly revolve around the states as the national government devolves more and more responsibility to them. States vary enormously. Their response to enlarged discretion affords a splendid opportunity to learn more about different forms of health policy implementation and the factors that shape it.

Second, we need to shine light on the implementation issues posed by the government's headlong rush toward managed care. Proponents of this approach believe that these plans can bring greater efficiency at no cost in access or quality to Medicaid and Medicare beneficiaries. Officials in both these programs have had experience with managed care in the past. But the implementation challenges posed by a much more massive commitment to this mode of health care delivery await dissection.

Third, the 1990s spawned administrative reform initiatives that promised to increase the capacity of administrative agencies, but may evolve in ways that corrode such capacity. The reinvention movement—with its emphasis on higher-quality, responsive service, internal deregulation of administrative agencies to exercise outmoded rules, the reliance on market competition, and other themes—injected important and positive ideas into the bloodstream of public administration. But the "R" phase of this reform period, with its emphasis on words like *reinvention, revitalization,* and *rejuvenation,* runs the risk of becoming a "D" phase, where the focus shifts to *downsizing, dismantling,* and *deinventing.*

Ironically, the federal government and many of its state and local counterparts have taken to downsizing at precisely the time when the fervor for this approach in the private sector has met with growing skepticism.[8] As many downsized companies have seen profits and growth shrink, management experts have increasingly questioned the wisdom of a strategy based on "shrinking to greatness" (Wysocki, 1995; see also Kettl & DiIulio, 1995). The possibility of the private sector diffusing its mistakes to the government cannot be dismissed, especially in a society with a strong antigovernment bias. In many cases, it seems likely that the government will continue health programs but with tax cuts and downsizing that erode the capacity of implementing agents to carry them out efficiently and effectively.

Fourth, as of the mid-1990s, the broader political context of policy implementation featured remarkably high levels of cynicism, mistrust, and partisan polarization. If well-performing government institutions in fact flourish more in a civic community built on a fabric of trust and cooperation, the United States has cause for concern (Putnam, 1993). Countless forces have contributed to this predicament. The media, for instance, has moved toward an adversarial and cynical (as distinct from skeptical) posture toward the government (Starobin, 1995). Among top policymakers in the national government and in many states, a pit-bull, win-at-any-procedural-price partisanship frequently prevails. Give-and-take gives way to non-negotiable demands. Comity, "the adherence to a set of norms that includes courtesy and reciprocity," becomes less evident (Uslaner, 1993, p. 1).

---

[8]Downsizing, as used here, refers to reducing the workforce of an agency in the absence of significant diminution in its statutory responsibilities. Obviously, downsizing can also follow in the wake of fundamental changes in law designed to withdraw the government from involvement in certain policy arenas.

All of these forces make efforts to sustain and enhance the capacity and performance of administrative agencies more arduous as public servants "become the scapegoats for other people's quarrels" (Wildavsky, 1987, p. 10). Perhaps the late 1990s will witness a period of Republican Party hegemony at all levels of the federal system that will mute the bite of this dissensus while reinforcing the emphasis on downsizing and dismantling administrative agencies. Whatever the case, those engaged in implementing health policy will face unprecedented challenges.

REFERENCES

Bardach, Eugene. (1977). *The implementation game*. Cambridge: MIT Press.

Barrilleaux, Charles J., & Mark E. Miller. (1988). The political economy of state Medicaid policy. *American Political Science Review, 82* (December), 1089–1108.

Brown, Lawrence D. (1983). *Politics and health care organization: HMOs as federal policy*. Washington, D.C.: The Brookings Institution.

Cohen, Michael D., James G. March, & Johan P. Olsen. (1972). A garbage can model of organizational choice. *Administrative Science Quarterly, 17* (March), 1–25.

Coughlin, Teresa A., Leighton Ku, & John Holahan. (1994). *Medicaid since 1980*. Washington, D.C.: Urban Institute.

Derthick, Martha. (1979). *Policymaking for Social Security*. Washington, D.C.: The Brookings Institution.

Derthick, Martha. (1990). *Agency under stress*. Washington, D.C.: The Brookings Institution.

DiIulio, John J., Jr., & Richard P. Nathan. (1994). *Making health reform work: The view from the states*. Washington, D.C.: The Brookings Institution.

Elmore, Richard F. (1987). Instruments and strategy in public policy. *Policy Studies Review, 7* (Autumn), 174–186.

Fact Finders. (1994). *American values and expectations for health care reform*. New York: Delmar.

Foltz, Anne-Marie. (1975). The development of ambiguous federal policy: Early and periodic screening, diagnosis and treatment (EPSDT). *Milbank Memorial Fund Quarterly/Health and Society, 53* (Winter), 35–64.

Goggin, Malcolm L. (1987). *Policy design and the politics of implementation*. Knoxville: University of Tennessee Press.

Goggin, Malcolm L., Ann O'M. Bowman, James P. Lester, & Laurence J. O'Toole Jr. (1990). *Implementation theory and practice:

Toward a third generation. Glenview, IL: Scott Foresman/Little, Brown.

Grogan, Colleen M., Roger D. Feldman, John A. Nyman, & Janet Shapiro. (1994). How will we use clinical guidelines? The experience of Medicare carriers. *Journal of Health Politics, Policy and Law, 19* (Spring), 7–26.

Heclo, Hugh, & Aaron Wildavsky. (1974). *The private government of public money*. Berkeley: University of California Press.

Holahan, John, Theresa Coughlin, Leighton Ku, Debra J. Lipson, & Shruti Rajan. (1995). Insuring the poor through Medicaid 1115 waivers. *Health Affairs, 14* (Spring), 200–217.

Ingram, Helen. (1990). Implementation: A review and suggested framework. In Naomi Lynn and Aaron Wildavsky (Eds.), *Public administration: The state of the discipline* (pp. 462–482). Chatham, NJ: Chatham House.

Institute of Medicine. (1988). *The future of public health*. Washington, D.C.: National Academy Press.

Jacobs, Lawrence R. (1993). Health reform impasse: The politics of American ambivalence toward government. *Journal of Health Politics, Policy and Law, 18* (Fall), 629–656.

Kettl, Donald F., & John J. DiIulio Jr. (1995). *Cutting government*. Washington, D.C.: Center for Public Management, The Brookings Institution.

Kingdon, John W. (1984). *Agendas, alternatives, and public policies*. Boston: Little, Brown.

Majone, Giandomenico, & Aaron Wildavsky. (1979). Implementation as evolution. In Jeffrey Pressman & Aaron Wildavsky (Eds.), *Implementation* (2nd ed., pp. 177–194). Berkeley: University of California Press.

March, James G. (1978). Bounded rationality: Ambiguity and the engineering of choice. *Bell Journal of Economics, 9* (March), 587–608.

Melnick, R. Shep. (1994). *Between the lines: Interpreting welfare rights*. Washington, D.C.: The Brookings Institution.

Moon, Marilyn. (1993). *Medicare now and in the future*. Washington, D.C.: Urban Institute.

Morone, James A. (1993). The health care bureaucracy: Small changes, big consequences. *Journal of Health Politics, Policy and Law, 18* (Fall), 723–739.

Murphy, Jerome T. (1981). The paradox of state government reform. *The Public Interest, 64* (Summer), 124–139.

National Commission on the State and Local Public Service. (1993a). *Hard truths/tough choices: An agenda for state and local reform*. Albany, NY: Rockefeller Institute of Government.

National Commission on the State and Local Public Service. (1993b). *Frustrated federalism: Rx for state and local health care reform*. Albany, NY: Rockefeller Institute of Government.

National Performance Review. (1993a). *Department of Health and Human Services*. Draft edition. Washington, D.C.

National Performance Review. (1993b). *From red tape to results: Creating a government that works better and costs less.* Washington, D.C.: U.S. Government Printing Office.

Pauly, Mark V., & John C. Goodman. (1995). Tax credits for health insurance and medical savings accounts. *Health Affairs, 14* (Spring), 125–139.

Peterson, Paul E., & Mark Rom. (1988). American federalism, welfare policy, and residential choices. *American Political Science Review, 83* (September), 711–728.

Peterson, Paul E., Mark C. Rom, & Kenneth F. Scheve Jr. (1995). *Social welfare policy: A race to the bottom?* Paper prepared for the National Association for Welfare Research and Statistics Annual Research Conference, Jackson, WY.

Pressman, Jeffrey, & Aaron Wildavsky. (1973). *Implementation.* Berkeley: University of California Press.

Putnam, Robert D. (1993). *Making democracy work.* Princeton: Princeton University Press.

Rivlin, Alice. (1992). *Reviving the American dream.* Washington, D.C.: The Brookings Institution.

Sabatier, Paul, & Daniel Mazmanian. (1979). The conditions of effective implementation: A guide to accomplishing policy objectives. *Policy Analysis, 5* (Fall), 481–504.

Salamon, Lester M. (Ed.). (1989). *Beyond privatization: The tools of government action.* Washington, D.C.: Urban Institute.

Schneider, Anne, & Helen Ingram. (1993). Social construction of target populations: Implications for politics and policy. *American Political Science Review, 87* (June), 334–347.

Sparer, Michael, & Lawrence D. Brown. (1993). Between a rock and a hard place: How public managers manage Medicaid. In Frank J. Thompson (Ed.), *Revitalizing state and local public service* (pp. 279–306). San Francisco: Jossey-Bass.

Starobin, Paul. (1995). A generation of vipers. *Columbia Journalism Review, 1* (March/April), 25–32.

Starr, Paul. (1995). What happened to health care reform? *The American Prospect, 20,* 20–31.

Tallon, James R., Jr., & Lawrence D. Brown. (1994). Health alliances: Functions, forms, and federalism. In John J. DiIulio Jr. & Richard P. Nathan (Eds.), *Making health reform work: The view from the states* (pp. 40–59). Washington, D.C.: The Brookings Institution.

Thompson, Frank J. (1981). *Health policy and the bureaucracy.* Cambridge: MIT Press.

Thompson, Frank J. (1993). *Revitalizing state and local public service.* San Francisco: Jossey-Bass.

Thompson, Frank J. (1994). The quest for quality care: Implementation issues. In John J. DiIulio Jr. & Richard P. Nathan (Eds.), *Making health reform work: The view from the states* (pp. 85–113). Washington, D.C.: The Brookings Institution.

U.S. Advisory Commission on Intergovernment Relations. (1985). *The question of state government capability.* Washington, D.C.: U.S. Government Printing Office.

U.S. General Accounting Office. (1993). *Health insurance regulation: Variation in states' authority, oversight, and resources* (GAO/HRD-94-26). Washington, D.C.

U.S. General Accounting Office. (1994). *Medicare Part B: Regional variation in denial rates for medical necessity* (GAO-PEMD-95-10). Washington: D.C.

U.S. General Accounting Office. (1995a). *Medicaid: Spending pressures drive states toward program reinvention* (GAO/HEHS-95-122). Washington, D.C.

U.S. General Accounting Office. (1995b). *VA health care: Challenges and options for the future* (GAO/HEHS-95-147). Washington, D.C.

U.S. House Committee on Appropriations. (1977). *Department of Labor and Health, Education, and Welfare appropriations for 1978: Part 6.* Washington, D.C.: U.S. Government Printing Office.

U.S. Office of Technology Assessment. (1994). *International comparisons of administrative costs in health care.* Washington, D.C.: U.S. Government Printing Office.

Uslaner, Eric M. (1993). *The decline of comity in Congress.* Ann Arbor: University of Michigan Press.

Waldo, Dwight. (1980). *The enterprise of public administration.* Novato, CA: Chandler and Sharp.

Weaver, R. Kent, & Bert A. Rockman. (Eds.). (1993). *Do institutions matter? Government capabilities in the United States and abroad.* Washington, D.C.: The Brookings Institution.

Wildavsky, Aaron. (1987). "Ubiquitous anomie" or public service in an era of ideological dissensus. In Larry M. Lane (Ed.), *The campus and the public service* (pp. 5–10). Washington, D.C.: National Academy of Public Administration.

Wolcott, Mark W., & Charles B. Smith. (1991). Can we learn from our own experience? The VA as national health care. In Robert B. Huefner & Margaret P. Battin (Eds.), *Changing to national health care* (pp. 139–162). Salt Lake City: University of Utah Press.

Wysocki, Bernard, Jr. (1995). Some companies cut costs too far, suffer "corporate anorexia." *Wall Street Journal* (July 5), A1.

CHAPTER

State Roles in Health Care Policy: Past as Prologue?

Debra J. Lipson

States have had primary responsibility for the development and implementation of health care policy, regulation, and program administration for most of this country's history. Yet, by virtue of financing and administering two of the largest programs in the entire federal government—Medicare and Medicaid—the federal government has a very large role in health policy as well. Given an increasingly complex health care system, neither level of government would seem to have the capacity to enact, implement, and enforce all the policies and programs needed to manage the health care system. Indeed, with large and growing proportions of the budgets of both federal and state governments (not to mention local governments) being consumed by health care costs, neither is prepared to bear the financing burdens alone.

If both are essential, then the more important question becomes how each level of government can best share their joint responsibilities for regulating, financing, and improving the efficiency of the nation's health care system. This chapter examines what roles the states have played in health policy and seeks to evaluate how well they have performed them. Such an assessment may help shed light on which roles states are best equipped to undertake as the nation begins to shift more responsibility to them.

Theoretically, the relationship of the federal government to states in the health arena could lie at any point along a continuum between a complete abdication of control to the states to a complete takeover of all responsibility by the federal government. Debates surrounding federalism in health policy over the past thirty to forty years have focused on where to place the fulcrum in this continuum. From the federal government's perspective, the question often has been framed as: Can the states be entrusted with broad powers and flexibility? When must the federal government set national standards and rules to assure equity and efficiency in the health care system? From the states' perspective, the question is often expressed as: When will the federal government give us the flexibility we need to structure our own cost-effective health care systems?

These issues have been the subject of intense national debate in the recent past. The nation's 1993–94 debate on health care reform presented an opportunity to reexamine states' roles (Chisman et al., 1994). The Clinton proposal would have given states substantial responsibilities to administer and finance a national health care system, while making dramatic improvements in national uniformity in health care coverage levels and benefits. A year later, in 1995, Congress was again debating how much authority and control to give to states, through its consideration of proposals to place numerous federal health programs, including the Medicaid program, into block grants to the states. This would shift the balance of power toward much greater state control.

Such debates are critical ones for a country that claims to be committed to equality yet is deeply suspicious of a large federal presence in state or local affairs. But to carry on an informed debate, it is important to understand the strengths and weaknesses of the states' capacities and willingness to undertake various roles and responsibilities in health policy.

This chapter reviews the experience of the states in performing a broad range of roles in health policy, including financing or paying for health care; assuring the public's health; regulating health professionals, facilities, and insurance arrangements; and experimenting with approaches to comprehensive health care reform. For each of these roles, emphasis is placed on state governments' relationships with the federal government and on variations among states in how they approach these roles. It also describes changes in the way states have carried out these roles in the past ten to fifteen years and points out some of the challenges facing states in performing these roles in the future. It concludes by discussing trade-offs between significant state flexibility versus greater federal involvement in performing these critical roles in health policy.

FEDERALISM AND HEALTH POLICY

Debates about the appropriate responsibility of each level of government for various functions in the health care system have a long legacy. Since the nation's founding, there has been a constant struggle to find the right balance between a strong central government and state and local autonomy. From the late 1700s to the early 1900s, local governments were clearly dominant, with neither the states nor the federal government having much involvement at all. That began to change in the 1930s. First, the Social Security Act (1935) authorized federal grants to states for maternal and child health care, and for care to disabled individuals. Second, the Food and Drug Administration (FDA) within the federal government was created in 1938 to assure the safety and efficacy of food and pharmaceutical products crossing state lines, drawing its authority from the commerce clause of the Constitution giving Congress the power to regulate commerce among the states.

From the 1930s through the 1950s, states' involvement in health care was limited to basic public health functions, such as control of communicable diseases, direct delivery of certain services such as care for the chronically mentally ill, and administration of federal grants-in-aid. With the start of the health insurance industry in the 1940s and 1950s, states also began to regulate both Blue Cross and Blue Shield plans and commercial policies. Meanwhile, Washington's role in and spending on domestic programs grew in response to the Great Depression that reinforced a belief that national institutions were needed to "strengthen the economy and perform functions that states could not be expected to perform on their own" (Rivlin, 1992). In other words, state and local health and welfare systems were not regarded as capable of addressing national economic hardships.

The 1960s marked a period of escalating influence of the federal government over health care policy. Here, as in many other arenas, states were viewed as performing their assigned responsibilities poorly. Like other programs that grew out of the administrations of Kennedy and Johnson, Medicare and Medicaid were created, in large measure, to address shortcomings in the states' abilities to serve the needs of the elderly, poor, urban residents, and minorities (Thompson, 1986).

The states' role in health care diminished considerably in the 1970s as Medicare and Medicaid grew well beyond most of their creators' predictions and as other federal programs, such as support for community health centers, expanded in scope. In 1965, state and local governments spent about the same amount ($5.2 billion) as the federal government on health and medical care. By 1980, the federal government was spending twice as much as state and local governments and two and a half times more in 1985 (U.S. Department of Health and Human Services, 1987). Continuing disparities among the states in the reach and effectiveness of various health and social service programs were quite apparent. For example, participants at a January 1980 conference on state and local government involvement in health care concluded that state governments were more vulnerable to political patronage and more inefficient than the federal government (Jain, 1981).

During the 1980s, President Reagan ushered in a new era characterized by an effort to return to the states greater control and discretion over the financing, delivery, and regulation of health care. In his first State of the Union Address in January 1982, the president promised cuts in taxes, cuts in federal spending, and a reduction in burdensome federal regulatory requirements by giving more decision-making authority to state and local governments (*Congressional Quarterly*, 1982). Block grants, which consolidate funds from many different categorical programs into one lump sum that is distributed to the states on a formula basis, became a key vehicle to achieve all three goals. While the Democratic-controlled Congress agreed to transfer some control to the states, it tried to cushion the blow by appropriating more money for block grants than the Reagan administration had requested. Nonetheless, federal grants to state and local governments (excluding payments for individuals) fell by 38 percent in inflation-adjusted dollars between 1980 and 1989 (U.S. Office of Manaagement and Budget, 1990).

Contrary to expectations, state governments responded by considerably expanding their own spending on health and social services. According to a U.S. General Accounting Office study (1995), state expenditures on health-related programs funded in part with federal block grant funds increased in 85 percent of the states studied. If the block grants represented a test of the states' political commitment to human service programs without federal mandates and with reduced federal funding, they "passed this test . . . to a greater degree than most observers anticipated," according to an analysis by the Urban Institute (Peterson, 1986).

Their ability to pass the test was possible because of an economic upswing that began in late 1982 and remained through the 1980s. That enabled more than half of the states to raise personal income or sales taxes from 1982 to 1986; state tax collections rose by 33 percent over this period. This infusion of funds allowed states not only to restore federal funds cut at the beginning of the decade, but to reduce taxes and even initiate new and innovative health programs toward the end of the decade.

At the start of the 1990s, the states' good fortunes came to an abrupt end. It began with regional economic recessions in New England in 1988, eventually hitting every region of the country by the end of 1992. State budgets took a beating. By 1992, most states were in their second and third years of "making painful spending cuts, raising taxes, imposing new fees and using all sorts of accounting gimmicks to squeeze their budgets into balance" (Lemov, 1992).

Despite these difficulties, states did not come to be viewed as "failing the test." This may be due to the fact that the federal government was in no position to make up for their deficiencies. But it may also be because of the creative ways in which they handled health care policy during the economic downturn. For example, even though more poor individuals were entitled by the federal government to Medicaid between 1986 and 1992, the states found the means to finance rapidly expanding Medicaid budgets. One of the more popular methods involved taxing hospitals and other health care providers and counting those revenues as state Medicaid funds that then qualified for federal matching dollars. This resulted in greater federal spending, with little or no increase in state outlays for Medicaid expansions. A few states also made the commitment to provide health care coverage to all of their residents, even though the federal government failed to make a similar promise (Lipson, 1994). Ironically, if states faced any barrier to doing even more, they blamed the mandates and rigid rules imposed by the federal government.

By the mid-1990s, states faced the prospect of gaining even greater control and flexibility for the administration and financing of health and human service programs. In 1995, Congress considered seriously a proposal to turn the entire Medicaid program over to state governments by giving them a block grant with very few federal strings attached. But the increased flexibility would come with a price: strict annual spending growth caps would be placed on them.

How would states handle increased responsibility with fewer dollars? Would they, as in the early 1980s, respond by increasing state allocations to health programs and using other creative methods to stretch existing funds? Or would they be forced to cut eligibility, services, or provider payments to make ends meet?

To predict how states would respond to a transfer of responsibility from the federal government and how they would use the additional flexibility, it is useful to examine how well they have performed previous and long-standing roles. Similarly, to gauge how well states are prepared to meet emerging roles that arise from a changing health care system, it is instructive to examine how they have addressed health care problems that arose in the past decade.

STATES AS PAYERS OF HEALTH CARE SERVICES

All states bear a large responsibility for financing health services for the poor, primarily through the Medicaid program, for which financing is shared with the federal government. States also pay the costs of providing health coverage to state employees and retirees, and sometimes for other publicly employed workers, such as teachers, police, and the like. In addition, most states also help subsidize some of the costs of delivering health services to those without any coverage at all, public or private. Significant changes have occurred in state financing of health services over the past decade, the

most notable being the tremendous rise in total spending. In response to the cost growth, states have undertaken a variety of measures to control the annual growth of such costs and to cover uninsured people in more cost-effective ways.

State Medicaid Programs

An estimated $125.2 billion was spent on the Medicaid program by both the federal and state governments in 1993, and served 32.1 million individuals (Kaiser Commission, 1995a). The Medicaid program is actually fifty-six programs (fifty states and six other jurisdictions) because each state is allowed to operate its own Medicaid program within relatively broad federal guidelines. These guidelines specify both required and allowed eligibility groups and health care benefits. Within these federal parameters, states have adopted more or less generous programs, depending on such factors as the state's economic capacity to finance Medicaid services, state or regional health care costs, the demographics of the state's population, influence of interest groups in the state political and budget processes, competing priorities with other state programs, and federal financial incentives or sanctions.

This flexibility has resulted in great variation in the Medicaid program from state to state. For example, in 1993, state expenditures per capita ranged from $1,275 in the District of Columbia and $1,104 in New York to $278 in Idaho and $276 in Utah (Kaiser Commission, 1995b).[1] Eligibility for Medicaid also has varied widely among the states. Federal Medicaid rules require that anyone eligible for cash welfare programs are also eligible for the program. But state Aid to Families with Dependent Children (AFDC) eligibility thresholds, for example, ranged from $1,440 in annual income for a family of three in Mississippi to $7,800 in Vermont as of February 1995 (National Governors Association, 1995). Less variation among state eligibility standards occurs in coverage of the aged and disabled because fed-

---

[1]These figures are per capita (covering all residents of each state), *not* per Medicaid beneficiary. Per beneficiary spending averaged $3,895 across all states, ranging from $2,380 in Mississippi to $9,700 in New Hampshire.

eral rules govern eligibility for Supplemental Security Income (SSI), the cash assistance program for low-income people in those groups.

Federal guidelines also have permitted coverage of several other groups of people at a state's option. Beginning in 1984, Congress enacted a series of laws that gradually expanded coverage for more low-income people who did not qualify for cash welfare programs. The Omnibus Budget Reconciliation Act of 1986 (OBRA-86) was the first in a series of laws to break the long-standing connection between eligibility for cash assistance (AFDC or SSI) and Medicaid. It permitted states to provide Medicaid coverage to all pregnant women and children up to age five in households with family incomes *above* the state's AFDC standard of need but below the federal poverty level. OBRA-86 also permitted states to cover the aged and disabled who made less than the federal poverty level but still had incomes above the SSI eligibility threshold.

Later, the Medicare Catastrophic Coverage Act of 1988 required all state Medicaid programs to pay for the Medicare premiums, deductibles, and co-payments for elderly and disabled Medicare beneficiaries who made less than 100 percent of the federal poverty level.[2] Then, OBRA-89 and -90 mandated that state Medicaid programs cover all pregnant women and children up to age six living in families with incomes below 133 percent of the poverty level. On a phased-in basis, all children below age nineteen living in poverty were required to be covered by Medicaid by the year 2002. States were still allowed to cover pregnant women and infants whose incomes were up to 185 percent of the poverty line and by July 1994, thirty-four states had set the level at some point above the 133 percent minimum.

In an attempt to reduce wide interstate variations, each state's "match rate," or the proportion of each state's Medicaid costs covered by the federal government has been determined on the basis of per capita personal income relative to the national average. As of 1995, those with less than the national average are entitled to greater federal funds; those with more than the national average get less. So, the federal matching rate varied from 80 percent in a state with the lowest per capita income (Mississippi) to 50 percent, which is the minimum match rate.[3]

Though the variable federal matching rate was intended to reallocate resources from the wealthier to the poorer states, this did not occur. According to a 1995 Kaiser Commission report,

> Medicaid spending per poor person is generally greater in higher income states than in lower income states. For example, Medicaid spending per person below 150% of the poverty line varied from $4,852 in New York and $4,007 in Connecticut [high-income states] to $958 in Idaho and $953 in Utah [low-income states]. Because of differences in program generosity, many higher income states have federal per capita contributions which are well above the national average, despite low federal matching rates. In contrast, many lower income states have federal per capita contributions which are well below the national average, despite much higher federal matching rates" (Kaiser Commission, 1995b).

Early studies of interstate spending variations attributed these differences to the tendency of lower-income states, particularly in the South, to spend very little on the poor, regardless of how much money the federal government offered to help them serve this group (Sundquist, 1969). Another study confirmed that differences in Medicaid coverage of the poor reflected variations in states' income standards used to determine welfare, and therefore Medicaid, eligibility as well as states' coverage of certain optional eligibility groups under the program (Holahan & Cohen, 1986).

By the mid-1990s, however, such explanations fell short. While state policies affecting welfare eligibility were influential in the 1970s and 1980s, the gradual delinking of Medicaid from welfare eligibility diminished the influence of state welfare policies on Medicaid spending variation. Increasingly, interstate spending differences have been better explained by a combination of factors: variations in the states' ability to pay, the

---

[2]While the Medicare Catastrophic Coverage Act was later repealed by Congress, the provisions pertaining to Medicaid eligibility expansions were retained.

[3]Major changes to the federal matching rate formula were the subject of considerable debate in the 104th Congress.

composition of Medicaid recipients in each state, cost of health care in the state, and provider payment policies, especially those concerning payments to disproportionate share hospitals (DSHs) that serve greater numbers of Medicaid and uninsured people.

The multiplicity of factors contributing to interstate spending variations highlight the shortcomings of the federal funding formula, which only accounts for differences in states' per capita income. Thus, many proposals for Medicaid reforms often suggest changes to the federal formula that would take into account each state's ability to pay, the cost of health care in each state, and differences in the number of poor, elderly, or disabled people (Kaiser Commission, 1995b). However, changes in the federal formula would produce winners and losers and "set off a battle royal among states about how to divide the dollars" (Fraley, 1995).

Why? Because a great deal of money is at stake. The expected federal–state tab of $170 billion in fiscal year 1996 is over three times what was spent just six years earlier in 1989 (Fraley, 1995). For the states, total state spending on Medicaid grew at rate much higher than nearly every other state spending category, except corrections, during this period of time. In 1993, 18.4 percent of state budgets on average was consumed by Medicaid expenditures, almost double the 10 percent figure in 1987 (National Association of State Budget Officers, 1994).

The growth in Medicaid spending in the past seven years was due in part to an increase in those eligible for Medicaid. Nationwide, approximately 32.1 million individuals were covered by Medicaid in 1993, compared to 23.2 million in 1987. Most of this growth reflects expanded coverage of pregnant women and young children, and increases in the number of blind and disabled beneficiaries. However, according to an analysis of the reasons for cost growth between 1988 and 1992, only 36 percent of the increase was attributable to greater enrollment (Coughlin et al., 1994). Health care inflation (the rise in medical care prices) played a major role in the rise in Medicaid spending, contributing another 26 percent of the cost growth. Increases in service utilization, which reflect greater amounts and intensity of care, as well as increased payments to providers in ex-

cess of the medical inflation rate contributed the last 33 percent of the cost growth during this period.

Generally speaking, states were able to absorb the increasing costs of the program at the beginning of the eligibility expansions in 1986 because state budgets were relatively healthy in the late 1980s. But as the economic recession of 1991–92 squeezed state revenues and caused Medicaid rolls to swell, states needed to employ a variety of techniques to reduce the annual rate of cost growth, or increase revenues to, the Medicaid program.

In some states, fiscal crises turned a casual search for alternative sources of Medicaid revenue into an economic imperative. Dozens of states decided to increase revenues to cover growing Medicaid costs, initially by requesting donations from, and later by imposing taxes on, hospitals and other providers. States then used these provider donations or taxes to generate additional federal matching funds and to pay hospitals higher rates than they would have otherwise received. States with high federal match rates found the strategy particularly attractive; by the end of 1991, nearly half the states had adopted either provider donation or tax schemes, or both.

Among thirty-two states with a provider tax or donation program in fiscal year 1992, the revenues represented on average 23.5 percent of states' nonfederal expenditures on Medicaid. In some states, however, the figure went much higher. Tennessee, for example, raised $1 billion, or nearly half of its total Medicaid budget, from provider fees and other revenues (Lipson, 1993).

By 1993, the cumulative effect of state Medicaid provider donations and taxes on the federal government was high. The provider taxes were cited as one of the major contributors to rapidly increasing Medicaid costs at the federal level. And because federal Medicaid reimbursements to states increased so dramatically between 1989 and 1993, the rise in federal payments served to transform the Medicaid program from its primary role in financing health care for the poor, elderly, and disabled into a major federal revenue sharing program for states (Miller, 1992). "Medicaid growth has reversed the decline in federal grants to state and local governments," wrote Miller. He based this conclusion on trends showing that federal grants to states dropped from 17 percent of total federal spending in the late 1970s to 11 percent throughout the 1980s. Due to the rise in Medicaid payments alone, these figures increased to 13 percent in 1993 and were projected to reach 16 percent by 1993. As a proportion of all federal grants to state and local governments, Medicaid payments rose from 15 percent in 1980 to 35 percent in 1991, with a possible rise to 55 percent in 1997 (Miller, 1992).

In response to very high annual growth rates in total Medicaid spending, Congress enacted a law designed to prevent states from repaying the provider taxes back to the hospitals in the form of increased rates. The law banned donation programs, set ground rules for provider tax programs, and set aggregate national and state limits on payments made to disproportionate share hospitals (DSHs), or those that serve greater than average numbers of Medicaid and uninsured patients.

States' use of provider taxes to generate federal Medicaid funds represented yet another battleground in an ongoing contest between federal and state governments over how much the federal Treasury will dispense to states for their Medicaid programs. The Medicaid financing system has always given states tremendous incentives to devise ways to maximize federal funds. Despite Congress's limitations on the states' use of provider taxes to finance their share of Medicaid, the solution represented a temporary "fix," deferring a decision on the real issue underlying the controversy: How should the federal government and the states divide responsibility for raising the funds necessary to pay for health care provided to poor and low-income people? As the most recent round of federal government attempts to rein in these costs plays itself out over the next several years, this question will undoubtedly surface again.

In response to rising Medicaid costs, states did more than just try to maximize federal funds. In fact, nearly all states implemented a variety of cost-cutting measures. Between 1984 and 1992, the vast majority of states changed their hospital reimbursement methods from cost-based to prospective payment based on diagnosis-related groups (DRGs), consistent with the federal Medicare program. Nursing home reimbursement has also switched to prospective payment methods, us-

ing case-mix adjusters to vary rates based on the intensity of care needed by each patient. And with the growing costs of pharmaceutical drugs—total Medicaid spending grew by 116 percent between 1989 and 1993—states have tried to limit expenditures by using formularies and requiring the use of generics, performing drug utilization reviews, and limiting quantities permitted to be dispensed. Federal law also required that drug manufacturers pay rebates to state Medicaid agencies for single-source drugs, to approximate the discounts provided to HMOs and large group purchasers.

But by far, the states' most significant effort to contain costs was to increase enrollment of Medicaid beneficiaries into HMOs and other managed care arrangements. "Expanding the use of managed care to improve access and contain costs is a central goal of virtually all Medicaid programs today and is a feature of Medicaid in 43 states and the District of Columbia" (Rowland et al., 1995). There is a great deal of variety in the types of managed care plans utilized—from HMOs paid on a fully capitated basis to partially capitated plans to primary care "gatekeeper" programs that continue to pay physicians on a fee-for-service basis, but dispense an extra monthly fee to them to coordinate and manage the care received by patients.

A review of studies on the effects of Medicaid managed care programs confirmed cost savings of 10 percent to 15 percent below those of the regular fee-for-service system (Rowland et al., 1995). However, such savings were more common in programs that rely on prepaid capitated plans, rather than on physician gatekeeper models. The review left open the question of whether such savings are due to more efficient care (i.e., substituting outpatient physician visits for emergency room use) or discounts to providers' rates. It also suggested that while access to primary care appeared to increase under such plans, use of preventive services may stay the same or even decline, and health outcomes were not significantly better (Rowland et al., 1995).

From the states' perspective, managed care does no harm and at least assures a lower rate of increase and more predictability in annual costs compared to the fee-for-service system. This explains why, in 1994, 23 percent of all Medicaid beneficiaries were enrolled in managed care arrangements, up from 14 percent in 1993 and just 3 percent in 1983. But these figures masked significant interstate variation. Arizona and Tennessee, for example, had enrolled virtually all Medicaid beneficiaries into managed care plans, through waivers from federal Medicaid rules that otherwise prevent mandatory enrollment into managed care. Oregon, Washington, Utah, and Massachusetts had over 40 percent of Medicaid beneficiaries in managed care plans. But some states had very little (i.e., less than 10 percent) or no managed care enrollment at all (Lewin-VHI, 1995).

With more and more of the privately insured population enrolled in managed care, states began to find it easier to interest HMOs and other managed care plans in serving the Medicaid population. In 1995, a third of all Medicaid recipients were projected to be enrolled in managed care arrangements of some type. However, states' ability to enroll all of their Medicaid population into managed care still depended on the willingness of the federal government to grant them permission to make managed care enrollment mandatory. And states continued to face big challenges in assuring that managed care plans would guarantee access and high quality, not to mention improved health outcomes, for groups that by definition—being poor, old, or disabled—have more serious health risks and problems than the rest of the population.

State Programs for the Uninsured

Although it is generally assumed that the Medicaid program provides health insurance protection for the nation's poor, it does not do so completely. The percentage of all poor people covered under Medicaid dropped from a high of 65 percent in 1976 to a low of about 40 percent in 1984, then rose to 58 percent in 1993 due to recent expansions that covered more low-income people ineligible for welfare. Medicaid's inability to cover all the poor is one reason that nearly one in six Americans under the age of sixty-five lacks health coverage. Approximately four of every five persons without health insurance are in poor and near-poor families in which one or both parents are working, but are not offered or cannot afford health insurance through their workplace.

Often, it falls to state governments, along with city and county governments, to help subsidize the costs of caring for those who lack health coverage. While many of these individuals are served by public health agencies or public hospitals that provide direct care to those without health insurance, many states also administer programs to provide coverage to such people.

State "indigent care" programs comprised one type of program. Often funded and administered jointly by the state and local governments, all but ten of the fifty states had medically indigent care programs in operation on a statewide basis in 1985. Even in states without such programs, most had nonuniform county-based programs in operation that may have covered some or all of the state's population (Desonia & King, 1985). Estimates of total state and county expenditures for health care services provided under these state indigent care programs ranged from $2.5 billion to over $15 billion annually (Butler, 1988, p. 39).

State indigent care programs are extremely diverse, and little data are available on the number of people covered or served. About twenty states have general assistance medical programs, which serve as a safety net for single adults or disabled people who have little or no income and are ineligible for federally supported welfare programs such as AFDC or SSI. Another twenty-five states have indigent care programs in addition to or instead of general assistance medical programs and are often operated in conjunction with county governments. Some states operate other small programs that cover very limited target populations or specialized services, such as pharmaceuticals for the elderly.

For many years, states met their obligation to assure care for the medically indigent by subsidizing providers—primarily hospitals—for the cost of delivering care to the uninsured. However, throughout the 1980s, it became increasingly apparent to policymakers that reimbursing hospitals for uncompensated care costs would not address access to primary care or other outpatient care that might prevent inappropriate use of hospitals by the uninsured. And no matter how much states gave to hospitals—even through Medicaid disproportionate share hospital (DSH) funds, for example—the growing numbers of uninsured people continued to overwhelm public hospitals.

State policymakers, tired of trying to fill a seemingly unending well of uncompensated care costs out of state general revenue funds, searched throughout the 1980s and early 1990s for a more broad-based financing strategy to pay for care of the uninsured. State governments experimented with a variety of insurance premium subsidy programs that targeted low-income workers and small companies, which are less likely to provide coverage to employees.

Several states, such as Hawaii, Maine, Massachusetts, Michigan, Minnesota, and Washington, established pilot programs that offered state subsidies to low- and moderate-income families to help them afford health insurance premiums. These programs typically restricted eligibility to individuals with incomes under 200 percent of federal poverty guidelines, and did not have access to an employer-sponsored group insurance plan. They also structured premium subsidies and co-payments according to a sliding fee scale based on income. In addition, several offered coverage primarily through managed care systems, such as HMOs, which would be less costly. Minnesota initially limited its program to children, but later expanded it to cover low-income families as well. A few of these programs were eliminated during the economic recession of the early 1990s (e.g., Maine and Massachusetts). But most of them were continued, or even expanded, when federal funds became available through Section 1115 waiver programs (see below).

The few states that made a commitment to assure health coverage to all or most of their residents in the early 1990s found that insurance premium subsidy programs were essential to make coverage affordable for low-income individuals (Lipson, 1994). But the cost to the states was high. By the mid-1990s, more and more states turned to the federal government to help pay for the subsidies to the uninsured.

Specifically, they asked for greater leeway to stretch existing Medicaid dollars to finance coverage for the uninsured. By the middle of 1995, nearly twenty states had applied for federal Medicaid waivers under Section 1115 of the Social Security Act that permits states to conduct special demonstration programs. For the most part, they were using the Section 1115 waivers to help pay for expanded coverage to low-income uninsured with dollars saved from enrolling all previous Medicaid enrollees into managed care plans, or by using disproportionate share hospital dollars to subsidize premiums for less costly care (Holahan et al., 1995). A few states, such as Tennessee and Florida, relied on new funds like premium contributions from low-income people to generate additional federal Medicaid match funds as well.

Meanwhile, many states supported other voluntary approaches to help make health insurance more affordable to employers, particularly small firms that had trouble gaining access to the private health insurance market. For example, Oregon and Massachusetts authorized tax credits for small businesses providing health care benefits for the first time. Many states enabled the formation of health insurance purchasing alliances and multiple employer trusts to encourage small businesses to buy health coverage as a large group at lower costs.

However, states came to realize very quickly that voluntary approaches would only solve part of the problem. Officials in several states believed that more drastic measures would be necessary to provide coverage to everyone, which was not only the equitable thing to do, but necessary to end cost shifting by providers and to gain greater control of health care costs. That brought several states to consider the possibility of mandating employers and individuals to purchase health insurance.

States have been generally reluctant to consider employer mandates, not just because businesses oppose it, but because of the economic implications: firms can leave the state if faced with higher costs. A few states, notably Massachusetts, Oregon, and Washington, overcame political objections by the business community in passing laws that would have eventually either required employers to provide coverage, or pay taxes if they did not. But none of these states was able to implement the mandates for two reasons. First, to enforce such laws, states needed federal exemption from the Employee Retirement Income Security Act (ERISA), which prohibits states from mandating employer coverage. Hawaii remains the only state that has received an ERISA exemption, which allows it to mandate that employers cover certain workers' health insurance premiums. But Congress has been unwilling to grant any further exemptions. Second, support for the employer mandates deteriorated in these states after Congress failed to enact national health care reform in 1994 and more politically conservative leaders were elected to both Congress and state legislatures that same year.

Clearly, states have a major role to play as payers of health care. While their relationships with the federal government in sharing the financial burden often have been strained, neither seems to be able to do without the other. For the most part, states have gone much further than the federal government in trying different approaches to saving costs, especially by enrolling Medicaid beneficiaries, public employees, and low-income uninsured people into managed care plans. This experience should serve the federal government well if it decides to enroll greater numbers of Medicare beneficiaries into managed care.

However, significant variations remain in state Medicaid programs, which contribute to continuing inequities in their coverage of the low-income population. Furthermore, not all states have the same capability to administer increasingly complex programs; for example, contracting, negotiating with, and monitoring managed care plans require an entirely different set of skills than those needed to pay provider claims.

Moreover, huge differences continue to exist among the states in their commitment and ability to subsidize health care for uninsured residents. While almost every state tries to assure access to emergency care, only those states with better economies and tax bases are generally willing and able to provide access to basic health care for most or all of their poor citizens. Virtually every state perceives limits on its ability to provide comprehensive health benefits to every resident because of political and economic realities that make it hard to impose taxes to support such services. One clear message from the states' efforts to expand the reach of Medicaid

and other programs for low-income people is that no state can do it without the financial help and legislative sanction of the federal government.

STATE ROLES IN ASSURING THE PUBLIC'S HEALTH

One of the oldest and most fundamental roles played by states in the health arena has been seeking to protect the public's health. Originally, this meant controlling the spread of communicable disease. The role has expanded exponentially over the past several decades to include protecting the environment, workplaces, housing, food, and water; preventing injuries and promoting healthy behaviors; responding to disasters and assisting communities in recovery efforts; assuring the quality, accessibility, and accountability of medical care, and providing basic health services when otherwise unavailable; monitoring population health status and changes in the health care system; and developing policies and plans that support individual and community health improvement. The Institute of Medicine (1988) condensed these various activities into three basic functions: assessment of health status and systems; policy development; and assurance of personal, educational, and environmental health services.

In some ways, states are more similar to each other in their approaches to these basic public health functions than the other roles they play in the health arena. However, their ability to perform all of their public health protection roles has been eroded by an increasing need to provide health services directly to those who cannot obtain them in the private sector. The biggest challenge facing state public health agencies today is how they can strengthen their capacity to protect and promote the public's health, while assuring that basic health services are still available to those who cannot pay.

Among the three levels of government—federal, state, and local—states have primary responsibility for public health functions. States have the constitutional authority to make laws that provide for public health and welfare. Even so, states must carry out certain public health protection responsibilities delegated to them by the federal government, such as monitoring and assuring that they meet environmental quality standards. At the same time, states have great incentives to encourage or require local governments to share responsibility for implementing various public health programs. They must also decide how much each locality should receive of available federal and state public health funds, based on their needs and capabilities.

Personal health services funded or provided by states, often in cooperation with local government, range from public health nursing and communicable disease control, to family planning and prenatal care, to nutritional counseling and home health services. States have long been involved in the direct provision of health care, though their role is sometimes overshadowed by local governments, which are more likely to own and operate expensive public hospitals. Many states, however, continue to operate mental institutions.

Total state health agency expenditures (excluding Medicaid) rose from $2.5 billion in 1976, to $6.8 billion in 1985, to $8.3 billion in 1988. Of all these dollars, the majority—about 75 percent—are devoted to personal health services, with an emphasis on maternal and child health services. Personal health program expenditures on services provided outside institutional settings showed the largest increase over this period. As of 1988, federal grant and contract funds contributed 36 percent of total spending (down from 56 percent in 1985) while state funds contributed 55 percent; fees and other sources made up the remaining 5 percent. Interestingly, most of the federal funds given to states for health programs come from the U.S. Department of Agriculture's Special Supplemental Food Program for Women, Infants, and Children (WIC). Local Health Departments spent another $1.6 billion in 1985, rising to $4 billion in 1988 (Public Health Foundation, 1990).

As important as these services have been to communities, state and local governments could barely keep up with the need to provide care to those who could not afford it in the private sector. The demand for services from public health agencies rose gradually during the 1980s, as more and more people lacked health insurance and had few other alternatives in the private sector to obtain free or low-cost care. By 1988, it had become increasingly clear that "many state governments [were] unwilling to provide a large amount of funding necessary for providing health care to all indigent people as well as support public health departments" (Institute of Medicine, 1988)

That the public health functions were neglected or sorely wanting, in order to provide care to those without the ability to pay, became painfully clear with the emergence of new diseases, especially AIDS, and the resurgence of "old" diseases, including typhoid, measles, and tuberculosis. The latter in particular "is a warning to public policy makers of the danger of neglecting the public health agencies and programs" (Gittler, 1994).

This does not mean that states were completely negligent. In fact, when human immunodeficiency virus (HIV) first appeared in the early 1980s, states filled an important gap left by the federal government in responding to one of the major public health crises of our age. Nearly 80 percent of the states formed an AIDS task force, commission, or other advisory group to review state policies and recommend changes to the governor or the legislature, long before the federal government organized such a commission (see Robins & Backstrom, Chapter 20).

Virtually every state government, especially those hit hardest by the epidemic (New York, California, New Jersey, Florida, and Texas), contended with a myriad of issues that the federal government largely avoided during the first several years of the epidemic (Shilts, 1987). They had to decide how to establish screening programs and whether to allow or require tests for HIV among various groups of the population; how to establish surveillance of HIV infection that protected the public's health while maintaining individuals' right to privacy; what legal actions would be necessary to reduce discrimination against persons with AIDS or HIV infection; what types of financing options could be used to pay for services needed by AIDS patients; how to provide comprehensive, coordinated medical care and support services to AIDS patients; what types of public education programs were needed; and how much to support research on the causes and treatment of AIDS (Rowe & Ryan, 1987).

There are numerous examples of states taking the initiative to address the AIDS epidemic, with the majority of them doing so in ways that helped reduce the panic and fear associated with AIDS. For example, in almost every state legislature where it was proposed, mandatory premarital testing for HIV was defeated, recognizing that this was among the least effective methods available for detection and control. Many states took explicit action to extend antidiscrimination protection to people with AIDS or HIV infection. And nearly every state established public health education programs aimed at health professionals, persons displaying high-risk behaviors, the general public, or all three groups.

As the Institute of Medicine observed, however, "public health officials at the state and local level are very much aware of their responsibility to make sure that AIDS is combated effectively. But they are hamstrung by the speed with which the problem has developed and the political heat it has generated, as well as by the difficulty of marshaling enough resources to do what they feel is needed" (1988, p. 134).

It became clear that public health was receiving an ever smaller share of the total health care spending pie. Between 1981 and 1993, total U.S. spending on health care rose by over 200 percent, while funding for public health activities dropped 25 percent. If the solution to the crumbling public health infrastructure simply involved increased funding, it might be possible to address the problem. But it was not that simple.

The deterioration of public health agencies was due only in part to insufficient funding for core public health activities. Public health agencies also had more difficulty recruiting and retaining qualified health professionals, in part due to lower salaries than those offered by the private sector. More seriously, the Institute of Medicine concluded that the public health system "is a hodgepodge of fractionated interests and programs, organizational turmoil among new agencies, and well-intended but unbalanced appropriations—without coherent direction by well-qualified professionals" (1988, p. 139). A follow-up report in 1992 found little change. In other words, to deal adequately with AIDS, tuberculosis, and other serious public health problems would take more than increased funds. It would also require stronger leadership, a more skilled public health work-

force, a comprehensive data collection system, and greater coordination between public and private sectors and among levels of government.

To their credit, state policymakers have started to explore ways to address this challenging agenda. In order to breathe new life into essential public health functions, states in the 1990s started the process of cutting back on their own involvement in providing direct services to individuals. But in some cases, they did so by shifting more responsibility back to city and county governments—in effect, dumping the problem on other public agencies.

Some states signaled a more fundamental change in their approach to the problem by providing greater incentives to the private sector to care for low-income people, as discussed previously. Such actions were spurred in great part by the belief that expanded insurance coverage—perhaps even universal coverage—was on the horizon as suggested by health care reform debates occurring in 1993 and 1994. Universal coverage would make it possible for states and local governments to completely withdraw from their role as providers of direct care to the indigent and operators of public hospitals since this care would be available in the private sector.

For example, states such as Washington and Minnesota, which were among those to make significant commitments to universal coverage, also made the improvement of public health an explicit goal of state health reform. To achieve this goal, they updated or redefined the core functions of their public health agencies and allocated some additional funds to strengthen the capacity of local health agencies in performing them (Washington State Department of Health, 1994; Minnesota Department of Health, 1995).

Few other states followed their lead, however. With the defeat of national health care reform proposals in 1994 and the slowing of state health care reform efforts in 1994 and 1995, the words "universal coverage" faded quickly from public dialogue and media attention. Even in the absence of universal coverage, however, some states continued to strengthen their public health systems and redefine their roles to deemphasize direct delivery. In states where private managed care companies found it more attractive to serve Medicaid clients than they had in the past, local Health Departments saw a decline in the amount of direct care provided to Medicaid patients. And as public hospitals realized it was in their interest to integrate inpatient with outpatient services, some local Health Departments found anxious buyers for their clinics.

The challenge before state public health agencies for the rest of this decade and into the next century becomes one of seeking such partnerships with the private sector or with local governments. The goal is not merely to decrease their role in direct care, but rather to engage private-sector and local government partners in efforts that will improve overall health status. One of the potential benefits of the emerging dominance of managed care organizations in the private health care market is their greater incentive to invest in prevention and ability to deliver population-based services, at least to their enrolled population. Indeed, some managed care organizations are becoming much more involved in activities once relegated solely to public health (*Medicine and Health*, 1995). Whether states are able to harness such ability for the good of the community at large, however, will be a much bigger test.

STATES AS REGULATORS OF THE HEALTH INDUSTRY

States are vested with broad legal authority to regulate almost every facet of the health care system. They license and regulate health care facilities and health professionals; restrict the content, marketing, and price of health insurance (including professional liability or malpractice insurance); set and enforce environmental quality standards; and enact a variety of controls on health care costs.

During the 1980s and early 1990s, states pursued two very different paths in the regulatory arena. For some industries or sectors, many states decided to eliminate or significantly reduce regulations in favor of allowing private market forces to achieve public policy objectives, such as cost control. But for other health care entities, most states strengthened regulations and gave state agencies more power to set rules for private

market behaviors. What were the motivations that drove these opposite trends, and what have been the results of states' actions so far?

Traditionally, states have focused much of their regulatory attention on health facility construction or expansion and equipment purchases. As a result of federal legislation passed in 1975 (the National Health Planning and Resources Development Act), states were mandated to establish state health planning and development agencies. Their purpose was to review and approve certificates-of-need (CONs) for new hospital and health facility construction, a condition required for Medicare reimbursement by the federal government.

When the Reagan administration reduced and later eliminated the health planning program in the mid-1980s, several states began to weaken or abolish their CON programs. In 1983, New Mexico and Idaho were the first two states to repeal their CON statutes. In the following two years, another four states allowed their CON programs to sunset.

Another traditional focus for state regulatory oversight of the health care industry was hospital costs. In 1981, nine states had mandatory hospital rate-setting programs and another eight asked hospitals to comply with voluntary budget reviews (Esposito et al., 1982). Among these states was New Jersey, which since 1976 had been involved in an experiment funded by the federal Health Care Financing Administration to develop a hospital prospective rate-setting system based on a patient's diagnosis. The case-mix system, using a set of diagnosis-related groups (DRGs), was adopted in 1980, and was used to set the rates paid by all payers, including Medicare, Medicaid, and all commercial and non-profit insurance plans in the state. This prospective payment, DRG-based rate-setting system was later adopted by the federal government to replace the former cost-based reimbursement system used to pay hospitals in the Medicare program.

But toward the end of the 1980s and the early 1990s, states swung back in the other direction. By 1995, only one state (Maryland) controlled the rates that all public and private payers could pay hospitals. One other state, New York, still had hospital rate setting in place for all commercial insurers, Blue Cross and Blue Shield,

HMOs, and Medicaid. The rest eliminated their hospital rate-setting programs, or made hospital budget review completely voluntary, and in 1995 New York seriously considered a major overhaul of its prospective hospital reimbursement methodology.

What drove these deregulation trends? The usual explanation is that states wanted to allow economic forces of supply and demand to reassert themselves. The antiregulatory, procompetition forces convinced a majority of legislators that excess supply would lead suppliers to drop their prices, according to basic economic principles. By getting states out of the business of price setting, buyers would be free to bargain with health providers to get lower prices.

The actual behavior of state policymakers indicates that in their role as purchasers of health services, they still preferred to protect their own financial interests by setting their own terms and prices. For example, while more states joined the CON deregulation bandwagon—twelve states repealed their programs after the federal government ended national health planning—the program hardly faded away. Efforts to repeal CON programs failed in several states. Furthermore, even states that deregulated the CON process still required some state review of newly constructed facilities, particularly nursing homes.

State officials understood that to permit unfettered construction of new nursing homes would strain their Medicaid long-term care budgets, since that program covers about half of all nursing home bills. The more beds built, the more would be filled and the more elderly and disabled people would eventually deplete their resources and come to rely on Medicaid. When it came to their own economic interests, states recognized great value in limiting health facility construction.

In a similar fashion, while states may have eschewed setting hospital rates for private payers, they were anxious to do so for their Medicaid programs. Between 1985 and 1995, nearly every state switched from a cost-based reimbursement system to pay hospitals to a Medicare-like DRG system in which states set the rates in advance. Granted, hospitals were allowed to keep any excess revenues if they could provide care at a cost less than the DRG rate for a given condition. But states also set limits on the profits that hospitals could make from Medicaid payments, and in most states, that amount is little to none. This suggests that state policymakers were far more comfortable letting private purchasers and payers fend for themselves in the market, than they were in trusting market forces to work in their own favor.

Nor did states give the market every opportunity to work by getting out of the way of competitive forces or loosening regulatory restrictions on the industry. This is best exemplified by reforms in the small group health insurance market. In the early 1990s, state policymakers came to recognize that those least able to secure affordable health insurance in the private market were small companies, generally those with fewer than fifty or so employees. Such companies are more subject to medical underwriting, which involves an assessment of employees' health status and their risk of needing health care. Because insurers based their premium rates on the health care experience of the group, rather than on community-wide rates, employers with older workers and those with even one worker who had a disabled child faced much higher premium rates. Some could not get insurance at any price. Small firms also lacked the leverage to bargain for better rates that larger companies with many more "covered lives" could obtain.

To level the playing field for small firms, all but five states had adopted what were collectively known as "small group insurance reforms" by the end of 1994 (Chollet & Paul, 1994). These included some of the following: (1) requiring all insurers that sell to small groups to guarantee issue of coverage, regardless of the groups' health risks, claims experience, and so on; (2) setting limits on the criteria that insurers could use to adjust rates, often restricted to age, geographic location, and family size; (3) setting bands around which rates could not vary (e.g., within 25% of the average premium for each class of individual or group); (4) allowing benefit packages sold to small groups to exclude some services that would otherwise be required; and (5) limiting preexisting condition exclusion periods to a certain amount of time, generally no more than six months to a year, and waiving such exclusions for people that formerly had coverage within the prior few months (referred to as portability). At least a dozen states also authorized the establishment of purchasing alliances for small groups to increase their ability to bargain for better rates as a larger group.

The combination of these restrictions on insurers and the number of states adopting them would suggest a veritable conversion to the regulatory gospel. Yet it is clear from the legislative history of these reforms that their primary purpose was not to regulate per se, but to increase the availability and affordability of health insurance for those who wanted it. The laws did not coerce small firms to buy coverage since the decision to purchase health insurance remained voluntary. And compared to other strategies that might increase coverage, such as direct subsidies, the insurance reforms were certainly less onerous to state budgets.

What effect have the insurance reforms had so far? While few studies have carefully examined their combined or separate effects, early experience of the small group insurance reforms suggests that they have very little net effect on how many people are insured (Morrisey & Jensen, 1994). However, community rating of the small group market appeared to have the greatest impact on the market, by forcing insurers to compete on the basis of their ability to manage costs, rather than through risk selection (Chollet & Paul, 1994). With respect to health insurance purchasing cooperatives for small business, the early experience is only a bit more positive. Those that have the ability to negotiate with carriers (not all do) appear to have a better chance of holding down the rise in health care premiums (U.S. General Accounting Office, 1994; Lipson & De Sa, 1995).

The fundamental puzzle remains: How does one reconcile the seeming contradiction between state actions that are promarket and procompetitive with those that are clearly regulatory? Many analysts characterize the past several years as a period in which the pendulum has swung back in favor of market-oriented approaches to health care cost control. Yet state actions indicate an equally, if not stronger, trend to reassert greater control over the health industry.

The explanation lies somewhere in state policymakers' genuine attempts to find the right balance between market forces and government regulation that will most effectively hold down health care cost increases while assuring consumers' (voters') rights are protected. It is often a difficult balancing point, but one for which some states continually search.

Minnesota may be the best example of a state that continues to refine its market-oriented approach to health care cost control and its government intervention in the market to afford equal access and coverage for its citizens. Over the past twelve to fifteen years, the state sometimes swung more in one direction or the other. But for the most part, it has also striven to find the right amount and type of government attempts to structure the health care market.

For example, the state repealed its CON program in 1984, in line with its preference for using market forces to improve the efficiency of health care services and reduce health care costs. However, in recognition of its position as having one of the highest rates of nursing home beds per capita of any state, Minnesota slapped an indefinite moratorium on nursing home construction—one that continues ten years later. While the state still has among the highest ratios of nursing home beds to population in the country, at least it has not become any worse. Minnesota was also among the leading states in fostering the development and growth of new health care plans—HMOs, PPOs, and other hybrid managed care plans. It did so both by restructuring the state employee benefits program to restrict workers' choices to managed care plans, and later, by codifying into law the types of organizations they would require all health care entities to become. Called integrated service networks, or ISNs, these were regarded by some as "next-generation HMOs," defined as publicly accountable, risk-bearing, integrated financing and delivery systems. At the same time, the state established several requirements for HMOs to assure that the plans would in fact be accountable to consumers. For example, HMOs must be non-for-profit (with minimum and maximum capital reserve limits), and they must collaborate with public health agencies to develop plans that will improve population health.

The health care regulatory changes in Minnesota over the past decade demonstrate the state's strong interest in promoting marketplace solutions with an equally strong willingness to step in to protect consumers. Its example sets a good one for other states struggling to find such a balance. But their exact actions are not necessarily ones that should be duplicated in every state. Health care markets are still essentially local. That is, the unique combination of provider supply, insurer types and market shares, purchaser sophistication in bargaining, and the ability of providers to guarantee care for the uninsured varies tremendously from state to state and from community to community.

Thus, the goal for each state is to determine how much leeway and how much protection to afford the players in each sector to make competition work and to make it work fairly in their state or local markets. One of the more difficult issues facing states in this arena concerns the appropriate type of regulation, if any, for one of the newest forms of managed care entities: physician/hospital organizations (PHOs). These organizations are alliances between hospital(s) and a group of physicians that join together for purposes of negotiating contracts with purchasers to provide health care services. In many cases, PHOs contract directly with insurance companies and HMOs. But in some instances, they are seeking to directly contract with employers; in the process the PHOs take on a level of financial risk that presents insurance regulators with some concerns.

State insurance regulators have just begun to formulate the questions that must be asked, even before they decide how to regulate these new organizations, if at all (Blankenau, 1994). For example, should PHOs be regulated as insurance plans if they assume financial risk? Does the answer depend on the degree of financial risk assumed? Or, is the relevant issue with whom the PHO contracts and whether state regulators can oversee their financial status? As a sign of their concern with promoting competition and delivery innovations that contain costs, state officials' biggest concern is how to regulate the financial risk borne by PHOs without thwarting the development of integrated delivery systems that are better able to control health care costs (Bureau of National Affairs, 1994).

States have an even more challenging task in determining whether those providers who cannot compete, or those the market will not include, will still be given a seat at the table. For example, what will happen if insurers regard academic health centers, public hospitals, and community health centers as too expensive to include in their provider networks? Will independent physicians, who wish to remain independent from large insurer or provider systems, be assured the right of contracting with all groups? Or will health plans be reserved the right to pick and choose the most cost-efficient providers, even if that means leaving out some that are the major providers of care to people in certain communities? As managed care continues to enroll an ever greater proportion of the population, these are questions that states will confront more frequently in the years ahead.

STATES AS LEADERS IN COMPREHENSIVE HEALTH REFORM

In 1993 and 1994, the nation debated proposals that would have changed its health care system in dramatic and fundamental ways. President Clinton was elected to office in part because of a campaign platform that emphasized the need for "health care that could never be taken away." In the aftermath of the defeat of his proposed Health Security Act, many commentators believed that the focus of the debate would shift to the states.

Perhaps a more accurate description of the direction of that focus, however, would have been a *returning* to the states. As this review of states' involvement in health care issues has shown, states have always been active in financing and regulating the health care system, and in seeking to promote or protect public health. But what often got lost in the glare of the spotlight on the national health care reform debate of 1993 and 1994 was that states were already undertaking comprehensive reforms of their own.

As already noted, several states have made important strides in expanding coverage to low-income uninsured groups through subsidy programs, Medicaid expansions, and insurance reforms. Many states have implemented effective cost-containment programs, such as hospital rate setting and setting limits on insurance premium increases. In the area of delivery system reforms, several states have enacted laws that actively encourage health care providers to form integrated systems that can achieve greater efficiencies and provide more coordinated patient care.

Moreover, a handful of states have even put together reforms addressing the triad of problems plaguing the health system—high costs, uneven access, and uncertain quality—in an integrated, cohesive fashion. Two states in particular—Oregon and Minnesota—stand out for their bold efforts to bring more rationality and equity to their health care systems.

The Oregon Health Plan

Oregon began its health care reform odyssey in 1989 with the passage of the Oregon Health Plan, an innovative program that would provide coverage to all individuals with incomes below the poverty line but limit covered benefits to those that had been proven cost-effective. The state's explicit attempt to ration services gained it much notoriety. According to the plan, if state funds were insufficient to cover all services to all poor individuals, services that fell lower on the "priority list" would be cut, rather than individuals or provider payments. While taking a step toward more rational allocation of resources, the plan remained vulnerable to charges of discrimination since the priority list has been limited to the poor.

Oregon coupled this plan with a mandate for employers to cover all qualified workers, tax incentives to encourage employers to provide coverage before the mandate would take effect, and concerted efforts to enroll Medicaid beneficiaries into managed care plans. The state was unable to get a federal ERISA exemption to implement its employer mandate, due to congressional resistance to tampering with large employers' benefit plans that are protected by ERISA. But because it obtained federal approval of its Section 1115 waiver application, over 125,000 individuals have been enrolled in the Oregon Health Plan thus far.

MinnesotaCare and Other Initiatives

Minnesota is also notable for its comprehensive approach to reform as well as its attempts to build on the successes of the private market in holding down costs in the larger health care system (U.S. Congress, Office of Technology Assessment, 1994). It folded its Children's Health Plan into a larger subsidy program, called Min-

nesotaCare, which has covered over 85,000 people. Although the state's uninsured rate remained fairly constant between 1992 and 1994, state officials believe the rate would have been higher if the program had not offset losses in private employer-sponsored coverage. The uninsured rate may even start to decline in the future when the state begins to implement its Medicaid 1115 waiver that will bring in more federal dollars to help finance coverage to even more uninsured people.

On the cost-containment side, Minnesota has sought to encourage more rapid formation of integrated service networks, which are systems that can accept capitated payments to deliver a comprehensive array of services. Although a law adopted in 1993 allows the state to limit annual increases in premium rates to these networks, the state has not needed to do so as cost increases have remained below the state-determined level. While intended as a backup mechanism, the state legislature nonetheless decided in 1995 to repeal this provision due to antiregulatory sentiment in the legislature.

To improve access and promote public health, the state adopted a set of reforms designed to increase the numbers of primary care physicians graduating from the state medical school, encourage the formation of rural health networks to make care more accessible in underserved areas, and ensure that managed care plans and public health agencies work together on projects that will improve overall population health.

It is still too early to evaluate the combined effects of these strategies on overall costs, insurance coverage levels, quality of care, and health outcomes in Oregon and Minnesota compared to those in other states. But these states give credence to the notion that in contrast to the national level, state-level political processes can produce consensus on a strategy that makes more than incremental change. This is not to say that states in general are better than the federal government at overcoming "craven politics, bureaucratic domination, or capture by special interests" (Brown, 1994). Nor does this mean that any state's approach should serve as *the* model for the nation; the country is simply too diverse to expect one model to serve the needs of every state.

Instead, the value of such attempts at comprehensive reform lies in the practical and political lessons they can offer to other states and to the federal government, even before the final results are known. For example, according to Governor Howard Dean of Vermont, the key lesson from Oregon is that the public will support limitations in coverage, as long as they "see a perceptible improvement in service alongside the financial constraints" (Neville, 1995). Minnesota showed that, at least for four years, provider taxes were regarded as politically acceptable sources of financing for covering the uninsured. Moreover, efforts by state employee benefit programs to structure premium contributions and negotiate with managed care plans could serve as useful models for the federal Medicare program. Many state employee health benefit plans aggressively negotiate with contracting health plans, limit the number of plans that can participate to encourage competition, and require strong cost management techniques for those plans that win the contracts (National Institute for Health Care Management, 1995).

In the end, the most important lesson that states can teach through their attempts at comprehensive reform is that they cannot solve the financing problem alone, although they may be the most appropriate level of government for dealing with local delivery system problems. As Lawrence Brown concluded, "financing, coverage and entitlement issues require central government rules that are clear and firm and that admit exceptions that are few, marginal and well-justified. Delivery system and, perhaps, cost containment mechanisms demand the reverse: a federal framework of 'rules' that are fairly broad and flexible and that permit localities to improvise arrangements—within national limits to be sure—that make sense for them" (Brown, 1994, p. 14).

STATE ROLES IN HEALTH CARE IN THE FUTURE

The end of the twentieth century presents a mixed picture for states. The economic recovery of 1994 and 1995 brightened prospects for state revenue projections. States' reserves—an important indicator of fiscal health—were at their highest levels in fifteen years. But state budgets may be in for a battering.

The 1994 election that gave Republicans control of both houses of Congress resulted in a set of proposals that are likely to reduce the federal flow of funds to states in all areas, but especially in health care services. Congressional bills under consideration in 1995 proposed to turn over even greater authority for health care programs to the states through transforming two entitlement programs—Medicaid and Aid to Families with Dependent Children (AFDC)—into block grants. These proposals represented a significant departure from previous policy by ending the entitlement nature of these programs. States would also receive less federal funding than they did before because the bills proposed to limit the annual growth in spending on these programs, regardless of the number of people in need. One study found that even if states successfully controlled costs in their Medicaid program through provider payment reductions, elimination of optional benefits, and greater use of managed care, some states would still have to reduce the number of eligible people to live within the caps proposed (4 percent growth rate annually, compared to 10 percent that is projected between 1996 and 2000; see Kaiser Commission on the Future of Medicaid, 1995c).

How might states respond to cuts in federal funding on this order of magnitude? The answer depends on several factors. The first is how much flexibility the federal government grants them. Another set of factors involves differences among the states themselves—their administrative and management capabilities, their capacity to absorb the cuts, and their willingness to raise additional funds for health and social services. Wide variations in the latter set of factors suggest that the effects of federal budget cuts will play out in the states in very different ways.

While the intent of block grants is to give states more freedom, it remains uncertain just how much control the federal government is willing to give up. The history of the 1981 block grants showed that "over time constraints were added which had the effect of 'recategorizing' them. These constraints often took the forms of set-asides, requiring a minimum portion of funds be used for a specific purpose, and cost ceilings, specifying the maximum portion of funds that could be used for other purposes" (U.S. General Accounting Office, 1995). If they have fewer resources with greater responsibilities and only a small increase in flexibility, states will face the worst of all possible scenarios. It would make it almost impossible for them to carry out long-standing responsibilities for overseeing the health care system and take on some of the new roles that are evolving from changes in the private health marketplace or in response to new public health problems. For example, if Medicaid funding is cut and eligibility is tightened, more people will be without health insurance. In turn, this will make it necessary for state and local public Health Departments to increase their resources devoted to direct patient care at the expense of critical public health activities needed to protect the general population.

With greater flexibility, states may be able to shield current Medicaid eligibles from being cut. Some believe that with increased flexibility to shift funds between programs and blend funds from different sources, efficiencies could be produced that will stretch dollars farther than they went before (National Health Policy Forum, 1995). Others believe that decisions about which programs to cut, how much to cut, and how the cuts should be targeted are likely to depend more on political choices. They argue that in the case of Medicaid program cuts, nursing home lobbyists will always win the day over advocates for poor children (National Health Policy Forum, 1995).

In terms of state administrative capacity, it appears that states have improved markedly over the past twenty years. Based on the growing number of staff in state legislatures, organizational restructuring of the executive branches, improved fiscal management practices, and other factors, "states have actually strengthened both their structures and functions and their finances to the point where they are quite capable of assuming full partnership in the federal system. Indeed, by almost every measure, states have improved their ability to govern, provide services, and meet the current and anticipated future needs of their constituents" (U.S. Advisory Committee on Intergovernmental Relations, 1980). Another report on the subject five years later found state governments to be "more representative, more responsive, more activist and more professional in their operations than they ever have been" (U.S. Advisory Committee on Intergovernmental Relations, 1985).

Other analysts have taken a less sanguine view of the report, arguing that there is not necessarily a direct relationship between large legislative staffs and enhanced effectiveness in governing (Thompson, 1986). Ten years after those reports were written, there remain large discrepancies among the states with respect to number and skill of legislative, policy analysis, and program management capability. New York and California, for instance, have much greater management capacity and legislative support staff than North Dakota and Alaska. So, some states will be better equipped to manage their own health and welfare programs, should Congress give them the flexibility to do so. Still, the scope of the changes and extraordinary increase in the states' responsibilities proposed by Congress suggest that every state will face significant administrative and technical challenges in designing and managing their own programs.

Each state's response to the massive turnover of responsibilities from the federal government will also depend on their capacity to absorb reductions in federal funds. If spending growth caps do not account adequately for variations in each state's demographic profile, for example, states with greater proportions of higher-cost elderly and disabled residents will be more hard-pressed than those with higher proportions of lower-cost children. States with fast-growing populations of poor and low-income residents will fare worse than those with steady or declining numbers of people in poverty.

Finally, one of the most important determinants of how each state reacts to federal funding cuts will be their fiscal systems and willingness to modify their tax structures to make up for lost federal dollars. Almost half the states have a limitation on the growth of state spending or revenue, usually tied to the increase in personal income (Gold, 1990). These measures could cause serious problems since none of them make an allowance for relaxing the limits when the federal government imposes new responsibilities on states or cuts in funding.

In addition, because most states rely heavily on personal/corporate income taxes and sales taxes, a recession could cause serious fiscal problems in nearly all states since economic downturns reduce the amounts raised from these sources. Without any guaranteed financial assistance from the federal government, a recession could cause large revenue shortfalls in those states affected. Because all states but one have constitutional requirements to balance their budgets, a revenue shortfall dictates that states either cut spending or increase taxes. Given taxpayer resistance to tax increases, the latter is not likely unless there is a perceived fiscal emergency. The size of the federal funding cuts and their impact on each state will determine whether and in what circumstances such emergencies are serious enough to warrant such an action.

Some states that eschew tax raises may instead take the opportunity to restructure their tax systems to bring in revenue that escapes current tax mechanisms. For example, during the recession of the early 1990s, a dozen states enacted changes in their income tax codes to make them more progressive; others broadened their sales tax base to capture growth in the service sector (Lemov, 1992). These strategies could be used by other states to compensate for federal funding cuts.

The outcome of this experiment in public policy and in federalism cannot be predicted with any certainty. As this chapter amply demonstrates, some states will rise to the challenges ahead while others will perform poorly. If the past can be regarded as prologue, states will continue to display wide variation in the manner they carry out both traditional health policy roles as well as new ones demanded by a changing health care system. It also indicates that if states bear even greater responsibility for Medicaid policy with fewer federal restrictions, the differences among states in both eligibility levels and range of services will likely grow even more extreme.

Conclusion

After fifteen years of experience with a shift in the locus of control to the states, it is important to ask whether the variation that inevitably results from a lack of federal standards leads to an unacceptable degree of inequity among citizens of different states. There will always be states that are slow to act in the face of crises, or unwilling to address glaring inequities in the health care system. These are the states that are often held up

as reasons for greater national involvement in health care issues of the day. And it is not always the "slow" or "unwilling" states that highlight the need for federal involvement in health policy. Sometimes the most innovative states illustrate the need for federal action by demonstrating the obstacles that federal law puts in the way of state efforts to make progress and the need for Congress to remove those constraints.

Occasionally, state government representatives argue that they would be happy to let the federal government take over any number of health programs, as long as states would not have to be financially obligated to help pay for them. But if the federal government expects states to help pay the bills, they argue, then state flexibility is essential due to variations in state economies and tax policies.

For now, this is the argument that seems to have won the day. In the immediate future, states are likely to continue to play a critical role in health policymaking, because the federal government is trying to reduce its responsibilities and would like the states to maintain their existing financial contributions to health services and long-term care. As long as the states' portion of the health care expenditures remains as high as it is, they will continue to retain substantial power in any national debate on health care issues.

Regardless of how much of the bill they pay, states are not likely to give up any of their other roles—as protectors and promoters of the public health and as regulators of the health industry. With the pendulum of federalism still swinging away from strong federal government control, states are likely to be first in line for taking on any new roles that the public decides are appropriate for government.

For now, the consensus appears to be that states have proven their ability to manage complex programs, successfully maneuver their way in and out of regulatory relationships with the private sector, and develop innovative strategies to deal with health care problems more quickly than the federal government in ways that respond to the unique set of political and economic factors and conditions in each state. As one review of the states' assumption of new roles during the 1980s concluded, "At its best, a renewed federalism—in which the states play a more active policy-making role than the national government—can produce innovative solutions to vexing problems, allowing states to test these remedies on a small scale, discarding what doesn't work and building on what does" (Hamilton, 1988).

Whether this remains the case, however, will hinge on how states meet the challenges of the next decade. If they do well in the eyes of the public, the scale of federalism that tilted in their favor in the 1980s and 1990s will continue on into the next century. Their failure is likely to see the pendulum swing back to a stronger federal role.

REFERENCES

Blankenau, Renee. (1994). The rules of the game: New solvency standards will govern health plans, capitation arrangements. *Hospitals and Health Networks, 68* (July 20), 44–46.

Brown, Lawrence D. (1994). Federalism and health reform: An introduction. In Forrest P. Chisman et al. (Eds.), *National health reform: What should the state role be?* Washington, D.C.: National Academy of Social Insurance.

Bureau of National Affairs. (1994). As PHOs assume financial risk, state regulators consider PHO-specific rules. *Health Care Policy Report, 2* (November 14), 1906–1907.

Butler, Patricia. (1988). *Too poor to be sick: Access to medical care for the uninsured.* Washington, D.C.: American Public Health Association.

Chisman, Forrest P., Lawrence D. Brown, & Pamela J. Larson. (Eds.). (1994). *National health reform: What should the state role be?* Washington, D.C.: National Academy of Social Insurance.

Chollet, Deborah J., & Rebecca R. Paul. (1994). *Community rating: Issues and experience.* Washington, D.C.: Alpha Center.

Congressional Quarterly. (1982). *Weekly Report, 40,* 178.

Coughlin, Teresa A., Leighton Ku, & John Holahan. (1994). *Medicaid since 1980: Costs, coverage, and the shifting alliance between the federal government and the states.* Washington, D.C.: Urban Institute Press.

Desonia, Randolph, & Kathleen M. King. (1985). *State programs of assistance for the medically indigent.* Washington, D.C.: Intergovernmental Health Policy Project, George Washington University.

Esposito, Alfonso, et al. (1982). Abstracts of state legislated hospital cost containment programs. *Health Care Financing Review, 4* (2), 129–158.

Fraley, Collette. (1995). States guard their borders as Medicaid talks begin. *Congressional Quarterly, 54* (223), 1637–1641.

Gittler, Josephine. (1994). Controlling resurgent tuberculosis: Public health agencies, public policy and law. *Journal of Health Politics, Policy and Law, 19* (1), 107–147.

Gold, Steven D. (1990). *The state fiscal agenda for the 1990s.* Denver, CO: National Conference of State Legislatures.

Hamilton, Martha. (1988). States assuming new powers as federal policy role ebbs. *Washington Post* (August 30).

Holahan, John, Teresa A Coughlin, Leighton Ku, Debra J. Lipson, & Shruti Rajan. (1995). Insuring the poor through Medicaid 1115 waivers. *Health Affairs, 14* (1), 199–216.

Holahan, John, & Joel Cohen. (1986). *Medicaid: The trade-off between cost containment and access to care.* Washington, D.C.: Urban Institute Press.

Institute of Medicine. (1988). *The future of public health.* Committee for the Study of the Future of Public Health. Washington, D.C.: National Academy of Sciences.

Jain, Sagar C. (Ed.). (1981). Introduction and summary to role of state and local governments in relation to personal health services. *American Journal of Public Health, 71* (Suppl.), 5–8.

Kaiser Commission on the Future of Medicaid. (1995a). *Medicaid expenditures and beneficiaries: National and state profiles and trends, 1984–1993.* Washington, D.C.

Kaiser Commission on the Future of Medicaid. (1995b). *State variations in Medicaid: Implications for block grants and expenditure growth caps.* Policy brief prepared by John Holahan & David Liska. Washington, D.C.: Urban Institute.

Kaiser Commission on the Future of Medicaid. (1995c). *Medicaid and federal, state and local budgets.* Policy brief, Washington, D.C.

Lemov, Penelope. (1992). The decade of red ink. *Governing, 5* (9), 22–26.

Lewin-VHI. (1995). *States as payers: Managed care for Medicaid populations.* Washington, D.C.: National Institute for Health Care Management.

Lipson, Debra J. (1993). *The question behind the Medicaid provider tax debate: What constitutes a state dollar?* (Issue Brief No. 625). Washington, D.C.: National Health Policy Forum.

Lipson, Debra J. (1994). *Keeping the promise? Achieving universal health coverage in six states.* Innovations in State Health Reform Series. Menlo Park, CA: Henry J. Kaiser Family Foundation.

Lipson, Debra J., & Jeanne De Sa. (1995). *The health insurance plan of California: First year results of a purchasing alliance.* Washington, D.C.: Alpha Center.

Medicine and Health. (1995). Public health and managed care find common ground perspectives. Washington, D.C.: Faulkner and Gray. (August 14).

Miller, Victor J. (1992). State Medicaid expansion in the early 1990s: Program growth in a period of fiscal stress, in Medicaid financing crisis: Balancing responsibilities, priorities, and dollars. Background Papers, July, Kaiser Commission on the Future of Medicaid, Washington, D.C.

Minnesota Department of Health. (1995). Building a solid foundation for health: A report on public health system development. Community Health Services Division, March.

Morrisey, Michael, & Gail Jensen. (1994). *State small group insurance reform.* Unpublished paper presented at a conference on "Health Care Reform and the Role of States," sponsored by the Institute of Government and Public Affairs, University of Illinois, April 28–29.

National Association of State Budget Officers. (1994). 1993 state expenditure report. Washington, D.C., March.

National Governors Association. (1995). State coverage of pregnant women and children—February 1995. Health Policy Studies Division, Washington, D.C.

National Health Policy Forum. (1995). Exploring the impact of Medicaid block grants and spending caps. (Issue Brief No. 672).

National Institute for Health Care Management. (1995). States as purchasers: Innovations in state employee health benefit programs. Prepared by Lewin-VHI, Washington, D.C.

Neville, Sarah. (1995). Oregon may hold the key to public acceptance of health care rationing. *Washington Post* (July 10).

Peterson, George E. (1986). *The Reagan block grants.* Washington, D.C.: Urban Institute.

Public Health Foundation. (1990). Public health agencies 1990: Inventory of programs. Washington, D.C.: Public Health Foundation.

Rivlin, Alice. (1992). *Reviving the American dream: The economy, the states, and the federal government.* Washington, D.C.: The Brookings Institution.

Rowe, Mona, & Caitlin Ryan. (1987). *AIDS: A public health challenge, state issues, policies and programs, intergovernmental health policy project.* Washington, D.C.: George Washington University.

Rowland, Diane, Sara Rosenbaum, Lois Simon, & Elizabeth Chait. (1995). *Medicaid and managed care: Lessons from the literature.* Washington, D.C.: Kaiser Commission on the Future of Medicaid.

Shilts, Randy. (1987). *And the band played on: Politics, people and the AIDS epidemic.* New York: St. Martin's Press.

Sundquist, James. (1969). *Making federalism work.* Washington, D.C.: The Brookings Institution.

Thompson, Frank J. (1986). New Federalism and health care policy: States and the old questions. *Journal of Health Politics, Policy and Law, 11* (4), 647–669.

U.S. Advisory Commission on Intergovernmental Relations. (1980). ACIR and the intergovernmental system: A 20-year report. *Intergovernmental Perspective, 6,* 20.

U.S. Advisory Commission on Intergovernmental Relations. (1985). The question of state government capability. Washington, D.C.

U.S. Congress, Office of Technology Assessment. (1994). Managed care and competitive health care markets: The Twin Cities experience (OTA-BP-H-130). Washington, D.C.: U.S. Government Printing Office.

U.S. Department of Health and Human Services, Health Care Financing Administration, Office of the Actuary. (1987). National health expenditures, 1986–2000. *Health Care Financing Review, 8* (4), 1–36.

U.S. General Accounting Office. (1994). Access to health insurance: Public and private employers' experience with purchasing cooperatives (GAO/HEHS-94-142). Washington, D.C.: U.S. Government Printing Office.

U.S. General Accounting Office. (1995). Block grants: Characteristics, experience, and lessons learned (GAO/HEHS-95-74). Washington, D.C.: U.S. Government Printing Office.

U.S. Office of Management and Budget. (1990). Budget of the United States government, fiscal year 1991. Washington, D.C.: U.S. Government Printing Office.

Washington State Department of Health. (1994). Public health improvement plan. Olympia, WA.

PART THREE

THE ROLE OF PUBLIC OPINION AND INTEREST GROUPS IN HEALTH POLICY

The significant role public opinion and special interest groups play in the formation of health policy and the legislative process is the subject of a series of three insightful chapters by Robert Blendon and Mollyann Brodie, Paul Feldstein, and Katherine Hinckley with Bette Hill.

Drawing on a rich and extensive body of survey and polling data, Blendon and Brodie explore the relationship between public opinion and health policy outcomes, noting the conflicting views that Americans hold toward their government and health policy and the problems this poses for reaching consensus regarding an acceptable approach to health care reform in this country.

The importance that economic self-interest plays in framing the positions taken by various health-related special interest groups is highlighted by Feldstein in his chapter on the demand for legislation.

Finally, how health interest groups behave in the political arena and why they act the way they do is the focus on the Hinckley–Hill analysis of the strategic behavior of five major health interest groups—the American Hospital Association, the Federation of American Health Systems, the American Medical Association, the American Nurses Association, and the Health Insurance Association of America—vis-à-vis their dealings with Congress and to a somewhat lesser extent the presidency over the issues of Medicare, Medicaid, and National Health Insurance. While demonstrating that the strategic choices of such groups tend to be shaped by the nature of the organization itself, its resources, the character of the institutions it targets, and the current issue agenda, they conclude that in an issue-area as convoluted and hotly contested as national health policy, the decision to pursue either an inside or outside strategy is fraught with danger as each path leads onto treacherous ground.

CHAPTER

Public Opinion and Health Policy

Robert J. Blendon and Mollyann Brodie

This chapter addresses the relationship between public opinion and health policy outcomes. Because health policy takes place within the broader political system, it is influenced by the same factors that affect policy and politics in general, including public opinion, electoral outcomes, and political-institutional structures.

Understanding the nature of public opinion in the health care context is important for a number of reasons. First, public opinion influences the outcomes of elections. Candidates who wish to be elected to public office must concern themselves with the perceived needs and preferences of the American public. Public opinion surveys capture the mood, values, and policy preferences of Americans, and therefore help predict election outcomes and set political agendas. Public opinion in the electoral context is reflected by more than just opinion surveys, however; it includes individual contacts with elected officials (mail, telephone, and electronic technologies) and voting patterns.

Second, studies have shown that public opinion influences public decision making on many issues beyond election outcomes (Page & Shapiro, 1983; Monroe, 1979; Jacobs & Shapiro, 1994). Researchers have shown that public opinion is associated both with policy change and with the actions and decisions of Congress, the executive branch, and the Supreme Court. Public opinion was found to be the second most influential factor on congressional decision making in the 1993–94 health care reform debate (Columbia Institute, 1995). Furthermore, the 1989 repeal of the Medicare Catastrophic Act just one year after its passage has been largely attributed to the public's (in this case senior citizens') response to the increase in taxes required to pay for the expanded benefits of the Medicare program (Schur et al., 1990; American Association for Retired Persons, 1989; Wirthlin, 1989).

Third, public opinion matters because Americans have very low levels of trust in government leaders and experts. In the absence of a clear-cut legitimacy for the views of leaders and experts, political decisions to determine the direction of public policies often give substantial weight to the views of the public over those of government officials and experts. Therefore, understanding the public's policy preferences and attitudes toward decisions on the governmental agenda helps us predict trends in legislative decision making.

Fourth, though public opinion may not directly influence all policy decisions, particularly those made away from the public spotlight, it is a measure of the political environment within which issues are debated and discussed. As we will show later, the mood of Americans often has a direct and profound impact on the policy solutions they will support. During periods of economic uncertainty Americans' willingness to spend resources on public programs falls. Similarly, during periods when Americans feel decidedly cynical and distrustful of government, their willingness to grant the federal government more powers declines, particularly for policies that would increase government regulation in various aspects of their daily lives.

Finally, we should recognize the unique role that public opinion plays in the health field. Health care is a service industry that directly touches the lives of most Americans. Therefore, the public's views on how well the health system works or on how well doctors and hospitals serve them acts as one indicator of the success of our health policies. Cross-national studies show that Americans express a greater degree of dissatisfaction with their health care system than Canadians or West Germans. While 29 percent of Canadians and 30 percent of West Germans thought their respective health care systems worked fairly well and needed only minor changes, only 18 percent of Americans expressed this level of satisfaction (Blendon et al., forthcoming).

Interpreting appropriately the role public opinion plays requires some understanding of the nature of the issues involved and the context in which individuals are considering these issues. Public opinion will have a stronger influence and effect on policymaking when certain conditions are met. Public opinion is likely to be most influential in publicly visible debates, for issues that could affect the outcomes of elections, and for is-

sues decided by initiative or referendum. On the other hand, public opinion will matter less in the case of more technical policymaking, where the public lacks knowledge, interest, and views regarding the possible policy outcomes. For example, the public's views on whether specific factors should be used in devising the resource-based relative value scale to pay physicians for services provided to Medicare patients will be decidedly less important than their views on whether Medicare program eligibility should be changed so that only retirees age seventy and older are eligible. Similarly, because these issues are technical and far removed from average people's lives, the public's preferences on how clinical labs should be regulated are likely to be irrelevant, whereas their views will be decidedly more influential in the issue of whether individuals should be limited in their choices of doctors.

To analyze the role public opinion plays in health care policy this chapter is divided into three sections. In the first we explore some of the key principles of public opinion as it relates to health care policy. In the second section, we turn our attention to the key values and beliefs Americans hold that directly influence the way they think about health care policies and that shape the way in which they answer public opinion survey questions. With these tools, underlying principles, and core beliefs, the ability of public opinion to influence health policy will be infinitely clearer, as will our ability to understand and strategically respond to the dynamics of public opinion. Finally, in the third section we apply all we have learned to two cases: (1) the case of national health insurance over the period from President Truman to President Clinton; and (2) the case of a single-payer ballot initiative in California's 1994 November election.

KEY PRINCIPLES OF PUBLIC OPINION AS THEY RELATE TO HEALTH CARE POLICY

In order to understand the nature of public opinion on health care issues, we must first understand the key principles that underlie public opinion. Understanding these principles will make us much better interpreters of public opinion surveys and more sophisticated analysts of the health policy process.

Public Lacks Knowledge, But Holds Strong Beliefs and Values

Americans do not know a great deal about the details of health policy, but they do hold a set of core beliefs and values that shape how they think about health policy choices. Given their importance and influence, the next section of this chapter explores these core beliefs in greater depth. For now, however, note that poor performance on knowledge-based questions does not mean that the public is unable to draw clear policy preferences and exert strong opinions. For example, although the public knew little about the key issues and terms in the 1993–94 health care reform debate, they had come to the judgment that they did not support the Clinton plan. After a year-long debate about health care reform, the public remained largely unaware of the major Democratic alternatives to President Clinton's health reform plan and even less aware of Republican options. Nor did most Americans (73%) know that President Clinton was the principal sponsor of an employer mandate. Furthermore, in spite of intense media coverage, only 34 percent of the American public knew that most of the uninsured come from families in which someone is employed; and but 35 percent knew that the United States spends more of its economic resources on health care than other countries (Henry J. Kaiser Family Foundation/Harvard School of Public Health/Princeton Survey Research Associates, 1994). However, polling results showed that Americans had strong policy preferences: people wanted health care reform but opposed (48%) the president's plan—the only plan they were aware of (Gallup/CNN/*USA Today*, 1994b).

The Public Prioritizes Their Opinions on Issues

Because the number of issues for public debate exceeds the number any individual is able to pay attention to and engage in at a given point in time, individuals prioritize their opinions on issues, with some being more or less important to them personally. The political system recognizes this and responds to public priorities. Therefore, it is crucial to understand the salience, that is, the importance that the public ascribes to issues, particularly health policy issues.

Salience of a given issue is assessed in comparison to other issues. Use of the "Most Important Problem" question is the most common method of determining how salient an issue is to the public at any given point in time. Americans are periodically asked in an open-ended way: "What are the two most important issues you think are facing the country?" Or, alternatively, "What are the two most important issues for the government to solve?" Policymakers and legislators consider the issues that rank anywhere between number one to four as the most important issues on the public agenda and the ones most likely to influence the outcomes of elections. Often there is a close correlation between these rankings and the issues that gain the most visible media coverage.

In reality, issues are only one part of why an individual votes for a particular candidate. And, even when people do vote based on issues, it is only on a small number of issues. In fact, between 1960 and 1988, the president who was elected came from the same political party that the public deemed best able to solve the issue that was named the most important problem facing the country. Furthermore, since 1956, with only two exceptions, the elected president came from the party the public deemed better for the nation's prosperity. In the only two exceptions, the 1968 (Nixon) and 1980 (Reagan) elections, the winning party trailed the chosen party by less than 3 percentage points on this measure (Gallup/CONUS/*Los Angeles Times*, 1989).

Public opinion on a given issue will matter significantly more when that issue is salient to the American public, and, therefore, the health policy community needs to be well aware of the salience to which the public ascribes to the health policy issue at hand. For example, in 1990 almost 60 percent of Americans ranked medical costs as a very serious economic and social concern, while only about 25 percent ranked smoking and 19 percent ranked improving race relations at the same level of concern (Conference Board, 1990). Ultimately, the potential impact of public opinion can be predicted by the salience that the public or particular segments of the public ascribe to a specific issue.

Three Definitions of Who Constitutes the Public

As noted above, health policy is made within the political context. The political system distinguishes among three different definitions of what is public opinion, and at any given time each of these groups may have a different set of views on health policy legislation than those held by the other groups.

First, at the most general level the term "public" refers to all Americans. The views and opinions of this public can be discerned by national random sample telephone surveys.

Second, at the next level "public" refers to voters or likely voters, that is, the subset of Americans who directly determine the outcomes of elections. During election periods (primary and general elections) the views and opinions of this subset become especially important to legislators and decision makers, particularly on the most salient issues. Note that only rarely does a health care issue make it to the "election agenda." Only rarely does a health care issue rank high enough on Americans' list of concerns for it to be an issue that candidates fear voters will cast their votes in relation to. For example, reform of the health care system ranked high enough to become an election issue in the 1989 Pennsylvania Senate race and the 1992 presidential election (Blendon et al., 1994a).

Third, the final level includes only those who are politically active as the "public." This group is made up of those Americans who communicate directly with their representatives, by either writing or calling, contributing money to politicians or political groups, attending protests or other forums on behalf of a particular interest or candidate, or in other ways make their voices and policy preferences heard. Legislators are most responsive to the views or wishes of these active Americans, particularly when they are constituents from within their legislative districts. Political activity is more likely

among those who are older, have more years of education, and have strong party identification (Verba & Nie, 1972).

It is important to determine which "public" is most pertinent for the issue at hand. In some cases when political leaders say they are responding to public opinion it is in reality to the opinions of those who are politically active; in others, to the general public as a whole as reflected in opinion surveys. For example, take the controversial issue of abortion. While there exists majority support among the *general* public for the principle of legally available abortion, a review of available data from 1984, 1988, and 1992 presidential election exit polls showed that the majority of those for whom abortion was important to their presidential vote were those who wanted abortion to be illegal in all circumstances or to see its availability in our society substantially restricted (Blendon et al., 1993a). That is, those who held the pro-life position were more likely to say the abortion issue was important in their vote than those who held the pro-choice position in these elections. Furthermore, more than 50 percent of the political activity directly related to the abortion issue, including protesting and contacting legislative representatives, came from the 30 percent of Americans who held pro-life positions (Verba et al., 1995). Therefore, these different "groups" of the public—voters versus non-voters, the politically active versus the non-active—hold different policy preferences on the legality of abortion and compose different groups for political decision makers to respond to.

Americans Often Hold Parallel and Conflicting Values When It Comes to Public Policy

In addressing public opinion on issue debates it is important to know that Americans often hold conflicting views. Until these conflicts are resolved we cannot accurately predict where the public actually stands on the specific health policy confronting them. For example, in 1992, 66 percent of the public (CBS News/*New York Times*, 1992) supported national health reform and named it as the number two issue for government to solve (Voter Research and Survey, 1992). At the same time, however, Americans simultaneously mistrusted the government and were cynical about the government's ability to do things right. Thus, while the public consistently supports the goal of national health insurance it also rejects the idea of the federal government running the health insurance system. Similarly, while the public wants the government to control health care costs, it also believes that the federal government already controls too much of our daily lives (Blendon et al., 1995c).

In each of these cases, the public's conflicting views lead them to support policies that oppose one another. Thus if asked about any one of these policies, in isolation, without an explicit comparison, Americans seem to support both conflicting policy options. Only by presenting the specific policy choices in comparison to one another can we see how Americans make trade-offs and resolve their conflicting views and values.

Americans Often Agree on Broad Goals for Our Society But Disagree on the Means to Achieve Them

These differences can be seen clearly only when survey questions are designed that explicitly separate the goals from the various means of achieving them. Public opinion textbooks talk at length about the importance of question wording. Here we note that the types of questions asked will fundamentally determine what the survey results really reflect about public opinion on a particular issue. For example, in March 1993, 85 percent said that everyone should have access to the same health insurance coverage (Gallup/Consumers Union, 1993), while 59 percent said they favored national health insurance as a means of guaranteeing universal coverage (CBS News/*New York Times*, 1993b). Sixty-five percent said they were willing to pay more in higher taxes or premiums for a national health care program (Harvard School of Public Health/Marttila & Kiley/ Robert Wood Johnson Foundation, 1993), but the average amount people were willing to pay was only $20 per month (Gallup/Consumers Union, 1993).

This can be further illustrated from an example from another issue debate: welfare reform. Although Americans support the concept that women should work for welfare benefits and should therefore be provided with job training and employment so that they can keep and be successful at jobs, they, once again, are not willing to pay taxes or have other programs cut in order to make sure that jobs and day care are actually available (Blendon et al., 1995a).

The main point from these examples is that the public often supports goals of public policies, but not the means of achieving them. This suggests an important caveat for public opinion research: do not mix up the goals and the means of achieving those goals in the same questions or else the real policy preferences of Americans will be misconstrued. Furthermore, an observed increase in support for a particular policy goal does not necessarily mean that there is consensus on the means of achieving that goal. Throughout policy debates it is often easier to get agreement on general principles and goals than it is to get consensus on the particular mechanisms and programs that would actually meet those goals.

Potential Consequences of a Policy Ultimately Affects Its Public Support

Americans' support for a particular policy often shifts when the potential consequences of that policy become more widely known. As a result, measures of public opinion gathered before a large-scale campaign or debate on an issue can be misleading and are often very different than measures taken at the end of the debate period. As Anthony Downs (1972), a prominent political economist at The Brookings Institution, makes clear, as a problem initially emerges on the public agenda, the public wants to see action. This desire to "do something" is often reflected in their answers to public opinion survey questions. However, as the public debate ensues, Americans become more aware of the potential consequences of each policy option, and support for large-scale changes falls. This was seen clearly over the course of the 1993–94 national health care reform debate. Throughout this one-year period, the president went from enjoying strong support for his proposal in its initial phase to seeing public attitudes turn decisively negative toward his plan at the end. (Blendon et al., 1995c).

Furthermore, simply providing respondents with more details regarding the potential effects of policies can change their initial support even in the absence of a lengthy public debate. For example, 69 percent of Americans said that they would be less likely to support national health care reform if they heard that the plan would hit the elderly the hardest, since the elderly would share in the tax hike and pay more for Medicare. Similarly, 64 percent said they would be less inclined to support reform if their ability to choose doctors and hospitals would be restricted, and 60 percent would not do so if they heard that there would be rationing, and some expensive treatments would no longer be available. On the other hand, providing "positive" consequences can increase respondents public support for a policy. In the case of health care reform, 83 percent said that they would be more inclined to support it if they heard the statement that if all Americans had access to health care, they would be more likely to get preventive treatment. Moreover, 81 percent would increase their support for comprehensive reform if they heard the statement that one in three uninsured Americans could not get needed medical care the previous year (Blendon et al., 1994b).

Overall, public support for health care policies can be dramatically affected by whether or not the potential consequences of the policy are either widely understood or explicitly stated in the survey question.

Public Opinion May Be Time-Dependent

Public opinion may not always be stable for particular policy preferences and may shift statements of support at one point in time to opposition at another as the result of specific national events or particular problems in the health care system. In certain public policy areas and for certain types of policy-related survey questions, researchers have shown that public opinion results can remain quite stable over time (Page & Shapiro, 1992). However, in other cases, particularly when looking at

debates over specific policy options, public opinion can change quite rapidly.

Support for national health insurance increases and decreases over time as does support for fundamental reform of the health care system. "Windows of opportunity" (Kingdon, 1986) exist when an issue such as health care reform moves to the top of the national agenda and presents an opportunity for mobilizing public support for comprehensive reform. But over time, public interest in the issue is often not sustainable. This can be seen in the results of the debate over health care reform. In September 1993, the health care issue was ranked third by Americans as one of the two most important problems facing the country, a clear "window of opportunity." But by April 1995, it declined in priority and was listed ninth, behind such issues as high taxes, family values, and the economy (Princeton Survey Research Associates/Times Mirror, 1995).

Unlike some areas of social science research where there are clear findings that remain constant over time, public opinion can vary significantly from one period to another. It can be affected by the outcomes of debates, political advertising, improved public knowledge, or the impact of events. Careful analysis of public opinion requires the monitoring of public preferences over time rather than relying on a single observation at any particular point in time.

KEY VALUES AND BELIEFS AMERICANS HOLD[1]

Health policy issues are often complex, involving numerous technical details, yet Americans manage to determine preferences and hold strong views on many of these issues. How does the public draw clear conclusions amidst many complex policy choices? Americans consider the health policy proposals within the broader context of their deeply held beliefs and values, and this allows them to reach firmly held policy preferences across a broad range of issues. Americans organize their responses to surveys and policy questions through a

---

[1]Much of this section comes directly from Blendon et al. (1994b). Adapted with permission from *Health Affairs* (1995).

framework of how they generally think about health policy and other social issues. The core beliefs that help make up this framework include beliefs about the relative importance of health care issues, attitudes toward equity, usefulness of new technologies, attitudes toward the role of government, and beliefs about the functioning of the health care system. In our view there are ten core beliefs that shape Americans' views on health policy. They are as follows.

Health Is an Important, But Second-Level Priority

To sick people getting well may be their most important priority, but to those who are well it is of lesser importance. As we discussed in the previous section, the salience with which Americans rank issues is important to understanding the role of public opinion. It is also important to note that generally Americans rate health care issues as a second-level concern, behind such issues as the economy, crime, inflation, and the deficit. Only rarely does the general issue of national health care reform attain a level of prominence among all other issues for Americans. What this means is that although polls may show support for increasing health care spending, such preference must be considered within the context of stronger preferences and higher priorities in other areas. For example, in many time periods Americans have been more concerned with increasing national defense spending than they were with increasing public spending on health care.

Americans' Romance with Technology

While experts are somewhat skeptical of how much new medical technologies contribute to improving health, Americans think they get tremendous benefits out of expensive new medical technologies and procedures. For instance, on surveys Americans rank biomedical research as one of the nation's highest research priorities and do not want to see its fruits "rationed" or unavailable. Moreover, polls show that few people (21%) support "rationing" high-cost medical equipment and procedures. Just how strongly this view is

held is revealed in a 1990 poll in which 75 percent of the public indicated that "health insurance should pay for any treatments which will save lives even if it costs one million dollars to save a life" and 90 percent agreed that "everyone should have the right to get the best possible health care—as good as the treatment a millionaire gets" (Louis Harris & Associates, 1990). Furthermore, about a fourth of those surveyed believe that insurers should pay for very expensive surgery even if the patient's doctor says it is unneeded—a sign of our belief about the underlying usefulness of medical technology (Taylor & Leitman, 1991).

Critical of the System, But Satisfied with Their Own Personal Health Care Arrangements

Americans continue to express conflicting views on how they perceive their health care. While they are satisfied with their *personal* health care arrangements and physicians, they believe that there is something wrong with the *national* health care system. For example, in 1994, 75 percent of the public said that our health care system required fundamental change (Princeton Survey Research Associates/Times Mirror, 1994) and 84 percent said there was a crisis in the health care system (Gallup/CNN/*USA Today*, 1994a). But, at the same time, 93 percent said they were somewhat or very satisfied with the medical care they received, 91 percent with the way the doctor explained things, and 81 percent with the amount of time they had to wait to see the doctor when thinking about their most recent visit to their medical doctor (Gallup/American Medical Association, 1994). These conflicting beliefs frame the way Americans think about reform debates—change the system, but do not interfere with my personal health care arrangements.

A Moral Concern for the Uninsured

Surveys show that moral concern for the uninsured is a strong public value. For example, 86 percent of Americans say everybody should get the care they need regardless of their ability to pay (Blendon et al., 1994a).

Furthermore, in 1995, 65 percent agreed that the government should do whatever is necessary, whatever the cost in taxes, to see that everyone gets the medical care they need (Harris, 1995). This fundamental concern for the uninsured remains a powerful factor in shaping public attitudes toward health care reform. Any proposal aimed at assuring universal access is likely to enjoy a great deal of political legitimacy, grounded in the moral convictions of the American people (Blendon et al., 1994a).

Desire for Security

Americans are, at least in part, motivated by worries that the problems of the uninsured may one day be their problems. Underlying many survey results is a clear sense of anxiety—the fear that one's own health coverage may at some time prove to be inadequate. To the extent that Americans see their own sense of security threatened, they will be far more likely to endorse significant actions to reform the health care system (Blendon et al., 1994a).

A Limited Willingness to Sacrifice

One of the most striking features of public opinion surveys is that while Americans frequently state support for a national goal, they are unwilling to make any sacrifice to reach it—whether paying higher taxes, cutting other programs, limiting their choices, or having more government interference in their health care arrangements. The fact that millions of Americans without health insurance may face rationing of health care on a daily basis does not motivate the majority of people who have insurance to share in that rationing or to pay higher taxes so that this situation could be remedied.

Americans are resistant to paying increased taxes needed to fund comprehensive health care reform. The reason for this appears to be embedded in our culture. Americans are less committed than citizens of European industrialized countries to the idea that it is the government's responsibility to even out differences in wealth between people of high and low incomes. In 1993, the progressive federal income tax was considered the worst of federal, state, or local taxes (Gallup, 1993a). Relatively flat taxes such as state sales taxes, the burden of which often falls disproportionately on the poor, are more widely favored by the public. In addition, they perceive themselves as overly taxed by the government. These views are somewhat surprising, given that the United States currently has one of the lowest levels of taxation among the eighteen wealthiest industrialized countries. Nearly six of ten Americans describe their federal income taxes as too high (Blendon & Donelan, 1990).

Ideological Orientation of Americans

Americans' views of what the legitimate role of government should be in health care is heavily influenced by their ideological orientation. Americans divide themselves across an ideological continuum, from liberal to conservative. Currently, about 39 percent self-identify themselves as conservative, 17 percent as liberal, and 39 percent as moderate (Gallup/CNN/*USA Today*, 1995).

In thinking about the expansion of the government's role in health care, in almost all cases those who see themselves as being liberal are more receptive to an enlarged government role, and those who see themselves as more conservative are more resistant to government intervention. Additionally, when it comes to how responsible individuals versus society should be on matters of health, conservatives are more likely to see individuals as much more accountable for their own situations and liberals are more likely to see the society as a whole take responsibility.

Lack of Confidence in and Distrust of Government

As is the case with virtually every major public policy issue, the public's pronounced reluctance to allow the federal government a more active role in their lives will influence their opinions on health care issues. Though Americans show strong support for national efforts to improve health, they have a deep suspicion of government (Blendon et al., 1995c). In 1993, only 23 percent of Americans said they trusted the federal government to do what is right most of the time (Gallup, 1993a). Similarly, 65 percent told pollsters that the federal government controlled too much of their daily lives, and 69 percent agreed that when something is run by the government it is usually inefficient or wasteful (Princeton Survey Research Associates/Times Mirror, 1993). Finally, 80 percent regarded the value they get from taxes paid to the federal government as only fair or poor, and 60 percent favored a smaller government with fewer services (Harris/*Business Week*, 1993; *Los Angeles Times*, 1993).

Distrust of "big government" is a long-established American political value, bolstered by the belief that the private sector is inherently more efficient than the government. This belief is tempered in health care, however, by distrust of the health insurance industry and suspicions that providers are taking financial advantage of them. Because of these beliefs and fears, Americans want the government to serve as a "referee" to protect them from insurers and other health care providers (Blendon et al., 1994a).

Cynicism about "The System"

Americans are cynical about the efficiency and ethical behavior of major institutions and professionals in our society. They believe that the most serious problems facing the health care system are those caused by the waste, inefficiency, and greed of the major institutions involved—insurance companies, hospitals, the medical profession, and malpractice lawyers. While there is clearly some truth in the public's perception of a system plagued by inefficiency, this view causes the public to overlook many more significant long-term problems, such as the aging of the population, the frequent use of expensive new technologies, and the cost of using highly trained medical specialists. Because Americans do not see these other factors as important, they are likely to be less willing to support proposals to address them if the proposals involve major sacrifices for themselves and their families (Blendon et al., 1994b).

This general cynicism becomes more complex when directed toward the medical profession. There is an ap-

parent dichotomy in the way the public views medicine. They see the profession and its leaders in a different light than they do their personal physicians (Blendon, 1988). Thus, although public confidence in medicine has declined since the late 1970s and although most Americans (68%) report that they have been increasingly losing faith in physicians, this has not affected the high level of satisfaction most people have with their most recent physician encounter (83%) or their positive feelings toward their own physician (80%) (Blendon, 1988). Thus, the public may react differently, depending on how a policy issue is framed—that is, whether the culprit is their own personal physician or the medical profession as a whole.

A Lack of Self-blame

Americans do not see the problems of the health care system as their own doing. When asked to assess responsibility for the nation's health care ills, only 4 percent of those surveyed named "patients" as among the one or two most blameworthy groups. While ready to cast blame on the major components of the health care system (including doctors, insurers, and hospitals), the public does not sense that many of the system's problems may be related to their own behavior as consumers of health care—or at least to the lack of incentive for consumers to be price-conscious. As a result, it seems clear that Americans look for reforms that affect primarily the behavior of the major institutions that make up the system, rather than their own behavior (Blendon et al., 1994b).

THE ROLE OF PUBLIC ATTITUDES AND BELIEFS IN HEALTH POLICY: SOME CASE EXAMPLES

When a health issue emerges the public examines it in the light of the broad core beliefs they hold. These, taken together, tend to favor specific incremental changes over more sweeping efforts led by the government. The relationship between our core beliefs and health policy choices, and the subsequent bias toward incrementalism, is best illustrated by the cases of national health care reform and California's single-payer ballot initiative.

Case 1: The Public and Health Care Reform[2]

These principles and core beliefs can be seen at work when exploring the results of major national debates on health care reform. For the fourth time since World War II, Congress has just completed a major debate over reforming the nation's health care system. While each past campaign for health care reform centered on a unique policy proposal, there are common features between the recent debate and the contests of the past. Prior to the introduction of each bill, there existed strong public interest in and expectation for reform. And after each plan was introduced, opposing interest groups spent millions of dollars to convince the public that enactment of the proposal would result in a health care delivery system even worse than the status quo. Examining these past contests provides important lessons on the role of public opinion and interest group activity in determining the outcome of the national health care reform debate.

Almost fifty years ago, President Truman proposed a comprehensive, prepaid national health insurance plan to be financed through the Social Security tax program. Initially, Truman's proposal had the support of an impressive array of legislators and organizations, prompting political analysts to predict that passage of the plan would proceed smoothly. In response, however, special interests mounted a public relations campaign unprecedented in scope and unparalleled in term of campaign expenditures spent fighting the plan (Starr, 1982). Unable to match their resources, President Truman ultimately lost out to the interest groups' exaggerated claims regarding the details of his plan, and his proposal failed to attract sufficient public or legislative support. (See Table 9-1.)

TABLE 9-1 Change in Public Support for the Truman Health Reform Plan over Time

Public Support for Truman Health Plan	March 1949	November– December 1949	November 1950
For	38%	33%	29%
Against	38	47	60
No opinion	25	20	11

SOURCE: Gallup Poll, 1949, 1950.

National health insurance was again hotly debated after President Johnson's election to office in 1964. Three distinct proposals were floated: one from the Johnson administration, one from the Republican Party, and one from the proponents of health care for the poor. Strategically merging these three plans, House Ways and Means Chairman Wilbur Mills created a comprehensive program that resulted in the 1965 enactment of Medicare and Medicaid (Marmor, 1973). While this reform covered only the nation's poor and elderly citizens, proponents of universal national health insurance supported these programs as a necessary first step toward achieving their ultimate goals (Fein, 1989).

In 1974, the Nixon White House proposed a more extensive national health program called the Comprehensive Health Insurance Program (CHIP). This program mandated health insurance coverage for workers through their employers, and provided a separate program to cover the unemployed (Thompson, 1980). Given the similarities between the Nixon bill and the Democratic (Kennedy–Mills) alternative proposal, compromise seemed likely. However, the Watergate scandal significantly reduced the president's influence with Congress and the American public, and dominated the political agenda at a time when health care reform might otherwise have been achieved (Peterson, 1992).

In 1993–94, the United States once again faced major questions regarding the need for major health care reform, with the introduction of President Clinton's plan and a variety of alternative proposals, both Democratic and Republican, being debated in Congress. Once again an administration was proposing compre-

---

[2]This section comes directly from Blendon et al. (1993b). Adapted from Volume III of the *Future of American Health Care* series, published by Faulkner & Gray's Healthcare Information Center, New York, New York.

hensive national health reform, including provision of health insurance coverage for every American citizen.

To many outside the health field, the reasons underlying the surge of interest in health reform were not immediately apparent. Some believed that the issue was high on the national agenda because the health care system has reached a state of crisis: a large number of Americans were either uninsured or underinsured, and many were threatened by high health costs. If these conditions were the sole drivers of reform, however, then a national health insurance bill would have been enacted in Truman's day, when a far greater percentage of Americans were uninsured and far more were seriously threatened by high medical costs.

The national debate over universal health insurance has never been a reflection of the severity of the aggregate problem. With only 15 percent of Americans lacking health insurance today (Employee Benefits Research Institute, 1995), and with Medicare and Medicaid covering many of the nation's poor and elderly citizens, the most recent campaign was largely driven by something else: *middle-class anxieties over the security of their health insurance coverage.*

Anxiety about health insurance extended far beyond the ranks of the uninsured. The inability of the United States to control sharply rising medical costs had created a situation where health coverage was beginning to disintegrate for average working families. Sixty-four percent of Americans said they were worried that their health insurance would become too expensive to afford, 52 percent feared that very large medical bills would not be covered, 52 percent were concerned that their health benefits would be cut, and 31 percent worried that their family might lose health insurance coverage in the future (Henry J. Kaiser Family Foundation/Commonwealth Fund/Louis Harris & Associates, 1993).

These anxieties were based on real problems Americans experience. One in four did lose their health insurance during any two-year period (U.S. Bureau of the Census, 1992). Nearly one-half of the nation's employed workers had had their health benefits cut during the previous two-year period (CBS News/*New York Times*, 1993a). One in eight households reported someone locked into a job for health insurance reasons (Henry J. Kaiser Family Foundation/Commonwealth Fund/Louis Harris & Associates, 1993), and one in five had had someone denied coverage for a preexisting medical condition (CBS News/*New York Times*, 1993a). Surveys showed that 20 percent of Americans had had a problem paying medical bills in a given year (Henry J. Kaiser Family Foundation/Harvard School of Public Health/National Opinion Research Center, 1993). Similarly, 10 percent of Americans reported that there was a time in the past year when they needed medical care, but did not get it for economic reasons (Henry J. Kaiser Family Foundation/Commonwealth Fund/Louis Harris & Associates, 1993).

It is not surprising, therefore, that health care moved to near the top of the national political agenda and became a much more salient issue politically. According to a 1990 survey conducted in ten industrialized countries, Americans were the least likely to say that their own country's health care system works fairly well (Blendon et al., 1990). Voters in the 1992 presidential election cited health care as the third most important issue, with 19 percent of voters naming it as one of the top two issues in deciding how they voted. Among those who voted for Clinton, health care was the number two issue, second only to the economy (Voter Research and Survey, 1992).

Given this level of public anxiety and interest, it would seem that enactment of a major health plan was inevitable. But history tells us that public support for health care reform can be fragile. While Americans expressed strong opinions on what they thought was wrong with the health care system, there were four key reasons why the public did not, and has never, reached consensus on health care reform. As in the past, interest groups have appealed to the following uniquely American values in their efforts to defeat national health care reform, and in fact were successful once more.

1. *Americans want the federal government to solve the health care problem, but don't trust the government to do things right.* Americans differ from citizens of most other industrialized countries in their views about the role of government in solving society's problems—the United States has a stronger tradition of reliance on

private-sector action. In a multinational survey conducted in 1985, only 36 percent of Americans said it should definitely be the government's responsibility to care for the sick, compared to 87 percent in Italy, 86 percent in Great Britain, and 54 percent in West Germany (International Social Survey Program, 1985).

In addition, Americans' trust in the federal government has never completely recovered from the cynicism of the Vietnam War and the Watergate era. In the late 1950s, three-quarters of Americans said they trusted the government in Washington to do the right thing (Opinion Roundup, 1985); in 1993, fewer than one in four (23%) expressed such trust (CBS News/*New York Times*, 1993b). Between 1972 and 1974, Americans' trust in the federal government dropped from 54 percent to 37 percent (Opinion Roundup, 1985). Similarly, President Nixon's approval ratings fell from 67 percent in January 1973 (Gallup, 1973) to 24 percent shortly before his resignation in 1974 (Gallup, 1974), likely contributing to the defeat of his national health reform plan. Likewise, at the time the Clintons were developing their health plan, less than one in four (23%) Americans expressed generic trust in the government in Washington (Gallup, 1993a). This cynicism toward the federal government haunted the Clinton administration throughout its extensive campaign to convince the public that its plan would be good for average Americans.

2. *There has never been a consensus among the American people regarding an acceptable approach to health care reform.* While Americans are willing to applaud the *goal* of national health reform, they do not agree on the *means* of achieving that goal. In a 1945 survey, 82 percent said that something should be done "to make it easier for people to pay for doctor and hospital care." When asked whether each of three different plans (group coverage through an insurance company, a federal government plan as part of Social Security, and a doctors' organization plan) was a good, fair, or poor idea, at least a plurality of Americans rated each plan as good, and at least two-thirds rated each plan as good or fair. But when asked to choose among the three plans, none came close to achieving majority support and the government option was preferred by only a third (34%) of the public (see Table 9-2) (Payne, 1946).

TABLE 9-2 Level of Support for Three Health Reform Plans, 1945

Type of Plan	Percent Saying "Good or Fair Idea"	Percent Favoring in Forced Three-way Choice
Insurance company plan	88%	39%
Federal government plan	72	34
Doctor organization plan	69	12

SOURCE: Opinion Research Corporation Poll, 1945, cited in S. Payne.

Similarly, during the debate over the Nixon health reform plan, 66 percent of Americans agreed that "we need a new nationwide federal health insurance plan." But when asked whether they preferred to receive health insurance from a private insurance company or through the government, the public was almost evenly split (Opinion Research Corporation, 1972).

Again, in the 1993–94 debate, there seemed at first glance to be strong support for a national health insurance program. Fifty-nine percent of Americans said they favored "national health insurance, which would be financed by tax money, paying for most forms of health care" (CBS/*New York Times*, 1993a). Yet by more than a two to one margin (57% to 26%), they believed that private industry could do a better job managing health care than the government (Fact Finders/Novalis Corporation, 1993). Similarly, when offered a choice among the three principal reform options (Figure 9-1), the public consistently was divided almost evenly: 32 percent preferred a plan similar to President Clinton's; 32 percent opted for a tax credit plan such as the Republican proposal; and 28 percent preferred a single-payer system like that proposed by Representative James McDermott (D-WA) and Senator Paul Wellstone (D-MN) (Henry J. Kaiser Family Foundation/Commonwealth Fund/Louis Harris & Associates, 1993). Thus, no matter which of the three options was actually being promoted, two-thirds of the American public believed that there was a better alternative plan proposed.

Each of these examples suggests that caution is necessary in interpreting the public's will. First, agreement on a goal does not necessarily imply agreement on the means of achieving that goal. Additionally, where opin-

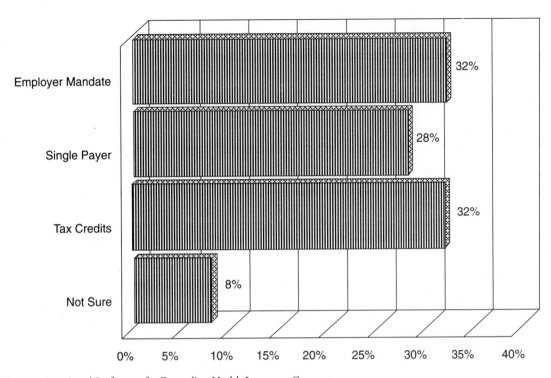

FIGURE 9-1 Americans' Preference for Expanding Health Insurance Coverage

SOURCE: Kaiser Family Foundation/Commonwealth/Harris, 1993.

ions on the means of achieving a goal are not strongly held, an idea presented alone receives higher approval than when it is presented along with alternative proposals that ultimately emerge in the course of the debate.

3. *While Americans are willing to spend a lot of money on health care, they have strong reservations about doing it through the tax system.* The longest continuous trend measuring public opinion on health care spending in this country shows that the public consistently believes that the United States is spending too little, rather than too much, on health (Davis & Smith, 1993). However, support for such spending does not necessarily translate into support for increased taxes. This pattern is evident as far back as 1944, when 68 percent of the public said they thought it would be a good idea for Social Security to cover doctor and hospital care. Support for the idea dropped to 41 percent, however, when respondents who opposed a payroll tax increase and those who preferred a private-sector plan were removed from the approval ratings (Payne, 1946).

In the months immediately after the 1992 election, Americans expressed some willingness to pay additional taxes dedicated to a national health reform plan. A March 1993 survey found that 65 percent of Americans were willing to pay either increased taxes or higher premiums for "a national health care program that would provide every American with access to health care." At the same time, however, only 40 percent were willing to pay as much as $30 more a month (Harvard School of Public Health/Marttila & Kiley/Robert Wood Johnson Foundation, 1993). Moreover, this willingness to pay even a small tax increase was on the decline. By late September 1993, support for higher taxes fell to 48 percent (Princeton Survey Research Associates/*Newsweek*, 1993), and by early October 1993, just 40 percent supported an increase in taxes to help pay for President Clinton's health reform plan (ABC News/*Washington Post*, 1993b).

4. *While Americans are dissatisfied with the health care system overall, they are quite satisfied with the quality of*

their own *health care.* Americans have consistently rejected significant health care reform because while they believe there may be problems with the aggregate system, they are highly satisfied with the care they personally receive. In 1993, 71 percent of Americans reported being satisfied with the quality of their medical care (CBS News/*New York Times*, 1993a); at the same time, 73 percent believed that our health care system is fundamentally unsound (Gallup/CNN/*USA Today*, 1993). This disparity makes it possible for opponents of health reform to advance the argument that changes made to the aggregate health care system might adversely affect the patient's own health care arrangements.

Even as far back as the 1940s, interest groups have been able to rally Americans against health reform by claiming that the quality of *their own* medical care would be worse under a reformed system. Political advertisements attacking President Truman's health insurance plan contrasted Norman Rockwell images of the doctor–patient relationship so valued by the public with the threat of government bureaucratic interference. The interest groups' campaign played on public anxieties by questioning whether in the future patients would be able to freely choose their own physicians (which was guaranteed by the Truman plan) with slogans such as, "Your Doctor, or Doctor X?" (Kelley, 1956).

Taken together, these four key public attitudes toward health care reform have historically served as constraints on policymakers' ability to restructure the U.S. health care system. The paramount lesson they provide for those interested in promoting health care reform is that early public enthusiasm for health reform ultimately may not translate into continuing public support for major changes in the health care system.

This is in fact what occurred in the case of the Clinton health care plan. The initial public support (in the range of 56 percent to 59 percent) for the president's plan declined over time (Gallup/CNN/*USA Today*, 1993; ABC News/*Washington Post*, 1993a; *Time*/CNN/Yankelovich Partners, 1993). As of spring 1994, public support stood at 43 percent, and surveys showed more public opposition than support (Gallup/CNN/*USA*

Today, 1994b). Although the Clinton plan contained several elements that had previously been shown to have considerable public support, Americans certainly ended up with a more negative view of the plan as a whole.

The opponents once again left the public fearful of the consequences of major change. A public that earlier had told pollsters of their desire for comprehensive reform later reported concerns that the amount they would have had to pay for health care would increase under the Clinton plan. Moreover, twice as many Americans thought the quality of health care they received would get worse rather than better. The majority (55%) of the public came to believe they would have less choice of physicians, and almost half (46%) believed the president's proposal would entail excessive government involvement in their health care (*Time*/CNN/Yankelovich Partners, 1994).

Given this level of public anxiety, it is not surprising that by June 1994 only 33 percent of the public saw the Clinton health plan as good for the country—down from 55 percent just a few months earlier (Princeton Survey Research/*Newsweek*, 1993, 1994). This once again illustrates how volatile public opinion can be in the midst of a heated debate and how early support for general principles may not result in majority support for a specific proposal.

Case 2: California's Single-Payer Debate[3]

On November 8, 1994, by a vote of 73 percent to 27 percent, California voters overwhelmingly rejected Proposition 186, which proposed a state-run single-payer health insurance system. Drawing on four independent surveys conducted before, during, and after the Proposition 186 debate, as well as an analysis of the media campaigns of both sides, it is clear that the proposition's defeat was largely the result of voters' attitudes against "big government" and higher taxes—attitudes effectively tapped by the opponents of Proposition 186. Opponents made strong negative statements about the initiative in the California voters pamphlet, a booklet

---

[3]This case is adapted with permission from Danelski et al. (1995).

describing the pros and cons of each proposition that is sent out to all registered California voters prior to the election, and waged a well-financed, sophisticated media campaign that the proposition's proponents could not counter. While it is possible that proponents might have done better with more money, Proposition 186 was an idea that found itself in the wrong place at the wrong time, given the rising antigovernment sentiment expressed so powerfully on election eve.

The single-payer measure proposed a health care system in which the California government would replace the private health insurance companies. All California residents would be covered by a defined standard benefit package that would include preventative and primary care, prescription drugs, long-term care, mental health coverage, and some dental coverage. The state system would be headed by an elected health commissioner whose responsibilities would include establishing a global budget, setting up provider fee schedules, and approving capital expansions. The system would be financed by new taxes levied on employers, individuals, and tobacco products. The taxes were designed to replace current health care premiums, co-payments, and out-of-pocket expenses of businesses and individuals. The authors of the initiative established a coalition called "Californians for Health Security." The coalition was successful in collecting one million signatures, which placed the initiative on the November 1994 ballot. Three-quarters of the dollars raised, a total of $600,000, was spent on the signature collection phase alone (California Secretary of State, 1994a).

In a July 1994 survey, less than one-third (29%) of California voters had as yet heard of Proposition 186. However, after being read paragraph-long arguments for and against enacting a single-payer system during a telephone survey, the support was somewhat mixed. Thirty-eight percent said they would vote for the proposition, 34 percent said they would vote against it, and one out of four Californians said they did not know how they would vote (Henry J. Kaiser Family Foundation/Harvard School of Public Health/KRC Communications, 1994).

Such results could be taken as an encouraging sign by the Californians for Health Security, as one might

conclude that—at worse—there was some serious support for a single-payer plan, and—at best—after the proponents' argument became more widely known there was the potential for victory. However, the same survey revealed some of the core beliefs that Californians held toward their state government and showed that they were troubled by the "big government" implications of a single-payer system. When asked about the state government running the health insurance system instead of private health insurance companies, 62 percent of respondents said there would be too much government involvement; 51 percent expected that they would have to spend more for medical coverage; 48 percent expected that they would have fewer choices of doctors; and 45 percent expected that their quality of care would decline. In addition, 37 percent believed that they would be worse off if the proposition passed as compared with the 25 percent who thought they would be better off and the 24 percent who expected no change.

The importance of getting beyond the simple policy choice questions is evident from this example. It is easy to see the potential shape of the opponents' campaign strategy. The antigovernment feeling provided an enormous window for the opponents, and any optimistic reading of the previous data from the proponents' perspective could be quickly set aside. While Californians were somewhat open to the arguments for a single-payer system, they clearly did not believe that their health care arrangements would be better off under the control of the California government. In fact, the opponents latched immediately onto this cynicism and mistrust of government. The opposing coalition's name, "Taxpayers against the Government Takeover," in and of itself, attests to this.

The opponents had three times more resources than the proponents and spent four times more than the proponents on paid media campaigns (California Secretary of State, 1994b). Media analysis showed that the opponents reached an estimated 96 percent of the state between September 1 and election day, with the frequency of their ads airing between nine and twenty-six times per day (Broadcast Data Systems, 1994). As if they had closely studied the results from the July 1994 survey, the opponents' media messages drew on the existing negative attitudes toward "big government" as the solution for health care reform. They vilified "big government" and capitalized on the anti-tax sentiment, concern over the economy and the potential for job losses, as well as the concern over the perceived loss of provider choice and diminished quality of care.

In contrast to this highly visible opposition campaign and because of their more limited resources, proponents could not begin their radio ads until October 15, just one month before the election, and their television ads until November 1, just one week before the election. The estimated frequency of proponents' ads per day was much less than that of their opponents, ranging between three and five times per day (Broadcast Data Systems, 1994). Moreover, the main message of the proponents was to make Proposition 186 a referendum on the insurance industry. Vilifying the insurance industry, their ads capitalized on public dislike for alleged industry practices such as denying coverage for certain health problems.

However, this tactic proved to overestimate the extent of public dissatisfaction with private insurers. The election day results show clearly that Californians' mistrust of the government's ability to run the health care system overshadowed any loathing of the insurance industry. The proposition lost big: 27 percent in favor and 73 percent opposed. In an election night survey, consistent with the earlier findings, the principal reason (57%) voters rejected the single-payer initiative was their concern that it would result in too much government involvement in the health care system. Another 15 percent voted against the initiative primarily because they believed it would decrease the quality of care they received, and 14 percent thought their costs would go up (Henry J. Kaiser Family Foundation/Harvard School of Public Health/KRC Communications, 1994).

On the other hand, only 15 percent of those who voted for the proposition did so primarily because it would eliminate the role of insurance companies, which was the primary media message of the proponents. The most frequently cited reason (39%) among those who voted for the proposition was that they did so because it would result in universal coverage, clearly a widely held policy goal. Another 16 percent supported the proposition primarily because they believed it would make the health care system fairer.

As could be predicted, ideology played a role in the voters' choice on the proposition. Eighty-two percent of conservatives voted against it, while 52 percent of liberals voted for it. In addition to this core belief, the unwillingness to sacrifice and risk the uncertainty of what a state-run single-payer plan might mean for individuals also played a role. For example, seniors, who already have in Medicare a type of single-payer system, voted three to one against the proposition. Also those voters from households where someone worked in a health care-related job voted three to one against the proposition. It is not clear whether these groups based their vote choices on an ideological concern or whether they believed that a state-run single-payer system might hurt their health care jobs or decrease the amount of services they, as Medicare beneficiaries in California, already receive.

This case also illustrates a phenomenon continually found in national public opinion surveys. Knowing that Americans, or in this case Californians, desire health care reform does not necessarily mean that they will favor an all-out government effort to run the health care system. The actors in any given policy debate need to know about the public attitudes not just to the policy option, but, even more important, about their attitudes toward the mechanism by which the policy will be enacted, much less implemented.

Conclusion

Public opinion is only one of the many factors that influence the development of health policies in the United States. However, monitoring and responding to public opinion are integral parts of our political system, and have taken on increasing importance with the rise of new communication technologies and the growth of direct democracy. The frequency of major government decisions influenced by direct voter referendum, talk radio, public opinion polling, and communication over the information highway has risen dramatically over the past few years. Increasingly, citizens' views, at a given moment, directly influence decision making that previously was the province of elected representatives and legions of experts and interest groups in Washington who influence them. These developments suggest that the role of public opinion in future health policy decisions will be greater than ever.

In thinking about public opinion in the future, a more sophisticated analysis of polls and surveys is required to understand the nature of public opinion and its potential influence in any given health policy debate. This analysis must reach across multiple surveys at multiple points in time, and should utilize the set of principles and the framework for analysis discussed in this chapter in order to draw accurate insights and conclusions. The key principles and core beliefs we have examined can be a baseline for designing an organizational framework.

A peculiar dilemma grows from the fact that the public does not hold the same beliefs and values as many experts in the health care field. The reasoning behind the way Americans think about issues is very different than that used by experts. The public does not reach the same conclusions using the same type of evidence or logic as would a given health policy expert. As a result, those who seek to influence public opinion on major health policy issues are going to have to develop their case and frame their policy options based on the public's core beliefs, priorities placed on solving health care problems, willingness to live with the consequences of various public policy actions, and level of trust and confidence in both government and interest groups that might be affected by the policy changes.

From the perspective of the health policy community, public opinion can be a double-edged sword. On the one hand, the public generally supports the many goals and policies that health care experts have advocated for years. On the other hand, Americans will be much less supportive of the means of achieving the goals than the experts who have proposed them. One of the major lessons from the 1993–94 health care reform debate is that, although a "window of opportunity" might exist for major government action to address a particular policy issue, the tendency is for experts to overestimate the willingness of Americans to sacrifice and risk the uncertain consequences of major changes on their lives.

Analysts must also be aware of the major influence actors in a debate can have on public opinion. What Americans believe at the beginning of any reform effort may be totally different than what they believe at the end of the process. In recent years a profession has grown and developed that is focused solely on trying to influence public opinion in the course of major debates. These political consultants, pollsters, and strategists use the very principles we discuss in this chapter to attempt to achieve the policy outcomes they desire. Health policy actors will have to become more skilled in these areas if they are to successfully champion their causes in the future.

REFERENCES

ABC News/*Washington Post* Poll. (1993a). Storrs, CT: Roper Center for Public Opinion Research. (September 22).

ABC News/*Washington Post* Poll. (1993b). Storrs, CT: Roper Center for Public Opinion Research. (October).

American Association of Retired Persons Research and Data Resources. (1989). *Opinion of Americans age 45 and over of the Medicare Catastrophic Coverage Act.* Washington, D.C.: American Association of Retired Persons.

Blendon, Robert J. (1988). The public's view of the future of health care. *Journal of the American Medical Association, 259* (24), 3587–3593.

Blendon, Robert J., Drew A. Altman, John M. Benson, Mollyann Brodie, Matt James, & Gerry Chervinsky. (1995a). The public and the welfare reform debate. *Archives of Pediatrics and Adolescent Medicine, 149* (October), 1059–1064.

Blendon, Robert J., John M. Benson, & Karen Donelan. (1993a). The public and the controversy over abortion. *Journal of the American Medical Association, 270* (23), 2871–2875.

Blendon, Robert J., John M. Benson, Karen Donelan, Robert Leitman, Humphrey Taylor, Christian Koeck, & Daniel Gitterman. (1995b). Who has the best health care system?: A second look. *Health Affairs, 14* (4), 220–230.

Blendon, Robert J., Mollyann Brodie, & John M. Benson. (1995c). What happened to Americans' support for the Clinton health plan? *Health Affairs, 14* (2), 7–23.

Blendon, Robert J., Mollyann Brodie, Tracey S. Hyams, & John M. Benson. (1994a). The American public and the critical choices for health system reform. *Journal of the American Medical Association, 271* (19), 1539–1544.

Blendon, Robert J., & Karen Donelan. (1990). The public and the emerging debate over national health insurance. *New England Journal of Medicine, 323* (3), 208–212.

Blendon, Robert J., Tracey S. Hyams, John M. Benson, & Mollyann Brodie (1993b). Introduction. In Richard M. Sorian (Ed.), *A new deal for American health care: How reform will reshape health care delivery and payment for a new century* (pp. 1–14). Washington, D.C.: Faulkner & Gray.

Blendon, Robert J., Robert Leitman, Ian Morrison, & Karen Donelan. (1990). Satisfaction with health systems in ten nations. *Health Affairs, 9* (2), 185–192.

Blendon, Robert J., John Marttila, John Benson, Matthew Shelter, Francis Connolly, & Tom Kiley. (1994b). The beliefs and values shaping today's health reform debate. *Health Affairs, 13* (1), 274–284.

Broadcast Data Systems. (1994). Unpublished data collected for the Henry J. Kaiser Family Foundation Single Payer Project. Menlo Park, CA: Henry J. Kaiser Family Foundation.

California Secretary of State. (1994a). Form 419 Financial Statements Submitted by "Californians for Health Security," December 1993–June 1994. Sacramento, CA.

California Secretary of State. (1994b). Form 419 Financial Statements Submitted by "Taxpayers against the Government Takeover," January–October 1994. Sacramento, CA.

CBS News/*New York Times* Poll. (1992). Storrs, CT: Roper Center for Public Opinion Research. (July 8).

CBS News/*New York Times* Poll. (1993a). Storrs, CT: Roper Center for Public Opinion Research. (January).

CBS News/*New York Times* Poll. (1993b). Storrs, CT: Roper Center for Public Opinion Research. (March 28).

CBS News/*New York Times* Poll. (1993c). Storrs, CT: Roper Center for Public Opinion Research. (September).

Columbia Institute. (1995). *What shapes lawmakers' views: A survey of members of Congress and key staff on health care reform.* Menlo Park, CA: Henry J. Kaiser Family Foundation.

Conference Board Poll. (1990). Storrs, CT: Roper Center for Public Opinion Research. (May).

Danelski, Ann E., Drew E. Altman, Jan Eldred, Matt James, & Diane Rowland. (1995). *The California single-payer debate: The defeat of Proposition 186.* Unpublished paper. Menlo Park, CA: Henry J. Kaiser Family Foundation.

Davis, J. A., & T. W. Smith. (1993). *General social surveys, 1972–1993: Cumulative codebook.* Storrs, CT: Roper Center for Public Opinion Research.

Downs, Anthony. (1972). Up and down with ecology—The "issue attention cycle." *The Public Interest, 28,* 38–50.

Employee Benefits Research Institute. (1995). Sources of health insurance and the characteristics of the uninsured: Analysis of the March 1994 CPS (Special Report and Issue Brief No. 158). Washington, D.C.: Employee Benefits Research Institution.

Fact Finders/Novalis Corporation Poll. (1993). Storrs, CT: Roper Center for Public Opinion Research. (January).

Fein, Rashi. (1989). *Medical care, medical costs: The search for a health insurance policy.* Cambridge, MA: Harvard University Press.

Gallup Organization, CONUS Communication, Inc., & *The Los Angeles Times Syndicate.* (1989). Election '88. Princeton, NJ: Gallup Organization.

Gallup Poll. (1949a). Storrs, CT: Roper Center for Public Opinion Research. (March).

Gallup Poll. (1949b). Storrs, CT: Roper Center for Public Opinion Research. (November/December).

Gallup Poll. (1950). Storrs, CT: Roper Center for Public Opinion Research. (November).

Gallup Poll. (1973). Storrs, CT: Roper Center for Public Opinion Research. (January).

Gallup Poll. (1974). Storrs, CT: Roper Center for Public Opinion Research. (August).

Gallup Poll. (1993a). Storrs, CT: Roper Center for Public Opinion Research. (March 22).

Gallup Poll. (1993b). Storrs, CT: Roper Center for Public Opinion Research. (June 25).

Gallup/American Medical Association Poll. (1994). Storrs, CT: Roper Center for Public Opinion Research. (January 20).

Gallup/CNN/*USA Today* Poll. (1993). Storrs, CT: Roper Center for Public Opinion Research. (September 24).

Gallup/CNN/*USA Today* Poll. (1994a). Storrs, CT: Roper Center for Public Opinion Research. (January 15).

Gallup/CNN/*USA Today* Poll. (1994b). Storrs, CT: Roper Center for Public Opinion Research. (February 26).

Gallup/CNN/*USA Today* Poll. (1995). Storrs, CT: Roper Center for Public Opinion Research. (July 20).

Gallup/Consumers Union Poll. (1993). Storrs, CT: Roper Center for Public Opinion Research. (March 26).

Harris Poll. (1995). Storrs, CT: Roper Center for Public Opinion Research. (April 14).

Harris/*Business Week* Poll. (1993). Storrs, CT: Roper Center for Public Opinion Research. (October 14).

Harvard School of Public Health/Marttila & Kiley/Robert Wood Johnson Foundation Poll. (1993). Storrs, CT: Roper Center for Public Opinion Research. (March).

Henry J. Kaiser Family Foundation/Commonwealth Fund/Louis Harris & Associates Poll. (1993). Storrs, CT: Roper Center for Public Opinion Research. (September).

Henry J. Kaiser Family Foundation/Harvard School of Public Health/KRC Communications, Inc. Poll. (1994a). California survey. Storrs, CT: Roper Center for Public Opinion Research. (July 27).

Henry J. Kaiser Family Foundation/Harvard School of Public Health/KRC Communications, Inc. Poll. (1994b). California survey. Storrs, CT: Roper Center for Public Opinion Research. (October 21).

Henry J. Kaiser Family Foundation/Harvard School of Public Health/KRC Communications Poll. (1994c). California election night survey. Storrs, CT: Roper Center for Public Opinion Research. (November 8).

Henry J. Kaiser Family Foundation/Harvard School of Public Health/National Opinion Research Center. (1993). Low income study. Unpublished data.

Henry J. Kaiser Family Foundation/Harvard School of Public Health/Princeton Survey Research Associates Poll. (1994). Storrs, CT: Roper Center for Public Opinion Research. (February 17).

International Social Survey Program Poll. (1985). Storrs, CT: Roper Center for Public Opinion Research.

Jacobs, Lawrence R., & Robert Y. Shapiro. (1994). Public opinion's tilt against private enterprise. *Health Affairs, 13* (1), 285–298.

Kelley, Stanley. (1956). *Professional public relations and political power*. Baltimore, MD: Johns Hopkins University Press.

Kingdon, John W. (1986). *Agendas, alternatives, and public policies*. Glenview, IL: Scott Foresman.

Los Angeles Times Poll. (1993). Storrs, CT: Roper Center for Public Opinion Research. (June 12).

Louis Harris & Associates. (1990). *Survey of health care consumers*. New York: Louis Harris & Associates.

Marmor, Theodore R. (1973). *The politics of Medicare*. Chicago, IL: Aldine Publishing Co.

Monroe, A. D. (1979). Consistency between public preferences and national policy decisions. *American Politics Quarterly, 7*, 3–19.

Opinion Research Corporation Poll. (1972). Storrs, CT: Roper Center for Public Opinion Research. (January).

Opinion Roundup: The State of the Nation. (1985). *Public Opinion, 8* (4), 21–40.

Page, Benjamin I., & Robert Y. Shapiro. (1983). Effects of public opinion on policy. *American Political Science Review, 77*, 175–190.

Page, Benjamin I., & Robert Y. Shapiro. (1992). *The rational public: Fifty years of trends in Americans' policy preference*. Chicago: University of Chicago Press.

Payne, Stanley. (1946). Some opinion research principles developed through studies of social medicine. *Public Opinion Quarterly, 10* (1), 93–98.

Peterson, Mark A. (1992). Leading our way to health: Entrepreneurship and leadership in the health care reform debate (Occasional Paper 92-6). Cambridge, MA: Center for American Political Studies.

Princeton Survey Research Associates/*Newsweek* Poll. (1993). Storrs, CT: Roper Center for Public Opinion Research. (September 23).

Princeton Survey Research Associates/*Newsweek* Poll. (1994). Storrs, CT: Roper Center for Public Opinion Research. (June 17).

Princeton Survey Research Associates/Times Mirror Center for People and the Press Poll. (1993). Storrs, CT: Roper Center for Public Opinion Research. (May 26).

Princeton Survey Research Associates/Times Mirror Center for People and the Press Poll. (1994). Storrs, CT: Roper Center for Public Opinion Research. (January 27).

Princeton Survey Research Associates/Times Mirror Center for People and the Press Poll. (1995). Storrs, CT: Roper Center for Public Opinion Research. (April 6).

Schur, C. L., M. L. Berk, & P. Mohr. (1990). Understanding the cost of a catastrophic drug benefit. *Health Affairs, 9* (3), 88–100.

Starr, Paul. (1982). *The social transformation of American medicine*. New York: Basic Books.

Taylor, Humphrey, & Robert Leitman. (1991). Consumers' satisfaction with their care. In Robert J. Blendon & Jennifer Edwards (Eds.), *System in crisis: The case for health care reform* (pp. 75–102). Washington, D.C.: Faulkner & Gray.

Time/CNN/Yankelovich Partners Poll. (1993). Storrs, CT: Roper Center for Public Opinion Research. (September 23).

Time/CNN/Yankelovich Partners Poll. (1994). Storrs, CT: Roper Center for Public Opinion Research. (March 2).

Thompson, M. C. (Ed.). (1980). *Health policy: The legislative agenda*. Washington, D.C.: Congressional Quarterly.

U.S. Bureau of the Census. (1974). *Statistical abstract of the United States: 1973*. Washington, D.C.: Bureau of the Census.

U.S. Bureau of the Census. (1992). *Current population survey*. Washington, D.C.: Bureau of the Census.

U.S. Department of Health, Education, and Welfare. (1967). *Medical care financing and administration* (Health Economics Series 1-A, Publication [PHS]947-1a). Washington, D.C.

Verba, Sidney, & Norman Nie. (1972). *Participation in America: Political democracy and social equality*. Chicago: University of Chicago Press.

Verba, Sidney, Kay Lehman Schlozman, & Henry E. Brady. (1995). *Voice and equality: Civic voluntarism in American politics*. Cambridge, MA: Harvard University Press.

Voter Research and Survey Election Day Exit Poll. (1992). Storrs, CT: Roper Center for Public Opinion Research. (November 3).

Wirthlin Group for the Coalition for Affordable Health Care. (1989). *Medicare Catastrophic Coverage Act Survey*. (May 15).

CHAPTER

10

The Demand for Legislation and National Health Care Reform

Paul J. Feldstein

THE ECONOMIC MOTIVATION UNDERLYING HEALTH LEGISLATION

Legislation and regulation redistribute wealth. Politically successful groups are able to receive net benefits by imposing net costs on those who are less politically powerful.[1] This fact has not escaped the attention of producer groups or organized population groups. When legislators seek the political support of population groups, such as the aged or the middle class, they are clearly proposing to provide these groups with benefits in excess of their costs. The proposed legislative benefits must be visible (obvious) to the population groups whose political support legislators are seeking; otherwise, the political support will not be forthcoming.[2]

An important reason for the failure of President Clinton's health care reform was the result of the middle class's perception that the president's extensive plan for revising the financing and delivery of medical services would not provide them with net benefits.

Most health legislation, however, is not publicly debated or visible in its effects on the public. The prime beneficiaries, hence demanders of legislation

---

[1]For a more complete discussion of the economic theory of regulation applied to health care, see Feldstein, Paul J. (1988). *The politics of health legislation: An economic perspective*. Ann Arbor, MI: Health Administration Press.

[2]The political support for means-tested programs, such as Medicaid, comes from the middle class and is based on how much they are willing to tax themselves. Means-tested programs, based on altruistic motivation, are a small portion of total government expenditures on explicit redistributive programs. According to the Congressional Budget Office, in 1994, $177 billion was spent on all means-tested programs as compared to $612 billion spent on non-means-tested programs, such as Medicare, farm price supports, and so on. Non-means-tested programs are also expected to have a greater absolute

and regulation less visible in its effects, are producer groups. Producer groups are said to have a "concentrated" interest, that is, the legislation has a sufficiently large impact on their revenues or costs as to make it worth their while to organize other producers, represent their economic interests before legislators, and provide them with political support. Whereas producers often receive their entire incomes from the services they produce, consumers rarely spend more than a small portion of their income on any one product; thus their economic interests are considered "diffuse." The costs imposed on the public from producer regulation are relatively small and indirect, such as higher prices for a physician office visit or a hospital admission. Further, the public is often unaware of the enactment of such laws.

The reason most legislation, particularly at the state level, benefits producer groups is that the economic interests of producers are concentrated whereas the economic interests of consumers are diffused over many areas of economic activity. The benefits to producers from legislation are potentially so large as to provide them with ample incentive to secure legislation on their behalf. The proponents of such legislation are rarely so bold as to admit that their incomes will be increased by imposing what is the equivalent of a tax on all consumers of their products and services. Instead, such legislation is presented as being in the public interest.

While health legislation may appear to be uncoordinated, promote provider inefficiencies, and be inequitable in its effects, it is the outcome of a rational policy process. The results are what were intended: the prevalence of concentrated interests over those with diffuse interests. Legislators are assumed to maximize their political support (necessary for reelection) by making cost–benefit calculations—namely, the political support gained by backing concentrated interests compared to the political support lost by opposing those with diffuse interests.

Until recently, the concentrated interests of health providers and the diffuse costs imposed on consumers explained much of the federal and state health legislation enacted. State practice acts define the tasks to be performed by different health professionals and establish the requirements for licensure. Methods of provider payment under Medicare and Medicaid, state restrictions on prepaid group practice, state appropriations for medical, dental, and other health professional educational institutions, and the "process" approach toward ensuring physician quality were all enacted based on the economic interests of providers, particularly physicians, who had a concentrated interest in their outcomes. These policies were too remote to consumers for them to be aware of the effects on their incomes.

Since the 1980s, much of the diminished political power and economic benefits enjoyed by organized medicine has been the result of the rise of opposing concentrated interests, in part because diffuse costs increased to where they became concentrated, and the applicability of the anti-trust laws to the health field prohibited any anticompetitive actions by physicians. For instance, the federal and state governments have developed a concentrated interest in reducing the rise in Medicare and Medicaid expenditures; otherwise taxes would have to be raised or politically popular programs cut back. Large employers and their unions have a concentrated interest in reducing the rise in their employees' health insurance premiums; otherwise their product prices must be increased and employee wages reduced.

A FRAMEWORK FOR ANALYZING LEGISLATIVE BEHAVIOR

Although the political power of health interest groups has diminished, these groups are still influential in the policy process. To understand why the structure of our financing and delivery system has evolved the way it has, it is necessary to understand the demands for legislation by health associations. A framework is therefore provided within which are described the types of

---

expenditure increase. (By the year 2000 both programs are expected to be $290 billion and $882 billion, respectively.) The beneficiaries of non-means-tested programs are primarily middle- and high-income groups. For a more complete discussion of the political support underlying Medicaid and Medicare, as well as examples of means and non-means-tested programs, see Feldstein, Chapters 8 and 9.

health legislation favored and opposed by health interest groups, since it is not always obvious how certain types of legislation promote the economic interests of association members. The political positions taken by various health interest groups during the most recent debate over health care reform are also discussed.

The Self-interest of Health Associations

Health associations demand legislation that serves their members' interests. Without a definition of those interests, however, it would not be obvious how specific legislation promotes their economic interests.

Health professionals and health organizations, such as hospitals, have many goals. Even within the same profession, individuals place different weights on what they perceive to be their self-interest. The tendency, therefore, is to make the definition of self-interest complex. However, if the definition attempts to encompass this diversity, or if different motivations are specified for each piece of legislation, then it is not possible to develop a good predictive model. It is easier to evaluate the effects of legislation using a simple one. Further, unless there is a common goal, one that the membership easily understands, the members may not provide their association with the support it needs. The true test of whether the simply defined goal accurately measures member self-interest is how well it predicts the association's legislative behavior.

The legislative goal of associations with individuals as members—physicians, dentists, nurses, optometrists—is assumed to be to *maximize the incomes of its current members*. Health professionals are no different than other individuals; they will say that they have many goals, of which income is only one. However, income is the only goal that all the members have in common. (Goals such as increased autonomy and control over their practice are highly correlated with increased incomes. Income is thus a more general goal.)

Nonprofit institutions—hospitals, Blue Cross, medical schools, and dental schools—cannot retain profits. Medical and dental schools are assumed to be interested in maximizing their prestige, such as a research-oriented faculty and a low student-to-faculty ratio. His-

torically, little prestige has accrued to a medical school that trains students to enter family practice or to practice in underserved areas.

Until the mid-1980s, when hospitals were reimbursed according to their costs, hospitals were also interested in maximizing their prestige, as indicated by their size and the number of facilities and services they offered. Administrators of large, prestigious hospitals were held in esteem by their peers; they were also able to earn higher incomes. Each hospital attempted to become a medical center.

Beginning in the early 1980s, hospital objectives began to change. The payment system for hospital care went from cost-based reimbursement to fixed prices; hospitals engaged in price competition to increase their volume of patients from insurers and health maintenance organizations (HMOs); low-cost substitutes for hospitals, such as outpatient surgery centers, began to reduce hospital utilization, as did utilization review programs. As these changes occurred, hospitals became more concerned with survival than with emulating major teaching institutions. Even teaching hospitals began to act as though their future was in doubt. To succeed in a more competitive environment, hospitals attempted to minimize their costs and to act as though they were trying to maximize their profits.

Blue Cross and Blue Shield plans were originally started by hospitals and physicians, respectively. Hospitals and medical societies provided the initial capital to Blue Cross and Blue Shield plans and controlled their organization. It was not until the 1970s that these nonprofit organizations separated from the providers that controlled them. Until they did, the objectives of Blue Cross and Blue Shield plans were in accordance with the economic interests of hospitals and physicians. These policies also coincided with the organizations' managers' own interests. The managers of nonprofit organizations want growth, which justifies additional personnel, larger facilities, and higher incomes.

As health care became more price-competitive in the 1980s, competition among health insurers and HMOs increased. The Blues' behavior became similar to for-profit insurance companies. They acted as though they were attempting to maximize profits. In analyzing the legislative behavior of Blue Cross and Blue Shield plans, it is important to keep in mind the periods when their objectives differed.

Although differences existed in the objectives of health associations representing health professionals, hospitals, medical schools, dental schools, and Blue Cross and Blue Shield plans, the members of these associations all tried to make as much money as possible. They would then retain it for themselves, as did health professionals, or spend it to achieve prestige goals, as did hospitals and medical schools. Thus the objective underlying the demand for legislation is the same for each health association. Each association attempts to achieve for its members through legislation what cannot be achieved through a competitive market, namely, a monopoly position. Increased monopoly power and the ability to price as a monopolist seller of services was, and is, the best way for the associations to achieve their members' goals.

There are five types of legislation demanded by health associations to enhance their members' economic interests. As government policy shifted from increasing to decreasing health expenditures (given the concern over the budget deficit), the emphasis devoted to each of these types of legislation by health interest groups has changed over time.

Demand-increasing Legislation

An increase in demand, with a given supply, will result in an increase in price, an increase in total revenues, and, consequently, an increase in incomes or net revenues. The most obvious way to increase the demand for the services of an association's members is to have the government subsidize the purchase of insurance for the provider's services. Health providers, however, have been opposed to the government insuring everyone, which would greatly increase the cost of the program to the government and result in the government developing a concentrated interest in controlling the provider's prices, utilization, and expenditures. Instead, providers want selective demand subsidies, since the greatest increase in demand would result from extending coverage to those unable to pay.

The American Medical Association (AMA) successfully defeated President Truman's national health insurance proposal in 1948 because subsidies would have been provided to all regardless of income level. The AMA's opposition to Medicare was also based on the fact that all aged, regardless of income, were to be subsidized. Instead, the AMA favored tax credits for the purchase of health insurance, which would decline as a person's income rose.

In more recent years as concern with the federal deficit has increased and federal funds to subsidize those with low incomes are unlikely to be available, the AMA has favored an employer mandate, whereby employers are required to purchase health insurance on behalf of their employees. An employer mandate would increase the demand for physician services by requiring the working uninsured to have private coverage. It would also move low-income employees and their families off Medicaid into private insurance, which reimburses providers at a higher rate. For the same reason, the American Hospital Association has also favored an employer mandate.

The Health Insurance Association of America (HIAA), promoter of the famous "Harry and Louise" television commercials opposing various aspects of President Clinton's health plan, also favored an employer mandate because it would increase the demand for private health insurance.

The financing mechanism relied upon by President Clinton in his health care reform proposal was an employer mandate, which would have shifted rapidly rising Medicaid expenditures onto the private sector. Federal and state governments developed a concentrated interest in reducing their Medicaid expenditures; otherwise these expenditures would have increased the federal deficit or necessitated reduced expenditures on politically popular programs.

Large unions also favored an employer mandate because it would have increased the cost of low-wage labor, with whom they were in competition.

Thus, an unlikely set of allies—the Clinton administration, the AMA, hospital associations, health insurers, and the unions—all favored an employer mandate because it was in each group's economic interest to do so.

Previously, the approach used by hospitals to increase the demand for their services was the establishment and control of Blue Cross. When hospitals started Blue Cross, Blue Cross only paid the costs of hospital care. Even if it was less expensive to perform diagnostic tests in an outpatient setting, for the patient with Blue Cross coverage it was less expensive to have it performed in the hospital. The patient with Blue Cross did not have to pay any additional hospital costs; thus high-cost hospitals were not at a price disadvantage with low-cost hospitals, thereby precluding price competition for Blue Cross patients.

Dental care is really not insurable, as are hospital or surgical services. Insurance is generally purchased for events that have a low probability of occurring and are very expensive, such as hospital care and in-hospital physician services. Dental expenditures are relatively small, expected, and not catastrophic. If special incentives to purchase dental insurance did not exist, most people would just pay for dental care when they needed it. The major reason for the growth in dental insurance has been the favorable tax treatment of employer-paid health insurance premiums. Such contributions are not considered part of the employee's income and the employee does not have to pay federal, Social Security, or state taxes on employer-paid health benefits.

For middle- and high-income people, the after-tax value of a $1,000 raise would be reduced by these three taxes, leaving the individual with perhaps one-half of that amount to spend on out-of-pocket medical payments, dental care, vision benefits, and so on. If instead the employer used the $1,000 to purchase more comprehensive health insurance for the employee, the employee could receive $1,000 worth of health benefits.

The lost federal, Social Security, and state tax revenue from the tax exclusion of employer-paid health benefits has been estimated to be in excess of $80 billion. The beneficiaries of this tax exclusion are clearly those in the higher-income tax brackets. If this tax subsidy for the purchase of health insurance were eliminated or reduced, it could raise sufficient revenues to finance health benefits for those with low incomes. Employees would also become more cost-conscious in

their choice of health plans, since more expensive health plans would be paid for with after-tax dollars.

Thus the American Dental Association's major demand-increasing effort has been to ensure that the tax subsidy for private health insurance is not changed; otherwise there would be a decrease in the demand for private dental insurance and consumers would be more inclined to "shop" among dentists for the lowest price.

Few politicians have been so bold as to propose eliminating or reducing this tax subsidy for the purchase of health insurance as part of health reform. This $80 billion tax subsidy is national health insurance for those with middle and high incomes.

The Association of American Medical Colleges has favored legislation, at both state and federal levels, which provides schools with unrestricted operating subsidies, enabling the schools to set tuition levels greatly below the actual costs of education. With artificially low tuition levels and limits on the number of students they accept, there is an excess demand for their spaces. Since these schools have a monopoly over the provision of medical and dental education, they are able to lengthen the educational requirements for entering the profession. These policies are also in the economic interest of physicians and dentists since they lead to higher incomes.

The American Nurses Association (ANA) has favored three types of demand-increasing legislation. The first are proposals that increase the demand for medical services. An example is the ANA's support for national health insurance. Increases in demand for medical services intensify the demand for institutions in which RNs are employed, thereby increasing the demand for RNs. However, since health insurance coverage for hospital care is more extensive than for any other delivery settings (and two-thirds of nurses work in hospitals), nurse associations have also favored other demand-increasing proposals as well.

For instance, the ANA has favored requiring minimum nurse staffing ratios in institutions for certification purposes, such as mandating that there be a minimum number of RNs on the staffs of nursing homes and home health agencies. Similar in its effect, nurse associations have opposed hospital attempts to permit lower-paid nurse aides to perform more of the RNs' tasks, which would decrease the demand for RNs.

Finally, nurse associations have proposed expanding the nurse's role, namely, increasing the number of tasks nurses are legally able to perform. As nurses are permitted to perform more, and higher-valued, tasks, the demand for their services will increase, with a consequent increase in their incomes. In attempting to increase their tasks, nurses have come in conflict with the AMA, which is fearful that broadening the role of nurses with advanced training would decrease the demand for physicians. The ANA viewed President Clinton's health plan as supportive of a broadening of their roles.

All health professional associations compete in the legislative marketplace to increase their role, while preventing other health professionals from encroaching upon their own tasks. Examples of the legislative conflict over state practice acts include the attempts by optometrists to increase their role at the expense of ophthalmologists—as well as the struggles of psychologists versus psychiatrists, obstetricians versus nurse midwives, and podiatrists versus orthopedists.

Securing the Highest Method of Reimbursement

The basic approach used by health associations to achieve the highest possible reimbursement for their members has been to eliminate price competition. The ability to engage in price competition is more important to new practitioners or firms entering a market. New competitors must be able to let potential patients know (through advertising) they are available and provide a financial incentive for patients to switch physicians.

To prevent price competition from occurring, health associations have termed its elements, such as advertising and fee splitting, "unethical behavior" and have prohibited such behavior in their state practice acts. The medical and dental professions have used strong sanctions against practitioners who have engaged in unethical behavior. Previously, a physician could have had his or her license suspended and be assessed financial penalties. Medical societies were also able to deny hospital privileges to physicians who advertised or engaged in price competition (Kessel, 1958). Since physicians new to an area had the greatest incentive to engage in such "unethical" behavior, they were given probationary membership in the local medical society. They were thereby placed on notice that they could lose their hospital privileges if they engaged in such behavior.

As a result of the Federal Trade Commission's (FTC) successful suit against the AMA (upheld by the U.S. Supreme Court in 1982), state medical and other professional societies such as dentistry can no longer penalize their members if they advertise or engage in other competitive activities. Anticompetitive behavior in health care is now subject to anti-trust laws.

A more recent approach used by many state medical and dental societies to limit price competition has been to enact "any willing provider" legislation to counter the provider of HMOs and preferred provider organizations (PPOs) of including in their closed panels only those providers who are willing to discount their fees and practice cost-effectively in return for receiving a greater volume of patients. Such closed panel providers are engaged in price competition with providers who are not in the closed panels, since those not in the panel do not have access to the HMOs' and PPOs' patient population.

"Any willing provider" legislation essentially eliminates the use of closed provider panels by opening them to all providers, thus removing their financial incentive to discount their fees in return for more patients. If providers in closed panels have to share their patients with providers who are not in closed panels, providers are unlikely to join closed panels and discount their fees.

The AMA, over strenuous opposition of the HMO industry, successfully lobbied to have "any willing provider" legislation included in both the Democratic House and Senate versions of President Clinton's health care reform proposal.

The American Nurses Association has lobbied for permitting advanced practice nurses to bill fee for service, which has been used with such success by physicians and dentists. By striving to have nurse practitioners and nurse midwives become independent practitioners, they will then be able to bill the patient fee for service. Fee-for-service payment to a health professional, which in most cases is reimbursed by the government (under Medicare and Medicaid) and private insurance, is the most direct way for a health professional to increase income and to work independently of physicians.

Subsidies to public medical and dental schools go directly to them, as do government funds to be distributed for loans and scholarships. The student receives a subsidy (tuition less than costs) only by attending a subsidized school. Thus students compete for admission to subsidized medical and dental schools. If, instead, the government gave these subsidies, loans, and scholarships directly to students, then the schools would have to compete for students. Students would then have an incentive to shop and select a school based on its tuition rates and reputation. Schools prefer to receive these funds directly so they can distribute them, thereby having a price advantage over private, non-government-subsidized schools.

Health associations, then, in negotiating with the government, in establishing their own insurance organizations, and in proposing legislation, have a clear appreciation for which pricing strategies are in their members' economic interest.

Legislation to Reduce the Price or Increase the Quantity of Complements

A registered nurse may be a substitute or a complement to the physician. It is difficult to determine when an input, such as a nurse, is a complement or a substitute based only on the task performed. A nurse may be as competent as a physician in performing certain tasks. If the nurse works for the physician and the physician receives the fee for the performance of that task, then the nurse has increased the physician's productivity and is a complement. If, however, the nurse performs the same task and is a nurse practitioner billing independently of the physician, then the nurse is a substitute. The essential element in determining whether an input is a complement or a substitute is who receives the payment for the services provided by that input. Whoever receives the payment controls the use of that input.

State practice acts are the legal basis for determining which tasks each health profession can perform and under whose direction health professionals must work. A major legislative activity for each health association is to ensure that the state practice acts work to their members' interests. Health associations that represent complements (e.g., nurses and denturists) attempt to have their members become substitutes. Health associations whose members control complements seek to retain the status quo.

Further, providers can increase their incomes if an increase in demand for their services is met through greater productivity than through an increase in the number of competing providers. Providers' income can be increased still further if they do not have to pay the full cost of the increased productivity.

Examples of legislation that have subsidized provider productivity are the American Hospital Association's successful lobbying for the Nurse Training Act to provide federal educational subsidies to increase the supply of RNs. With a larger supply of nurses, nurses' wages would be lower than they otherwise would have been. For similar reasons, the AHA favored educational subsidies to increase the supply of allied health professionals. The AHA was a strong proponent of the Hill–Burton program, which provided capital subsidies to modernize hospitals. The AHA opposed legislation that would have increased the cost of inputs to hospitals, such as the extension of minimum wage legislation to hospital employees, and has called for a moratorium on the separate licensing of each health professional. (Separate licensing limits the hospital's ability to use such personnel in a more flexible manner.) Conversely, separate licensing is demanded by each health profession so as to increase the demand for its members' services by restricting the tasks that other professions can perform.

The AMA has opposed educational subsidies for graduate-level training of nurses, since such training increases the nurses' qualifications to be physician substitutes.

The AMA has favored internship and residency programs in hospitals, since they are excellent complements for physicians. It is the physician who bills for the service. Residents can take care of the physician's hospitalized patients and relieve the physician from serving in the hospital emergency room and from being on call. The more advanced the resident is, the more productive he or she is. Similarly, the AMA has favored foreign medical graduates as residents; however, lest they become substitutes, the AMA has favored their return to their home country once their residencies are completed.

One of the AMA's and state medical society's highest legislative priorities today is for limits on increases in malpractice premiums. This legislative attempt by physicians to lower the cost of their inputs does not address the real reasons for the rise in malpractice premiums, one of which is physician incompetence (Danzon, 1985). "There have been estimates that as many as 5 to 15 percent of doctors are not fully competent to practice medicine, either from a deficiency of medical skills or because of impairment from drugs, alcohol, or mental illness" (Feinstein, 1985). Professional associations have been more willing to seek legislation to place limits on the size of malpractice awards than to make a concerted effort to eliminate unqualified practitioners.

Health associations are not the only interest groups to seek legislative relief to reduce input costs. An important reason why the auto companies and their unions were staunch supporters of the Clinton health plan was because it would have capped employee health benefits at 12 percent of total wages. The difference between the 12 percent and what the auto companies currently spend (15% to 18%), would have been shared by the union members and the companies. Further, the Clinton health plan would also have relieved businesses of many billions of dollars of their early retirees' medical liabilities by having the government pick up 80 percent of those costs.

Legislation to Decrease the Availability or Increase the Price of Substitutes

All health associations try to increase the price of services that are substitutes to those provided by their members. (Similar to increasing the price of a substitute is decreasing its availability.) If the health association is successful in achieving this, then the demand for its members' services will be increased.

One approach to accomplish this is to simply have the substitute declared illegal. If substitute health professionals are not permitted to practice, or if substitutes are severely restricted in the tasks they are legally permitted to perform, then there will be a shift in demand away from the substitute service. The second approach, used when the first approach is unsuccessful, is to exclude the substitute service from payment by any third party, including government health programs. This approach raises the price of the substitute to patients. The third approach is to try and raise the costs of substitute providers, who must then raise their own prices if they are to remain in business. The following are examples of these tactics.

Optometrists and chiropractors are potential substitutes for ophthalmologists and family physicians. By opposing the inclusion of optometrists and chiropractors as providers under Medicare Part B, the prices of their services to the aged are effectively increased relative to those of physicians. An aged person with Medicare Part B pays less for a physician's services. The AMA has also opposed direct payment of nurse anesthetists under Medicare.

In one case the intervention of the courts prevented physicians from artificially raising the price of a substitute. In Virginia, Blue Shield did not reimburse psychologists as providers of psychotherapy. Psychiatrists' services were therefore less expensive than psychologists' to a patient with Blue Shield. The psychologists brought a successful anti-trust case against Blue Shield in 1980, claiming discrimination against nonphysician providers.

Similarly, the AMA opposed payment for chiropractic services under veterans' benefits and under CHAMPUS, the government's military dependents' health plan, thereby making those services more expensive to veterans and CHAMPUS eligibles.

Foreign-trained registered nurses are substitutes for U.S. registered nurses. Nurses' salaries are considerably higher in the United States than in other countries, providing a financial incentive for foreign nurses to enter this country. The ANA has been successful in decreasing the availability of low-cost substitutes for U.S. registered nurses by making it more difficult for foreign-trained RNs to enter the country. Both the U.S. Department of Labor and the Immigration and Naturalization Service require that foreign nurse graduates pass a screening exam—in English—that measures proficiency in both language and nursing before a work permit and a labor preference visa will be issued. Unless they pass the exam, they are unlikely to emigrate. If the screening exam were administered only in the United States, then foreign-trained RNs could keep retaking the exam and still work in some nursing capacity even if they did not pass the exam.

An additional legislative approach used by the ANA to raise the cost of substitutes to RNs has been to prevent other personnel from performing tasks performed by RNs. The ANA has opposed permitting LPNs to be in charge of skilled nursing homes; otherwise there would be substitution away from RNs (who receive higher wages) currently performing such functions. The ANA has also opposed permitting physicians to decide which personnel can perform nursing tasks.

Denying Blue Cross reimbursement to freestanding surgicenters and including them under certificate-of-need (CON) legislation have been approaches favored by hospital associations to raise the cost of and decrease the availability of a low-cost substitute. Although Congress repealed the federal CON law in 1979, after HMOs were able to persuade Congress that CON legislation was inhibiting their ability to compete, many states still use CON to limit entry by new health facilities. Even new home health agencies have been opposed, because existing facilities do not want competition.

Nonprofit and for-profit hospitals have each tried to increase the cost of the other. For-profit hospitals have attempted to remove the tax-exempt status of nonprofit hospitals, thereby raising their costs. Nonprofit hospitals, in turn, have successfully lobbied for reducing the return on equity of for-profit hospitals under Medicare reimbursement and have opposed Blue Cross payment of for-profit hospitals.

Substitutes for American medical and dental schools are foreign schools whose graduates (who may be U.S. citizens) want to practice in the United States. To re-

duce the likelihood that foreign medical schools will substitute for U.S. medical schools, the Association of American Medical Colleges (AAMC) has favored strong restrictions on the number of foreign medical graduates who can enter the country.

Legislation to Limit Increases in Supply

Essential to the creation of a monopoly are limits on the number of providers of a service. Health associations, however, have justified supply control policies on grounds of quality. Restrictions on entry, they maintain, ensure high quality of care to the public. These same health associations, however, oppose quality measures that would have an adverse economic effect on existing providers (their members). This apparent anomaly—stringent entry requirements and then virtually no quality assurance programs directed at existing providers—is only consistent with a policy that seeks to establish a monopoly for existing providers.

If health associations were consistent in their desire to improve and maintain high quality standards, then they should favor all policies that ensure quality of care, regardless of the effect on their members. However, quality control measures directed at existing providers, such as reexamination, relicensure, and monitoring of the care actually provided, would adversely affect the incomes of some providers. More important, such "outcome" measures of quality assurance would make entry or "process" measures less necessary, thereby permitting entry of a larger number of providers.

A test of the hypothesis that entry barriers are primarily directed toward developing a monopoly position rather than improving quality of care would be as follows: Does the health association favor quality measures, regardless of the effect on its members' incomes, or does it only favor those quality measures that increase members' incomes? If the health association only favors those quality measures that have a favorable impact on its members' economic position, then it can be concluded that the real intent of those quality measures is the improvement of its members' competitive position rather than the assurance of quality care in the most efficient manner.

The following examples illustrate health associations' positions on quality. Health associations have typically controlled the licensure process by having their own members appointed to the licensing board and by having them establish the requirements for licensure. Since licensure, by itself, is not a sufficiently strong barrier to entry, an educational requirement is imposed, stating that before taking the licensing exam a person must have had a minimum number of years of education in an educational institution approved by the profession or by its representatives. (The number of years of training is continuously increased while no additional requirements are placed on existing practitioners.)

The number of educational institutions is kept limited so that, as in medicine and dentistry, there is a continual excess demand for admission. (Medical and dental schools, as well as optometric, veterinary, and similar schools, favor such supply control policies since it provides them with an education monopoly.) Placing limits on the number of educational spaces and specifying educational requirements in excess of the skills necessary to practice reduce the number of persons that can take the licensing exam.

If the licensure requirements merely specified passing an examination, then potential applicants for the exam could receive the necessary knowledge in a number of ways, in different institutions, and in different lengths of time. The number of persons taking and passing the exam would be much greater than if those applying were limited by the number of approved educational spaces. The above approach to quality has been used by both the AMA and the ADA, as well as other health professions.

Nursing is also moving toward requiring more stringent educational requirements. Previously, most nurses graduated from diploma schools of nursing (90 percent in 1955). These programs were operated in conjunction with hospitals and generally lasted two years. The demand for a diploma school education declined and most nursing education then occurred in two-year colleges, with the RNs receiving an associate arts degree.

The growth in demand for an associate arts degree was related to its high rate of return relative to the four-year bachelor of arts degree. Nurses with two- and four-year degrees received similar incomes. Since the four-year degree did not result in sufficiently higher wages to offset the additional two years, the ANA has proposed that nursing education take place only in colleges that offer a bachelor of arts. The ANA proposed that only four-year nurse graduates would be referred to as professional nurses; the others would be "technical" nurses. Nurse associations have lobbied their state legislatures for these increased educational requirements.

An increase in the educational requirement of two-thirds of the nurse graduates (who do not have a bachelor of arts degree) will result in a much smaller supply of registered nurses and increased wages for RNs. The ANA will also use the increased educational requirement to justify an increase in tasks that nurses are able to perform. Existing nurses, with lower educational requirements, would be grandfathered in as professional nurses.

It is unlikely one would ever observe a situation where a health association proposes increased educational requirements that are then applied to its existing members. Rather, a health association would favor additional training requirements for its existing members only to forestall more stringent requirements proposed by others. Health associations do not favor relicensure or reexamination requirements for their current members, even though increased knowledge is the basis for requiring additional training for those entering the profession. Reexamination and relicensure would lower the incomes of their members, since they may not be able to pass the exam. Longer educational requirements increase the cost of entering a profession; thus, no health association proposes that the time required to prepare individuals to enter their profession be reduced. The American Dental Association (ADA), for example, has proposed that each dental graduate take an additional one-year postdoctoral program, which includes hospital experience.

Health associations have opposed any attempts by others to monitor the quality of care practiced by their members. Health associations that have proposed continuing education for their members have done so in response to demands by those outside the profession. These requirements are made easy to achieve and at low cost to the members of the profession.

The current method of quality assurance for health professionals is aimed solely at entry into the profession rather than at monitoring the quality of care given. The inadequate performance of state licensing boards in disciplining their members is evidence of this practice. Further, little communication exists between state licensing boards to check the credentials and status of a physician moving from one state to another. The public is less protected against unethical and incompetent practitioners than it has been led to believe. The public will become better protected, not as a result of the good intentions of the profession, but when the health professions are forced to respond to the demands for quality from those outside the professions.

Conclusion

The political activities of health associations should be viewed in their proper perspective, namely, to benefit their members while imposing a cost on the rest of society. Past reliance on professional regulation to protect the patient has resulted in health care prices being higher than they would be otherwise. These higher prices, which are not visibly attributed to these legislative policies, are borne by patients and by taxpayers who finance government programs.

Further, the legislative success of health associations has resulted in the public being provided with a false assurance with respect to the quality of the medical care it receives.

The movement toward a competitive market in medical services has resulted in a new emphasis on quality of care. Large employers are pressuring HMOs to provide information on their enrollees' medical outcomes, preventive measures undertaken, and health status indicators of their subscriber population. It is through actions by such large purchasers that HMOs are developing "report cards." Employer emphasis on "outcome" measures is forcing HMOs and medical groups to reexamine how medical care is provided. If it were not for large purchasers and market competition, this new approach toward quality would not have occurred.

The movement toward market competition in health services is bringing about change in areas previously considered in the domain of health professionals and subject to government regulation. For example, as part of the Clinton health plan, government regulation was proposed to change the specialty distribution of physicians. Medical schools and residency programs favored specialty programs, resulting in too great a proportion of specialists. Market pressures are currently forcing residency programs to change and also decreasing the number of specialists more rapidly than could be achieved by government.

Health associations are now competing in the political marketplace with employers, government, insurers, and HMOs, all of whom have a concentrated interest in health legislation. The outcome is likely to be greater efficiency and equity in the economic marketplace.

REFERENCES

Danzon, Patricia M. (1985). *Medical malpractice: Theory, evidence and public policy.* Cambridge, MA: Harvard University Press.

Federal Trade Commission v. AMA. United States Reports, *455* (October Term 1981).

Feinstein, Richard J. (1985). The ethics of professional regulation. *New England Journal of Medicine, 312* (March 21), 801–804.

Kessel, Reuben. (1985). Price discrimination in medicine. *Journal of Law and Economics, 1* (October), 20–53.

CHAPTER

On Treacherous Ground: The Strategic Choices of Health Interest Groups

Katherine A. Hinckley
with Bette S. Hill

How do health interest groups behave in the political arena, and why do they act as they do? Although these are apparently simple questions, like most simple questions they are far easier to ask than to answer. In fact, since they have not been answered very well for any set of interest groups, this study begins with a short review and a bit of theoretical exploration.

In answer to the first question—how groups behave politically—we may distinguish between tactical and strategic actions. Tactics typically refer to fairly narrow, short-range activities in pursuit of some specific, preestablished goal. Providing political campaign contributions is one example. Strategies, on the other hand, are normally longer-range and broader in scope, and sometimes very close to the goals themselves. For in-

stance, a decision to help elect as many liberal or conservative candidates as possible is clearly a strategic decision; how one goes about it constitutes the tactics. The primary interest here is in strategic behavior, although some information on health group tactics is also provided.

Interest groups make a variety of strategic decisions, ranging from the decision to enter politics in the first place to the choice of specific targets on which to concentrate. They must also decide whether to use "hired guns" or their own in-house personnel for lobbying, the breadth of the agenda they want to pursue, and their top issue priorities (Hinckley & Hill, 1995). But two other types of strategic decisions are especially vital. One is the group's definition of the issues and the stances it takes on them. The other is whether to concentrate on an "inside" or an "outside" strategy of influence.

The way in which an issue is defined pushes toward a particular type of solution. For instance, if the primary health issue is defined as making sure that the quality of care is never compromised, one set of options comes to mind (e.g., building well-equipped hospitals, training better personnel). If cost is the primary issue, quite another set of options appears. So as interest groups offer different issue definitions to decision makers, they are simultaneously advocating different policy directions.

Further, groups need to decide how strong and uncompromising a stance they will take with regard to their definitions and preferred solutions. If they do not admit other possibilities, they may win big. They may also lose big. The amount of flexibility a group displays is thus a vital aspect of its strategic behavior, and may have a lot to do with its success.

The choice of an "inside" versus an "outside" strategy essentially is the choice between direct and indirect lobbying. In the first strategy, groups approach policymakers directly—lobbying Congress, seeking access to the White House, filing court briefs. The second strategy, in contrast, relies largely on bringing third-party pressure to bear on decision makers. Although the distinction is not fully developed, and in fact many groups use both strategies simultaneously, it is generally agreed that enlisting media and public opinion in the battle for influence represents the classic outside strategy. (Attempts to influence elections are less easily categorized; Hinckley & Hill [1995] consider them outside strategies, while Walker [1991] treats them as inside-oriented.) In any case, while groups have bolstered their inside lobbying, they have increasingly added outside strategies to their arsenal (Schlozman & Tierney, 1986)—a pattern that has become quite evident in the activities of health care groups during recent years.

SOURCES OF STRATEGIC BEHAVIOR

What kinds of factors might account for differences in these two central aspects of group strategy? There are four major possibilities: group resources, the character

of the organization itself, the nature of the target system it seeks to influence, and the nature of the current issue agenda. These four factors often interact with each other in determining group strategies.

Group Resources

Resources have generally been examined for their tactical rather than strategic possibilities, and in truth, such resources as money or technical expertise do not seem very much related to its issue stances. They are, however, importantly related to the use of inside as opposed to outside strategies (Hinckley & Hill, 1995). Strong expertise, high credibility and prestige, and good contacts should incline a group to inside lobbying; so does a sizable staff (Walker, 1991). On the other hand, a large and active membership, and a particularly appealing cause, can be turned to good account with an outside strategy.

Organizational Character

The nature of the interest group organization also affects strategic choice. It is particularly important for basic issue stands. An interest group suffering from internal divisions—quite likely with a highly heterogeneous membership and a structure of semiautonomous subunits—may find it difficult to reach any clear-cut position at all on an issue, much less communicate it forcefully to politicians.

The flexibility of issue stands will be affected by other organizational characteristics, most notably style, incentives for membership, and whether decisions are made from the top down or the bottom up. A group composed of members who are ideologically inclined, and in fact joined the organization to pursue policy goals, will probably find itself constrained to a fairly rigid set of issue positions. This is especially true if the membership is very influential in making the group's decisions—that is, if the flow of decision making is from the bottom up.

Finally, the choice of an inside versus an outside strategy will also be partly a function of organizational characteristics. Probably the most important are how long the group has been politically active, and whether it is accepted as legitimate by other actors. Hayes (1981) suggests that newer groups will be inclined to follow more radical "outsider" strategies, partly because they tend to lack legitimacy. Even having gained political experience and legitimacy, however, an organization may still habitually follow an outsider strategy if it was previously successful. The nature of both members and leaders will have an influence here; as Walker (1991) found, profit-based occupational groups tend strongly toward inside strategies, in contrast to "citizen" groups, which are much more inclined to go outside. In short, a group's political behavior is determined not just by its resources, but also by its general way of doing things.

Target System Characteristics

The importance of target system characteristics is widely recognized in the classic interest group literature (Truman, 1951; Zeigler, 1964). Any given system may offer very expansive or very limited opportunities for different groups. Congress, for example, has generally offered a rich set of strategic and tactical opportunities to interest groups in comparison with those afforded by the federal courts and even the White House.

While interest groups are generally thought to be highly skilled at matching strategies to opportunities, this is not necessarily the case. After all, political systems are moving targets, not stationary ones. They change—sometimes rather rapidly—with "windows of opportunity" for groups, legislators, and bureaucrats opening and shutting in an irregular way (Kingdon, 1984). Whether groups in fact respond by altering basic strategies is very much an empirical question. The answer may depend at least in part on their own organizational character.

Nature of the Agenda

Much the same argument could be made concerning the nature of the agenda, the last class of variables potentially affecting interest group behavior. Of course, groups themselves have a hand in setting agendas. But prominent issues arise from other sources too—executive or legislative entrepreneurs, the media, judicial action, and especially, unexpected or unplanned-for developments in the outside world. We need to know how groups "read" the political agenda at any given moment, and to what extent they alter their behavior in response.

STUDY DESIGN

Developments in national health policy since the mid-1980s provide an excellent opportunity for investigating the impact of all four of these classes of variables—group resources, organizational character, target system characteristics, and nature of the agenda—on health interest group strategies. To permit some detail in analysis, a limited number of such groups are examined here. The focus is primarily on their dealings with Congress, and secondarily the presidency, in relation to the major issues of Medicare, Medicaid, and national health insurance (NHI).

Four of the groups are major providers of health services. The American Hospital Association and the Federation of American Health Systems represent hospitals as institutional providers. The American Medical Association is of course a prominent professional group, while the American Nurses Association is a combination professional association and trade union. A fifth, the Health Insurance Association of America, is basically a trade association for small and medium-size insurance companies.

Congress is emphasized as a target for two reasons. First, as the primary player in the formation of broad health care policy, it is the primary target of the groups themselves. And second, it has undergone remarkable changes in recent years, severely altering the nature of the playing field for interest groups. It therefore gives us a focal point for understanding a highly complex policy system. The White House also deserves consideration, though, because the strategic actions of recent presidents have affected interest groups both directly and through Congress.

Medicare, Medicaid, and NHI proposals certainly do not begin to encompass all the federal health issues on which interest groups take stands; in fact, they are somewhat unrepresentative of day-to-day interest group activities. They are, however, very high-profile, high-stakes issues, on which groups must carefully consider strategic choices. And they have become a central part of the biggest agenda item of all—the federal budget deficit.

Health Interest Groups: Resources and Organizational Character

Our examination of the five health interest groups begins with a discussion of their resources and organizational character. As will be seen, they differ from each other in a variety of interesting ways.

American Hospital Association (AHA)

Founded in 1893 as an eight-man organization of hospital superintendents, the AHA today has a combined membership of approximately 54,500 individuals, hospitals, and other institutions (Daniels & Schwartz, 1994). Individual members are affiliated through sixteen professional groups and the subsidiary American Organization of Nurse Executives. Institutional members range from health care corporations and HMOs to substance abuse centers, hospices, and all types of hospitals—urban and rural, nonprofit and investor-owned, secular and religious (Hill & Hinckley, 1995). This diversity, which extends to geography, services offered, and patient mixtures (American Hospital Association, 1985), provides both individual and institutional representation in virtually every congressional district.

The fiscal resources of AHA include an annual budget (as of 1991) of $86 million (American Hospital Association, 1991–92). There are over eight hundred employees in its Chicago headquarters, and a sixty-four-person staff in Washington (Hill & Hinckley, 1995), headed since 1991 by Richard Davidson, former president of the Maryland Hospital Association. Its political action committee, PAC of AHA, was only founded in 1976, but grew quite rapidly, more than doubling its

total federal contributions from $227,000 in 1983–84 to over $500,000 in 1991–92.

However, the AHA is hampered by a complex and rather cumbersome governing structure. While a board of trustees governs on a day-to-day basis, a 218-member house of delegates is the highest authority for approving AHA policy. Below that is a complex set of regional advisory boards, which debate policy stands at length at the grassroots level before they even come to the house of delegates. Because of this sizable structure and the diverse interests it represents, the AHA has some problems in maintaining organizational cohesion and credibly representing a membership majority, especially since cuts in the federal budget have forced hospitals to compete for limited funds. Still, some observers have noted that the AHA is adept at reinforcing its message with appeals from state associations and local hospitals, which have considerable local economic importance (Pear, 1986; Rhein, 1978).

Federation of American Health Systems (FAHS)

The AHA's diversity problem is exemplified by the Federation of American Health Systems, which was formed in 1966 by a small group of physician-owned hospitals that felt the AHA was not adequately representing their interests. Originally called the Federation of American Hospitals, it was renamed in 1986, and today represents 1,300 investor-owned hospitals and some sixty parent companies, such as Humana, Inc., and Hospital Corporation of America. It in essence is the trade association for the investor-owned hospital industry (Zuckerman, 1994). Some additional members are in health insurance, home health care services, and nursing homes, accounting for the change of name. Though the FAHS membership is concentrated in the Sunbelt, it does extend across all fifty states, Puerto Rico, and eleven foreign nations (Federation of American Health Systems, 1992).

In terms of financial resources the FAHS is rather small compared to the AHA; its budget is only $4 million, with 80 percent coming from hospital member dues. Its staff of twenty-six is split almost evenly between the national office in Washington, which attends to legislative and regulatory matters, and the administrative headquarters in Little Rock, Arkansas, whose duties include publications and membership (Federation of American Health Systems, 1992). It has sponsored a political action committee since the early 1970s; contributions over the 1983–92 period hovered around $160,000 for each election cycle, though there have been some ups and downs.

Despite its relatively small size, FAHS has enjoyed high-quality professional leadership. Michael Bromberg, a lawyer and former congressional aide, served as the federation's executive director from 1969 to 1995 and was rated one of the best health lobbyists in Washington (Rhein, 1978; Pressman, 1984). Highly knowledgeable about health policymaking processes, he is credited with having developed an excellent staff and particularly for being able to generate strong grassroots pressure from members. Of course, he was greatly helped in the latter by the fact that many FAHS hospital board members are prominent people with good access to lawmakers (Pressman, 1984).

The organizational structure of the Federation consists of a six-member executive committee, a twenty-member board of directors, and a 161-member board of governors; in addition, there are standing committees, special committees, and occasional task forces (Federation of American Health Systems, 1992). As befits a trade association, its organization is more streamlined and business-oriented than that of the AHA. With smaller size and more homogeneous membership, the FAHS has a high level of cohesion, representational credibility, and the flexibility needed for quick negotiations. Observers have noted that Bromberg could make compromises and bring them quickly to his group's membership for ratification. He once said, "I can call 10 people [representing large corporate members] and get a decision" (Rhein, 1978, p. 78).

The FAHS probably has the highest credibility of the four provider groups with Congress, largely because of the leadership skills of Bromberg. But it has also gained status by piling up a number of small wins, taking an honest approach to the proprietary hospitals' image

(e.g., admitting they "skim" the best patients), and showing support for broader, sometimes liberal, health issues.

American Medical Association (AMA)

The AMA is composed of over 290,000 physician members and fifty-four state groups (Hilts, 1993; Daniels & Schwartz, 1994). It represents over 40 percent of all U.S. physicians, but this is considerably less than the 70 percent it enjoyed in the 1960s. Moreover, most of its members are over forty-five years old (Alston, 1989). Many young doctors are apathetic about joining the AMA, perhaps partly because it is seen in some quarters as not especially forward-looking and more concerned with doctors' pocketbooks than the nation's health (Pear, 1986; Pressman, 1984). In addition, while it certainly can mobilize influential members to testify before Congress, its grassroots resources are limited because its members, though of high status, are often too busy to exert widespread political pressure. It also faces increasing competition from specialty societies.

The AMA's financial resources are quite impressive, however. The annual budget of approximately $200 million supports a staff of one thousand; about a third of its revenues come from membership dues, another quarter from advertising, and an additional 10 percent from subscriptions to publications. Though national headquarters are in Chicago—a slight disadvantage for federal lobbying—about $4 million is provided for its fifty-eight-person Washington office (Hill & Hinckley, 1995).

In addition, the AMA has a very sizable political action committee, AMPAC, which was founded in 1961. AMPAC regularly ranks among the top five contributors to national political campaigns. Its contributions have steadily risen. In the 1991–92 federal election cycle, for instance, it gave $2.94 million, up from $1.84 million only eight years earlier (Zuckerman, 1994). It has become a leader in developing and testing new contribution techniques, such as conducting surveys for favored candidates and then holding the results for sixty days so that they will be treated by the Federal Election

Commission as having a low in-kind contribution value. It is also one of a half dozen PACs that make large independent expenditures (i.e., outside candidate donations). Such independent expenditures serve as a supplement to candidate contributions, an opportunity to target some candidates for defeat, and a way of putting issues directly to the public (Sorauf, 1988). Clearly AMPAC has become a major element in the AMA's strategy of influence, as will be seen.

In general, then, the AMA is extraordinarily rich in resources, especially when the prestige, contacts, and policy expertise of its members are added to its financial strength. Its only real resource weakness may lie in the intangible areas of image and credibility, and these are in large part a result of the nature of the organization.

Like that of the AHA, the AMA's governing structure presents something of an obstacle to flexibility and effective action. Final authority to take policy stands rests with a 371-member house of delegates. The board of trustees, which governs the organization on a day-to-day basis, can adopt positions in the interim between meetings of the house of delegates, but it tries to match these positions to "the tenor of past and current action" of its parent body (American Medical Association, 1985). As a result of these decision processes and the organization's distinctly conservative bent, AMA positions on legislative proposals tend to be rather inflexible, leaving its lobbyists very little room for the give and take necessary in the drafting of legislation (Pressman, 1984). One writer refers to the organization's "cumbersome machinery" (Alston, 1989, p. 2606). A former AMA lobbyist has admitted that one of the big problems he faced was "Chicago headquarters' unyielding opposition to legislation" (Rhein, 1978), but this is understandable in light of membership relations. In its December 1993 meeting, for instance, AMA leaders had to plead with the delegates not to "tie the trustees' hands" in developing its strategy vis-à-vis the Clinton health plan ("AMA Assails," 1994).

They have also had problems at the top. In 1990, the executive vice president of the organization, Dr. James H. Sammons, was replaced by Dr. James S. Todd in the wake of controversy over Sammons' approval of loans to two former AMA officials without following "the usual fiscal policies and procedures" ("AMA Executive," 1989, p. B13).

Finally, the AMA has experienced some difficulties with internal cohesion. Cohesion was not difficult to sustain in an age when most doctors were like small businessmen, engaged in individual practices or partnerships. Today, however, with the rise of group practices and other new financial structures, political consensus among physicians has become more problematic. One long-term House member noted that both the AMA and AHA have a problem as "umbrella organizations trying to represent a diverse membership" (Pear, 1986, p. A24). As we shall see, this was reflected in splits with specialty societies, and even breakaway groups.

American Nurses Association (ANA)

The ANA, established in 1896, represents some two hundred thousand registered nurses (Daniels & Schwartz, 1994). It "functions primarily as a professional society at the national level" (Zuckerman, 1994, p. 170), but its fifty-three state associations and 860 local affiliates act as collective bargaining units for pay and working conditions. Like the other provider groups, its membership is located in every congressional district.

The ANA operates with a budget of some $17 million and a staff of about 175 (Daniels & Schwartz, 1994). It did not really become active in national lobbying until the 1980s, though by 1978 it had developed a lobbying staff and at least one policy analyst (Holleran, 1978). Headquarters were in Kansas City, Missouri, until 1992, when like so many other groups, the ANA moved them to Washington. According to its president, the shift was intended to increase visibility and effectiveness with lawmakers, funding agencies, and other health-related associations. In addition, the ANA hoped to increase its ability to work with non-health associations and labor unions ("ANA Opens," 1992), and presumably, with the specialty nursing organizations for whom it does some contract lobbying work (Goldwater & Zusy, 1990).

The ANA sponsors a PAC, originally called N-CAP but now renamed ANA-PAC, which is different from the other groups' PACs in several respects. First, it is the only one classified as a labor PAC; the others are listed among trade/membership/health committees. Second, it is the most partisan in its contribution patterns, contributing heavily to Democrats. Befitting its membership, ANA-PAC is one of the few national PACs that make special efforts to support female candidates (Symons, 1984). Compared to the AMA and AHA, the ANA has fewer resources and less national lobbying experience. Moreover, nursing interests are not particularly well entrenched in federal legislation. Nonetheless, it clearly has moved fairly rapidly in a short time, no doubt encouraged by legislators' increasing sensitivity to the women's vote.

The ANA has also altered its organizational structure to help its political efforts. In 1982, it adopted its existing federated structure of state, territorial, and district associations. According to its national headquarters, the move has resulted in organizational growth through more action at the state level. Yet it may also create problems for national leadership, since internal disagreements are a classic characteristic of federated structures (Wilson, 1973). And indeed, nurses are divided over at least one central issue: the educational credentials necessary for professional entry. The ANA has sought since 1965 to make a bachelor's degree the minimum requirement for licensing registered nurses, arguing that those with less training should be designated "technical nurses." But there is still sharp disagreement on the matter, contributing to a "widespread belief that nursing is unable to get its own house in order" (Inglehart, 1987, p. 649).

Still, nurses have demonstrated an ability to unite on other issues, particularly with regard to their own status vis-à-vis physicians. And they have long been on the more liberal side of the question of government involvement in health care.

Health Insurance Association of America (HIAA)

Formed in 1956 with the merger of two older underwriters' organizations, HIAA is the primary trade association for private health and disability insurance companies. From the beginning it stressed political representation before state and federal governments to ensure a strong private-sector role in health policy. Its membership of over 260 companies was quite diverse in size until 1992–93, when five of the largest companies departed to form a separate Alliance for Managed Competition, representing managed care operators in contrast to traditional health insurers (Thompson, 1995).

The departure of these insurers cost HIAA close to $5 million in annual dues, leaving it with a budget of around $25 million. It has 150 full-time employees in its national headquarters in Washington, with six registered lobbyists and additional lobbyists at the state level (Thompson, 1995). In addition, it has a PAC that grew with remarkable rapidity; from a total of $45,000 in contributions in 1983–84, it rose to $130,000, $176,000, and $156,000 over the next three elections, and then leapt again to $232,000 in 1991–92. Its pattern of contributions by party varied sharply over this period, but in general tended to favor Republican candidates, sometimes by sizable margins (Zuckerman, 1994).

HIAA's organizational structure follows a fairly standard format for business and trade organizations—that is, a board of directors, an elected executive committee for interim governance and policy proposal development, and a number of departments for major administrative functions. It is headed by Willis Gradison, former ranking minority member (R-OH) on the House Ways and Means Health Subcommittee, who left Congress to take the position following the resignation of its previous president, Carl Schramm, in early 1993. HIAA soon undertook an unusually visible foray into an "outside" political strategy, which will be discussed later.

Target Systems: Congress and the President

Congress has always been regarded as a splendid target for interest groups. This basically stems from its power as the "first branch of government" under the Constitution. Despite the enhancement of presidential status in the twentieth century, Congress retains a vital, often primary, role in the policy process. Interest groups go where the power lies, and indeed, the organizations examined by Schlozman and Tierney (1986) reported that Congress was their primary target.

Its attractiveness is further enhanced by the excellent access it affords groups. Development of legislation in each chamber centers around the standing committees, whose jurisdictions and membership virtually offer an open invitation to interest group activity.

Nonetheless, Congress has undergone a series of profound changes in the past twenty years—some rather gradual, others shockingly sudden. Among those most relevant for health care interest groups are the following.

Group Competition and Conflict

As every textbook notes, there has been a tremendous rise in the number of interest groups operating at the federal level (Berry, 1989; Loomis & Cigler, 1995). Though most scholarly attention has been devoted to the increase in certain kinds of groups, such as citizen organizations, growth has also reverberated through every policy area. While in 1979 there were only about a hundred health lobbies active in Washington, by 1994 the number had climbed to over seven hundred (Rauch, 1994; Berry, 1994). Craig Ramsay (1995) has edited a volume of over four hundred pages describing just the major ones. Some of this growth results from the establishment of truly new groups; much of it represents the development of independent Washington lobby operations by older organizations. For instance, specialty physician groups such as the American Society of Internal Medicine have expanded their offices in Washington or moved there to improve their political clout (Rhein, 1978). Though the AMA long laid claim to being "the" representative of organized medicine, these groups are contacting Congress directly rather than allowing the AMA to assume leadership. Similarly, there are now different types of hospital associations representing particular interests—for example, the National Association of Public Hospitals, and in fact the FAHS. Both emerged because their member hospitals felt the AHA could not adequately represent their particular concerns (Ramsay, 1995).

Older health groups thus face more and more competition for congressional access. They also face more opposition than before. Based on data from the early 1980s, Salisbury et al. (1987) found relatively low levels of conflict within the health field, particularly compared with labor or energy policy. Today, however, there is rich evidence of conflict, even among provider groups. A 1,200-member group, Physicians for a National Health Program, formed for the express purpose of touting the kind of single-payer national health insurance system vehemently opposed by the AMA. Testimony on physician payment reform before the House Energy and Commerce Health Subcommittee hearings in 1989 found the AMA, urologists, radiologists, internists, family practitioners, and surgeons all staking out "widely variant positions" (Alston, 1989, p. 2606).

It should not be thought, of course, that intergroup relations are purely matters of competition and conflict. Scholars have documented a sizable rise in the use of group coalitions, at least in part because coalitional activity enables the groups to pool their resources and exchange important information (Berry, 1989). Nonetheless, coalition members are often only interested in a few specific provisions (Hula, 1995); not infrequently a major organization will go off on its own.

Committees

Two sets of committees are central to health legislation, and their jurisdictions overlap. General health bills typically go to the House Commerce Committee (formerly, until 1995, the House Energy and Commerce Committee) and the Senate Labor and Human Resources Committee. But any revenue legislation—and therefore anything involving a payroll tax such as Medicare—must go to the House Ways and Means Committee and the Senate Finance Committee. To complicate matters further, the House Commerce Committee has complete jurisdiction over Medicaid and joint jurisdiction with Ways and Means over Medicare Part B, which pays for physician services. The Senate Labor and Human Resources Committee, on the other hand, lacks jurisdiction over either.

From 1987 through 1994, both the House and Senate, and thus all the committees, were controlled by the majority Democrats, and all were fairly partisan; but that did not necessarily mean they agreed on health issues. There were also differences between the health subcommittees of each. In the House, the Health and Environment Subcommittee of Energy and Commerce was chaired by Henry A. Waxman of California, a strong (and largely successful) advocate for the expansion of Medicaid, but not particularly hostile to health providers. The Ways and Means Health Subcommittee, however, was under the gavel of Fortney H. ("Pete") Stark, also of California, and a particular nemesis of the AMA. He regularly referred to physicians as "troglodytes," was the target of a major independent expenditure campaign by AMPAC in 1986, and subsequently filed a complaint with the Federal Election Commission on grounds of illegal AMPAC contributions to his opponent (Rovner, 1989g). Though both parent committees had particularly powerful chairs—John Dingell (D-MI) on Energy and Commerce and Dan Rostenkowski (D-IL) on Ways and Means—the subcommittees had a fair amount of autonomy as the result of internal House reforms dating back to the mid-1970s.

On the Senate side, Labor and Human Resources was headed by Edward Kennedy (D-MA), a long-time supporter of national health insurance, while the considerably more conservative Lloyd Bentsen (D-TX) chaired the Finance Committee until 1993, when he was appointed secretary of the treasury and Daniel Patrick Moynihan (D-NY) took over. However, the particular composition and leadership of the Senate committees are not quite so vital to interest groups as those in the House, because the Senate operates in a much more individualistic fashion, granting less deference and control over issues to its committees and subcommittees (Sinclair, 1989).

Even before the Republican electoral victories of 1994, then, health interest groups faced a wide variety of committee situations in planning strategy, as well as the necessity of dealing with many more participants in the process than had been the case in an earlier era. The election of President Clinton in 1992, and the shift of control of Congress to the Republicans two years later, changed committee roles still further.

Congressional Leadership

The personnel and practices of the congressional leadership, and its relations with the president, were in fairly constant flux throughout this period. Since the start of 1981, there have been four different Speakers of the House, three House minority leaders, four Senate majority leaders, and three Senate minority leaders. While admittedly this is partly a matter of leaders exchanging positions as party control has changed, it still creates real difficulties for maintaining stable congressional relationships.

Changes in House leaders were accompanied by changes in leadership methods. During the 1980s, Speakers began recentralizing power in their own hands. To try to gain unity and advantage for the fractious Democratic majority, they manipulated the referral of bills to committee, the rules for debate on bills coming to the floor, and a variety of other procedural and internal party powers (Smith, 1989).

Changes in the Senate leadership, on the other hand, have had far less effect, largely because its leaders, like its committees, have far fewer power resources than in the House. In addition, the majority party margin has typically been smaller in the Senate—often not even enough to break a filibuster—so that a good deal of compromise and cooperation with minority party members is usually necessary. Senate majority leaders have struggled valiantly for legislative success, but most would probably agree with the comment of Howard Baker (TN), Republican majority leader in the early 1980s, that "leading the Senate is like pushing a wet noodle." For interest groups, even those with the best of access to leaders or committees, the Senate is an uncertain and perilous terrain.

The Electoral Connection

But life is increasingly uncertain and perilous for members of Congress, too. They have always been deeply concerned with keeping their constituents happy in the interests of reelection. Thus any groups representing important elements of their constituencies, or able to assist their campaigns, have been highly welcome on Capitol Hill. But in recent years it appears that electoral sensitivity has been heightened, so that members are increasingly "running scared." This increased emphasis on reelection was noted almost two decades ago, and surely has not declined since; in fact, lower winning margins and significant numbers of incumbent defeats in the 1990s have no doubt exacerbated the phenomenon.

It might be thought that this would further advantage interest groups, and in some ways it has. Campaign contributions are more vital today; members are more concerned about casting votes that might be displeasing to constituents. Interest groups may well be able to take advantage of these concerns. On the other hand, there are indications that direct "inside" lobbying may not be as effective as in the past. With more extensive media coverage of Congress, fewer votes are of the low-profile sort that classically advantage interest groups. Members of Congress may key their behavior to opinion in the district or state at large, rather than to organization representatives. In fact, one study of agricultural policy finds that members are turning for information not to Washington lobbyists, but to well-placed individuals in their districts (Browne, 1995). To the extent this is true more generally, it has major implications for interest group strategy.

The Budget Process

Finally, changes in congressional budgeting practices have also been highly significant for interest groups. The Budget and Impoundment Control Act of 1974 set in motion a new budget process, whereby Congress was to develop each year a concurrent resolution setting targets for revenues, expenditures, and the overall deficit for the coming fiscal year. The standing committees were to complete their own work in line with the resolution. After some wobbly first years, the new House and Senate Budget Committees developed real "teeth" in the form of direct "reconciliation" instructions to the other committees, forcing them to change federal law if necessary to meet their budgetary targets.

Though interest groups were originally not much concerned with budget reform, they soon discovered that it affected them deeply. For one thing, the process eventually reduced the autonomy of the standing committees. Moreover, as Fuchs and Hoadley (1987) noted, the meetings in which all the reconciliation changes were packaged for final floor consideration were generally controlled by the party leadership and closed to the public. As a result, interest groups often could not tell what was happening until the deals were done and a complete package emerged.

The Presidency

Finally, there is the occupant of the White House to consider. Interest groups have never had the kind of easy access to the president that most of them enjoy with Congress, although recent administrations have developed institutionalized forms of access through the Office of Public Liaison as well as some White House personnel (Pika, 1991). Different presidents have granted access to different groups, reflecting their electoral constituencies and policy ambitions (Peterson, 1992). Partisan considerations enter into the equation, too, with the situation for groups changing as different parties control Congress and the presidency.

But there are two factors affecting interest groups that have been relatively constant for all presidents, beginning at least with Jimmy Carter. One is the obsession with the budget, which is as strong in the White House as it is on the Hill. The other is the tendency of presidents to "go public"—to appeal to the mass of the citizenry as a primary strategy in dealing with Congress (Kernell, 1986). Presidents Carter and Reagan are often seen as having been particularly inclined to use this method of arousing support for their policy proposals, but Clinton has also certainly employed it. While there is some dispute about the extent to which going public has really replaced quieter bargaining, and certainly about its efficacy (Brace and Hinckley, 1993), it does appear that presidents are much more oriented to media messages and polls than was true in an earlier era. Like members of Congress, they seem to be acting with at least one eye fixed firmly on larger public opinion. Thus a variety of changes have occurred at both ends of

Pennsylvania Avenue that affect interest group prospects and that might encourage them to rethink older strategies.

Changing Agendas

Meanwhile, the nature of the national issue agenda—the final variable affecting interest group stances and strategies—also changed, and in ways that proved quite painful for health fiscal groups. As budget problems rose in importance over the course of the 1980s, so health policy rose in importance; indeed, it became the central budget issue.

The basic problem was very simple: it would be virtually impossible to control the burgeoning federal budget deficits without controlling the costs of federal health care programs. These costs were rising much faster than wages, inflation, or revenues, with the result that their shares of both federal and state budgets expanded.

As Congress, the administration, and the public increasingly focused on budgets and deficits, the pressures for restraining Medicare and Medicaid costs mounted, regularly placing health interest groups on the defensive and often dividing them from one another. A brief chronicle of major developments serves as a background for the strategies and stances these groups took at different times.

Medicare and Hospitals

Congress began struggling with Medicare cost problems as early as the Nixon administration, though without notable success; an attempt at hospital cost containment during the Carter administration similarly came to grief. By 1982, however, overall deficits were soaring, fueled both by health program costs and by the tax cuts and increases in defense spending pushed by the Reagan administration. Congress had become thoroughly obsessed by the budget issue, and with the new reconciliation mechanism in place, was able to make about $15.5 billion in spending reductions for Medicare and another $1.1 billion for Medicaid under the Tax Equity and Fiscal Responsibility Act (TEFRA). About two-thirds of this fell on hospitals, whose Part A

services accounted for about 70 percent of Medicare spending. The following year Congress enacted a new and radically different system for reimbursing hospital costs. Rather than paying hospitals retrospectively for services to Medicare patients, the new prospective payment system (PPS) would grant a flat sum for each type of illness, or diagnosis-related group (Hinckley & Hill, 1992).

It should not be thought that this solved the hospital cost problem. For one thing, Congress needed to make regular adjustments to the payment rates under PPS in the face of continued hospital inflation. Furthermore, it had to contend with the differential effects of the system on inner-city hospitals, which tended to have a disproportionate number of the poor and very ill, and on rural hospitals, whose costs per patient were higher. Another problem soon surfaced in the form of reports that hospitals were discharging Medicare patients "quicker and sicker" in an effort to keep actual costs of treatment at the reimbursement level. And, finally, there were inevitable complaints about the appropriateness of particular DRGs, the question of continued allowances for hospitals' capital costs, and sizable rises in the Part A hospital deductible paid by beneficiaries (Hook, 1986).

As a result, Congress in the reconciliation bill for fiscal year 1987 directed the secretary of health and human services to prepare legislation modifying the DRG system to take into account illness severity and case complexity; it also allowed a 1.15 percent increase in Medicare hospital payments (considerably under inflation). At the same time, however, it capped the hospital deductible at $520 instead of the scheduled $587, and in light of complaints about hospitals' discharge practices, required them to have discharge planners (Calmes, 1986).

In subsequent years, Congress continued the practice of holding increases in hospital reimbursement rates under inflation as measured by a "market basket" of hospital goods and services, although rural and inner-city hospitals suffered less. The provisions of the multiyear reconciliation bills passed in 1990 and 1993 read like a litany—inflation minus 2.5 percent, minus 2 percent, minus 1 percent, and so on. The 1993 bill even reduced the payments for fiscal years 1994 and

1995 that had been agreed upon in the five-year 1990 bill, a double cut. In addition, there were reductions in the growth of reimbursement for most hospital outpatient services and capital costs.

Physician Payments

The larger problem, however, lay in payments to physicians under Part B of Medicare, which had actually been growing faster than Part A costs ever since 1974 (Hinckley & Hill, 1992). Continuing to pay "usual, customary, and reasonable" physicians' charges, as had been done since the beginning of Medicare, was a recipe for financial disaster. But cutting payments did not prevent doctors from charging the balance directly to the patient; and there were fears that stopping balance billing might lead physicians to reject Medicare patients altogether, for doctors depended on them for income far less than did hospitals. Congress did seek to encourage physicians to accept assignment of Medicare reimbursement as payment in full for services, and by 1984 decided to offer higher rates to "participating physicians," who would accept assignment for all Medicare patients. In addition, with Reagan administration support, it instituted a freeze on physician fees beginning July 1, 1984, with stiff fines for doctors who accepted Medicare patients but raised their fees (*Congress and the Nation*, 1985).

In its fiscal year 1987 reconciliation bill, passed in October 1986, Congress ended the freeze and granted a 3.2 percent increase in fees ("Health," 1986). But it was becoming evident that doctors had responded to the price freeze in good part by simply increasing the volume of services. In 1989, therefore, Congress tackled the physician payment problem on a triple front: (1) reform of the reimbursement system to reflect the time, training, and skill required for a given service—a "resource-based relative value scale"; (2) control over balance billing, so that by 1993, doctors could not charge Medicare patients more than 115 percent of the fee schedule amount; and (3) creation of national volume standards for physician services, with the intent to reduce inflation adjustments in fees if the volume goals were exceeded (Hook, 1989). This last precipitated a

particularly hot fight with the AMA. A ban on physicians' referral of bills to clinical labs in which they had financial interests was also included in the bill.

The reconciliation bills of 1990 and 1993 generally followed the pattern described for hospitals—that is, freezing reimbursement rates or keeping them below medical inflation (though not general inflation). The 1993 bill continued the ban on referrals to clinical labs in which physicians or their immediate families had a financial interest, and extended it to referrals for physical and occupational therapy, radiology, durable medical equipment, home health agencies, outpatient prescription drugs, and hospital services (Budget, 1993). Clearly physicians, like hospitals, were gradually being squeezed tighter and tighter in the effort to control Medicare costs.

Medicaid

Meanwhile, thanks in large part to the efforts of Representative Waxman (D-CA), Medicaid eligibility was actually expanded. Without specifying the provisions in detail, we can see a fairly consistent pattern in the legislation from 1986 through 1989. In one year the states would be permitted to expand eligibility (for instance, to pregnant women who did not qualify for welfare, or those whose income was slightly above the poverty line, or children up to a given age). A year or so later the optional expansion would become mandatory on the states. The highwater mark was probably reached in the 1990 reconciliation bill, which required states gradually to increase coverage for children up to age eighteen in families below the poverty line, and created two new "capped" entitlements, one for home care for the frail elderly and another for services to the mentally retarded. It also allowed for expansion of Medicaid "cost sharing" of Medicare premiums, co-insurance, and deductibles for those not quite poor enough to qualify for straight Medicaid (Hook, 1990).

The 1990 bill's provisions covered two years, however, eliminating the need for another reconciliation bill in 1991; furthermore, it specified that any program additions had to be offset by cuts elsewhere in the budget. In reaction to the increasing burden of Medicaid on state budgets, the National Governors Association even asked Congress to delay putting the 1990 Medicaid mandates into effect (Rovner, 1991b). In short, the political environment was beginning to be distinctly less favorable to Medicaid; soon events would be moving in quite a different direction.

Access and National Health Insurance

As must be evident from the above description, payments under Medicare and Medicaid were not covering the costs of servicing their poor and elderly clienteles. Service providers, who previously might shift costs to Medicare bills, now were shifting unreimbursed Medicare costs to private patients. The federal government might be saving money, but charges went higher and higher in the private market. This, in turn, raised insurance rates, pricing both individuals and employers out of the market. Millions of Americans—spouses, other dependents, unemployed workers, employees of small businesses—had no health insurance at all, and even those covered by employer group insurance found access to medical services increasingly constrained.

The initial congressional response was to nibble around the edges of the problem. In the fiscal year 1986 legislation, it required larger employers to continue to offer group rate coverage to laid-off workers and various categories of current and former dependents. Attempts were made in both the fiscal year 1987 and 1988 bills to require establishment of state "risk pools" for those not normally insurable, but were ultimately quashed in conference ("Health," 1986, 1987).

Some members of Congress, however, were taking a broader view. Senator Kennedy introduced legislation in 1987 requiring all employers to provide at least minimum health insurance benefits, though it was never acted on by the full Senate in the face of adamant opposition from both small business and the Republican presidential candidate, George Bush (Hook, 1988). Kennedy and Waxman introduced similar legislation in 1989, adding Bush's proposal to let the unemployed buy into Medicaid, but with no success.

By the start of 1991, the health care system was widely regarded as broken, but there was no agreement on how to fix it. Although President Bush offered a plan, it was largely focused on subjects like medical malpractice, infant mortality, and childhood immunization. His Medicaid buy-in proposal was considered highly unlikely to go anywhere, not the least reason being doubt that Medicaid was worth buying into (Rovner, 1991e). In truth, the president was not really that much interested in the matter, and also was leery that Congress might pump up a modest proposal to unsustainable proportions (Rovner, 1991b). Voters were unhappy, but not inclined to pay more for health care. Absent major voter demand, Congress would not do much either. As Representative Gradison (later to become HIAA president) said, "My hunch is that 1991 and federal health-care legislation will be all talk and virtually no action" (Rovner, 1991b, p. 415).

And so it was, until Harris Wofford, running on a platform focused on the need for health care reform, unexpectedly won the special November 1991 election in Pennsylvania to replace the deceased Senator John Heinz. Suddenly Congress seemed galvanized. The overhaul proposal that Majority Leader George Mitchell (D-ME) had been working on for much of the year abruptly took center stage. The House Democratic caucus unanimously approved a resolution calling for comprehensive national health care legislation, though there were severe internal divisions over the specifics. A number of groups, including the AHA, weighed in with their own plans (Rovner, 1991c).

But Gradison's prediction ultimately proved correct. Internal divisions on the proper course of action were so great that the 102nd Congress closed in fall 1992 without health care reform reaching the floor of either chamber. Congress could not even manage to pass a bipartisan bill to ease the health insurance situation for small business (Donovan, 1992).

However, the election of Bill Clinton as president on a platform that included major health care reform insured its continued prominence. A self-professed "policy wonk," Clinton delegated the drafting of legislation to a large task force of experts from Congress, the administration, and the private sector chaired by his wife, Hillary Rodham Clinton, with Ira Magaziner as staff director. The final plan was built around the principle of universal coverage; employers would pay 80 percent of health insurance premiums, with government subsidies for low-income workers and some small businesses. The delivery system would be thoroughly revamped; each state could either develop its own single-payer system or set up one or more "health alliances" to serve as middlemen in the large-scale purchase of health insurance plans from groups of doctors and hospitals. Larger corporations could bypass the health alliances and purchase insurance directly, but would pay an additional one percent tax for doing so. Other provisions included a cap on insurance premiums, increased cigarette taxes, and limits on the growth of Medicare and Medicaid (Hook, 1993).

The administration clearly followed a strategy of "going public" in an effort to gain congressional approval of the plan. The Democratic National Committee mounted a major grassroots effort, headed by Richard Celeste, a former Ohio governor and strong Clinton supporter; many from the 1992 Clinton campaign team were also involved. Activities included development of state-level teams to argue the case, ads to answer criticism, bumper stickers, an 800 telephone number, and five hundred house parties across the country on the night of Clinton's health care speech to Congress (Connolly, 1993a). In July 1994, "Health Security" buses, modeled after the 1992 Clinton–Gore campaign buses, toured various parts of the country (Connolly, 1994). Clinton himself, in his 1994 State of the Union Address, resorted to tough rhetoric: "If you send me legislation that does not guarantee every American private health insurance . . . you will force me to take this pen [brandishing it], veto the legislation, and we'll come right back here and start all over again" (Rubin & Donovan, 1994, p. 174).

As it turned out, Clinton never got a chance to use his veto pen. Neither the House nor the Senate passed any version of health reform. The factors responsible have been much debated, and no doubt are complex and multiple: the sheer complexity of the proposal, which made it difficult for even experts to understand; the fact that it was delayed until September 1993, losing the advantage of the early "honeymoon" period ac-

corded a new president; and Clinton's own uncertain signals about exactly what compromises he would be willing to make. Borger (1994) argues that the secrecy of the task force deliberations and the unwillingness of the administration to listen to practical political advice were extremely damaging. Others commented on Clinton's mistakes in dealing with public opinion, particularly in alienating congressional Republicans and moderate Democrats (Zaldivar, 1994).

In retrospect, it appears that there was *never* any consensus among Congress and interest groups on health reform in general, and equally important, no real constituency for the Clinton plan in particular. The president had not much more than presented his reform proposal than other plans were being introduced. In the House, the legislation was referred in full to three different committees, each of which produced its own version; the final version assembled by Majority Leader Richard Gephardt was withheld from floor debate until it was clear what the Senate would do. But in the Senate even a modified, bipartisan version of health reform could not gain the support of enough members to break a threatened filibuster and bring the measure up for debate ("Health Care Overhaul," 1994).

Exactly what role interest groups played in the collapse of health reform is, as always, difficult to estimate precisely. But it is evident that the major concern here—their strategies and stances—came in the context of the president's actions, the congressional situation, and their own outlook and resources, just as in other health policy issues of recent years. It is to those strategic choices that we now turn.

AHA Strategies and Stances

Between 1986 and 1992, the AHA took fairly predictable positions on the major health policy issues discussed previously. It defended itself and the basic prospective payment system (PPS) against charges that hospitals were discharging patients too early, "or that the entire industry is adopting practices that jeopardize the quality of care available to Medicare beneficiaries" (Hook, 1986, p. 120). It supported provisions to modify the diagnosis-related group (DRG) specifications (Rovner, 1986b); and, of course, it pleaded vehemently for higher hospital reimbursement rates, pointing out that 46 percent of urban hospitals, and 63 percent of rural ones, were losing money on Medicare patients (Rovner, 1989b). Indeed, along with the AMA, it was outraged by the 1990 budget summit proposal (Rovner, 1990).

But it also was active on issues more tied to professional autonomy than to economic problems. For instance, it joined with the AMA in bringing an ultimately successful suit against HHS regulations requiring the treatment of all handicapped infants, regardless of the wishes of the parents—the "Baby Doe" regulations (Witt, 1986a, 1986b). In legislation barring discrimination in federally supported institutions, it supported a guarantee that would ensure that no hospital would be forced to perform abortions. As Executive Vice President Jack Owen noted, the association firmly believed that a hospital should be free to choose whether to provide such services (Cohodas, 1988, p. 161).

The AHA's stances often represented attempts to deal with the diversity of its membership. For instance, it opposed legislation granting states money to develop regional trauma care systems, largely because the proposed guidelines might restrict the number of centers qualifying in a given area; the association argued that any hospital devoting the necessary resources should be able to qualify (Rovner, 1988d). But straddling the full range of membership needs was not always easy. The question of differential payments to inner-city and rural hospitals had posed particular problems for them during negotiations over the 1984 reconciliation bill. At that time they asked for the rate differentials; by 1992, they were asking for a single base rate, but adjusted for patient characteristics and resource prices (American Hospital Association, 1992).

It is worth noting that almost all of the AHA's activity represented an inside strategy—gaining direct access to decision makers. One mark of this was the pattern of donations by the PAC of AHA. About two-thirds of its contributions went to Democratic congressional candidates, which is in line with the general tendencies of

PACs seeking access to the majority party. Moreover, heavy contributions were made to the committees with jurisdiction over the AHA's priority issues. In the two election cycles from 1989 through 1992, the PAC of AHA gave $107,000 to members of the Ways and Means Committee, $144,000 to members of House Energy and Commerce, and $71,000 and $67,000 to members of Senate Finance and Senate Labor and Human Resources, respectively ("Top Givers," 1993). These amounts represented about 40 percent of their total contributions during that period.

Another clear indicator of the AHA's inside strategy tendencies was its participation in lobbying partnerships or coalitions with other groups, some of which are not even in the health field. For instance, it joined with the National Right to Life Committee and the U.S. Catholic Conference in supporting hospital choice on performing abortions. In addition to its cooperation with the AMA noted earlier, it joined with the AMA and ANA in supporting a bill by Kennedy and Waxman to provide federal funds for voluntary AIDS testing and counseling (Hook, 1987), vehemently opposing amendments for expanded mandatory testing (Rovner, 1988a, 1988b). In 1991, the AHA, HIAA, AMA, and Blue Cross and Blue Shield Association "issued a joint statement of principles endorsing universal access to health care services" (Thompson, 1995, p. 232). The AHA favored employer-sponsored programs and "a consolidated public program combining and expanding Medicare and Medicaid," but opposed a single-payer system (Hill & Hinckley, 1995, p. 83).

The preference for working inside the system was evident in AHA's dealings with the Clinton administration. Supporting the principles of universal access and mandates for employer-paid insurance, it agreed to some less attractive aspects of the developing health reform package (Cloud & Rubin, 1993; "Two Years," 1993). However, it was deeply disappointed in the outcome of the 1993 reconciliation act. The cuts in Medicare had to be deepened because, despite heavy lobbying by AHA and over twenty other groups, energy interests and producer-state senators succeeded in eliminating a revenue-raising energy tax. AHA felt the president had caved in. Herb Kuhn, AHA vice president for congressional relations, said, "We worked very hard with this administration, and we certainly will be more cautious in the future" (Rubin, 1993a, p. 2227).

So while the AHA went along with the basic task force process, it clearly did not wish to alienate congressional Republicans. In spring 1993, the Democratic National Committee (DNC) attempted to establish a bipartisan health care team separate from the political party, hoping to raise millions of dollars for a grassroots campaign in support of the president's efforts. The AHA was wary of the project. According to Richard Wade, vice president of communications, it feared the campaign would inevitably be viewed purely as an arm of the Democratic Party. It therefore declined participation, along with many other groups (Connolly, 1993a).

Moreover, the final Clinton health proposal proved highly unsatisfactory to the AHA in a number of respects. Although the association liked the principle of universal access, it was dubious about the size and potential power of the health alliances. As its chief executive officer, Richard Davidson, had said earlier, combining a payroll tax with mandatory purchasing of insurance through the alliances would make them resemble single-payer systems ("Two Years," 1993). But the AHA's deepest concerns were the proposals for a global budget in health care spending and a cap on insurance premiums. The AHA was very much afraid that caps would mean a decline in salaries for hospital personnel, as insurers cut their reimbursement rates.

Asked before the Clinton health plan was completed what would be the "line in the sand" for the AHA, Davidson had replied, "It's always dangerous to say, 'Here are the lines in the sand, and there will be no compromise.'" But he went on to remark, "If you conceive of a global budget by just pulling a number out of the sky, we would react strongly to that" ("Two Years," 1993, p. 60). Throughout the spring and summer of 1994, then, the AHA fought the caps and the scope of the health alliances—two central points of the Clinton plan.

Moreover, in a somewhat unusual departure from its usual practices, the AHA did not confine its activities to inside lobbying. In February 1994, Davidson announced to members that the AHA was putting the final touches on a national campaign "designed to position hospitals and their communities to take charge of the coming changes, rather than having those changes dictated to them." The campaign, he said, "will help Congress understand that to truly achieve reform" the AHA's proposals would have to be part of any bill. These included universal access through pluralistic financing, limits on the scope of health purchasing alliances, broad-based financing without rigid, formula-driven global budgets, and prevention of further Medicare spending reductions (Davidson, 1994, p. 8). In May, when the House Ways and Means Committee was trying to construct a bill, the AHA was running radio ads in the districts of some committee members; by July, *Congressional Quarterly* was reporting that hospitals and insurers were waging a massive television and advertising campaign (Rubin, 1994). Furthermore, in the 1993–94 election cycle, the AHA made over $100,000 worth of independent expenditures (Federal Election Commission, 1993–94).

That the AHA, normally a rather staid and cooperative inside lobby group, would have been driven to mount a campaign to "ignite grassroots action in targeted congressional districts and states" (Davidson, 1994, p. 8) is indicative of just how high it believed the stakes were for its members. It may also have represented the culmination of long years of frustration at the squeezing of Medicare and Medicaid reimbursements to hospitals. But perhaps more important, it was a sign of the change in the presidential and congressional systems that make outside strategies increasingly important.

FAHS Stances and Strategies

The for-profit, tax-paying character of the FAHS membership produces a distinctly more business-oriented outlook than is true of the AHA. This has been the case from the beginning; in fact, it underlay the breakaway of the original FAH from the AHA in 1966, and has been consistently reflected in their stances on health policy.

There have been three major, interlocking strands in the FAHS approach. One has been basic opposition to government regulation of health care. The Federation adamantly opposed Carter's hospital cost-containment plan in 1977 as, among other things, perpetuating inefficiencies. Though it cooperated in the formation of the PPS system, it objected strongly to Medicare cuts throughout the 1980s, because the arbitrary lowering of reimbursement levels failed to reward those hospitals that had instituted competitive efficiencies. Furthermore, it regarded Medicaid, like Medicare, as underfunded, and asked for federal minimum standards for reimbursement levels (Federation of American Health Systems, 1992).

Naturally, it strongly opposed the Clinton health plan. As Bromberg said to Vice President Albert Gore, at the one public hearing held on the plan, "The ultimate issue is who is going to control one-seventh of this economy—the government or the people?" (Connell, 1993, p. A8). But it had also opposed earlier, less extensive "play or pay" proposals as well. In 1992, Bromberg declared, "While some may support the concept of mandated employer coverage or a play-or-pay approach, these plans will lead straight to a single-payer system if they are tied in any way to government price controls" (Federation of American Health Systems, 1992, pp. 4–5).

Second, as part of its preference for marketplace strategies, the Federation has argued for increased use of private insurance. In its ten-point health reform plan of 1992, it advocated not only the expansion of employer-based insurance coverage, but also the conversion of Medicare to a program offering private insurance options to beneficiaries, with the federal government paying a fixed amount for each person. It also asked for federal preemption of state insurance mandates (Federation of American Health Systems, 1992).

Finally, the FAHS believed that an essential part of cost control was restraint of consumer demand for health services, and many of its stances were directly or indirectly aimed at this. Its ten-point plan called for a cap on the amount of employer-paid health insurance that would be tax-free, arguing that under the present system, there were no incentives for cost-effective coverage. In addition, it supported reforms aiding small business, changes in malpractice laws, and taxation of the actuarial value of Medicare benefits (Federation of American Health Systems, 1992).

Perhaps because of Bromberg's extensive congressional experience, the FAHS has always emphasized an inside, access-oriented strategy. The pattern of its PAC donations is one indication. While its campaign contributions went disproportionately to Republicans in 1983–84 and 1985–86, after that the bulk of them were given to candidates of the incumbent Democratic majority (Zuckerman, 1994). Another sign is its emphasis on working with other interest groups. "United we stand; divided we fall" has always been a good rule for approaching Congress, which likes to see proposals supported as widely as possible. The Federation's 1992 annual report had several comments about the importance of providers responding to the health reform issue in a unified manner (Federation of American Health Systems, 1992). Although it parted company with the AHA on the question of employer mandates, it cooperated on several other issues. Equally important, the Federation moved to unite with its natural ally, business. It joined the Healthcare Leadership Council (HLC), an organization of executives of health insurers, providers, and suppliers, and in late 1991, the council and the Federation joined the Healthcare Equity Action League (HEAL) (Federation of American Health Systems, 1992). This latter organization, representing some three hundred small and large employers and employer associations (with a total of more than 35 million workers), was spearheaded by the National Federation of Independent Businesses, which was particularly incensed over employer mandate proposals and, later, the Clinton plan (Ramsay, 1995).

Yet given the changes in the political environment, even the Washington-oriented FAHS realized that inside lobbying was not enough. Beginning in 1992, the Federation put grassroots programs into action at the community level, collaborating with the HLC and HEAL (Federation of American Health Systems, 1992). By the start of the Clinton administration, the strategy had developed further. As Bromberg said in February 1993, in response to Clinton's public campaign for his budget proposals and the prospects for health reform, "Lobbying is not standing at the corridors of power with bags full of money. It's at the grass roots. We're going to do the same thing [Clinton is] doing—go to the grass roots." Adding that the FAHS planned to invite members of Congress to tour member hospitals, which employed millions of people, he declared, "We're going to ask them: 'Which ones of our employees do you want us to lay off?'" (Kuntz, 1993, p. 382).

AMA Strategies and Stances

Historically, the AMA has opposed almost all government intervention in the health care field. It opposed the original Medicare program; it opposed government sponsorship of HMOs; it opposed the DRG system; it opposed the participating physicians program; it of course opposed the physician fee freeze. Often this opposition was rigid indeed, as was suggested in the earlier description of the workings of the organization.

The appeals and issue definitions used by the AMA have varied quite widely, from the danger of untried techniques to questions of promises made and basic fairness. Most commonly, however, the AMA has cast its stances in one of two molds—the importance of professional expertise and autonomy in decision making, or the importance of maintaining public health and the quality of care. What is usually missing is the construction most of the AMA's critics would put on its actions—the pursuit of bald economic interest. In the discussion that follows we can see all of these interpretations of AMA behavior, as well as the way in which its strategic choices reflect the congressional environment, changing agendas, and the organization's own resources and needs.

Professional Concerns

A really quite remarkable number of the AMA's stances in this period clearly reflected its professional concerns, and they were by no means always conservative. It consistently rejected both congressional and administrative attempts to restrict abortion counseling by entities receiving federal funds, arguing that medical and ethical obligations to the patient would be violated (Rovner, 1987b). In 1988, it joined in a suit to block implementation of new regulations on the subject (Rovner, 1988c), and though losing the case, continued in opposition. In 1991, though not mentioning abortion specifically, the AMA annual meeting urged repeal of all laws and regulations that "prevent physicians from freely discussing or providing information to patients about medical care and procedure or interfere with the physician–patient relationship" (Rovner, 1991d, p. 1766). Professional autonomy also seems to have been a major concern in joining with the AHA to bring suit against the "Baby Doe regulations."

The AMA defended its professional members in other ways, too, calling in 1990 for the resignation of Richard Kusserow, inspector general of HHS. Kusserow, who zealously pursued fraud and abuse in the Medicare and Medicaid programs, was seen by the AMA as less interested in the actual guilt or innocence of the accused physicians than in the generation of impressive conviction statistics. Though others did not necessarily agree (Sidney Wolfe, director of Public Citizen's Health Research Group, called the AMA's attacks a "mark of distinction" for Kusserow), the AMA stuck to its guns (MacPherson, 1992).

Public Health Issues

The AMA also regularly intervened in public health questions, some of which were quite controversial. For instance, its 1987 annual meeting flatly rejected the Reagan administration's proposals for expanding mandatory AIDS testing, which it argued would drive those at high risk underground and produce needless alarm among those at low risk because of false positives. It called for increased funding for AIDS research, as well as confidentiality and antidiscrimination legislation, and thereafter supported the Kennedy–Waxman bill (Rovner, 1987a, 1987c). In 1991, it supported the plans of the Centers for Disease Control to develop a list of exposure-prone procedures that doctors and dentists infected with the HIV virus should not perform, although it seems to have been the only medical group to have done so (Altman, 1991).

In other public health matters, the AMA filed an amicus brief before the Supreme Court involving a Florida schoolteacher who was fired because she had tuberculosis (Witt, 1986c); supported legislation requiring notification of workers exposed to toxic substances in the workplace (Morehouse, 1988); and issued guidelines saying physicians should routinely question female patients about domestic abuse (Rudavsky, 1992).

Internal Affairs

At least some AMA stands seemed to reflect internal organizational considerations. It came out strongly for a smoke-free society, and in 1986 made banning cigarette advertising the top item on its public health agenda. The Tobacco Institute charged that its stance was "a thinly disguised effort to try to attract young doctors," which the AMA did not deny. Said one association spokesman, "The AMA opened its doors about 10 years ago to medical students and residents and they've been relentless about this issue" (Rovner, 1986a, p. 3050). Curiously, however, a study by Scharfstein and Scharfstein (1994) found that the AMA, through AMPAC, actually contributed significantly more to House candidates from 1989–92 who *opposed* the AMA's stands on tobacco exports, the "gag rule" on abortion counseling, and a mandatory waiting period for handgun purchases than to those who supported them. This raises the real possibility that AMA concerns were more centered on a fourth area, the economic interests of physicians.

Economic Interests

Certainly, in the face of the enormous changes going on in the health care field, the AMA has devoted a great deal of time to matters clearly affecting doctors' economic interests. Here it has been torn between its classic oppositional posture and the sense that some image burnishing and more positive approaches were necessary.

For instance, by 1986, pressures had developed for overhauling the system of physician reimbursement. One possibility was a DRG system for physicians, but the AMA strongly objected to assignment, which would be necessary for the system to work. It *was*, however, interested in restructuring fee schedules to reflect the "relative value" of training and expertise required in treating patients. So while it was complaining vigorously about the differential fees for participating physicians (Hook, 1986, 1987), it was also participating as a subcontractor in the study by Harvard economist William C. Hsiao, who essentially developed the relative value scale. Indeed, the AMA house of delegates tentatively endorsed the RVS in late 1988 (Rovner, 1989c).

But from the AMA's point of view, rising medical costs were not basically the fault of physicians. It blamed the advent of new and more expensive technologies, high patient expectations, and, perhaps most bitterly, attorneys whose suits had raised the costs of malpractice insurance and forced doctors into "defensive" testing and treatment. It therefore objected strongly to legislative proposals barring physicians from referring patients to clinical labs in which they held a financial interest (Rovner & staff, 1988). Dr. James Todd, then the AMA senior deputy executive vice president, told the Ways and Means Health Subcommittee that the issue was not ownership, but "appropriate use," and contended that there were plenty of existing laws to deal with the problems (Rovner, 1989g, p. 460).

Its real wrath, though, was reserved for proposals to establish "expenditure targets" controlling the volume of physician services. In fact, the "ETs" issue became the great health care battle of 1989. Responding to the report of the Physician Payment Reform Commission, which recommended both the targets and balance billing controls, Todd told the Senate Finance Committee, "The AMA believes that both concepts will lead to rationing of health care" (Rovner, 1989h, p. 588). A week later, Joseph T. Painter, the vice chairman of the AMA board of trustees, told the Ways and Means Health Subcommittee that expenditure targets in Canada had been connected with delays and lack of service.

These remarks brought on a tirade from subcommittee chairman Pete Stark: "That's always been the AMA's position: 'If we don't get what we want, we won't treat people.' . . . I haven't heard one word about the doctors being willing to take a little less." After warning that there *would* be a volume cap, Stark asked Painter, "Does the AMA want to participate [in negotiations] or does it want to toddle off in its usual 19th-century mind-set and have no part?" (Rovner, 1989a, p. 654).

Nor was that the end of the AMA's troubles. There was no solace from the Bush administration, which supported expenditure targets in the interests of deficit reduction (Rovner, 1989f). Worse yet, the American College of Surgeons and ten specialty surgical societies broke away from the AMA's position and cut its own deal with the subcommittee for a special set of surgery expenditure targets (Rovner, 1989a). "Never in my life," said Princeton health economist Uwe E. Reinhardt in reviewing the debacle, "have I seen pure economic theory predict human behavior more accurately. . . . In the old game, health-care providers stood together and Congress forked over more money. The new game in Congress seems to be divide and rule" (Alston, 1989, p. 2605).

The AMA thus suffered from the combination of a hostile environment and the breakdown of physician unity in trying to combat the expenditure targets. But it also suffered from its own rigidity and rhetoric, as Stark's comments illustrate. Alston notes that the surgeons' move badly undercut the AMA's position, isolating it as "events overtook its original position and its cumbersome machinery ground toward a new one. For most of the spring, it could do little more than say no" (Alston, 1989, p. 2607). By the time it turned to research and guidelines on effective treatment as an alternative, momentum for expenditure targets had already built up, with political cover for congressmen provided by the Payment Commission report and the Bush administration.

The AMA was not insensitive to the general problems of the health care system, though. In March 1990, the Association offered its own plan for health care reform, requiring employers to provide health insurance for full-time workers and families, expanding Medicaid

to nationally uniform coverage, creating "risk pools" for the normally uninsurable, and revamping the malpractice system. In December 1992, the AMA house of delegates voted to support a modified version of the plan calling for universal coverage (West, 1992). But apart from supporting tax incentives to make insurance more affordable, the original plan did not suggest how the program should be financed or what it would cost (Rovner, 1991b). In fact, the final version drew opposition from the American College of Physicians for failure to live within a budget (West, 1992). And the AMA still disliked managed competition because the authorizations, preclearances, and reviews of doctors and their decisions by managed care companies were viewed as both administrative burdens and professional insults.

But as the Clinton task force began its labors, the AMA began to fear that it would be left out of the negotiations entirely. On March 3, 1993, Todd wrote a letter to Ira Magaziner, offering to join in the "shared sacrifice," and accept managed care. It conceded the idea of a National Health Board to review prices and practices in medicine, as well as a cap plan on spending, though not the "global budget approach." In return, the AMA asked for participation in the planning sessions and consideration of such proposals as malpractice reform, anti-trust relief for doctors to negotiate fees, and guarantees of patient choice of physicians (Hilts, 1993). Despite this rather abrupt about-face in approach, the Clinton administration rebuffed the Association "with only minimal courtesy." Said Clinton, "That would be like opening the White House at every staff meeting we have. . . . [The team] would never get anything done" (Clift & Hager, 1993, p. 37).

Inside and Outside Strategies

In pursuing its various goals, the AMA has clearly engaged in a predominantly inside strategy—targeting not only Congress, but also the administration and the courts. It has regularly engaged in coalition work with other organizations, particularly the AHA. Furthermore, much of its election effort should be seen as an inside strategy designed to gain and maintain access to important congressional decision makers. Although in the 1977–86 period, AMPAC gave very heavily to Republicans compared with Democrats, beginning in 1988 its contributions were much more balanced (Hinckley & Hill, 1990). In fact, it openly adhered to a strategy of giving to "friendly incumbents," and in some cases contributed after the election to winning candidates whom it had not originally supported (Gaunt, 1987).

Nevertheless, it has never been shy about going outside to appeal to the public. Historically it is noted for hiring the Whitaker and Baxter advertising agency to campaign against President Truman's national health insurance proposal—a first in modern group history. And, as noted earlier, it is among the few groups to engage in extensive independent expenditures, working not through the candidate's campaign but directly on the public.

These tendencies were quite evident in the AMA's actions in the late 1980s and early 1990s. It engaged in a massive (over $500,000) but unsuccessful effort in 1986 to unseat Representative Stark and his predecessor in the Ways and Means Health Subcommittee position, Andrew Jacobs of Indiana. Then, in April 1987, angry at Democratic sponsorship of a campaign finance reform bill with strong limits on PACs, it boycotted a fundraising dinner for the party's congressional and senatorial campaign committees. An AMA spokesman said, "We're getting a little tired of sitting there and being part of the team, and being told, 'Thanks for your money, but we . . . don't want your advice'" (Watson, 1987, pp. 782–84).

The AMA also continued its independent expenditures, though in a somewhat uneven fashion. It racked up $850,000 worth in 1988, largely in television advertising (Alston, 1988), before dropping off to around $200,000 in the 1990 elections. In 1991–92, its independent expenditures came to over $1 million, though none were made in 1993–94 (Federal Election Commission, 1989–90, 1991–92, 1993–94).

Independent expenditures were not the only outside strategic activities the AMA engaged in, however. In June 1989, after the Ways and Means Health Subcommittee had approved expenditure targets but before the full committee markup, the association launched a full-scale lobbying and newspaper advertising campaign. A particularly impressive ad featured an elderly woman and the headline, "How do you tell someone on Medicare she's an Expenditure Target?" (Rovner, 1989d, p. 1551). It went on to say that such targets would lead to rationing of medical care, though in later versions the word "would" was changed to "could" (Alston, 1989).

Simultaneously, the AMA encouraged House members to give special one-minute speeches opposing expenditure targets (ETs). Their lobbyists wore buttons with the international bar signifying "prohibited" across the words, "ETs (rationing!)" (Rovner, 1989d, p. 1551), and physicians called on congressmen in both Washington and the District (Alston, 1989). While this campaign was primarily directed at Congress, its rhetoric also had a distinct public coloration. After the full committee approved the targets, Painter said, "What committee members have voted for, without public debate and behind closed doors, is nothing less than a national health-care rationing scheme for senior citizens and the disabled covered by Medicare. Furthermore, what they are trying to do is make physicians do the dirty work of deciding which services to cut" (Rovner, 1989i, p. 1627).

Although this was probably the high point of the AMA's "outside" efforts, it did continue the strategy with a somewhat lower profile. In April 1993, more than one thousand "grassroots" members converged on Washington to apprise Congress of their objection to more cuts in Medicare fee payments. Further national advertising was undertaken, including a series in the *Washington Post* early in 1993 making clear the AMA's positions on the proper contents of national health reform. Later that year, at the time of the Clinton plan's release, another ad showed a doctor's hand touching a child's hand in a manner distinctly reminiscent of Michelangelo's "The Creation of Adam" on the Sistine ceiling. It raised three fundamental questions about the Clinton plan for the public:

1. Will you continue to be free to choose your own physician and health care plan?
2. Will you and your physician be free to make medical decisions . . . without interference from government

bureaucrats, insurance companies, or your employer?

3. Will health plan administrators assume the physicians' responsibility for establishing medical treatment policies and standards of care? (American Medical Association, 1993, p. 75)

If, as Dr. James Todd said, "There's a mentality that you have to take a pound of flesh out of the medical profession" ("Doctors Under," 1993, p. 28), the AMA intended to fight back on all fronts. According to West and Heith (1994), the association spent about $2 million on health care ads in 1993–94.

How successful have these efforts been? Most of the candidates the AMA has heavily supported have won; but not all have. Independent expenditure campaigns are costly, and furthermore they may make enemies— not just the opposing candidate, but his or her supporters as well. Stark pointed out that the AMA's campaign against him in 1986 galvanized the nurses in his district *for* him. Even one's own membership may be soured. In the 1988 South Carolina race between incumbent Democrat Liz Patterson and Republican Knox White, prominent local physicians in Greenville who had formed a White fundraising committee were quite angry about the AMA's intervention (Alston, 1988). The expenditures also received front-page coverage in the Greenville paper—presumably of a sort the AMA did not particularly enjoy.

The efficacy of the campaign against expenditure targets was even more dubious. Some felt it did more harm than good. Congressman Gradison (who later was to become president of HIAA), normally sympathetic to provider interests, angrily denounced the AMA ad (Alston, 1989, p. 2609). Waxman, whose own subcommittee version of the physician payment bill had rejected ETs as hurting all doctors, said, "I hold my point of view in spite of their ad campaign, not because of it" (Rovner, 1989i, p. 1627). Members of Congress were not the only unhappy ones. White House Chief of Staff John Sununu was also annoyed, and let AMA officials know it (Alston, 1989).

This raises a paradoxical point. Dr. Robert Graham, executive vice president of the American Academy of Family Physicians, has observed that the AMA "has taken successively ill-tempered, ill-thought-out and extreme positions on public policy issues that have hurt their credibility with legislators" (Alston, 1989, p. 1608). Yet in view of the budget-cutting drives of the Reagan and Bush administrations, the AMA actually has preferred to see Congress, with its greater constituency sensitivity, in charge of physician payment policy. One revealing incident along this line occurred in August 1991, when the Bush administration released its proposed regulations on the RVS payment system, not merely reallocating payments but actually reducing them by $7 billion between 1992 and 1996. Not unexpectedly, the AMA was infuriated: "If these proposals are finalized in their present form, physicians can only conclude that the federal government has broken faith with the medical profession and its patients" (Rovner, 1991a, p. 2256). But the congressional committees of jurisdiction were also furious. Even Stark immediately introduced legislation to remove the cuts if the administration did not back down (Rovner, 1991a).

Thus the AMA must rely to a considerable extent on Congress to protect its interests, even in Republican administrations. Yet the outside strategy, which is increasingly seen as the most effective way to pressure an electorally sensitive body, may cause resentments that hinder the group's direct lobbying efforts. It is worth remembering that while the public campaign to sway the House on expenditure targets did not have much favorable impact, the AMA's hard "inside" bargaining with senators did ameliorate the final provisions. It is clear that in the modern political context, groups often must perform a delicate strategic balancing act.

ANA Actions

The ANA is an interesting contrast to the AMA. The differences stem partly from its organization and membership, but above all, from its political and professional position.

On one hand, the ANA has been much more supportive of liberal initiatives in the health care field, as might be expected from its dual nature as a labor union. It has been a strong advocate of federal health insurance for the elderly dating back to the original Medicare legislation. It adamantly objected to increases in Medicare beneficiaries' out-of-pocket costs during the Reagan administration, arguing that they were both unfair and injurious to the elderly. It made AIDS policy one of its top priorities between 1987 and 1992, supporting the Kennedy–Waxman bill on funds for voluntary AIDS testing and acting with AHA as one of the co-leaders in opposition to mandatory test expansion and reporting (Hill & Hinckley, 1995; Hook, 1987; Rovner, 1988a, 1988b).

On the other hand, it is much less wealthy, prestigious, experienced, and entrenched than the AMA. In consequence, most of its energies have been spent trying to establish itself professionally and politically, though quite naturally it tries to define these issues in terms of larger public concerns.

Over the course of the 1980s, the ANA sought more nursing education funds, the right of nurse anesthetists to receive direct Medicare payment, and development of new categories of nurse caregivers (Hill & Hinckley, 1995). It also supported legislation providing for "portable" pension plans for nurses. In the private sector, the ANA has been particularly worried about the loss of nursing jobs occasioned by hospital restructuring and about inroads on nursing functions by unlicensed assistants ("ANA Delegates," 1993). More generally, it has pushed hard for greater autonomy for nurses and a broader scope for the health services they can offer. Its argument is that advanced practice nurses could provide most primary care services at a level equal in quality to that of physicians and at considerably lower cost ("Nurses Gain," 1993). Naturally, this brings them in direct conflict with the AMA, which takes a very different view. The exchanges on this question have at times been quite acrimonious.

All of these tendencies—liberalism, the push for professional independence, and conflict with physicians—were manifested in the ANA's actions and stances on the Clinton health plan. It formally endorsed Clinton in the 1992 campaign, and ANA President Virginia Trotter Betts served on the Clinton campaign's health advisory council. An RN was placed on the Clinton transition team before the inauguration; the ANA also

developed a project to get more nurses in federal policymaking positions ("Nurses Gain," 1993.) Finally, and most important, it was in on the drafting of the Clinton reform plan, meeting several times with Ira Magaziner ("Nurses Help," 1993).

The specifics it sought were very much in line with the 1991 *Nursing's Agenda for Health Care Reform*, ratified by over sixty national nursing groups. This agenda called for universal access to a basic core of health services, employer mandates, and a government-sponsored plan for the poor—all part of the original Clinton campaign stance ("Nurses Gain," 1993). But the key elements the ANA wanted, and the ones on which it conditioned its support, basically centered on the advancement of nursing. One of the major points was inclusion of advanced practice nurses among providers whose services would be covered as part of the basic benefit package; another was a guarantee that APNs would play an equal role in provider networks and the new health alliances. In addition, it wanted a Nurse Education and Training Trust fund as a new entitlement program and loan forgiveness programs. A final, and central, provision sought was elimination of requirements for physician supervision of APNs, so that the latter could provide primary care services and be paid directly for them ("Nurses Help," 1993; "Doctors," 1993).

This last brought a blast from the AMA house of delegates, which approved in December 1993 a "stinging report" questioning APN qualifications and the supposed cost advantages of allowing them to provide primary care. It is "irrational," the report said, "to jeopardize patient safety by allowing unsupervised APN practice." ANA President Betts retorted that the report used "inaccuracy and innuendo" to undermine APN performance, and added that it was "disappointed" by the AMA's whole approach to health care reform ("AMA Assails," 1994, p. 76).

In actuality, the ANA was also rather disappointed by the Clinton plan. Some points they thought they had successfully negotiated were either omitted or left unclear, such as eliminating requirements for physician supervision, specifying APN services in the benefit package, establishing the trust fund, and limiting state restrictions ("RNs Aim," 1994). Although some of these were amended in later drafts, close inspection suggests that the plan did not in fact include much of the ANA's core agenda.

It is plain that in regard to general health reform, the ANA relied very heavily on an inside access strategy, with the Clinton administration as its primary target. It offered both electoral and policy support to Clinton, and as a result, obtained recognition of its interests and a certain degree of political status. In addition to granting advisory appointments and participation in the drafting process, both the president and Mrs. Clinton addressed the ANA during 1994 (*Weekly Compilation of Presidential Documents*, 1994; "Clinton," 1994). But there is often a trade-off for this sort of recognition; presidents frequently choose to use the groups for policy advancement or reelection purposes (Peterson, 1992). It appears that this is what happened to the ANA.

Of course, the White House was not the ANA's typical target; it had been lobbying Congress well before Clinton assumed the presidency. There it followed standard procedures—testifying, working with other groups in coalitions, making fairly sizable campaign donations. Its actions with regard to the latter are rather interesting; of the $306,000 ANA-PAC gave to federal candidates in 1986, 90 percent went to Democrats (Zuckerman, 1994). Such heavily Democratic giving is standard for labor union PACs, though, and furthermore coincides with the incumbent bias shown by most PACs.

In addition, the ANA has engaged in fairly vigorous efforts to stimulate member participation. By the mid-1980s, it had established a network of several hundred congressional district coordinators (CDCs), whose functions were to develop campaign organizations for nurses within their districts, register nurses to vote, and distribute literature on endorsed candidates. Motivating more members to become active in politics was the goal of a special project, "Nurses Visible in Politics (N:VIP)," which developed a National Nursing Agenda and held regional workshops (Symons, 1984). The association also attempted to target the political parties; it was one of fifteen women's organizations caucusing together as Women's Central each day at the 1988 Democratic National Convention (Freeman, 1988). In early 1994, it geared up for a grassroots drive in support of the pending health reform legislation ("AMA Assails," 1994).

In one sense, these grassroots efforts are ideal for influencing decision makers. Firsthand constituent participation is much more effective than secondhand reaction to media campaigns. In another sense, though, they often create their own problems for organizations, chief of which is the danger of losing control. Activism is valued, but must be channeled, for members often do not recognize on their own what is politically possible or tactically smart. The ANA has apparently already experienced some mild versions of this difficulty. In August 1993, on learning of the Senate Finance Committee's vote against expanded Medicare reimbursements for nurse practitioners, the ANA house of delegates meeting "erupted in anger." Only with some difficulty were members persuaded to send two of their number to each senator's office instead of instituting a mass march on the Capitol ("ANA Delegates," 1993, p. 71). A year later, a vigorous argument was made by several of the large state delegations for endorsement of a single-payer plan; again, it was necessary to convince members the association should not commit itself to an exclusive and politically unfeasible course of action ("Clinton," 1994). As we have already seen with the AMA, outside strategies often are used at a cost.

HIAA and the Clinton Plan

Historically, much of HIAA's action has been centered on state governments, as they, rather than the federal government, have been the major insurance regulators. But federal health proposals also naturally draw HIAA's attention to that level.

HIAA has regularly used inside strategies in pursuit of its goals, employing standard lobbying tactics and coalitional work. In 1988, it joined with other organizations such as the U.S. Chamber of Commerce and the American Health Care Association (representing the nursing home industry) in opposing the Pepper bill to provide a full program of long-term care for the elderly (Rovner, 1988e). It also strongly opposed the Kennedy–Waxman legislation requiring employer insurance coverage and permitting Medicare buy-ins by the unemployed; its president at that time, Carl

Schramm, said that without a way to control costs, expenses under such a program would skyrocket (Rovner, 1989e). And it lobbied hard against proposals to give states more power to set benefit program standards and to ease the way for suits against insurance companies by those whose health claims had been denied (Palmer, 1992). In both cases it was worried about having to deal with fifty different state standards.

Of the groups examined here, however, the HIAA seems to have the strongest penchant for employing outside strategies. Its pattern of donations, which clearly favored Republicans even in a period of Democratic control, suggests that it may be following a "replacement" strategy typical of ideological groups and those recently experiencing regulation (Conway & Green, 1995). In 1991–92, for instance, it gave only about $89,000 to Democratic candidates, but $143,000 to Republicans (Zuckerman, 1994). In common with a number of corporations, it has found paid media a useful device for getting its views across to the public. In opposing the Pepper bill, for instance, HIAA ran a large ad in the *Washington Post*, charging that "Haste Makes Waste" (Rovner, 1988e, p. 1492).

But it was the Clinton health plan that elicited the strongest "outside" strategic response from HIAA—an advertising campaign that landed it national publicity. There seem to have been two major factors behind its reaction. One was simply that the stakes for the organization were extremely high—much more than for any other group. The problem was not universal coverage, nor even the employer mandate in the plan; scenting an expanded market, HIAA had joined with the AMA and AHA in endorsing the first in 1991, and it had changed its mind on the second in 1992 (Thompson, 1995). Rather, the major difficulties were the national health budget and its accompanying premium caps, and most especially, the proposed health alliances. These would be fine for the big HMO insurers, but a disaster for smaller companies, which would essentially be displaced by the alliances (Rubin, 1993b). Indeed, HIAA feared that many of its members simply could not survive under the Clinton system (Rubin & Connolly, 1993).

The second factor was the apparent decision of the White House and the Democratic National Committee to sharpen the debate on this very complex plan by pointing up a number of symbolic "enemies"—specifically, insurers, physicians, pharmaceutical manufacturers, and the promoters of an alternative health plan in Congress. According to Gradison, this was known to the targets quite early on (West & Heith, 1994).

In May 1993, as the preliminary content of the draft plan leaked out of the task force, HIAA took out a full-page ad in the *New York Times* on behalf of the Coalition for Health Insurance Choices (basically an insurance group) to tout its own proposal (Rubin, 1993b). By fall, it had undertaken two major advertising campaigns at a cost of $3.7 million, more than was budgeted for the entire DNC effort (Connolly, 1993a). These included the famous "Harry and Louise" television ads, in which a young couple discussed the potential problems of the Clinton health plan. The campaigns also featured newspaper advertisements and a toll-free number to which more than three hundred thousand calls were made between September 1993 and April 1994 (West & Heith, September, 1994).

The HIAA campaigns were not truly national; they were aimed at key congressional districts, large states, and elite opinion in Washington (Connolly, 1993a, 1994). But they did receive national newspaper and television coverage, and the administration reacted sharply. DNC chairman David Wilhelm attacked the ads as being misleading; HIAA responded that the DNC had launched "incessant, incendiary attacks against the health insurance industry" (Connolly, 1993a, p. 2810). In November, Mrs. Clinton also attacked the industry and appealed to citizens: "It is time for you and for every American to stand up and say to the insurance industry: 'Enough is enough.'" The HIAA response was another new commercial (Connolly, 1993b, p. 3052). It has been estimated that the combined costs of all the HIAA campaigns came to something over $14 million (Connolly, 1994).

How much damage did the HIAA campaign (and that of the Pharmaceutical Research and Manufacturers Association, which spent even more) do to the prospects for the Clinton health plan? Many reporters and administration officials felt it had a very broad and destructive effect. Gradison himself suggested that the impact was broader than was actually planned. "We tried to use a rifle shot," he said, "but we struck a chord in the public, their concern about government control and bureaucracy" (Donovan, 1994a, p. 1706). Certainly it seems to have had an impact in Congress; Representative Dan Rostenkowski, before he was forced to resign the Ways and Means chairmanship under criminal indictment, actually traded concessions on the committee bill for a HIAA promise not to run ads in particular states (Donovan, 1994b; West & Heith, 1994). The effects on general public opinion, however, are much more doubtful. West and Heith (1994) contend that while general viewing of health ads had some negative impact, the "Harry and Louise" ads specifically were not granted much credibility and had almost no effect on opinions about the plan. Yet whatever conclusion one reaches about the matter, one thing is clear: interest groups as well as presidents can play the "going public" game.

The Republican Congress

After the 1994 midterm elections, the situation for interest groups was once again altered dramatically. The most obvious and important changes, of course, were the new Republican majorities in both Senate and House—in the latter case, for the first time in forty years. The Republicans controlled all the committees and their chairmanships, and were the primary architects of floor action. But their ascension meant more than just numerical control, especially in the House; it also meant structural and procedural changes. Committee staff were cut, and some jurisdictions were partially rearranged. More important, the new Speaker, Newt Gingrich (GA), thoroughly dominated his party and the committees, choosing some chairs out of the line of seniority, installing loyal newcomers in unusually important positions, and further undercutting the standing committees by means of special task forces for major issue areas (Bruck, 1995). Access to the committees, the mainstay of group influence for so many years, became relatively less important than access to the temporary task forces and party leadership.

Furthermore, although health policy remained high on the congressional agenda under the Republicans, the tenor of the agenda was altered. The GOP was not interested in revisiting the national health insurance issue. Rather, its primary goal was balancing the federal budget by the year 2002, while simultaneously cutting taxes. And the only way this could be done, as everyone knew all along, was through extremely large reductions in the future growth of Medicare and Medicaid.

The Republicans basically approached the Medicare problem by seeking to allot a fixed sum to each Medicare recipient, with a choice of using the money to either stay in the traditional program, join a managed care organization or a newly established network sponsored by doctors and hospitals, or use a "medical savings account" to buy a high-deductible insurance policy and bank the remainder for future use. These options, along with scheduled increases in Part B premiums, especially for the wealthier, were meant to encourage cost-consciousness and the migration of beneficiaries out of the standard program (Fraley, 1995a). In addition, there would be significant reimbursement cuts in that standard program. Medicaid was also to be revamped, primarily by turning the program over to the states as a block grant and giving them great flexibility to design benefit and eligibility standards. It should be noted that the House was the primary leader in pushing these plans, though the Senate generally went along.

How were our five interest groups affected by these changes? First, with the exception of the ANA, they were all basically more in tune with the Republicans' approach to health policy. In that respect their situation was improved. Second, they faced a congressional majority that was remarkably united in its determination to cut back on health care costs, and which on the House side had also become remarkably centralized in the person of the Speaker. Under these circumstances, the best strategy was to remain reasonably flexible, engage in classic "inside" negotiations with the leadership, and see how things would turn out.

And that, in essence, is what they did. The first step was to repair any holes in the web of access. PAC of AHA made almost $40,000 in campaign contributions in the first two months of 1995, 81 percent of which went to congressional Republicans—a sharp increase from 53 percent in the comparable period in 1993. It was by no means the only group to have second thoughts; Speaker Gingrich made it quite plain that contributions were henceforth expected to go disproportionately to Republicans, and even labor groups such as the Teamsters and United Auto Workers reacted accordingly (Salant & Cloud, 1995).

Next was to get in on policy development. This was helped along in the House by the Republican leadership's strategy of working as closely as possible with as many groups as possible, trying to meet their concerns and angling for their support. As AHA lobbyist Michael Rock said, "They've been very receptive to our ideas; we send them [legislative] language; they send us language, we send them language" (Rubin, 1995, p. 2897).

Naturally, not all was sweetness and light. FAHS lobbied vigorously against the Medicare reimbursement cuts, and actually had a multimillion-dollar ad campaign planned against the House provisions. But, as FAHS President Tom Scully noted in September, "Now we're not going to launch it, given how much Newt and the leadership have worked with us. We're not thrilled, but at least we're neutral" (Rubin, 1995, p. 2895). In addition, FAHS found the Republicans' proposed voucher plan quite appealing. According to Scully, "Only by eventually moving all seniors to privately managed systems operating under a defined federal contribution can the federal government truly restrain cost growth and drive efficiency into the system" (Fraley, 1995b, p. 2189).

The AHA was not quite so content with the end result, largely because it would be more strongly affected by the reimbursement cuts. It liked the idea of provider networks and the relaxation of anti-trust regulations that would make it possible to create such entities, along with exemptions from state licensing requirements. But even the persuasive tongue of the Speaker could not get the AHA to actually endorse the House package—only to refrain from actively opposing it (Taylor, 1995). And elimination of the anti-trust regulations and licensing exemptions in conference made the AHA even less happy. Their president, Richard Davidson, complained, "Instead of handing it over to health experts, they've given it over to the state insurance commissioners." Yet these changes were precisely

the ones that were gratifying to the HIAA, which felt all health insurance organizations should be under the same rules (Fraley, 1995a, p. 3538). HIAA certainly also was pleased with the general thrust of the GOP legislation in favor of the private market.

By any calculation, however, the AMA fared best. The House Republican leadership worked hard until October to get its support, and finally succeeded only after a special meeting in Gingrich's office elicited some changes in the reimbursement formula for physicians and a promise that the payments would not be cut in the future. Yet the AMA had already obtained some of its most cherished desires: options for provider networks exempted from anti-trust and state licensing requirements, which would give physicians the chance to escape the loss of authority and income endemic to managed care; repeal of the ban on clinical referrals; repeal of the limits on balanced billing; and limits on both "pain and suffering" and punitive awards in malpractice suits (Fraley & Taylor, 1995; Gottlieb, 1995).

Democrats were, to say the least, incensed by the agreement. Stark called it "unethical, despicable, underhanded"—a "bribe" from the Speaker. President Clinton waxed eloquent: "In the dark of night, the Republican leadership cut a deal with the AMA that once again put their interests ahead of the interests of the patients. It may help the Republicans to pass their plan, but the rest of America needs to know who's going to pay for the payoff to the AMA" (Fraley & Taylor, 1995, p. 3143). The AMA was attacked by the reformist Physicians for a National Health Program, and even by some of its own members, who felt "it was a deal over money" rather than health policy, though AMA President Dr. Lonnie R. Bristow was later to say, "There was no deal. What we did was to go in and explain that an unintended problem in access was about to be recreated, and once the House leadership saw that, they made an appropriate adjustment" (Pear, 1995, p. A1).

Of course, not all of what the AMA got in the House survived the conference agreement, but overall it did remarkably well. It is therefore a little odd to note that on December 4, 1995, the AMA board of trustees announced that it had never endorsed the Medicaid portion of the Republican health plan, and argued that

Congress should preserve Medicaid as a federal entitlement, with uniform national standards and a minimum package of benefits. The fear appeared to be that the states would reduce already low Medicaid payments even further under block grants (Pear, 1995). House Republican leaders were clearly not pleased with the defection of a chief supporter, and it seemed the AMA might have overreached once again, but two days later the question was mooted, at least for the time being, when Clinton vetoed the entire reconciliation bill.

Conclusion

The foregoing account amply demonstrates that interest groups' strategic choices are indeed shaped by all four of the variables initially described: the nature of the organization itself, its resources, the character of the institutions it targets, and the current issue agenda. Of the four, the latter two seem most vital for interest groups' stances and the flexibility with which they approach issues. The changes that have taken place in Congress and the presidency in recent years, and the implications for health policy of treating federal budget deficits as the nation's foremost problem, have tended to force groups to modify their positions. Though they may lose ground by doing so, they fear they will lose even more by appearing intransigent.

Yet interest groups do not always adapt adequately. They are constrained in important ways by their own structures and membership, as the experiences of the AHA, and particularly the AMA, indicate. And of course their resources are limited; they cannot fight on every front simultaneously. Yet they are tempted to overreach, particularly if pressured by their members.

There is another way in which the changed environment has affected group stances. With the scope of conflict increased as more and more groups enter the health policy field, it has become vital for groups to join forces in coalitions—to present a united front. But coalitions come at a cost, most often in compromise of one's positions. Throughout this period, the five groups frequently found themselves at odds with each other, even though their basic ideological interests often coincided. Perhaps they have been fortunate that their opposition

and congressional decision makers have been equally fragmented.

If adaptations in group stances are often subtle and difficult to track, changes in groups' choices regarding inside and outside strategies are much less so. There has been an unmistakable rise in the use of outside strategies by groups of all stripes, particularly in the forms of grassroots agitation and use of the paid media for advocacy purposes. As Cigler and Loomis (1995) point out, these have always been employed to some extent, but their increased use not only in health reform, but also with issues like NAFTA and abortion, amounts to a change in kind rather than degree. Certainly the availability of group resources has a major effect on choosing an outside strategy, but the decision is again conditioned by changes in behavior and electoral calculations by presidential and congressional targets.

Yet in the end, the experiences of these groups suggest that an outside strategy is not sufficient, and may in some instances even be counterproductive. Members of Congress are not passive in the face of such campaigns; they are quite capable of developing their own sources of information about what the public "really" thinks. And having done so, they may choose to discount or even ignore what the groups have to say about the specific aspects of policy. In short, the use of an outside strategy may make an inside strategy less successful.

As in the case of stances and flexibility, then, decisions to go inside or outside each carry dangers with them. Though external conditions and the group's own nature may point them in certain directions, the choice of path is finally their own. In an issue area as convoluted and hotly contended as national health policy, each path leads onto treacherous ground.

REFERENCES

Alston, Chuck. (1988). PACs' independent expenditures slow down. *Congressional Quarterly Weekly Report* (November 5), 3185–3187.

Alston, Chuck. (1989). Belt-tightening in Medicare pits doctor vs. doctor. *Congressional Quarterly Weekly Report* (October 7), 2605–2609.

Altman, Lawrence K. (1991). Agency faulted on list to show AIDS risks. *New York Times* (November 5), C2.

AMA assails broader role for RNs; ANA sees "inaccuracy and innuendo." (1994). *American Journal of Nursing, 94* (February), 76, 81.

AMA executive leaving amid rift. (1989). *New York Times* (December 6), B13.

American Hospital Association. (1985). *Annual report.* Chicago: American Hospital Association.

American Hospital Association. (1991–92). *Report to members.* Chicago: American Hospital Association.

American Hospital Association. (1992). *Public policy priority summary.* Chicago: American Hospital Association.

American Medical Association. (1985). *Reference guide to policy and official statements.* Chicago: American Medical Association.

American Medical Association. (1993). This is the moment of truth. *Newsweek* (September 13), 75.

ANA delegates act to prepare nurses for their future in a reformed system. (1993). *American Journal of Nursing* (August), 71–73.

ANA opens for business in D.C.; sees growing role in legislation. (1992). *American Journal of Nursing, 92* (April), 104.

Berry, Jeffrey M. (1989). *The interest group society* (2nd ed.). New York: HarperCollins.

Berry, Jeffrey M. (1994). *The dynamic qualities of issue networks.* Paper presented at the annual meeting of the American Political Science Association, New York City, September.

Borger, Gloria. (1994). Poor diagnosis, bad prescription. *U.S. News and World Report* (October 5), 44–47.

Brace, Paul, and Barbara Hinckley. (1993). Presidential activities from Truman through Reagan: Timing and impact. *Journal of Politics, 55,* 382–398.

Browne, William P. (1995). Organized interests, grassroots confidants, and Congress. In Allan J. Cigler and Burdett A. Loomis (Eds.), *Interest group politics* (4th ed., pp. 281–298). Washington, D.C.: Congressional Quarterly.

Bruck, Connie. (1995). The politics of perception. *The New Yorker* (October 9), 50–76.

Calmes, Jacqueline. (1986). The 99th Congress: A mixed record of success. *Congressional Quarterly Weekly Report* (October 25), 2661–2662.

Cigler, Allan J., and Burdett A. Loomis. (1995). Contemporary interest group politics: More than "more of the same." In Allan J. Cigler and Burdett A. Loomis (Eds.), *Interest group politics* (4th ed., pp. 393–406). Washington, D.C.: Congressional Quarterly.

Clift, Eleanor, and Mary Hager. (1993). Health care: Covert operation. *Newsweek* (March 15), 37.

Clinton "gives 'em health" as ANA faces reform fallout. (1994). *American Journal of Nursing, 94* (August), 69, 72–73.

Cloud, David S., and Alissa J. Rubin. (1993). Energy tax, Medicare cuts focus of Senate battle. *Congressional Quarterly Weekly Report* (June 12), 1458–1464.

Cohodas, Nadine. (1988). Sponsors plan early 1988 push for Grove City, housing bills. *Congressional Quarterly Weekly Report* (January 23), 160–163.

Congress and the Nation. (1985). Washington, D.C.: Congressional Quarterly.

Connell, Christopher. (1993). Fear of cost controls grips medical lobby. *Akron Beacon Journal* (March 31), A8.

Connolly, Ceci. (1993a). DNC aims to approach Hill from ground up. *Congressional Quarterly Weekly Report* (October 16), 2809–2812.

Connolly, Ceci. (1993b). Mrs. Clinton strikes back. *Congressional Quarterly Weekly Report* (November 6), 3052.

Connolly, Ceci. (1994). Storming the capital. *Congressional Quarterly Weekly Report* (July 23), 2042.

Conway, Margaret M., and Joanne Connor Green. (1995). Political action committees and the political process in the 1990s. In Allan J. Cigler and Burdett A. Loomis (Eds.), *Interest group politics* (4th ed., pp. 155–174). Washington, D.C.: Congressional Quarterly.

Daniels, Peggy Kneffel, and Carol A. Schwartz. (Eds.). (1994). *Encyclopedia of Associations* (Vol. 1). Detroit, MI: Gale Research, Inc.

Davidson, Dick. (1994). Moving forward to shape the debate. *Hospitals and Health Networks* (February 20), 8.

Doctors under the knife. (1993). *Newsweek* (April 5), 28–40.

The doctors vs. the nurses. (1993). *U.S. News and World Report* (December 20), 12.

Donovan, Beth. (1994a). Betting big on public backing, Clinton stands firm on veto. *Congressional Quarterly Weekly Report* (June 25), 1703–1706.

Donovan, Beth. (1994b). Leaders to forge new bill from committee efforts. *Congressional Quarterly Weekly Report* (July 2), 1792–1798.

Donovan, Beth, and *Congressional Quarterly* staff. (1992). Partisanship, purse strings hobbled the 102nd. *Congressional Quarterly Weekly Report* (October 31), 3476.

Federal Election Commission. (1989–90). *Committee summary reports (K Index).* Washington, D.C.

Federal Election Commission. (1991–92). *Committee summary reports (K Index).* Washington, D.C.

Federal Election Commission. (1993–94). *Committee summary reports (K Index).* Washington, D.C.

Federation of American Health Systems. (1992). *Forging partnerships for health care reform: Annual report.* Washington, D.C.: Federation of American Health Systems.

Fraley, Colette. (1995a). GOP scores on Medicare, but foes aren't done. *Congressional Quarterly Weekly Report* (November 18), 3535–3538.

Fraley, Colette. (1995b). Using vouchers for Medicare may help GOP cut costs. *Congressional Quarterly Weekly Report* (July 22), 2189–2190.

Fraley, Colette, and Andrew Taylor. (1995). House Republicans poised for Medicare showdown. *Congressional Quarterly Weekly Report* (October 14), 3142–3146.

Freeman, Jo. (1988). Women at the 1988 Democratic Convention. *Political Science and Politics, 21*, 875–881.

Fuchs, Beth C., and John F. Hoadley. (1987). Reflections from inside the Beltway: How Congress and the president grapple with health policy. *Political Science and Politics, 20*, 212–220.

Gaunt, Jeremy, with Andra H. Armstrong. (1987). Senate freshmen rewarded by post-election PAC giving. *Congressional Quarterly Weekly Report* (September 5), 2134–2136.

Goldwater, Marilyn, and Mary Jane Lloyd Zusy. (1990). *Prescription for nurses: Effective political action.* St. Louis: C. V. Mosby Company.

Gottlieb, Martin. (1995). Plan would give doctors new ways to make money. *New York Times* (October 31), A1, A16.

Hayes, Michael T. (1981). *Lobbyists and legislators.* New Brunswick, NJ: Rutgers University Press.

Health. (1986). *Congressional Quarterly Weekly Report* (October 25), 2661–2662.

Health. (1987). *Congressional Quarterly Weekly Report* (December 26), 3223–3225.

Health care overhaul. (1994). *Congressional Quarterly Weekly Report* (November 5), 3178–3179.

Hill, Bette S., & Katherine A. Hinckley. (1995). American Hospital Association; American Medical Association; American Nurses Association; Federation of American Health Systems. In Craig Ramsay (Ed.), *U.S. health policy groups: Institutional profiles* (pp. 79–84, 95–101, 109–115, 212–215). Westport, CT: Greenwood Press.

Hilts, Philip J. (1993). Doctors softening stand on changes in health system. *New York Times* (March 4), A1, A10.

Hinckley, Katherine A., and Bette S. Hill. (1990). *A new American Medical Association? Adaptive interest group behavior in the 1980s.* Paper presented at the annual meeting of the Southern Political Science Association, Atlanta, GA, November.

Hinckley, Katherine A., & Bette S. Hill. (1992). Biting the bullet? Post-1980 congressional processes and Medicare decisions. In Miriam K. Mills & Robert H. Blank (Eds.), *Health insurance and public policy: Risk, allocation, and equity* (pp. 25–49). Westport, CT: Greenwood Press.

Hinckley, Katherine A., & Bette S. Hill. (1995). Organizational character and interest group strategies. *National Political Science Review, 5*, 57–74.

Holleran, Constance. (1978). Nursing unity—political power. *Washington State Journal of Nursing, 50*, 18–21.

Hook, Janet. (1986). Medicare budget facing "Triple Jeopardy." *Congressional Quarterly Weekly Report* (January 18), 115–120.

Hook, Janet. (1987). More deep cuts in Medicare approved by Ways and Means. *Congressional Quarterly Weekly Report* (August 1), 1721–1722.

Hook, Janet. (1988). 100th Congress wraps up surprisingly busy year. *Congressional Quarterly Weekly Report* (October 29), 3130.

Hook, Janet. (1989). New leaders felt their way gingerly through session. *Congressional Quarterly Weekly Report* (December 2), 3302.

Hook, Janet. (1990). 101st Congress leaves behind plenty of laws, criticism. *Congressional Quarterly Weekly Report* (November 3), 3700–3701.

Hook, Janet. (1993). Democrats hail "productivity," but image problems remain. *Congressional Quarterly Weekly Report* (December 11), 3388–3389.

Hula, Kevin. (1995). Rounding up the usual suspects: Forging interest group coalitions in Washington. In Allan J. Cigler & Burdett A. Loomis (Eds.), *Interest group politics* (4th ed., pp. 239–258). Washington, D.C.: Congressional Quarterly.

Inglehart, John K. (1987). Health policy report: Problems facing the nursing profession. *New England Journal of Medicine, 317* (September 3), 646–651.

Kernell, Samuel. (1986). *Going public: New strategies of presidential leadership.* Washington, D.C.: Congressional Quarterly.

Kingdon, John W. (1984). *Agendas, alternatives, and public policies.* Boston: Little, Brown.

Kuntz, Phil. (1993). Special interest groups mobilize, prepare for show of force. *Congressional Quarterly Weekly Report* (February 20), 382–383.

Loomis, Burdett A., & Allan J. Cigler. (1995). Introduction: The changing nature of interest group politics. In Allan J. Cigler & Burdett A. Loomis (Eds.), *Interest group politics* (4th ed., pp. 1–31). Washington, D.C.: Congressional Quarterly.

MacPherson, Peter. (1992). Controversial watchdog steps down. *Washington Post* (June 30), 7.

Morehouse, Macon. (1988). Risk-notification measure derailed by GOP filibuster. *Congressional Quarterly Weekly Report* (April 2), 842.

1993 Budget Reconciliation Act. (1993). *Congressional Quarterly Weekly Report* (September 18), 2482–2497.

Nurses gain new policy clout as the fight to reform health care begins; ANA sees a "mandate" for change. (1993). *American Journal of Nursing, 93* (February), 83, 86.

Nurses help reshape Clinton's evolving plan for reform. (1993). *American Journal of Nursing, 93* (November), 85, 89.

Palmer, Elizabeth A. (1992). Revision of ERISA supports states' rights on contracts. *Congressional Quarterly Weekly Report* (June 13), 1706–1707.

Pear, Robert. (1986). The medical lobbies: Differing opinions. *New York Times* (August 19), A24.

Pear, Robert. (1995). Doctors part company with GOP on Medicaid. *Akron Beacon Journal* (December 5), A1.

Peterson, Mark A. (1992). The presidency and organized interests: White House patterns of interest group liaison. *American Journal of Political Science, 86*, 612–625.

Pika, Joseph A. (1991). Opening doors for kindred souls: The White House office of public liaison. In Allan J. Cigler & Burdett A. Loomis (Eds.), *Interest group politics* (3rd ed., pp. 277–298). Washington, D.C.: Congressional Quarterly.

Pressman, Steven. (1984). Physicians' lobbying machine showing signs of wear. *Congressional Quarterly Weekly Report* (January 7), 15–19.

Ramsay, Craig. (Ed.). (1995). *U.S. health policy groups: Institutional profiles*. Westport, CT: Greenwood Press.

Rauch, Jonathan. (1994). *Demisclerosis*. New York: Times Books.

Rhein, Reginald W., Jr. (1978). Health lobbyists: Clout in the corridors of power. *Medical World News, 19* (June 12), 65–81.

RNs aim to mend gaps in Clinton plan; AMA attacks advanced practice roles. (1994). *American Journal of Nursing, 94* (January), 83, 88–89.

Rovner, Julie. (1986a). Anti-smoking forces stoke legislative fires. *Congressional Quarterly Weekly Report* (December 13), 3049–3054.

Rovner, Julie. (1986b). Lawmakers moving to address Medicare quality concerns. *Congressional Quarterly Weekly Report* (April 26), 938–939.

Rovner, Julie. (1987a). House panel completes work on catastrophic-insurance bill. *Congressional Quarterly Weekly Report* (June 27), 1380–1381.

Rovner, Julie. (1987b). Senate Labor OKs family-planning legislation. *Congressional Quarterly Weekly Report* (November 14), 2821–2822.

Rovner, Julie. (1987c). Waxman, Kennedy offer bills ensuring privacy of AIDS tests. *Congressional Quarterly Weekly Report* (August 1), 1744.

Rovner, Julie. (1988a). AIDS-testing bill OK'd, minus anti-bias clause. *Congressional Quarterly Weekly Report* (June 25), 1732–1734.

Rovner, Julie. (1988b). House passes bill setting federal AIDS policy. *Congressional Quarterly Weekly Report* (September 24), 2652–2653.

Rovner, Julie. (1988c). New family-planning rules draw lawsuits. *Congressional Quarterly Weekly Report* (February 6), 269.

Rovner, Julie. (1988d). Panel seeks stiffer review of medical devices. *Congressional Quarterly Weekly Report* (May 21), 1403.

Rovner, Julie. (1988e). "Pepper Bill" pits politics against process. *Congressional Quarterly Weekly Report* (June 4), 1491–1493.

Rovner, Julie. (1989a). AMA, other groups target physician-fee proposal. *Congressional Quarterly Weekly Report* (March 25), 654.

Rovner, Julie. (1989b). Coalition seeks to overcome rural health-care woes. *Congressional Quarterly Weekly Report* (April 1), 695–697.

Rovner, Julie. (1989c). Doctor bills are next target for cost-control efforts. *Congressional Quarterly Weekly Report* (February 25), 386–393.

Rovner, Julie. (1989d). House panel votes increases for WIC, other programs. *Congressional Quarterly Weekly Report* (June 24), 1551.

Rovner, Julie. (1989e). Kennedy, Waxman introduce insurance-for-all proposal. *Congressional Quarterly Weekly Report* (April 15), 826–827.

Rovner, Julie. (1989f). Medicare's physician fees revised by house panel. *Congressional Quarterly Weekly Report* (June 17), 1470–1472.

Rovner, Julie. (1989g). Members may target referrals to doctor-owned facilities. *Congressional Quarterly Weekly Report* (March 4), 458–460.

Rovner, Julie. (1989h). Physician-fee schedule urged for the Medicare program. *Congressional Quarterly Weekly Report* (March 18), 588–589.

Rovner, Julie. (1989i). Ways and Means OKs overhaul of Medicare payment plan. *Congressional Quarterly Weekly Report* (July 1), 1626–1628.

Rovner, Julie. (1990). Proposed cuts in Medicare provoke outcry on Hill. *Congressional Quarterly Weekly Report* (October 6), 3217–3222.

Rovner, Julie. (1991a). Bush plan for doctors' fees is criticized as wrong Rx. *Congressional Quarterly Weekly Report* (August 10), 2256–2257.

Rovner, Julie. (1991b). Congress feels the pressure of health-care squeeze. *Congressional Quarterly Weekly Report* (February 16), 414–421.

Rovner, Julie. (1991c). Growing health-care debate widens partisan divisions. *Congressional Quarterly Weekly Report* (November 16), 3377–3382.

Rovner, Julie. (1991d). House passes LHHS measure; Abortion foes bank on veto. *Congressional Quarterly Weekly Report* (June 29), 1766–1767.

Rovner, Julie. (1991e). White House, on defensive, highlights its agenda. *Congressional Quarterly Weekly Report* (May 18), 1285.

Rovner, Julie, and staff. (1988). Bush, Congress face some familiar problems. *Congressional Quarterly Weekly Report* (December 24), 3560–3575.

Rubin, Alissa J. (1993a). Budget war casts shadow on overhaul plans. *Congressional Quarterly Weekly Report* (August 14), 2225–2227.

Rubin, Alissa J. (1993b). Special interests stampede to be heard on overhaul. *Congressional Quarterly Weekly Report* (May 1), 1081–1084.

Rubin, Alissa J. (1994). Cost containment next hurdle as overhaul moves to floor. *Congressional Quarterly Weekly Report* (July 23), 1043–2045.

Rubin, Alissa J. (1995). Spadework on Medicare pays off for GOP. *Congressional Quarterly Weekly Report* (September 23), 2895–2897.

Rubin, Alissa, J., & Ceci Connolly. (1993). Clinton delivers health bill, all 1,342 pages of it. *Congressional Quarterly Weekly Report* (October 30), 2968–2969.

Rubin, Alissa J., & Beth Donovan (1994). Clinton uses his "veto pen" to draw line in debate. *Congressional Quarterly Weekly Report* (January 29), 174–175.

Rudavsky, Shari. (1992). AMA urges questioning on abuse. *New York Times* (June 17), A1, A21.

Salant, Jonathan D., & David S. Cloud. (1995). To the '94 election victors go the fundraising spoils. *Congressional Quarterly Weekly Report* (April 15), 1055–1059.

Salisbury, Robert H., John P. Heinz, Edward O. Laumann, & Robert L. Nelson. (1987). Who works with whom? Interest group alliances and opposition. *American Political Science Review, 81*, 1217–1234.

Scharfstein, Joshua M., & Steven S. Scharfstein. (1994). Campaign contributions from the American Medical Political Action Committee to members of Congress: For or against the public health? *New England Journal of Medicine, 330* (January 6), 32–37.

Schlozman, Kay Lehman, & John T. Tierney. (1986). *Organized interests and American democracy.* New York: Harper & Row.

Sinclair, Barbara Deckard. (1989). *The transformation of the U.S. Senate.* Baltimore, MD: Johns Hopkins University Press.

Smith, Steven S. (1989). *Call to order: Floor politics in the House and Senate.* Washington, D.C.: The Brookings Institution.

Sorauf, Frank J. (1988). *Money in American elections.* Glenview, IL: Scott, Foresman.

Symons, Joanne L. (1984). Political education—political action. *Nursing Administration Quarterly, 8* (Summer), 2–36.

Taylor, Andrew. (1995). Interest groups take sides. *Congressional Quarterly Weekly Report* (October 14), 3144.

Thompson, Carolyn R. (1995). Health Insurance Association of America (HIAA). In C. Ramsay (Ed.), *U.S. health policy groups:*
Institutional profiles (pp. 230–233). Westport, CT: Greenwood Press.

Top givers. (1993). *Congressional Quarterly Weekly Report* (July 31), 2051.

Truman, David B. (1951). *The governmental process.* New York: Alfred A. Knopf.

Two years . . . and counting. (1993). *Hospitals and Health Networks* (August 5), 56–60.

Walker, Jack L., Jr. (1991). *Mobilizing interest groups in America: Patrons, professionals and social movements.* Ann Arbor: University of Michigan Press.

Watson, Tom. (1987). Business PACs wary of campaign finance bill. *Congressional Quarterly Weekly Report* (April 25), 782–784.

Weekly compilation of presidential documents. (1994). *30* (May 16), 1044–1050.

West, Darrell M., & Diane J. Heith (1994). *Harry and Louise go to Washington: Political advertising and health care reform.* Paper presented at the annual meeting of the American Political Science Association, New York City, September.

West, Phil. (1992). Doctors OK AMA plan for health reform. *Akron Beacon Journal* (December 9), A3.

Wilson, James Q. (1973). *Political organizations.* New York: Basic Books.

Witt, Elder. (1986a). Array of death penalty issues awaits resolution by Court. *Congressional Quarterly Weekly Report* (January 4), 28–29.

Witt, Elder. (1986b). Court renews abortion rights, strikes "baby doe" regulations. *Congressional Quarterly Weekly Report* (June 14), 1334–1336.

Witt, Elder. (1986c). "Creation-science" debate tops December arguments. *Congressional Quarterly Weekly Report* (November 29), 2992–2995.

Zaldivar, R. A. (1994). Critics say Clinton's error is overplaying his hand. *Akron Beacon Journal* (September 28), A2.

Zeigler, Harmon. (1964). *Interest groups in American society.* Englewood Cliffs, NJ: Prentice-Hall.

Zuckerman, Edward. (1994). *Almanac of federal PACs, 1994–95.* Arlington, VA: Amward Publications.

PART FOUR

HEALTH POLICY AND THE POLITICAL PROCESS

This section is explicitly devoted to health policy. Its primary mode of analysis, however, is not the comparison of costs and benefits, which lies at the core of much of policy analysis. Instead, it examines health policy from a political perspective.

An example should help make clear the benefits of a political perspective. Sole reliance on cost–benefit analysis would suggest that the poor would most benefit from programs like Medicaid that are particularly targeted to them. Under these programs the poor receive all of the program's benefits. Conversely, universalistic programs like Medicare, which cover all older people whether rich or poor, seem to "waste" money if measured by the criterion of the percentage of a program's expenditures that goes to the poor.

Yet advocates for the poor are often among the most ardent backers of universalistic programs. The reason is that universalistic programs are usually much more effective for political reasons. Medicare, for example, by benefiting all the elderly is supported by all the elderly (and those who prefer becoming elderly to the alternative), not just the poor elderly who are not likely to have much political clout. Moreover, service providers are much more likely to treat their clients with dignity and the clients are much more likely to demand respect when the program is given to what is perceived as a "deserving" population (Medicare) rather than an "undeserving" one (Medicaid).

While all the chapters in this section approach their subjects from a political perspective, it is important to reiterate the point made in the Preface to this volume that it would be a mistake to assume that all health policies have the same type of politics. Thus, no attempt has been made to impress upon the authors a single theoretical frame of reference (e.g., public choice theory, systems theory, group theory, etc.).

What might prove useful, however, is to distinguish between those chapters that deal with the medical care system as a whole and those that focus on specialized topics within it. The chapters on health finance by Evans, access by Fraser, and national health insurance by Marmor deal with the politics of the health system as a whole. Conversely, the chapters on mental health by Rochefort, disability by Albrecht, environmental health (only a subset of environmental issues) by Rabe, rural health by Mueller, and AIDS by Robins and Backstrom involve a more narrowly focused health politics. (While the chapter on health and the elderly by Brandon is a specialized one, its significance within the medical care system is of such magnitude that it is more properly grouped with the chapters dealing with the system as a whole.)

At first glance it appears that the macro-issues of cost containment and access are both more interesting and important than the various micro-topics covered in this section. But health professionals (or health professors, for that matter) rarely have the direct power or ability to influence medical care costs and have not been able to bring about national health insurance. In their capacities as health care providers, environmental public health workers, and AIDS case managers, however, they are much more likely to have some influence in their areas of expertise. Yet without a good understanding of the health system as a whole, their efforts are likely to prove counterproductive. The generalist reader is, therefore, urged to also give attention to the specialty chapters and the specialist reader to the chapters dealing with the system as a whole.

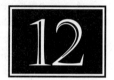

CHAPTER 12

Sharing the Burden, Containing the Cost: Fundamental Conflicts in Health Care Finance

Robert G. Evans

THE UNIVERSALITY OF COLLECTIVE FINANCE

In all developed societies, the financing of health care is a collective process. Pools of funds, described by White (1995) as "shared savings," are assembled through more or less compulsory levies on the general population, within or outside the formal tax system. These funds are then transferred to the providers of care through institutional structures and processes that vary considerably from one country to another. But in no developed society does direct payment by the user of services account for more than a small fraction of the total cost of health care.

Care is not, of course, "free"; the residents of each country must bear, one way or another, the cost of that country's health care system. But the amount that each must contribute is largely unrelated to his or her own personal use. The political struggles over who pays, and who gets what, are played out through the collective funding processes specific to each country.

The results determine how much care is provided, of what types, and for whom. But they also determine who must pay—how the costs will be distributed over the population—as well as who will be paid, and how much, for providing care. This distribution of economic benefits and burdens, through the political process, is at least as contentious as the process of health care provision itself.

One might expect the United States, with its emphasis on "private" funding, to be an exception to this generalization. But it is not. Direct payments by users of care made up (in 1993) just under 18 percent of total health spending in the United States (Levit et al., 1994). The rest flowed through collective channels. One would have to go back to the end of the 1950s to find a time when out-of-pocket payment accounted for as much as half of the total; the collective share has been stable or rising for decades.[1]

The assembly of these collective funds, however, is to a considerable extent carried out by private institutions. A substantial majority of Americans (64% in 1992) report that they rely primarily on private insurance against health care costs, more than three times those (20.6%) relying on public plans.[2] But the proportion of *costs* covered by private insurance is much less, about one-third. This is because private insurers try to avoid offering coverage to people in poor health or otherwise at high risk, and place a variety of limitations on the coverage they do offer. Any shortfalls must be paid out of pocket by beneficiaries, or shifted to the public sector.

The public sector accounts for about 44 percent (in 1993) of health care financing in the United States (Levit et al., 1994). This is still a remarkably low proportion, well below that in other developed countries. The average public share in the other countries of the Organization for Economic Cooperation and Development (OECD) is about three-quarters, with the lowest outside the United States being in the neighborhood of

two-thirds (Organization for Economic Cooperation and Development, 1994, Table 4.2).[3]

But the U.S. government also provides a large public subsidy for private health insurance, in the form of a tax expenditure for coverage bought by employers.[4] This subsidy was estimated at $75 billion in fiscal 1994, or roughly 8 percent of total health care expenditure. If it were recorded on the federal government's books as an expenditure, the public share of total health care costs would be over 50 percent.[5]

What is perhaps remarkable, then, is the predominant role that private insurers play both in Americans' (and others') perceptions of their health care system and in the formulation of health care policy, despite raising a relatively small share of the money. This role sharply distinguishes the United States from all other developed countries—at least in the OECD statistics. What does it mean in reality?

What it does *not* mean is that "private" insurance coverage in the United States is a commodity bought over the counter by individual consumers, along with boxes of breakfast cereal or cans of beans. Although it is often treated as a private consumption purchase in national statistics, and particularly in economic analyses, this is in fact nonsense. The public subsidy to employment-based insurance, plus the problems of information flow in insurance markets, the well-known process of "adverse selection" (Fein, 1986), result in a minimal market for individual private coverage.[6] Health insurance comes with the job—and goes with it.

---

[1]Remarkably, however, out-of-pocket payments *as a share of GDP* have changed very little: 2.48 percent of GDP in 1993, down from 2.60 percent in 1960, and the ratio has fluctuated within a very narrow band. Meanwhile, the share covered through collective mechanisms has more than quadrupled, from 2.7 percent to 11.5 percent of GDP.

[2]The remaining 15.4 percent were uninsured. Here and elsewhere we draw on a very useful assemblage by White (1995) of recent data on the U.S. financing system from a number of public and private sources.

[3]Organization for Economic Cooperation and Development (OECD): Europe, Canada, the United States, Japan, Australia, and New Zealand. The one exception within the organization is Turkey, with about the same public-sector share as in the United States, and about half of health care costs paid out of pocket (Organization for Economic Cooperation and Development, 1994, Table 21.6).

[4]The premiums are deductible from the employer's taxable income, but not taxed as income in the hands of the employee. This public subsidy provides the greatest benefits to people in the highest tax brackets; those with no taxable income receive no support from the general taxpayer. This "reverse Robin Hood," or "Sheriff of Nottingham," feature no doubt accounts for its political resilience.

[5]It is not obvious whether private health insurance could survive in the United States without this "life support" from the public Treasury.

[6]There is a market for individual coverage, but in these contracts only about one dollar in two is actually paid out in benefits. Marketing expenses eat up

Private health insurance is not only collectively purchased and heavily subsidized; it is also subject to considerable public regulation. In these respects it is similar to the social insurance systems in several European countries. There are, however, critical differences between private health insurance in the United States and the various insurance organizations in each of the countries conforming to what White (1995) calls the "international standard." These latter have public roles and responsibilities that are quite foreign to American experience.

First, private insurers bear no collective responsibility for the population as a whole. About 15 percent of Americans have no coverage, and an even larger number may have grossly inadequate coverage. In other developed countries the public requirement of universal, comprehensive coverage implies that all residents must have adequate coverage from *some* agency. Insurers collectively cannot simply wash their hands of a substantial part of the population as "not our problem." But for-profit firms, competing in private markets, cannot take on such public functions, and the United States is correspondingly unique in the incompleteness of its coverage.

Second, private insurance premiums are explicitly risk-based. People at higher risk pay more. If the resulting premiums are beyond their means, they must "go bare," or try to find some form of public assistance specific to their circumstances. Social insurance premiums, by contrast, are largely or wholly unrelated to risk status. Moreover, they typically bear some relation to wage or income level. Thus wealthier people pay a larger share of total health care costs, and sicker people pay less, than under private health insurance.

On the other hand, the premiums levied in social insurance systems are themselves less closely related to income than are the taxes in tax-financed systems. The latter thus distribute the overall burden of health care

costs still more closely in accordance with ability to pay. But regardless of how, and from whom, the "shared savings" are raised, public systems do not impose higher costs on individuals with higher risk of illness.[7] Private insurance does.

Third, private insurers cannot be involved in the management of the health care system itself.[8] In other countries, control of the payment process is a critical lever whereby governments try to influence the evolution of system capacity, costs, and coverage. Payments may come directly from governments, as in Canada, the United Kingdom, or Sweden, or flow through a large (Germany, Switzerland) or small (France, Belgium) number of health insurers that are nonprofit and closely regulated. Such organizations occupy a middle ground between the strictly "private" (for-profit, commercial) and strictly "public" (line civil service) sectors. They are being subjected to increasing public regulation and accountability, largely in response to cost pressures. But a large and fluctuating group of private insurers, competing in a private marketplace, cannot be coordinated to manage the system as a whole.

The impossibility of global system management in the United States lies behind the increasing divergence between expenditure patterns in the United States and the rest of the OECD. Figure 12.1 shows comparative data, from the OECD Health Data File, on health expenditures relative to gross domestic product, from 1960 to 1993. The (unweighted) average of this ratio

---

much of the rest, since bad products take a lot of selling. Only about 14 percent of people covered primarily by private insurance—7.3 percent of the population—had individual contracts in 1992. There is, of course, an active individual market for "medigap" insurance to cover the holes in the public Medicare program for the elderly, but this is a low-risk product precisely because it is only supplementary.

[7]All generalizations are false. Individuals at higher risk do not make larger contributions. But in employment-based systems, of which Germany is a leading example, people (and their employers) do contribute a larger or smaller proportion of their earnings for coverage, depending upon the overall income and health status of the membership of the sickness fund to which they belong. Within each fund, however, the contribution percentage is the same for all, so higher-income people pay more, and sicker people do not.

But the range of variation among funds is limited by law, and there is enforced cross-subsidization. A portion of the contributions of members of "healthier" funds is transferred to "sicker" funds to reduce the burden on their membership. In particular, retired members are supported from a separate pool, drawn from the contributions of working members of all sickness funds. Such cross-subsidization is found in all systems of social insurance built up from separate funds.

[8]They may become heavily involved, through setting criteria for reimbursement, in the standards of care for individual patients. But the implications, if any, for system-wide behavior are far from clear.

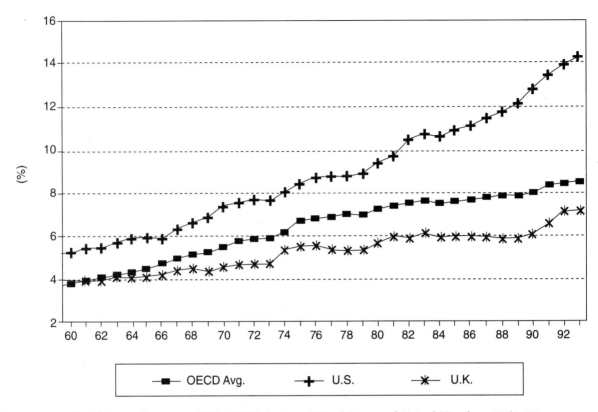

Figure 12-1 Health Expenditure over GDP, OECD Average, United States and United Kingdom, 1960–93

SOURCES: OECD Health Data File, 1995.

(for countries with continuous data available) is bracketed by the United States on the high side, and the United Kingdom on the low. (Canada is included because of its similarity in other respects to the United States.)

From 1960 until the mid-1970s, the OECD average ratio rises in parallel with that of the United States; from then on it flattens out and moves more or less parallel to the United Kingdom. The United States diverges from the OECD more and more on the high side. It was during the mid- to late 1970s that governments in most European countries became concerned over the rate of escalation of health costs, and began developing mechanisms to control them (Abel-Smith, 1992; Abel-Smith & Mossialos, 1994). Such concerns were being expressed in the United States as early as

1970, but they could not be translated into effective policy.

Thus the U.S. health care system is the "odd man out," as Abel-Smith (1985) pointed out ten years ago. White (1995) reaches the same conclusion, referring to an "international standard" in health care finance from which the United States alone deviates.

The United States, like every other developed country, raises by far the bulk of the revenue for health care through collective institutions. Moreover, although the role of private funding is much greater in the United States than in other developed countries, private insurance (after accounting for the public tax expenditure subsidy) only raises about half as much money as the public sector. Yet this mix of financial sources has been sufficient to prevent the United States from developing public mechanisms for management and control similar to those that were worked out throughout the OECD during the 1970s, and have been progressively refined since.

The result has been a health care system that is, relative to White's "international standard," inequitable, inefficient, unpopular, and spectacularly expensive—but enormously profitable for *some* Americans. The latter feature is, of course, the key to its survival.

PLANES OF CLEAVAGE

The collective financing of health care services is marked by a number of planes of cleavage or conflicts of interest among key participants. These include the following.

Providers versus Payers

The revenues raised to pay for health care, whether through taxes, private insurance premiums, or out-of-pocket payments, make up one component of a fundamental three-part accounting identity that must always hold, by definition, over all systems of health care finance. The total revenues raised to pay for health care in any society must be equal to the expenditures on health care, and each in turn must exactly equal the total incomes earned from its provision:[9]

TOTAL REVENUE ≡ TOTAL EXPENDITURE ≡ TOTAL INCOME

These can then be factored as

$$T + R + C \equiv P \times Q \equiv W \times Z$$

where T or taxes represents revenue raised through the public sector, R represents private insurance premiums,

and C is direct charges to patients. Total expenditures, in turn, are the product of the quantities of health care services provided, Q, and their average prices, P, while total incomes earned can be factored into average rates of pay, W, and the total volumes of "factor inputs" used—person-hours, for example, or capital services—which we label Z.

The incomes earned from health care may be salaries or net incomes from professional practice; they also include interest on hospital bonds or dividends from private pharmaceutical or equipment companies. They are earned by doctors and nurses, dentists and pharmacists, but also by employees of firms selling health insurance or providing management consulting services to hospitals or ministries of health. The channels through which funds flow may be multiple and complex, but at the end of the day every dollar that someone has paid out must have been received by someone else. And if the goods or services which that dollar of expenditure bought were defined (albeit somewhat arbitrarily) as health care, then the corresponding dollar of income was by the same definition earned by providing health care. And someone, somehow, had to contribute an equal amount of revenue to pay for it.

This elementary accounting fact underlies the primary political conflict in every health care system, that between the payers for care and the providers of care.[10] There are also secondary conflicts on each side of this divide, among providers and among payers. But the most prominent division follows the income–expenditure distinction.

This political struggle is most evident in the universal discussions, even lamentations, over "cost containment." In political rhetoric, "cost explosions" in health care are commonly presented as if they were some elemental force of nature, like tides or earthquakes, against

[9]Strictly speaking, in an open economy the identity must be extended to account for external purchasers and suppliers of health care—exports and imports. It would also require an explicit intertemporal structure to allow for changes in asset levels. But these additional complications are well known from national income accounting, and add no further enlightenment to compensate for the extra notation.

[10]Not "buyers" and "sellers." The dominance of collective funding, combined with professional self-regulation and external public regulation, and rooted ultimately in the obvious fact that most users of health care are not able to define their own needs without professional help, implies that the images of the "free market," with voluntary exchange of goods/services for money, between fully informed, self-interested, autonomous, and unconstrained transactors, exist only in the dreamworld of neoclassical economic theory.

which all those concerned with health policy struggle as best they can. This image, assiduously promoted by providers—and some economists—is false (Evans, 1985, 1986). The real dynamic at work was expressed succinctly by Aaron Wildavsky (1977) as the Law of Medical Money: "costs will increase to the level of available funds. . . . That level must be limited to keep costs down."

Those who *pay* for care are to a greater or lesser degree concerned to limit the escalation of costs. Those who *are paid* for care, however, are engaged in discouraging or avoiding such controls, and in trying to keep the costs rising. For the sake of political credibility they may wish to be seen to share in the general hand-wringing about the relentless pressure of health care costs. But in actual fact, many if not most providers of health care believe that the adoption of appropriate priorities would lead to *more* spending, not less—at least on those services in which they have a professional interest. This in turn would necessarily increase the total of incomes earned from health care, making a larger total pie to share. When $P \times Q$ rises, so does $W \times Z$—that is what an identity means. Successful cost containment, on the other hand, means that someone in the system takes a wage or fee cut (W falls), or loses a job (Z falls).

Meeting Needs or Marketing Services— How Much Care Is Enough?

In making their case to the rest of society for more resources, and resisting pressures for cost containment, those who are paid for providing care focus primarily on the quantity of services. No matter what the current level of provision, there are always alleged to be unmet needs, and more money is needed to meet them. Furthermore these needs are constantly being increased by external forces of one sort or another, such as the aging of the population, the progress of technology, public expectations, AIDS, or violence.

Specific "explanations" of increased need may in fact be refuted empirically, sometimes quite conclusively. But they continue to be asserted, because they are in reality not offered as a testable account of causality, but as a form of product advertising. They are the classic

"Your money or your life!" argument; if enough resources are not forthcoming people will die, or at least suffer, unnecessarily. We *must* "meet the needs."

Such an argument is probably as old as medicine itself. At the individual level, it is the standard method whereby the therapist exerts power over the patient—which may well be in the patient's best interest. "Doctor's orders" are most effective when combined with an explanation of the beneficial results of compliance—and the ill effects of noncompliance. The relationship has a fundamental political dimension—"orders" are the exercise of power backed up by the perception of superior knowledge, and thus the ability to make credible, if not always specific, threats: "do this, or else." Again one must emphasize that, in the individual clinical encounter, both the language and the intent may be entirely benevolent.

But since in developed societies the financing of health care is collectivized, providers must influence the controllers of those collective funds and induce them to spend more, on more different types of services. Political pressure is therefore brought to bear by convincing the relevant constituency (voters, employees, or premium payers) of the adverse consequences of refusal. "Heartless" bureaucrats, politicians, employers, even economists, are placing dollars above people's lives. Such claims, supported by human-interest anecdotes, are politically very powerful, and also sell newspapers.

Of course, as Williams (1978) has pointed out, if there is no natural limit to the scope of medicine, and if there is always some small benefit that might be gained, through sufficiently large expense, then logically it is impossible for any society to "meet all the needs" in a technical sense. Needs are infinite. It is then fundamentally a political question as to which needs—and whose—are "worth" meeting. Technical expertise may be necessary to determine what the payoffs to further expenditure in a particular situation might be, but the expert is no more qualified than any other citizen to state whether the benefits are worth paying for. In a democratic society everyone gets one vote.[11]

---

[11]Some might wonder why the question of "What is worth paying for?" is treated as political rather than economic. For many commodities we appeal

Providers accordingly seek to persuade their fellow citizens that the benefits of further expenditures are large (i.e., more "medical miracles"). But they emphasize especially the catastrophic consequences, in health and human happiness, of any (successful) attempt to restrain the escalation of costs. In other fields of endeavor this activity would be recognized immediately as marketing.

In the United States in particular, the technique has been refined into the specter of "rationing." Ever-advancing technology is portrayed as constantly enhancing the ability to extend life and maintain function, but at ever greater cost. Sooner or later, it is argued, we shall be forced to "ration"—deny people access to effective services, let them suffer or die—for sheer lack of the necessary resources (the "Painful Prescription" of Aaron & Schwartz, 1984). But in the meantime, and to postpone the evil day—send more money![12]

But unnecessary or harmful services add to costs—and generate employment and incomes—without yielding any corresponding health payoff. Health care is, after all, valued not for itself but for its anticipated (positive) impact on health. Absent this payoff, most health care services are "bads," not "goods." Furthermore, effective or ineffective care may be provided at different levels of technical efficiency. One country may spend more, not because it is getting more health benefits or even more health care, but simply because its in-stitutions for providing care are less efficient and more wasteful of human and physical resources.

Those who argue the inevitability of rationing must necessarily assume away the existence, on any significant scale, of either inefficient or ineffective care—and they do. They thus slide smoothly past a large and steadily growing body of contrary evidence—in effect ignoring what they cannot refute. But if the "rationing" story in health care is, at its core, not an intellectual investigation but rather part of a propaganda campaign to try to secure more resources and incomes for the health care sector, there is no reason to expect its advocates to take account of contrary evidence.

The specter of "rationing" may possibly become reality at some time in the indefinite future. But it is not now, and may never be, in any of the wealthier industrialized countries. There is, at present, no direct linkage between levels of expenditure on health care and the achievement of health outcomes in any health care system in the industrialized world (Mackenbach, 1991).[13] We are all a long way from the grim trade-off of "Your money or your life."

Less for Some, More for Others: The Oregon Experience

The highly publicized efforts by the legislature of the state of Oregon to establish explicit rationing criteria for Medicaid services, and to deny funding for certain life-prolonging but very expensive procedures, illustrate precisely what is really at issue in the "rationing" debate. In the first place, these efforts were not motivated by resource constraints in Oregon, much less in the U.S. system as a whole. Rather, they expressed the unwillingness of the better-off majority of the population to contribute more to the care of people in the lowest-income groups. What was "rationed" was willingness to pay—for others.

---

to the principle of consumer sovereignty, and rely on individuals to indicate, in the marketplace, what commodities each of them believes is worth paying for. The choice process is decentralized. But the decision to leave that process to the free market—where among other things people's preferences are weighted by their wealth, not by their needs—is itself a political choice. For a variety of reasons, no country in the world has seen fit to do this for health care. In the United States, however, the very strong ideological commitment to free markets as ends in themselves is in continuous tension with powerful humanitarian values. These make citizens very uncomfortable with the results inevitably generated by markets in health care. The result has been a form of schizophrenia in health policy, and a lurching back and forth from one approach to another.

[12]It may seem strange that we have grouped those who call for ever more money to "meet the needs" with those who argue that ultimately there will not *be* more money, because ever-growing demands will run into fundamental resource constraints. The critical linkage is that both assume that "more is better," and dismiss or simply ignore extensive evidence to the contrary. Thus in the near term, the "rationing" rhetoric serves to promote the further expansion of health care.

[13]Maynard (1981, p. 145) puts the point bluntly: "It is foolish to believe that increases in health care inputs and throughputs lead to increases in health status outcomes." But it is not at all foolish to try to persuade others to this belief, if one can thereby enhance the willingness to pay for one's own services and avoid awkward questions.

Second, such explicit rationing for a particular sub-group can coexist with overfunding and overprovision for other segments of the population—and apparently did in Oregon. Fisher et al. (1992) demonstrated that if discretionary hospital admissions in high-use areas could be brought down to the levels found in other parts of the state, enough money could be saved that there would be no need to ration Medicaid services. Apparently inappropriate—unnecessary—hospital use by the general population was being left untouched, while specific services were being denied, "rationed," for those dependent on Medicaid.[14]

The assumption that all care currently being provided is effective, and that any reductions must represent a threat to health, is not taken seriously by any student of health services in any country, least of all in the United States. But the specter of "rationing" plays the very important political role of diverting public attention from the question of whether the services now being provided are effective and appropriate. Instead, we are led back into the familiar bog: "How else will we meet the needs? We *must* have more money!"

Paying for More Care, or Just Paying Higher Prices?

But a moment's reflection should also remind us that more money does not necessarily buy more services, effective or otherwise. It may simply support higher prices. This point emerges very clearly from an analysis of OECD data by Gerdtham and Jönsson (1991b), in which they were able to isolate the effects of differences in the *relative* prices of health care services, from one country to another, on international comparisons of total health care costs.

Gerdtham and Jönsson began with a very common calculation, converting health care expenditures *per capita* in each of the OECD countries from domestic currency into U.S. dollars. Typically this is done using purchasing power parities (PPPs) rather than exchange rates.[15] When PPPs are based on comparisons of the relative prices of all the commodities in the GDP, one finds very large differences between *per capita* spending in the United States and in all other countries. Americans spend about 50 percent more than the next two most expensive countries, Canada and Switzerland, 75 percent more than France and Germany, and more than twice as much as any of the rest.

But if one converts other countries' currency into U.S. dollars using PPPs specific to the health care sector, Gerdtham and Jönsson found that much of this differential disappeared. In this alternative comparison, Canada spent as much *per capita* as the United States, Japan spent almost as much, and Sweden spent substantially more. Every country in the OECD moves up relative to the United States—some by a small amount and others by a great deal.

This finding implies that a large part of the differential is due to higher *relative prices* of health care in the United States, not to higher levels of services.[16] Americans receive, on average, no more care than Canadians, very little more than Japanese, and much less than Swedes. But they pay much more, relatively, for what they get. In terms of the identity above, P (price) is higher in the United States than anywhere else.

Other studies support this inference. Schieber et al. (1994) also show significantly higher rates of relative inflation of health sector prices in the United States than in other OECD countries. Several comparisons of the Canadian and American health care systems have shown rates of service use that are on average very similar, with Canadians receiving more of some forms of

---

[14]Note the parallel of interests between the "expansionists" and the "rationers." When rationing was attempted in Oregon, it was applied to the politically and economically weakest in the population, without raising any awkward questions about how effectively the health care system itself was functioning. Since, by assumption, that system is already both efficient and effective, what point would there be to such questions? And since we cannot do everything for everybody, we are with deep regret and much soul-searching forced to do less for *you*. Meanwhile the health care system as a whole expands along its merry way.

[15]These are less volatile than exchange rates, not being sensitive to short-term capital movements. They attempt to compare the relative costs of similar baskets of commodities in each country.

[16]The point is not that prices for health care goods and services are higher in the United States than elsewhere. They are; but what Figure 12-2 (p. 279) reflects is that the ratio of health care prices to the general price level is higher in the United States than in other countries.

care and less of others (Fuchs & Hahn, 1990; Nair et al., 1992; Redelmeier & Fuchs, 1993).

Why should care be so much more expensive in the United States? Apologists for the status quo either avoid the question entirely, or try to argue that the quantity comparisons are invalid. Americans pay more because they get higher "quality." But this alleged higher quality is not reflected in better outcomes, or better population health status, or even greater public satisfaction. So what is it?

Apologists trained in economics may then shift into theological arguments that reduce in essence to such comments as: "The quality *must* be higher, or else rational patients making informed choices in free markets would not have paid for it. Objective data are irrelevant; it is my *theory* that is decisive." Those whose religious faith is weaker refer instead to the excellence of the care received and the outcomes achieved by *some* Americans—and nobody can deny that these are indeed excellent. But systems must be judged on their total performance, bad as well as good, and it is hard to find any justification for higher prices in the United States.

Bargaining over Incomes— How Much Are Providers Worth?

High prices have two possible sources: high incomes or low efficiency. Gerdtham and Jönsson's data show the powerful effect of these factors taken together, but do not disentangle them.

Taking the first point first, much of health policy is taken up with, in Reinhardt's (1987) phrase, "the allocation of life-styles to providers." How much shall providers earn, relative to the rest of the community, or more generally how shall this be decided? Although this is obviously a critical factor in determining the costs of health care, it is not one that health care providers typically wish to discuss explicitly—at least not the highest-earning ones. They would rather talk about unmet needs and the escalating costs of providing quality care.

In a competitive marketplace, relative incomes are determined by "demand and supply" and are not amenable to political bargaining. In the real world of health care, however, the boundaries set by market forces tend to be broad and indistinct, and to leave a wide band of discretion. International comparisons of physicians' incomes, for example, show that their skills and long education periods lead to correspondingly high incomes everywhere, just as "demand and supply" would predict. But the *size* of their income advantage relative to the rest of the community is highly variable, both from country to country and over time within countries. It is relatively low in the Nordic countries, and particularly high in the United States. Physicians were in the past very well off in both Germany and Canada, but have lost some ground (in Germany quite a lot) relative to the general income level (Organization for Economic Cooperation and Development, 1987, p. 76; Gerdtham & Jönsson, 1991a; Groenewegen et al., 1991; Fein, 1992).

Much less attention has been given to international comparisons of incomes for other classes of health care personnel. Redelmeier and Fuchs (1993), however, found that overall the average rates of income of hospital workers were very similar in Canada and the United States—about 4 percent higher in the United States. But the wages of more highly skilled workers—head and general duty nurses—were about 20 percent higher in the United States, while wages of housekeepers and aides were about 20 percent lower. This may well reflect the greater role of unions in Canadian hospitals; if so, European countries may show patterns more similar to that in Canada.

The point for our purposes, however, is simply to emphasize the variability in worker incomes in the health care sector, across countries and over time, relative to the rest of the community. They are not dictated by "the market"; institutional environments matter. Accordingly, efforts by payers to control rates of pay—wages, salaries, fees, and prices—in the face of counterpressures from providers make up a large part of the process of cost containment in national health care systems. The political dimension of this process of bargaining over provider incomes is quite overt, in negotiations over the level of fees or salaries that will be paid by public or quasi-public insurers, and over the opportunities that physicians in particular will or will not have to increase their incomes by charging patients directly.

The process of bargaining over provider incomes varies with the structure of the delivery system in each country. In a number of countries physicians may be independent practitioners who are paid by fees for service. In Canada this is true of both generalists and specialists. In several of the European countries specialists may be hospital-based and on salary.[17] Most other health workers are salaried employees of hospitals or clinics that are themselves typically funded through some form of budgetary process. As a general observation, however, bargaining tends to evolve from specific items to more comprehensive budgets.

One may begin by negotiating fees with physicians. But payers rapidly discover that, depending upon the rules for payment, the total volume of billings per physician can be quite elastic. Hillman et al. (1990), for instance, found that for patients with clinically equivalent problems physicians who owned their own diagnostic radiology facilities took on average four times as many films, and charged 40 percent more, for a total cost over six times higher, than physicians who referred to arm's-length radiologists. Such observations rather undercut the claim that the volume of services provided is simply a response to patient needs—or, for that matter, demands. Which items are in the fee schedule (does it cover all diagnostic tests, for example?) and who can be reimbursed for particular services (all practitioners, or only selected ones?) may be as important for the evolution of total costs as the actual level of fees.

The same problem emerges for pharmaceuticals, where again prescriptions are typically reimbursed on an item of service basis. The price of any given drug may be stable or falling over time, but the constant introduction of "new" drugs, real or apparent, keeps increasing both the number of prescriptions per capita and the average price per prescription.

Thus, the attempt to control provider incomes leads payers through increasing restrictions on service volumes, toward some form of global budget within which the negotiation of prices for individual items of service may continue. Physicians—and drug companies—respond by trying to open up or expand access to the private funds of patients. A number of OECD countries are employing the currently fashionable rhetoric of the marketplace. But that rhetoric—privatization, competition, efficiency, and so on—is simply window dressing behind which providers are still following Wildavsky's law. They are trying to keep their health care systems expanding, in the face of relatively successful cost control in the public sector, by seeking other sources of funds to absorb.

In terms of the balancing identity, they are trying to expand the revenue side by increasing direct charges (C) and then private insurance (R) to compensate for the restrictions on public funding through various forms of taxes (T). This would then permit continuing increases in either or both of average prices (P) and volumes of services (Q), and correspondingly increased provider incomes. Demands for extra billing, and for expanded private "markets" more generally, in all public systems of health care finance, are thus quite understandable attempts to subvert cost *containment*, which threatens provider incomes, and replace it with cost *shifting*, which does not.

In the past five years the U.S. Medicare system has moved quite rapidly through the common stages of fee negotiation, establishing a resource-based relative value scale (fee schedule), and introducing measures both to encourage "assignment" (discourage extra billing) and to discourage multiplication of services (volume performance standards).[18]

But the principal difficulty is that Medicare operates alongside a private insurance system that has no such controls and much less potential for introducing them. This alternative, uncontrolled "market"—which is in reality quite unlike any "normal" market—weakens the bargaining power of the public program. Accordingly one finds that although Medicare pays markedly lower

---

[17]But if salaried practitioners are also permitted to engage in some level of private fee practice, the level of effort (not) devoted to the salaried service and the steering of patients become continuing problems that seem beyond the reach of negotiation or monitoring.

[18]There has always been a fee schedule for services paid for by Medicaid, but this is generally viewed as "welfare medicine," outside the American mainstream. Not all practitioners accept Medicaid patients, because the fees are considerably lower than those of Medicare, let alone private insurance.

fees than private insurers, it still pays very high fees by international standards. Thus the preservation of private insurance has been of vital importance to physicians in maintaining their fees and incomes, even though it pays only one-third of total health care costs.[19]

In contrast, physician incomes, and where relevant, fees, have been more or less restrained—though often with bruising political struggles—in most of the other countries of the OECD. More detailed comparisons with Canada have shown quite clearly that the centralization of bargaining over physicians' fees resulted in a slowing in the escalation both of fees and of overall outlays on physicians' services (Barer et al., 1988; Evans, 1986). This slowing is observed relative to both previous patterns in Canada, prior to the establishment of the public universal insurance plans, and contemporaneous experience in the United States. The private insurance sector in the United States has thus played precisely the "safety valve" role that Canadian physicians have identified for it in Canada—a way of protecting their incomes in the public plan and thus resisting cost containment.

"Interfering in the Practice of Medicine"

As noted above, health care—or anything else—can be expensive either because the people who produce it are paid a lot or because they are not very productive. High levels of W (rates of payment), or of Z/Q (inputs per unit of output), are both reflected in higher prices (P). The latter we may call technical inefficiency—more resources than necessary used up in production. Such inefficiency can show up either in the provision of health care per se, or in the operation of the payment system. This section focuses on health care; the organization of the payment process will be considered later.

Traditionally the payers for care, whether public or private, have avoided "interfering in the practice of medicine." They have not enquired into the details of servicing patterns, or how or why providers made their diagnostic and therapeutic decisions. Political and administrative negotiations or conflicts have focused on financial issues—fees, salaries, and budgets.

Payers in virtually every country have also tried to exert some control over the total capacity in the health care system, particularly hospital and major equipment capacity. There is general understanding that utilization of health care is predominantly capacity-driven, heavily influenced by the availability of facilities and personnel, independent of the "needs" (however defined) of the populations served.

Capacity control contributes to, but is not sufficient for, overall cost control, as American health planners have learned. Culyer (1988) argues that Canada and the European countries have been more successful because they have also placed global restraints on total financing rather than relying only on controls of "demand," "supply," or capacity.

Such global controls leave the maximum scope for provider autonomy within the overall physical and financial limits. The process of determining those limits, however, becomes rather arbitrary. Providers can always allege that the limits are too tight, and that serious needs are going unmet (people on the waiting lists dying). Payers counter with the rhetoric of cost explosions (more than the country can afford). The general public, in its various roles as actual or potential patient, taxpayer, or voter, is unlikely to find the facts of the case significantly clarified by either side.

For a number of years, however, researchers have been observing that there are large and unexplained variations between patterns of practice and servicing rates, between countries, between regions in the same country, or between practitioners, which seem to bear no identifiable relation to the needs of the populations served (Bunker, 1970; Vayda, 1973; McPherson et al., 1982; Roos et al., 1986; Chassin et al., 1986; Ham,

---

[19]Private insurers, rather than trying to develop negotiated fee systems paralleling that of Medicare, seem still to be putting their faith in "managed care" systems (White, 1995). This might seem irrational, given the unrelieved record of failure of managed care, over twenty-five years, to make any impression on the system-level problems of American health care. On the other hand, the payment systems in place in other countries have only two roles for private insurance: much reduced or none. Managed care offers a continuing, and indeed much expanded, role for insurers as system managers. Against this enormous advantage, the fact that it does not work—or at least never has yet—is a trivial objection.

1988). These variations show up in the fine structure of care—in particular procedures, not just aggregate utilization rates.[20]

At the same time, a considerable proportion of diagnostic and therapeutic interventions are carried out in the absence of any scientific evidence that they actually benefit patients, and in a nontrivial number of cases have been shown to do actual harm. A still more important problem, quantitatively, are those interventions that *have* been shown to benefit certain patients with particular conditions, but are offered to a much wider range of patients for whom no such evidence is available (Banta et al., 1981; Feeny et al., 1986).

Such observations have for a long time indicated that there was considerable potential for containing or reducing health care costs, with no harm or even benefit to patients. Realization of this potential depends, however, on improving the management of the health care system. More specifically, the system must be managed explicitly to achieve health outcomes, and to identify and eliminate ineffective and wasteful practices and procedures, rather than just to sustain traditional practices plus whatever other new ideas attract the attention of clinicians (Wennberg, 1984, 1988).[21] But only in the past decade has this realization begun to emerge in serious political debate (*The Economist*, 1988; Roper et al., 1988; Andersen & Mooney, 1989).

The principal reason for virtually universal political reluctance to tackle this issue is that such management directly challenges the professional prerogatives of providers. Practitioners have always insisted that the "best" medicine was practiced by trained and experienced clinicians relying on their own clinical judgment. The threat of accountability to others, who may draw on statistical and experimental evidence in evaluating and even directing their performance, strikes directly at professional autonomy. It is likely to excite even more severe political counterattacks than attempts at economic control, and may elicit substantially less support among the general public.

"Cost control" and fee/income bargaining seem to be viewed by the public, in most countries, as legitimate roles for payers. But it is not clear whether there is sufficient political support for more detailed intrusion into the way care is provided. Even if there is widespread and very solid evidence that a great deal of inappropriate and unnecessary care is being provided, members of the general public are not familiar with that evidence. As users of that care, they believe their needs are being met.

Thus it is probably not accidental that it is in the United States that the political debate has most clearly turned to the evidence of specific inefficiencies in the provision of health care and the need for detailed utilization review (Roper et al., 1988). Other countries have managed to contain their overall costs at an acceptable level, without taking on the political dangers inherent in appearing to attack professional autonomy. But the United States has thus far completely failed to achieve such control, while simultaneously failing to provide adequate coverage for its population. There appears to be widespread agreement among the American population that major reform is called for (Blendon, 1989), but as President Clinton discovered, no agreement at all on what form it should take.

Desperate times call for desperate measures. In these circumstances the United States has developed a high degree of sophistication in the technical aspects of health care management. The rapid spread of payer-enforced "guidelines" for patient treatment—de facto constraints—in the private sector amounts to precisely the direct "rationing" that Americans have been led to fear from state-financed systems. The ironic result has been that, in successfully fighting off "socialized medicine," American physicians now find themselves confronted with far more intrusion from payers than would be imaginable in any other country. And American patients

---

[20]The distinction between inefficient production and ineffective care becomes fuzzy here. If a stay in hospital is unnecessarily prolonged, is this the inefficient production of an episode of care, or the production of ineffective hospital days? At the most aggregated level, all ineffective care represents the inefficient production of health.

[21]Such evidence provides further reasons to reject the allegation that cost containment at present levels must lead to "rationing" of effective care. "Rationing" of *ineffective* care may well occur, but that is a solution, not a problem.

find their choice of provider increasingly restricted, again in a way unlike any other national system.

This is not to say that providers are not restricted in other countries. Budgets are never large enough; there is never enough equipment, sufficiently up to date, or enough support staff, to do all the things physicians would like to do—especially if they are paid fees for their services. Canadian physicians feel particularly put upon, as they compare themselves with their colleagues in the United States. But nowhere else do payers require physicians to justify and seek approval for their proposed care plans for individual patients, in order to ensure reimbursement. Payer-imposed guidelines constitute precisely the "cookbook medicine" that clinicians regard as unprofessional and dangerous for patients.

It is, of course, conceivable that if the guidelines are both valid and flexible, the care of patients could actually be improved. When there are wide variations in patterns of practice, it seems highly unlikely that *all* represent best practice—that "everything is optimal in its own way." But the private agencies now developing and enforcing guidelines are trying to limit their own outlays, not reform the practice of medicine. What they want are defensibly cheaper patterns of care; there is no reason why these should necessarily be better for patients.

It may be that the vigilance—and economic and professional interests—of providers, combined with the natural emotional bias against those who "sacrifice lives for dollars," will provide sufficient checks on the stinginess of payers to prevent patients from being put at risk. But there is no guarantee of this. There may be a real need for "political entrepreneurship" to design institutions and assemble coalitions capable of offsetting payer interests, as the balance of power swings in their direction.

In any case, there is as yet no indication that the rationing of care by private payers has had any impact on the global problems of the American health care system—uncontrolled costs, incomplete and inequitable coverage, and public dissatisfaction. There have been large changes in patterns of care, including major declines in the use of inpatient hospital care, in the past decade. But any savings appear to have been absorbed by increased costs of management.

How Do We Split the Bill?

Foreign experience indicates that these global problems can only be successfully addressed by coordinating the behavior of payers while making them politically accountable. Most other OECD countries have passed this stage, and have either a unitary payment system, or tight regulation and coordination of multiple payment agencies.

That unity or coordination, however, is not a once-for-all achievement. It must be maintained in the face of continuing pressures from providers who recognize very clearly the connection between "sole source funding" and overall cost control—and who reject both. In the debates over privatization in Canada and Western Europe, providers have always been quite explicit in their attempts to expand the flow of resources to allegedly "underfunded" health care systems by diversifying the sources of funding (Weller & Manga, 1983).

The assembly or maintenance of payer coalitions is made difficult not only by the efforts of providers, but also by the natural conflicts of interest among payers for and users of services. However a society determines the share of its economic resources to be given to the providers of care, it must still allocate that burden among its various members. At the same time, the terms and conditions of access to the health care goods and services provided, that is, "Who gets what, when and how," will also depend on the structural and administrative framework.

As noted above, in a tax-financed system the distribution of economic burden is related to ability to pay, with the closeness of the relationship depending on the overall tax structure. Taxes on income tend to be somewhat progressive, taking a larger share of income from those with higher incomes. Payroll taxes or "social insurance" premiums result in a more regressive distribution of burden, since they tend to take a higher proportion of lower incomes, and to exempt income from nonlabor sources. But in either case an individual's share of total health care costs does not depend on his or her health status.[22]

Private insurance systems, by contrast, set premiums on the basis of expected losses, as indicated by past experience. People with chronic illnesses, or elderly people, will carry a larger share of health expenditures, in the form of significantly higher premiums for coverage. Competition among insurers dictates this result; a company that tried to cover all comers at the same premium ("community rating") would find that it attracted all the worst risks.[23] Direct charges to patients distribute costs according to actual illness/care experience, rather than prior expectation of expense.

Which pattern of distribution is "fairer" is a political value judgment. As an empirical matter there does appear to be a broad consensus that people should contribute to the cost of health care in proportion to their ability to pay, and should receive care according to their needs (van Doorslaer et al., 1993).

Since illness and income are negatively correlated, a truly private financing system would assign the largest share of cost to those with the least resources. But it is manifestly impossible to finance a modern health care system solely on the basis of such a distribution. The unhealthy and unwealthy would simply not get care at all. The use of health care is highly concentrated on a small proportion of the population, who are predominantly elderly or chronically ill. Berk and Monheit (1992) found that among the noninstitutionalized U.S. population in 1987, the highest-using one percent accounted for 30 percent of all health expenditures, while the top 10 percent accounted for 72 percent of costs. The lowest-using half of the population, on the other hand, accounted for only 3 percent.

Hence the universal predominance of public payment, even in the United States. Unless a new political consensus emerges that would simply exclude a significant proportion of the population from access to health care—let 'em die—it is hard to see how that predominance could be challenged. On the other hand, the fact that at any one point in time a majority of the population is very little touched by health care costs means that most people would not immediately be hurt by a reduction in public funding. Some would be hurt a great deal, but they are a minority.

Maintenance of the political consensus for public payment thus depends on a combination of a sense of solidarity with the less fortunate, and a prudential realization that most of us will become old, if we are not already, and many of us, or those close to us, will develop chronic illnesses. Only the very well-off can be confident that they will never need some form of collective support, and that they can afford top priority in a private system. For them, shrinking the public sector is a rational agenda.

In most countries, individual contributions to collective financing are simply detached from health status. The United States, however, provides public programs for those with the greatest needs and least resources (Medicare and Medicaid), and public subsidies (through income tax exemptions) for the private insurance system. The resulting distribution of burden is shown in Figure 12-2. In total, health expenditures in the United States take a much smaller share of income from the highest-income groups than from the lowest, even though higher-income people contribute a substantially larger amount per capita.[24] The key observation, however, is that private insurance and self-payment have very similar distributions of burden—highly regressive—while tax-financed health spending is mildly progressive.

This observation frames the debate, in every country, over direct charges or private insurance. Shifting costs from public to private budgets implies shifting them down the income distribution, and conversely.

---

[22]Of course, total financial outlays are only one component of cost. Being ill or injured is a significant burden in itself; it may also result in loss of income or other additions to living expenses. The direct burden is inevitably borne by the patient; other economic losses are partially compensated at best.

[23]The nonprofit "Blue" plans in the United States began in the 1930s by community rating, with exactly this result. Competition from for-profit sector forced a shift to experience rating, or charging different premiums to different groups on the basis of estimated risk (Fein, 1986).

[24]Families in the top 5 percent of the income distribution contributed $13,234 to health care in 1987, but this was only 10.2 percent of their incomes, while the $960 contributed by families in the lowest decile was 26.9 percent of their much smaller incomes. Taxation to support health care funded through the public sector accounted for most of the difference in

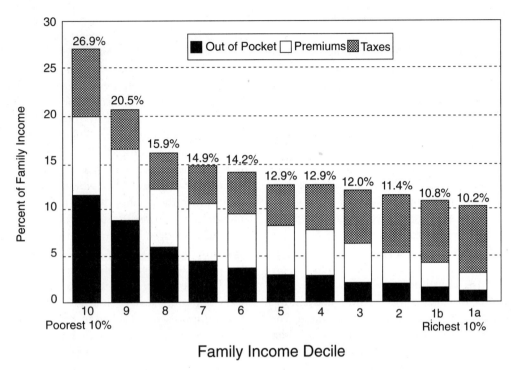

Figure 12-2 Family Expenditures for Health Care, 1987, by Family Income Decile

SOURCE: Rasell et al., n.d. [1993]. Used by permission of the Economic Policy Institute.

How the shared savings are assembled determines, to a considerable extent, how much each of us has to contribute. Thus the current debates over the relative mix of public and private financing, in every country, are to a large extent about how to shift the cost of care onto someone else.

But these struggles divert attention from the primary questions of how much to spend, and on what. It is as if a group of diners at a restaurant, greatly disturbed at the size of the bill and very suspicious about its contents, nevertheless spent all their energy debating who was to pay what share, rather than calling in the manager to demand an accounting for the overall cost.

Needless to say, the restaurant manager would prefer that the guests argue among themselves, rather than presenting him with a united front. The simplest summary explanation for the failure of cost control in the United States is that the institutional framework of health finance makes it easy and natural for the payers to try to pass the costs on to someone else, and very difficult for them to confront providers directly.

The intellectual framework provided by the rhetoric of the marketplace also tends to focus attention on the distribution among payers. The American economic literature perpetuates endless discussion of "deterrent charges" and the almost universal conviction that cost escalation results from low or zero "prices" to "consumers" at point of service, in spite of the obvious counterexamples in the rest of the world. Thus efforts by employers to shift the burden of health care costs to their workers—an understandable but unhelpful response to unchecked escalation—are applauded as

---

dollar amounts. The top 5 percent contributed $9,650 in taxes or 7.3 percent of their incomes; the bottom 10 percent were taxed only $214 per family or 6.8 percent of income. But their average payment of $746 for insurance and direct charges was 20.2 percent of income, compared with the 3 percent ($3,584) paid out by the 5 percent of families at the top (Rasell et al., 1993, Table 1).

"welfare-improving" despite their obvious lack of effect on overall costs (Manning et al., 1987).[25]

Tax-financed systems, in which the principle of universal coverage has long been accepted, are less vulnerable to these diversions. They do, however, show increasing conflict over access to care. If the community as payer controls outlays by limiting its overall "willingness to pay," there will remain individuals who, perhaps encouraged by their physicians, want more. Or they may want care on more favorable terms (e.g., shorter waiting lists, more convenient bookings, nicer surroundings). Pressure from unsatisfied users generates cleavages of two kinds, between users and payers and among users themselves.

The split between users and payers is quite straightforward. As noted above, payers are ultimately responsible to some user constituency, whether it be voters, premium payers, or workers. (In the final analysis, in a democratic society, they are always responsible to voters.) If the relevant constituency comes to believe that payers' efforts to limit cost escalation are threatening their own health, the controls will fail.

A delicate balance must thus be maintained between the voter-as-payer and the voter-as-patient. Much of the political activity by both payers and providers is intended to elicit from voters the identification favorable to their cause. People who think of themselves as actual or potential patients are likely to support increased health care spending; people who think of themselves as taxpayers or premium payers are more likely to support efforts to control costs.

But the more contentious question concerns the treatment of those who want more services, even though there is a well-established political consensus for restraint. Should they be able to pay for more, separately from the collective system?

The affirmative argument is usually presented as an alleged "natural" right to spend one's own resources as one sees fit, spiced with anecdotes of patients dying for lack of care. But the issue is, in reality, more complicated. Very few people are really willing or able to cover the full costs of medical care for serious illness out of their own pockets. Rather, those who are relatively healthy and wealthy are more likely to favor "moderate" deterrent charges, co-payments, which enable them to purchase better access by screening out some of those with lower incomes. They would like the right to buy their way to the front of the queue by a small extra payment, but not to pay the full price of additional services.

And providers, of course, would like the power to enhance their incomes by charging additional amounts for preferential treatment, as has been the practice in the U.K. for years. Very few providers, if any, imagine that they could survive in a system where more than a small minority of users had to pay the full cost of their own care. But a "multiclass" system not only enables providers to charge extra for preferred access to care that is predominantly collectively financed; it also permits them to "whipsaw" payers and undermine global restraints. A perception that those who pay extra are getting therapeutically superior care, that is, better outcomes, not just better amenities, will in a democratic society eventually lead to "more" for everybody.

All such discussion sidesteps the more fundamental issue of whether the services currently provided are medically necessary or efficiently produced. As noted, there is substantial evidence that the short answer is "No," and that even the health care systems of Canada and Western Europe are in fact overfunded. In these circumstances, further expenditures, whether individual or collective, would seem ill-advised, to say the least.[26]

But the specter of "rationing," the threat that some will be denied "needed" services, is a very potent mechanism for undermining the unity of users. The least sick,

---

[25]There is also a very strong ideological component to the conflict among payers and users (Weller and Manga, 1983). Since illness is inversely correlated with social class, whether measured by income, education, or looser measures of status, the detachment of economic burden from either actual or expected illness results in a corresponding redistribution of income from higher to lower levels in the social hierarchy. To some this egalitarian effect is offensive per se, even if it is associated with a lower overall burden.

[26]Rachlis and Kushner (1989) have written a comprehensive and very accessible survey of that evidence for the Canadian system. The Western European systems show a similar pattern (Maynard, 1981; Enthoven, 1985; Culyer et al., 1988). Yet Canada and the major European nations spend between 8 percent and 10 percent of their national income on health care, while the United States spends about 14 percent.

and most well-off, whether as voters or as patients, may be persuaded that they might fare better in a fragmented financing system with a greater element of user-pay.

And indeed some of them would. A shift from public to private funding definitely *will* move money, on average, from the less to the more wealthy as well as from the less to the more healthy—that is the message of Figure 12-2. The losers will be those, whether poor or moderately well-off, who have the misfortune to become seriously ill. Thus, providers who seek to fragment the sources of funding, and to increase the overall flow of funds by drawing in more private money, have natural allies in those toward the top of the income distribution. The unique American outcome of uncontrolled overall costs and a highly regressive distribution of burden—plus much better access for the wealthy and unhealthy—reflects the success of this political coalition.

How Many Spoons in the Dish?

The fragmentation of financing systems, under various justifications, is accordingly a common objective of providers the world over. They look for greater ability to negotiate increased resources from the rest of society, and to protect their own autonomy from external accountability. From a professional perspective, a multiplicity of funders with deep pockets and few questions represents the ideal environment both for doing good and for doing well. But can such conditions last? Again, the U.S. experience is critical, though the results are by no means all in yet, and may not be for years. Certain generalizations, however, seem secure.

First, economic success brings competitors. Large and rapidly growing pies attract others who would like to share. The normal reaction of a competitive marketplace to a "growth industry" is that new suppliers offer the same or better products at lower prices. The customer benefits from improved quality and falling costs—consider the case of personal computers, for example. But health care is not and never has been a competitive marketplace. The growth of the total revenues of the industry—health expenditures and incomes—has indeed drawn in new sharers, but the process and the re-

sults have been quite different from the predictions of hypothetical models of the competitive marketplace.

The first form of potential competition, starting in the 1960s, came from substitute personnel—nurse practitioners, midwives, dental therapists, chiropractors, denturists, and the like. In some cases these practitioners could offer the same or better services at lower cost; in others, the question of quality and servicing patterns was more open. But extensive research (Record, 1981; Spitzer, 1984) has left no room for doubt that, technically, such persons could significantly reduce the costs of health care services by substituting for the services of the peak professionals, physicians and dentists.

Unfortunately they would in the process also reduce the income streams of such personnel—the expenditure–income identity again. Accordingly, during the 1970s, professionals in all countries, including the "highly competitive" United States, used their political control of the self-regulatory process to suppress the development and deployment of their potential competitors. New forms of practitioners *did* emerge, but only under the economic control of the established professions. A potentially significant form of interprovider conflict was thus strangled at birth. The victory of the peak professionals was swift and complete (Spitzer, 1984).

Learning from this experience, alternative practitioners have in subsequent years tried to present themselves as complementary to rather than substitutes for the established professions. They offer new and different product lines, thus trying to add to the total flow of income and costs, rather than competing for a share of the existing flow. But it is obvious to payers that adding still more income claimants—increasing the factor inputs (Z) in the balancing identity—is unlikely to mitigate cost pressures.

Lawyers, on the other hand, have in the United States been relatively successful in appropriating a share of the gross revenues of the health care system, through malpractice litigation.[27] In terms of the overall identity,

---

[27]The lawyer's fees are paid from the plaintiff's award, which is paid by the malpractice insurer, who in turn collects a share of the physician's gross receipts as malpractice premiums. The physician passes on this cost in higher

the prices (*P*) of health services are increased to cover the costs of legal services—both plaintiffs and defendants—used up in association with health care delivery and paid for from health budgets. Lawyers have inserted themselves among the *Z*, raising the *Z*/*Q* ratio.

Physicians are particularly bitter about this incursion, and commonly attribute rising health care costs to the pressures placed on them by the tort system.[28] The direct costs of the tort system, however, as reflected in malpractice premiums, are far too small a part of overall health care costs to provide any explanation for their escalation. Lurid anecdotes about particular specialties, regions, or individual practitioners grossly misrepresent the overall picture.

Faced with such data, clinicians emphasize the addition to servicing made necessary by "defensive medicine," a cost allegedly several times greater than malpractice premiums themselves. Such an argument implicitly concedes that a considerable proportion of servicing is "medically unnecessary," but shifts the blame from clinicians to lawyers. The solution to inappropriate care and escalating costs is tort reform!

But do those who make this argument really believe that in the absence of the malpractice threat, rates of servicing—and costs—would fall sharply? How, then, would provider incomes be maintained, if they were *not* providing, and being paid for, the additional services that make up "defensive medicine"? In reality, the lawyers provide a justification for the increase in servicing, even as they skim off a (relatively small) share of the gross revenue and subject physicians to the miseries of litigation. Blaming the lawyers is simply another diversionary tactic to shift attention away from providers themselves.

The really serious challenge to clinicians, however, has arisen from management. By the end of the 1980s,

payment administrators and system managers had in the United States become established as the most potent new competitors for a share of health budgets (Lee & Etheredge, 1989). They will be difficult for providers to dislodge, because they have successfully integrated their services with the delivery of health care. Their relationship is not competition, but a complex combination of symbiosis and parasitism.

The fragmented funding system that prevents the containment of overall expenditures also costs a great deal to administer. The difference between premium or tax payments *to* insurance agencies, public or private, and claims or benefits paid *by* such agencies, is an overhead cost of the payment system. It is the cost of pushing paper rather than of providing services. Some such cost is unavoidable; complex institutions are not self-administering. But these costs in the United States are much larger than anywhere else for which data are available, and add literally tens of billions of dollars to American health care costs. Moreover, they have risen dramatically over the past three decades.

Corresponding to these costs of the insurance and prepayment process are large and increasing administrative costs within care institutions—hospitals and physicians' offices—made necessary by the process of complying with an increasingly complex payment system. These internal costs, which appear to be part of the cost of providing care but again are simply "paper pushing," add further tens of billions to expense without corresponding benefit to patients (Himmelstein & Woolhandler, 1986).

By the early 1990s, estimates of the extra costs generated by the private insurance system, in both payment agencies and provider institutions, relative to the corresponding costs in a unitary, universal payment system, was in the neighborhood of $100 billion, or about 15 percent of total U.S. health care costs (Woolhandler & Himmelstein, 1991). This monumental inefficiency of the payment process goes far to explain the relatively high prices of health care in the United States noted by Gerdtham and Jönsson.

No other country incurs administrative costs on this scale, to support what Reinhardt (1988) has identified as a huge private bureaucracy. Yet the simplified payment systems of other countries also permit direct

---

fees, or increased rates of servicing, to the patient or the patient's insurer. The latter, government or employer, passes on the cost to taxpayers or customers. At no point is there an agency with the authority or the incentive to control the process.

[28]Hence the bumper sticker: "Support a lawyer; send your child to medical school." Defenders of the tort system argue that the increase in legal inputs "buys" an improvement in the quality of output, keeping doctors on their toes in a way that regulation—especially self-regulation—never could. But this argument appears to be largely a prioristic, presented by interested parties operating in a data-free environment.

negotiations between providers and payers, and resulting overall control of expenditures.

The insurance bureaucracy was built up in the course of increasingly sophisticated efforts to shift costs from one payer to another. Relatively limited efforts were made by private payers to influence the costs of care themselves, and none at all to manage system-wide costs. The American payment system was a gigantic game of "Old Maid." But in the past decade, and particularly in the past five years, payers have become much more aggressive in trying to influence the patterns of care provided to their own beneficiaries.

Again, however, they have been unwilling or unable to combine and act at the system level. So far, the result seems to be the addition of yet another managerial layer that has absorbed any savings that may have been achieved in costs of clinical services.[29]

In terms of our restaurant analogy, the embattled diners have each called in their own accountants and lawyers to help them minimize their share of the bill. The total cost of the meal is predictably escalating even more rapidly, and the restaurant is now quite noisy and crowded. The manager is becoming somewhat nervous. These new participants are disturbing the smooth functioning of the restaurant—and they do not order anything to eat! Furthermore, they are taking a share of his customers' money, threatening to reduce the amount available to pay his bill.

American providers are caught in a dilemma. The financing system that by its diversity and complexity has protected them from external financial control is absorbing a larger and larger share of health system incomes just to keep it running. And, to add insult to injury, pressures from payers are leading to greatly increased attempts to influence the practice patterns of individual physicians. Physicians' autonomy is under threat from the payment system itself. Their former allies are becoming increasingly expensive, and are becoming ever more aggressive in grabbing the levers of power (Webber & Goldbeck, 1984; Roper et al., 1988;

Lee & Etheredge, 1989). Machiavelli would have appreciated the irony of the situation.

CONFLICT MANAGEMENT? OR, *SAUVE QUI PEUT?*[30]

The planes of cleavage described above are universal. The management of these fundamental conflicts of interest—particularly that between payers and providers—makes up a large part of the politics of health care finance in all developed countries. In no system can the conflict be avoided, but how it is managed makes a great deal of difference both to the balance of gains and losses and to the amount of "collateral damage" generated in the process.

Most countries have created collective institutions for negotiating between payers and providers. In the United States, however, the conflict remains largely decentralized even though the financing is collective. The results appear to be more advantageous to providers. Individual American physicians refusing to accept Medicaid patients are "withdrawing services" to drive up fees, just as are French physicians striking for a higher fee schedule. But the latter incur much higher costs and mobilize much more opposition, while the former can appeal to the rhetoric of the market to justify their pressure tactics. In any case American fees are much higher.

Similarly, the decentralization of the shared saving process, and its embedding in the institutions and rhetoric of "insurance," supports a pattern of distribution of the burden of health care costs that is much more favorable to those with higher incomes. It seems highly unlikely that any explicit political process for distribution would result in the pattern of generosity toward providers and regressivity of contributions, observed in the United States; certainly none has.

Quite apart from the distributional outcomes, however, different processes of conflict management may be more or less costly to operate, in both financial and nonfinancial terms. The extent of "collateral damage" provides an additional basis for comparison.

The most striking features of the American health care system are: (1) its costs are high, and escalating

---

[29]Nor is the United States unique in this regard. The National Health Service in Great Britain has greatly increased the role of professional managers, and the same complaints are emerging that a new layer of bureaucracy is simply transferring resources from health care to overhead.

[30]"Everyman for Himself."

quickly, compared with all other national systems; and (2) an extraordinarily large proportion of those costs are taken up with administrative overhead, bureaucratic waste motion. Driven by the first, and drawing on the second, administrative intrusion into clinical practice is creating a more and more restrictive, adversarial, and financially threatening environment for individual practitioners and patients.

These features, as argued above, are direct consequences of the failure to develop collective processes for managing fundamental conflicts of interest. They are the price paid for the distributional benefits—relative to other national systems— enjoyed by providers and upper-income payers/users in the American system. Needless to say, the beneficiaries find that price acceptable.

If this interpretation is correct, the really interesting political questions have to do with what happens when the escalation process ends. The recent experience with health care reform in the United States shows that opposition to White's "international standard" of collective institutions of management is still overwhelming. But the various proposals for new and better decentralized institutions—under the labels of managed care and competition—have yet to show any sign of success.

So what next? Continuing cost escalation, which has already gone on far longer than anyone twenty years ago would have imagined possible? Faith rewarded, as managed care systems finally begin to deliver on the ancient promise of market-based efficiency, effectiveness, and cost control? A sudden U-turn toward the single payer or closely coordinated multiple payers as in other national systems?

Or are Americans now willing to accept a radical reduction in the extent of collective finance, as right-wing economists have long advocated? Has the political climate finally changed to the point that one can simply throw people overboard and watch them drown? Less dramatically, will those who become sick or injured have to bear, in the future, a much higher level of economic loss as well—or simply do without?

The public sector in the United States funds a much lower proportion of total health care costs than in other developed countries, but it still covers about half. It follows that there is still a good deal of opportunity for

shifting costs from taxpayers to the sick by shrinking public programs and increasing the amount of private financing. Since people are taxed (roughly) in proportion to their incomes, and use health care (roughly) in proportion to their illness, this *would transfer money from the less to the more healthy and wealthy.* The less healthy and wealthy would have to pay a larger share of health care costs, or simply not get care at all.

The failure of the latest effort at health care reform, combined with ever-escalating costs projected into the indefinite future, now appears to provide an opportunity for this wealth redistribution under the banner of cost control. Advocates of the private marketplace have put a great deal of effort, over many years, into convincing Americans that cost escalation is the result of too much insurance coverage, particularly of government coverage. In this they have been remarkably successful, remarkable because the international experience makes it clear that this proposition is not only false, but completely backwards.[31]

The stage is thus set for an assault on the major public programs—Medicare and Medicaid. A variety of proposals are under discussion, but the core idea of each is to transfer more of the cost burden from government to individuals. In terms of the identity above, tax contributions (T) will be reduced and user charges (C) increased. The greater the share of each person's illness burden that must be borne by himself or herself, whether contemporaneously or from savings or borrowing, the greater the advantage to the wealthy and healthy.[32]

---

[31]Economists have been particularly energetic and effective in promoting this nonsense. Chalmers Johnson suggests in another context that if the United States were a properly run country, neoclassical economists would be hanged from the Capitol dome for consistently giving bad advice to those in charge of public policy, with disastrous consequences.

[32]Advocates of user charges place great emphasis on their putative impact on the use, and perhaps the price, of care. In the identity, if C goes up, Q, and perhaps P, will fall so total costs will go down. Unfortunately this "demand response," borrowed from the economics textbooks, has never been observed in any real-world health care system. It shows up in particular services and subpopulations, but is always damped out at a system-wide level. The distributional effects of a shift in funding sources from T to C are, by contrast, automatic and noncontroversial, and follow from basic accounting. Advocates of user fees simply avoid discussing them.

Two basic options appear to be on the table: moving more seniors into capitated, managed care plans, and offering "catastrophic" health insurance coverage, with a very high deductible, along with some system of "medical savings accounts" to assist people in meeting the deductible.[33] The former approach is old news, as is the claim that "it is finally starting to work!" The principal effect is likely to be a much greater variation in care provided to seniors. If costs grow faster than the government's contribution, the better-off elderly can buy into better plans with their own resources. The rest will make do with what is left.

"Catastrophic" insurance plus medical savings accounts looks new, but is really just the very high deductible coverage that right-wing economists have been advocating for twenty-five years. Adding some form of "medical savings account" encourages or forces people to save or borrow to cover these large deductibles, thus spreading their impact out over time.

The details of such schemes can be varied ad lib, but their interesting aspects fall under three heads.

First, all such plans are at root elaborate forms of user charges, in that participants are always worse off financially if they have to use health care than if they do not. But how much worse off are users, under a particular proposal, and what is the corresponding opportunity for reduced taxes? How much money is thus transferred from ill to well, and from less to more wealthy people?

Second, is there a tax advantage to participation? If, for example, account contributions or their cumulative earnings are untaxed, then the plan embodies the same "Sheriff of Nottingham" feature as the present subsidy for employer-paid insurance premiums. The greatest benefits go to those in the highest tax brackets.

Third, what happens when your account runs out? The distribution of expenditures is extremely skewed (Berk & Monheit, 1992). No change in funding policy will have much impact unless it affects the heavy users of care. But many of these are elderly, chronically ill,

and not very well-off. Such people typically do not have, and have not had, the opportunity to amass large savings. (The answer may be medical savings accounts will be an option, to be chosen only by the relatively well-off, who can thereby avoid wasting their money in paying for other people's care.)

Conclusion

In sum, the interesting question about American health care policy in the near term is whether those at the upper end of the income distribution—who would unquestionably gain from a major reduction in the share of public funding—can convince those in the middle that they should support radical changes, at the expense of those at the bottom. Many, perhaps most, of those in the middle will *not* come out ahead as a result. But it may well be possible, in the present political climate, to distract them from taking the long view. "You can fool all of the people some of the time, and some of the people all of the time . . . and that is often sufficient."

REFERENCES

Aaron, Henry J., & William B. Schwartz. (1984). *The painful prescription: Rationing in health care.* Washington, D.C.: The Brookings Institution.

Abel-Smith, Brian. (1985). Who is the odd man out: The experience of Western Europe in containing the costs of health care. *Milbank Memorial Fund Quarterly, 63* (1), 1–17.

Abel-Smith, Brian. (1992). Cost containment and new priorities in the European community. *Milbank Quarterly, 70* (3), 393–416.

Abel-Smith, Brian, & Elias Mossialos. (1994). Cost containment and health care reform: A study of the European union. *Health Policy, 28* (May), 89–132.

Andersen, Tavs Folmer, & Gavin Mooney. (Eds.). (1989). *The challenges of medical practice variations.* London: Macmillan.

Banta, H. David, Clyde Behney, & Jane S. Willems. (1981). *Toward rational technology in medicine: Considerations for health policy.* New York: Springer.

Barer, Morris L., Robert G. Evans, & Roberta J. Labelle. (1988). Fee controls as cost control: Tales from the frozen north. *Milbank Quarterly, 66* (1), 1–64.

Baumol, William J. (1988). *Price controls for medical services and the medical needs of the nation's elderly.* Paper prepared with the financial support of the American Medical Association and pre-

---

[33]The deductible is the amount an insured individual or family must pay out of pocket, in a given time period, before receiving any insurance reimbursement; co-insurance is the proportion of subsequent covered expenditure that must also be paid out of pocket.

sented before the Physician Payment Review Commission, Washington, D.C., February 11.

Berk, Marc L., & Alan C. Monheit. (1992). The concentration of health expenditures: An update. *Health Affairs, 11* (Winter), 145–149.

Blendon, Robert J. (1989). Three systems: A comparative survey. *Health Management Quarterly, 11*, 2–10.

Bunker, John P. (1970). Surgical manpower: A comparison of operations and surgeons in the United States and in England and Wales. *New England Journal of Medicine, 282* (January 15), 135–144.

Chassin, Mark R., Robert H. Brook, R. E. Park, et al. (1986). Variations in the use of medical and surgical services by the Medicare population. *New England Journal of Medicine, 314* (January 30), 285–290.

Culyer, Antony J. (1988). *Health expenditures in Canada: Myth and reality, past and future.* Toronto: Canadian Tax Foundation.

Culyer, Antony J., J. E. Brazier, & Owen O'Donnell. (1988). *Organizing health service provision: Drawing on experience* (Working Paper No. 2, Working Party on Alternative Delivery and Funding of Health Services). London: Institute of Health Services Management.

Economist, The. (1988). Fallible doctors: Patient's dilemma. *309* (December 17), 19–21.

Enthoven, Alain C. (1985). *Reflections on the management of the national health service* (Occasional Paper No. 5). London: The Nuffield Provincial Hospitals Trust.

Evans, Robert G. (1985). Illusions of necessity: Evading responsibility for choice in health care. *Journal of Health Politics, Policy and Law, 10* (Fall), 439–467.

Evans, Robert G. (1986). Finding the levers, finding the courage: Lessons from cost containment in North America. *Journal of Health Politics, Policy and Law, 11* (Tenth Anniversary Issue, Winter), 585–616.

Evans, Robert G., Morris L. Barer, & Gregory L. Stoddart. (1994). *Charging Peter to pay Paul: Accounting for the financial effects of user charges.* Toronto: The Premier's Council on Health, Wellbeing and Social Justice.

Feeny, David, Gordon Guyatt, & Peter Tugwell. (1986). *Health care technology: Effectiveness, efficiency and public policy.* Montreal: Institute for Research on Public Policy.

Fein, Rashi. (1986). *Medical care, medical costs: The search for a national health policy.* Cambridge, MA: Harvard University Press.

Fein, Rashi. (1992). Health care reform. *Scientific American, 267* (November), 46–53.

Fisher, Elliot S., H. Gilbert Welch, & John E. Wennberg. (1992). Prioritizing Oregon's hospital resources: An example based on variations in discretionary medical utilization. *Journal of the American Medical Association, 267* (April 8), 1925–1931.

Fuchs, Victor R., & James S. Hahn. (1990). How does Canada do it? A comparison of expenditures for physicians' services in the United States and Canada. *New England Journal of Medicine, 323* (September 27), 884–890.

Gerdtham, Ulf-G., & Bengt Jönsson. (1991a). Health care expenditure in Sweden—An international comparison. *Health Policy, 19* (December), 211–228.

Gerdtham, Ulf-G., & Bengt Jönsson. (1991b). Price and quantity in international comparisons of health care expenditure. *Applied Economics , 23* (September), 1519–1528.

Groenewegen, Peter P., Jouke van der Zee, & Rene van Haaften. (1991). *Remunerating general practitioners in Western Europe.* Aldershot: Avebury.

Ham, Chris. (Ed.). (1988). *Health care variations: Assessing the evidence* (Research Report No. 2). London: The King's Fund Institute.

Hillman, Bruce J., et al. (1990). Frequency and costs of diagnostic imaging in office practice—a comparison of self-referring and radiologist-referring physicians. *New England Journal of Medicine, 323* (December), 1604–1608.

Himmelstein David U., & Steffie Woolhandler. (1986). Cost without benefit: Administrative waste in U.S. health care. *New England Journal of Medicine, 314* (February 13), 441–445.

Lee, Philip R., & Lynn Etheredge. (1989). Clinical freedom: Two lessons for the UK from US experience with privatisation of health care. *The Lancet* (February 4), 263–266.

Levit, Katharine R., et al. (1994). National health spending trends, 1960–1993. *Health Affairs, 13* (Winter), 124–136.

Mackenbach, Johan P. (1991). Health care expenditure and mortality from amenable conditions in the European community. *Health Policy, 19* (2–3), 245–255.

Manning, Willard G., Joseph P. Newhouse, & N. Duan, et al. (1987). Health insurance and the demand for medical care. *American Economic Review, 77* (June), 251–277.

Marmor, Theodore R. (1983). *Political analysis and American medical care: Essays.* Cambridge: Cambridge University Press.

Maynard, Alan. (1981). The inefficiency and inequalities of the health care systems of Western Europe. *Social Policy and Administration, 15* (Summer), 145–163.

McPherson, Klim, John E. Wennberg, Oleb B. Hovind, & Peter Clifford. (1982). Small area variations in the use of common surgical procedures: An international comparison of New England, England and Norway. *New England Journal of Medicine, 307* (November 18), 1310–1314.

Nair, Cyril, R. Karim, & C. Nyers. (1992). Health care and health status: A Canada–United States statistical comparison. *Health Reports, 4* (October), 175–183.

Organization for Economic Cooperation and Development. (1987). *Financing and delivering health care: A comparative analysis of OECD countries* (Social Policy Studies No. 4). Paris: Organization for Economic Cooperation and Development.

Organization for Economic Cooperation and Development. (1994). *The reform of health care systems: A review of seventeen OECD countries* (Health Policy Studies No. 5). Paris: Organization for Economic Cooperation and Development.

Rachlis, Michael, & Carol Kushner. (1989). *Second opinion: What's wrong with Canada's health-care system and how to fix it.* Toronto: Collins.

Rasell, M. Edith, Jared Bernstein, & Kai Tang. (1993). *The impact of health care financing on family budgets* (Economic Policy Institute Briefing Paper, April). Washington, D.C.: Economic Policy Institute.

Record, Jane Cassels. (Ed.). (1981). *Staffing primary care in 1990: Physician replacement and cost savings.* New York: Springer.

Redelmeier, Donald A., & Victor R. Fuchs. (1993). Hospital expenditures in the United States and Canada. *New England Journal of Medicine, 328* (March 18), 772–778.

Reinhardt, Uwe E. (1987). Resource allocation in health care: The allocation of lifestyles to providers. *Milbank Quarterly, 65* (June), 153–176.

Reinhardt, Uwe E. (1988). On the B-Factor in American health care. *Washington Post* (August 9), 20.

Roos, Noralou P., Gordon Flowerdew, Andre Wajda, & Robert B. Tate. (1986). Variations in physicians' hospitalization practices: A population-based study in Manitoba, Canada. *American Journal of Public Health, 76* (January), 45–51.

Roper, William L., William Winkenwerder, Glenn M. Hackbarth, & Henry Krakauer. (1988). Effectiveness in health care: An initiative to evaluate and improve medical practice. *New England Journal of Medicine, 319* (November 3), 1197–1202.

Schieber, George J., Jean-Pierre Poullier, & Leslie M. Greenwald. (1994). Health system performance in OECD countries, 1980–1992. *Health Affairs, 13* (Fall), 100–112.

Spitzer, Walter O. (1984). The nurse practitioner revisited: Slow death of a good idea. *New England Journal of Medicine, 310* (April 19), 1049–1051.

Van Doorslaer, Eddy, Adam Wagstaff, & Frans Rutten. (Eds.). (1993). *Equity in the finance and delivery of health care: An international perspective.* Oxford: Oxford University Press.

Vayda, Eugene. (1973). A comparison of surgical rates in Canada and in England and Wales. *New England Journal of Medicine, 289* (December 6), 1224–1229.

Webber, Andrew, & Willis B. Goldbeck. (1984). Utilization review. In Peter D. Fox, Willis B. Goldbeck, & Jacob J. Spies (Eds.), *Health care cost management: Private sector initiatives* (pp. 69–90). Ann Arbor, MI: Health Administration Press.

Weller, Geoffrey R., & Pran Manga. (1983). The push for reprivatization of health care services in Canada, Britain and the United States. *Journal of Health Politics, Policy and Law, 8* (Fall), 495–518.

Wennberg, John E. (1984). Dealing with medical practice variations: A proposal for action. *Health Affairs, 3* (Summer), 6–32.

Wennberg, John E. (1988). Practice variations and the need for outcomes research. In Chris Ham (Ed.), *Health care variations: Assessing the evidence* (Research Report No. 2) (pp. 32–35). London: The King's Fund Institute.

White, Joseph. (1995). *Competing solutions: American health care proposals and international experience.* Washington, D.C.: The Brookings Institution.

Wildavsky, Aaron. (1977). Doing better and feeling worse: The political pathology of health policy. *Daedalus, 106* (1), 105–124.

Williams, Alan. (1978). Need: An economic exegesis. In Antony J. Culyer & Kenneth G. Wright (Eds.), *Economic aspects of health services* (pp. 32–45). London: Martin Robertson.

Woolhandler, Steffie, & David U. Himmelstein. (1991). The deteriorating administrative efficiency of the U.S. health care system. *New England Journal of Medicine, 324* (May 2), 1253–1258.

CHAPTER

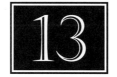

Access to Health Care

Irene Fraser

Although health care is not considered a basic right of citizenship in this country, the broadly shared social expectation is that people should be able to receive care when they need it, regardless of their ability to pay. In typical American fashion, the policy response to this expectation has combined private initiatives with public programs at many levels of government. Most people receive their health insurance through the workplace, while others purchase private coverage on their own. The federal government finances care through Medicare, the Veterans Administration, and a variety of other federal programs, and through a tax policy that subsidizes employer coverage. In cooperation with the states, it also provides care to the poor and near-poor through the Medicaid program. For their part, state and local governments have provided many direct services, and they also subsidize public hospitals and other providers of care for the poor. Despite these efforts, many people fall outside these systems. The ex-

pectation has been that these uninsured would either pay for their own care or receive charity care, and that the costs of charity care would simply be absorbed into the overhead costs of providers.

Beginning in the early 1980s, however, this pluralistic system began to unravel. Increases in the number of poor, greater competition in the health care industry, and concerted cost-containment efforts in the public and private sectors led to both a growing number of uninsured and a disruption of the traditional ways of financing their care. At the same time, the cost of this care continued to grow, creating severe budget problems at all levels of government and escalating payroll expenses for employers. By 1992, public concern with the twin problems of access and cost was so high that health care reform became a central issue in the presidential election.

When President Clinton's health reform proposal failed, the issue of access temporarily dropped from the national political agenda. But the number of uninsured has continued to grow, and Americans have very strong concerns about their continued access to coverage and health care. For example, a July 1995 survey by Louis Harris & Associates found that health insurance was the single greatest worry among American adults. Two-thirds of the respondents indicated that they worry about having enough health insurance to cover their medical bills, and almost four out of ten worry a great deal about this problem. Overall, they were more worried about losing coverage than about dying, losing their health, losing a loved one, being the victim of a crime, losing a job, or having insufficient income (American Health Line, August 29, 1995).

TRENDS IN ACCESS

In a world of perfect access, people would receive the services they need, at the appropriate site and at the appropriate time. Because we live in an insurance-based system (rather than a system where health care is financed by the state), possession of public or private health insurance coverage is the first and most important step to achieving access, though it is not the only one.

To translate coverage into access, consumers must know what services they need and what their plan or policy will pay for. They must identify providers willing and able to meet their particular needs, and be able to arrange the transportation, child care, and time off from work to seek care. However, this often does not happen. As a result, even Americans with private health insurance often do not receive necessary preventive and primary care services, and this access problem is even more pronounced among the poor, ethnic minorities, and vulnerable populations (Bashshur et al., 1994; Newacheck, 1988; Perez-Stable et al., 1994; Butler et al., 1987).

But in recent years, we have seen a continuing increase in the number of people who lack even the first prerequisite for access: coverage under a private policy or public plan. As shown in Figure 13-1, the number of uninsured grew by about a million per year between 1988 and 1993. By 1993, about 41 million people—

18.1 percent of the nonelderly population—lacked coverage. Matters were even worse in thirteen states and the District of Columbia, where at least one in five were uninsured (Employee Benefits Research Institute, 1995a). Finally, there was an additional group who were insured at the time of the survey but had been uninsured for some period of time in the previous two years. All in all, one-third of nonelderly adults were uninsured for some period of time between 1991 and 1993 (Davis, et al., 1995).

The 41 million uninsured are a diverse group, but many share three characteristics. Over half are poor or near-poor; about one-quarter are children; and 85 percent live in families headed by a worker (Employee Benefits Research Institute, 1995a, 1995b). Taken together, these facts say a great deal about the origins of the problem, and also about where one should look for solutions. Assuming the continued lack of a comprehensive solution at the national level, any real reduction in the number of uninsured is going to require an expansion of the Medicaid program, a substantial boost in employer-based health insurance, or both. In the short term, such actions may also have to be coupled with direct efforts to prop up financially stressed "safety net" hospitals, which serve large numbers of uninsured.

ACCESS ISSUES

The growing gap in our pluralistic health insurance system creates two access problems, one indirect and one direct. The indirect threat is that the surge in the ranks of the uninsured, and the resultant increase in the volume of uncompensated care, is occurring at a time when changes in the medical care financing system are dismantling long-standing mechanisms for financing this care and threatening the viability of traditional "safety net" hospitals to continue to serve the poor. The direct threat is that those without health insurance are less likely to seek care at all.

Indirect Threats to Access

Because of their mission, community expectations, and legal requirements, hospitals and other providers

Source of Coverage	1989	1990	1991	1992	1992 (revised)	1993
	Weight Based on 1980 Census[a]				Weight Based on 1990 Census[a]	
	Coverage in Millions					
Total population	213.7	215.9	218.1	220.8	223.8	226.2
Total with private health insurance	160.4	158.3	157.7	156.6	157.5	157.7
Employer coverage	140.8	138.7	139.8	138.0	138.7	137.4
Other private coverage	19.7	19.7	18.0	18.8	19.0	20.8
Total with public health insurance	26.2	29.2	31.7	33.4	34.3	36.3
Medicare	3.2	3.5	3.5	4.0	3.9	3.7
Medicaid	18.5	21.6	23.9	25.6	26.5	28.9
CHAMPUS/CHAMPVA[b]	5.9	5.9	5.9	5.7	5.8	5.6
No health insurance	34.4	35.7	36.3	38.5	39.8	40.9
	Percentage Covered					
Total population	100%	100%	100%	100%	100%	100%
Total with private health insurance	75.0	73.3	72.3	70.9	70.4	69.7
Employer coverage	65.9	64.2	64.1	62.5	62.0	60.8
Other private coverage	9.2	9.1	8.2	8.5	8.5	9.2
Total with public health insurance	12.2	13.5	14.5	15.1	15.3	16.1
Medicare	1.5	1.6	1.6	1.8	1.8	1.6
Medicaid	8.7	10.0	11.0	11.6	11.8	12.8
CHAMPUS/CHAMPVA[b]	2.8	2.7	2.7	2.6	2.6	2.5
No health insurance	16.1	16.6	16.6	17.4	17.8	18.1

FIGURE 13-1 Nonelderly Americans with Selected Sources of Health Insurance, 1989–93

SOURCE: Employee Benefits Research Institute (1995a) analysis of the March, 1990, 1991, 1992, 1993, and 1994 Current Population Survey. Used by permission of the Employee Benefits Research Institute.

[a]The 1989 data through the first set of 1992 data are based on 1980 census-based population controls. The second set of 1992 data (as revised) and 1993 data are based on 1990 census-based population controls. While the change in weighting has little effect on the percentage distributions, it does affect levels. Thus, by reweighting the 1992 data, these numbers may more accurately be compared with the more recent 1993 data.

[b]Includes only the retired military and members of their families provided coverage through the Civilian Health and Medical Program for the Uniformed Services and the Civilian Health and Medical Program of the Veterans Administration. Excludes active duty military personnel and members of their families.

historically have provided care to some patients without charge or at reduced charges. These reductions can take many forms, ranging from negotiated discounts for particular insurer or employer groups, to less voluntary reductions for public payers, to what traditionally has been termed charity care or bad debt. In theory, bad debt is care for which an individual could have paid but did not, while charity care is defined as care for which a hospital decides not to bill because the patient cannot pay. But studies in Indiana (Zollinger, 1991), Florida (Campbell, 1992; Duncan et al., 1986), and North Carolina (Duke University, 1986) indicate that most

uncompensated care, whether labeled "charity care" or "bad debt," results from care to those who are poor or near-poor, uninsured, or both. For this reason, most analyses of hospital care for the poor focus on uncompensated care costs, that is, the total cost of charity care and bad debt to the hospital.

Uncompensated care costs have increased substantially in recent years, rising from $3.9 billion in 1980 to $16.0 billion in 1993 (see Figure 13-2). During the early years of this period, uncompensated care also represented an increasing share of hospital cost. In 1980, uncompensated care accounted for 5.1 percent of hos-

Year	Hospitals	Total Expenses[a]	Gross Patient Revenue[a]	Uncompensated Care				Unsponsored Care	
				Charge-based[a]	Percent of Gross Patient Revenue	Cost-based[a]	Cost-based as a Percent of Total Expenses	Cost-based[a]	Cost-based as a Percent of Total Expenses
1980	5828	$76.8	$89.5	$4.6	5.2%	$3.9	5.1%	$2.8	3.7%
1981	5812	90.6	106.3	5.6	5.2	4.7	5.2	3.5	3.8
1982	5796	104.8	126.0	6.5	5.2	5.3	5.1	4.1	3.9
1983	5782	116.4	145.1	7.8	5.4	6.1	5.3	4.8	4.1
1984	5757	123.3	155.8	9.5	6.1	7.4	6.0	5.6	4.6
1985	5729	130.5	163.3	9.9	5.8	7.4	5.7	6.1	4.7
1986	5676	140.6	178.4	11.7	6.5	8.9	6.4	6.9	4.9
1987	5597	152.2	196.1	12.6	6.4	9.5	6.2	7.2	4.7
1988	5499	168.0	224.8	14.2	6.3	10.4	6.2	8.1	4.8
1989	5448	184.6	275.9	15.6	6.0	11.1	6.0	8.9	4.8
1990	5370	203.2	297.4	17.9	6.0	12.1	6.0	9.5	4.7
1991	5329	224.5	343.4	20.5	6.0	13.4	6.0	10.8	4.8
1992	5287	247.8	394.0	23.2	5.9	14.7	5.9	11.9	4.8
1993	5252	263.7	431.3	25.6	5.9	15.7	6.0	12.6	4.8

FIGURE 13-2   National Uncompensated and Unsponsored Care: 1980–93 (in Billions), Registered Community Hospitals

SOURCE: American Hospital Association Annual Survey of Hospitals, 1980–93 (includes estimated data). Uncompensated care cost figures are calculated for each hospital by multiplying uncompensated care charge data by the ratio of total expenses to gross patient revenues. Unsponsored care costs are derived by subtracting state and local governmental tax appropriations from uncompensated care costs. Uncompensated and unsponsored care figures do not include the cases of a small number of hospitals that derive the majority of their income from the tax appropriations, grants, and contributions and have no gross patient revenue.

[a]Dollar figures are in billions.

pital expenses, rising to 6.0 percent in 1984 and subsequent years. Although some uncompensated care costs are defrayed by state and local tax appropriations, these allocations have been growing much more slowly than the cost of uncompensated care. State and local taxes covered 27 percent of the cost of uncompensated care in 1980, but only 19 percent of these costs in 1993. As a result, a greater and greater proportion of the care to the poor remains truly "unsponsored"—not paid for by the patient or insurer, and not covered by state and local tax appropriations. In 1980, for instance, unsponsored care totaled $1.8 billion or 3.7 percent of hospital expenses. By 1993, it reached $12.9 billion or 4.8 percent of hospital expenses.

While the trend data show that uncompensated and unsponsored care levels are no longer growing as a percentage of hospital expenses (at least through 1993), the indirect threat to access is still growing, for three reasons. First, because of hospital differences in location,

mission, and a myriad of other factors, the distribution of uncompensated care tends to be very uneven across hospitals, resulting in severe financial stress for many. In 1993, for example, unsponsored care represented 5 percent of hospital costs nationwide, but 1,150 hospitals provided unsponsored care exceeding 6 percent of their costs, and 237 of these provided unsponsored care totaling more than 11 percent of their costs (American Hospital Association, 1993).

Second, many state Medicaid programs pay hospitals at a rate substantially below cost, and the resulting payment shortfalls have been growing both in absolute terms and as a percentage of total expenses. For instance, Medicaid shortfalls represented only $0.7 billion or 0.9 percent of hospital expenses in 1980, but rose to $3.7 billion or 1.4 percent of hospital expenses in 1991 (American Hospital Association, 1993).

Third, hospitals have a declining ability to shift costs, and those with high indigent care burdens have less ability than others. Traditionally, hospitals have been able to subsidize the cost of care provided to the medically indigent by increasing charges to insured patients and those able to pay their own bills. But changes in reimbursement under public and private insurance programs are making this arrangement more and more difficult to sustain. The principal sources of government financing, Medicare and Medicaid, provide no subsidies for costs incurred by indigent nonbeneficiaries. In fact, as discussed above, these programs often fail to cover the costs of their own beneficiaries. Insurers or large employers frequently are able to negotiate reduced rates and thereby exempt themselves from cost shifts as well. Hospitals that continue to provide large amounts of unsponsored care are at a severe disadvantage in an increasingly price-driven payment environment.

Direct Threats to Access

But these trends in uncompensated, unsponsored, and undercompensated care, no matter how serious, are only a small part of the broader access problem. The $12.9 billion in unsponsored care does not include, for example, the sizable amount of uncompensated care provided outside the hospital setting (Dunham et al., 1991; American Medical Association, 1988; Kilbane & Blacksin, 1988). It does not include out-of-pocket expenditures by the poor and middle-class uninsured who do manage to pay at least part of their bills, or out-of-pocket expenditures by the "underinsured," the approximately 29 million people who have coverage but who would still have catastrophic out-of-pocket costs in the event of a major illness (Short & Banthin, 1995). Finally, and most important, unsponsored care figures only take account of care that was received, and therefore do not reflect the enormous human, social, and economic costs resulting from unmet needs—care that the uninsured either did not seek or did not receive. Study after study (Freeman et al., 1987; Hendershot, 1988; Freeman et al., 1990) have shown that the uninsured are less likely to seek and receive timely and appropriate care. For example, a 1992 survey conducted by the Commonwealth Fund and the Henry J. Kaiser Family Foundation (Davis et al., 1995) found that 71

percent of the uninsured delayed seeking needed health services for financial reasons, and one-third did not receive needed services at all (see also Berk et al., 1995).

Other surveys (Long & Marquis, 1994) have shown that adults who are uncovered for a complete year have 60 percent as many ambulatory care visits and 70 percent of the inpatient hospital days they would have had if insured.

While the uninsured eventually receive critically needed services, they tend to seek too little, too late. They go to hospitals to have their babies, but often without benefit of prenatal care; they arrive in hospital emergency rooms with serious illnesses that could have been treated less expensively, and more successfully, a year earlier. As a result, they tend to have higher rates of hospitalization for preventable or controllable conditions such as asthma. For example, a survey of uninsured patients admitted to Washington, D.C. hospitals found that 23.5 percent of the admissions could have been prevented through appropriate and timely primary care (District of Columbia Hospital Association, 1988). As might be expected, studies have shown that the uninsured report poorer health than those with private coverage (Hahn & Flood, 1995).[1]

DYNAMICS OF COVERAGE

Given our pluralistic system of financing health care coverage, there is no single or simple explanation for the growing number of uninsured. Those without insurance are in a residual category, falling outside the cov-

---

[1]More unexpected is the finding that the uninsured report better health than those covered under the Medicaid program, even when sociodemographic factors, health care use, and other factors are taken into account (Hahn & Flood, 1995). One explanation may be that poor health is likely to precipitate public program enrollment, even when one controls for this effect by taking into account sociodemographic factors, health care use, and other such factors. Another explanation may be that the Hahn & Flood study measures perceptions rather than health status per se, and that public program enrollees may evaluate the same health status factors differently. Regardless of the other factors at work here, the finding of poor perceived health among the Medicaid population suggests that health care coverage is not a panacea, and that the type of coverage can be as important as the mere presence of coverage when it comes to predicting health. This finding is particularly significant in light of the fact that the past decade has seen a shift from private to public coverage as well as declines in the extent of coverage.

erage boundaries of a multiplicity of public and private insurers. These boundaries have shifted over the past decade, in two interrelated ways. First, the extent of private coverage has declined, especially for children. Second, the Medicaid program has expanded to pick up some, but not all of those squeezed out of the private market.

Private Coverage

The workplace has long been the predominant source of health insurance in the United States. Encouraged by a federal tax structure that subsidizes health insurance and other fringe benefits by permitting employers to purchase them with pretax dollars, most businesses offer health insurance coverage to at least some of their workers, and most businesses with health plans make at least some arrangement for dependent coverage. The result has been extensive private coverage of workers and their families. As shown in Figure 13-1, about 137 million of the 226 million nonelderly Americans receive health care coverage, directly or indirectly, through the workplace (Employee Benefits Research Institute, 1995a).

Despite this strong link between insurance and work, there also is a strong, growing, paradoxical link between noncoverage and work. That is, while the vast majority of the insured are receiving their coverage at the workplace, the vast majority of the uninsured also are workers, or dependents of workers, for whom the current system somehow is not operating. Figure 13-3 shows, for example, that three-quarters of the uninsured live in

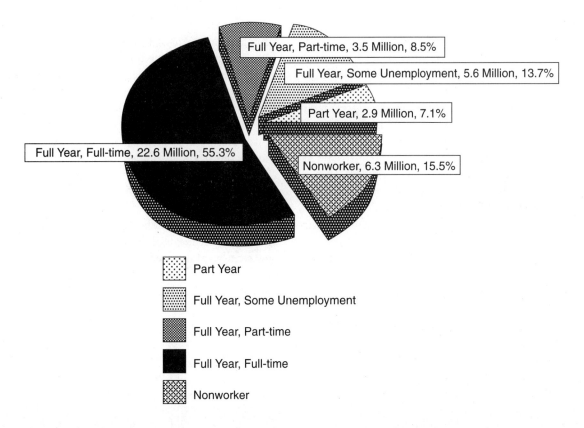

Figure 13-3   Nonelderly Population without Health Insurance, by Work Status of Family Head, 1993

SOURCE: Employee Benefits Research Institute (1995a) analysis of the March 1994 CPS. Used by permission of the Employee Benefits Research Institute.

families with a strong, fairly consistent link to the workplace and 55 percent live in families of full-year, full-time workers. Only 15.5 percent of the uninsured have no connection to the workplace. While getting a job may be the most common way to obtain insurance coverage, it is not a certain route.

In recent years, the link between employment and insurance has been steadily eroding, particularly for dependents. As shown in Figure 13-1, 65.9 percent of the nonelderly population had employer-sponsored coverage in 1989. By 1993, this percentage had dropped to 60.8. Over a million people lost employer coverage between 1992 and 1993 alone. The reasons for this decline are not clear. Conventional wisdom holds that lower coverage rates result from systemic trends in employment, including shifts from industrial to service employment and from full-time jobs to part-time jobs or self-employment. However, recent analyses (Long & Rodgers, 1995; Acs, 1995) indicate that these systemic factors explain little of the decline. Instead, what appears to be happening is that the decline in employer-sponsored coverage results from falling coverage rates in all industries. Across the board, fewer employers are offering health coverage and workers are finding it more difficult to pay their share of the premium or to purchase nongroup insurance.

As the prevalence of private coverage continues to decline, employees are becoming increasingly aware that it is not a benefit they can count on. The result is a broad level of nervousness reflected in the Harris survey cited earlier, and in particular a concern that a change in job could lead to loss of coverage—the so-called job lock phenomenon (Cooper & Monheit, 1993).

The nature of employer-sponsored coverage is also changing. In an effort to control escalating health care costs, employers have been shifting their employees into managed care, forging direct contractual arrangements with providers and networks, and taking a proactive approach to monitoring the cost and quality of care for employees and their families. Most large employers and many medium-sized employers are now self-insured. Under the Employee Retirement Income Security Act (ERISA), states cannot regulate the employee health plans of self-insured businesses, who are responsible for a large and growing proportion of the privately insured population. As a result, these self-insured businesses are outside the reach of state agencies who might wish to regulate or tax them. This limitation makes it very difficult for states to design comprehensive insurance-based solutions to access.

It is not yet clear whether the move to self-insurance, managed care, and direct contracting will expand, diminish, or simply maintain current levels of access for employees and their families, although the move to managed care and selective contracting certainly changes the rules of access. As discussed later, these employer practices can have an impact on access in the broader community, though again the direction of such change may vary from one situation to another. To the extent that value-based purchasing lowers the cost of care throughout the community, insurance rates could drop and more small employers could afford coverage. On the other hand, the immediate impact of managed care and selective contracting may be that large employers can escape their share of the hospital cost shift, thereby concentrating the burden of uncompensated care on small employers and others with less bargaining power, and perhaps pricing some of these marginal employers out of the insurance market altogether.

Medicaid

Medicaid is the public program designed to address the health care needs of the poor, just as Medicare serves the elderly, blind, and disabled. Since its inception, Medicaid has been a joint federal and state program, although there has been pressure from Republicans to turn the program over to the states under a block grant program.

While the prevalence of employer-based coverage has declined in recent years, the number of Medicaid enrollees has been growing. As shown in Figure 13-1, the Medicaid program covered 18.5 million people in 1989; by 1993, enrollment had grown to 28.9 million. Some of this growth resulted from federal mandates to cover pregnant women and children, some resulted from state exercise of options to cover new groups, and some resulted from a variety of state efforts to tap federal matching dollars for state initiatives. As a result, Medicaid is now a major insurer in most states. The program pays for a third of all births, finances care for one in four American children, and covers 60 percent of the poor. Medicaid also pays for half of all nursing home care, subsidizes acute care for poor Medicare enrollees, and has a large and increasing responsibility for people with disabilities and AIDS (Rowland, 1995a).

Despite this substantial increase in Medicaid enrollment, however, the number of uninsured has continued to grow as well, meaning that the growth of Medicaid has not been able to keep pace with declines in private coverage.

In actuality, the Medicaid program always has provided an insecure safety net, for four reasons. First, the program has some serious eligibility gaps and state inequities, because eligibility for the most part hinges on eligibility for welfare programs and these programs only apply to certain categories of the poor. Unless they are elderly or disabled, for example, single adults and childless couples are ineligible at any income level and in any state. Moreover, even for those who do fit the general demographic profile to qualify for Medicaid, eligibility levels can show considerable variation from state to state. For children and their families, for example, Medicaid eligibility ceilings historically have been linked to Aid to Families with Dependent Children (AFDC) payment levels, and these AFDC payment levels, in turn, show both tremendous interstate variation and a steep decline over time. Many of these inequalities persist despite legislation in the 1980s (the Omnibus Budget Reconciliation Acts of 1986 and 1987) extending eligibility to other poor or near-poor children and pregnant women. As a result of all of these factors, Medicaid only covered 58 percent of the nonelderly poor in 1994 (Nolan et al., 1995, citing Rowland, 1995b).

Enrollment rules and procedures have provided a second barrier to coverage. Historically, a sizable number of people eligible for Medicaid coverage have not in fact enrolled (Hill, 1988; Brown, 1988; Rymer, 1984). One recent state-by-state analysis (Winterbottom et al., 1995) estimated that about 73 percent of the people eligible for Medicaid were in fact enrolled, and that the ratio of enrollees to eligibles varied from a low of 49 percent in New Hampshire to a high of 92.8 percent in West Virginia. This gap exists even for the welfare-linked groups, and it can be very large for newer, state-option groups. The reasons are many: lack of adequate publicity regarding the availability of benefits for new groups, complicated eligibility criteria and enrollment procedures, eligibility rules that cause an individual or family to move in and out of eligibility with some frequency, an incentive system that penalizes states for errors in favor of applicants but not against applicants, and personnel shortages in Medicaid offices. Individuals who are eligible but not enrolled may incur sizable out-of-pocket costs, generate uncompensated care costs for hospitals, or delay necessary care.

Many of the technical and administrative problems that limit enrollment could be remedied. For example, eliminating the assets test for some or all groups would streamline the enrollment process considerably. While little data on the subject exist, there is considerable reason to believe that the main function of the assets test is to serve as a procedural hurdle. Applicants fail the test, or drop out, not because their assets are too great but because they cannot successfully document how few possessions they actually have (Shuptrine & Grant, 1988).

The political difficulty with all of these solutions is that, in a time of strong budget concerns at the federal as well as state levels, finding the money to extend eligibility to new politically photogenic groups such as young poor children or near-poor pregnant women is easier than finding the funds to assure greater enrollment of groups that presumably already have been taken care of.

A third problem area for Medicaid has been service coverage. Because it is a joint federal–state program, with states free to operate within general federal guidelines, state programs can and do vary considerably not only on the extent but also on the content of coverage. Federal rules mandate coverage of certain services, with other coverage decisions left to the states' discretion. This patchwork Medicaid system results in gaps and voids in which necessary and cost-effective services are not covered. The law also permits states to limit the amount and scope of required as well as optional services. Many states have sought to contain costs by drastically limiting the number of inpatient days that the program will cover, even when such services might be medically necessary. On the other hand, it should be noted that Medicaid's service package often includes some benefits—certain preventive services, for example—not generally available under private insurance.

A fourth issue for Medicaid has been finding the money to assure adequate reimbursement. In the past several years, states have been struggling to finance Medicaid expansion or, in some cases, straining simply to maintain the current level of commitment. One way states have reacted to the financing problem has been by holding down provider reimbursement—an opportunity ushered in by the so-called Boren amendment of the 1981 Omnibus Budget Reconciliation Act. Before 1981, states were required to reimburse hospitals based on Medicare reasonable cost criteria. Under the Boren amendment, states are free to establish their own reimbursement methodologies, as long as the rates they pay are reasonable and adequate to meet the costs that must be incurred by efficiently and economically operated facilities to provide care and services in conformity with applicable state and federal laws, regulations, and quality and safety standards. In addition, payment must be adequate enough to ensure that individuals eligible for medical assistance have reasonable access to inpatient hospital services of adequate quality (Section 1902[a][13][A] of the Social Security Act). Section 1902(A)(30) of the act requires that payments be consistent with efficiency, economy, and quality of care.

Because each state dollar must be matched by at least one federal dollar, the Health Care Financing Administration has not had a strong incentive to enforce this provision, and lack of clarity about key terms under Boren—"efficiently and economically operated", "reasonable," and so on—would make this a difficult task in any case. As a result, hospitals in many states have found that Medicaid payments fall short of meeting costs.

In recent years, issues of eligibility, enrollment, service, and reimbursement levels have taken on added urgency because of rapidly escalating costs. Up until the late 1980s, Medicaid costs grew more slowly than private-sector health care costs. Costs began to soar beginning in the late 1980s and early 1990s, however. Between 1988 and 1993, annual federal and state Medicaid expenditures rose from $51 billion to $125 billion. Care for aged, blind, and disabled beneficiaries—about a quarter of all beneficiaries—accounted for about 60 percent of these expenditures (Rowland, 1995a). There were many reasons for this increase: rapid eligibility expansion, a national recession, inflation in health care spending, and—most important—state use of disproportionate share hospital (DSH) funding and other statutory loopholes to leverage federal dollars. During the late 1980s and early 1990s, many states set up pooling arrangements that collected moneys from hospitals and combined these with state funds to obtain federal matching dollars. These new funds in turn were redistributed to hospitals, usually in the form of disproportionate share payments to hospitals serving large numbers of Medicaid and uninsured patients. This practice caused a rapid escalation in federal expenditures. In 1993, payments through these special financing schemes generated $17 billion of federal DSH payments, and accounted for about one-seventh of the money spent in the Medicaid program (see Ku & Coughlin, 1995).

Finding a way to control Medicaid costs has provided a growing challenge for both federal and state policymakers. One early federal response under the 1991 Medicaid Voluntary Contribution and Provider-Specific Tax Amendment was to place a cap on disproportionate share hospital (DSH) expenditures and to restrict states' ability to receive a federal match for provider taxes and donations. For their part, states have responded by moving enrollees into managed care. Section 1915(b) of the 1981 Omnibus Budget Reconciliation Act gave states greater flexibility to design managed care health plans, and Section 1115 of the Social Security Act allows states to experiment with innovative approaches to managing Medicaid through research and demonstration programs. As of December 1995, thirteen states had 1115 waivers, and another eleven had been submitted (Health Care Financing Administration, 1995). While the programs show considerable variation from state to state, the main format for most of them is to provide mandatory enrollment of certain

Medicaid eligibles (primarily pregnant women and children) in managed care, and to use the savings to provide coverage to the uninsured poor. The result is that states can receive a federal match for certain new programs to cover the uninsured.

APPROACHES TO THE COVERAGE PROBLEM

Because the indigent care problem's recent growth has occurred during a period of attempted federal disengagement from many domestic policy problems under the "New Federalism" banner, much of the responsibility for designing and financing a solution is being borne by the states—sometimes willingly, and sometimes in response to federal mandates. During the past several years, states have seen a quantum increase in their opportunity, and their responsibility, to extend health care protection to target groups of the poor. State and local experimentation and innovation in private-sector programs also has been extensive. As discussed below, these state approaches have taken three forms: assuring that providers have the financial capacity to provide free care to the uninsured, attempting to extend private coverage, and expanding Medicaid and other public programs.

Provider-focused Approaches

As noted earlier, the traditional way to shift costs was within the hospital. Unpaid bills from one patient would simply be added to charges for those who were paying. But for many hospitals, and in particular those with a high volume of care to uninsured or public-pay patients, this solution is no longer viable. Private payers account for a declining portion of hospital revenue, and increased market competition has enabled many of these private payers to avoid the cost shift. As a result, hospitals with a large number of unsponsored care patients have been at an increasing disadvantage.

To address this problem of competitive disadvantage, some states have designed programs to institutionalize and broaden the cost shift through uncompensated care pools. In an uncompensated care pool, the cost shift occurs among as well as within hospitals.

Although the funding in theory could come from many sources, it generally takes the form of a hospital payment add-on, with funds distributed to reimburse hospitals for unsponsored care (Fraser et al., 1990; Fraser, 1995). Until recently, as noted earlier, hospital taxes or "voluntary" contributions have provided a second way to fund pooling arrangements. But the phase-in of 1991 legislation limiting use of these arrangements is now virtually complete, so these funds can no longer be matched with federal dollars.

Depending on how it is designed, an uncompensated care pool has several disadvantages. First, it may reward some inefficient hospitals as well as efficient ones. Second, because the add-on generally is applied to hospital services only, it fixes responsibility for financing on a shrinking portion of the health care system. Third, this add-on may or may not be passed on equally to all employers enrolled in a particular plan. Fourth, the method is difficult to use without rate setting, and most states have moved away from rate setting in recent years (McDonough, 1995). Fifth, it directs funds to hospital care rather than preventive and primary care (though some states have begun to use pool funds to finance insurance expansion). Finally, because it directs money to institutions rather than individuals, it does not create in the patient a sense of entitlement to care, and this lack of empowerment, in turn, is likely to discourage patients from seeking needed services. Because of one or more of these disadvantages, most states have abandoned their use of uncompensated care pools; only New York and Maryland continue to use this approach.

On the other hand, this approach has some important advantages that may prompt a second look from states in the future. First, such pools provide a reasonably broad and stable source of funding. Second, they address the indirect access problem by assuring the continued existence of hospitals vital to care for the poor. Third, the approach is politically feasible because it is an off-budget and invisible tax. Fourth, pools appear to be one of the few ways states can legally involve all private payers in a comprehensive solution to the indigent care problem, given the constraints of the federal Employee Retirement Security Act (ERISA). In New York, insurers challenged the use of uncompensated care pools for this purpose, but a 1995 Supreme Court decision (*New*

York Conference of Blue Cross and Blue Shield Plans et al. v. Travelers Insurance Co. et al.) ruled that the state's hospital rate surcharges did not violate ERISA (Polzer, 1995; Butler, 1995.) In light of this ruling and the continuing fear of an ERISA challenge to some of the alternative approaches discussed below, some states may revisit the possibility of using an uncompensated care pool approach.

Private Insurance-based Approaches

An alternative way to address the problem of access is to build on and bolster the employment-based insurance system. This approach makes a great deal of sense for many political, financial, and philosophical reasons. Most of the uninsured are in working families, and much of the growth in the number of uninsured has resulted from an erosion in employer-sponsored coverage. Those employers who still do insure their workers cross-subsidize (through cost shifts) business competitors who do not.

At the national level, recognition of the decline in private coverage has led many to propose a variety of ways to expand private coverage, whether through tax incentives, market reforms, or mandates. For example, President Clinton's National Security Act proposal would have required most employers to sponsor coverage for their employees and their families, and it would have offered a variety of incentives and subsidies to enable them to do so.

To date, however, the only concrete actions resulting from this growing national concern with private health insurance issues have taken place at the state and local levels. The general thrust of all of these programs is to create mechanisms to enable businesses currently disadvantaged by the private health insurance system (small unincorporated firms, for example) to purchase health insurance more easily and more cheaply. The following sections describe six of these approaches.

Creating Large Groups and Purchasing Pools

Small firms, in particular, small unincorporated firms, are the least likely to cover their workers. For ex-

ample, one recent ten-state study (Kantor et al., 1995) found that only a third of small firms (with one to four workers) offered coverage, compared with 93 percent of large firms (with fifty or more workers). There are many reasons for this. Small firms are likely to be newer and more insecure financially than larger firms. More important, small firms are at a substantial disadvantage when it comes to buying health insurance, lacking large firms' purchasing clout, economies of scale, and ability to perform administrative services in-house. They are, or are perceived to be, less stable as businesses, more likely to have high employee turnover, and more likely to change insurance carriers. Since they lack a large base over which risks can be spread, insurers fear that any given company may have one or more high-risk employees or dependents who could elevate costs for the group. Partially in response to these concerns, insurers may "redline" entire industries or exclude preexisting conditions from coverage (Fraser & Hooper, 1988; McLaughlin & Zellers, 1994).

Given these problems, one logical approach for expanding private coverage has been to convert small groups into larger ones and thereby give small employers the advantages of big ones. One of the most common mechanisms is the grouping of employers in a multiple-employer plan or purchasing cooperative, sometimes called a purchasing alliance. These arrangements can be sponsored by labor unions, trade associations, business associations or coalitions, financial institutions, and insurers themselves. State governments have also used public cooperatives to purchase insurance for state employees, and sometimes for county and municipal workers as well.

In recent years, states have begun to establish, or at least actively encourage, the development of health purchasing cooperatives for small firms as part of the state's private insurance reform strategy. In addition to performing the core insurance functions of enrollment, premium collection, and contracting with health plans, some cooperatives also develop standard benefits packages and negotiate with carriers (U.S. General Accounting Office, 1994).

The Health Insurance Plan of California (HIPC) provides an example of a particularly active state-established purchasing cooperative for small businesses with between five and fifty employees. The HIPC operates on a state-wide basis, dividing the state into six different premium rating areas, with a minimum of four plans operating in each region. In the first eight months of its operation, the HIPC enrolled 2,500 small employers covering 40,000 persons. About 15 percent of these enrollees were previously uninsured.

These numbers do not represent a large share of the California small-group market (where there are about 8 million employees of small firms), but the HIPC has been credited with lowering prices in the overall market by about 15 percent, thereby making it somewhat easier for employers and employees throughout the state to purchase coverage (Jacobson, et al., 1994).

While purchasing cooperatives clearly have the potential to lower costs and broaden access for participating small businesses, they are not a panacea. First, their reduction in premium rates may still be insufficient to attract most employers and employees without a subsidy. Second, unless the playing field is first leveled through broader insurance market reforms, these pools may find themselves subject to adverse selection, attracting only those businesses who for one reason or another cannot obtain a better rate on their own.

Small-group Market Reforms

A second approach, often used in conjunction with others, is to make it easier for small groups and individuals to obtain affordable insurance by changing the rules of the insurance marketplace. For example, states can require that coverage be available to all groups meeting certain definitions, at least during "open enrollment" periods; prohibit the cancellation of coverage by the insurer; limit the use of waiting periods for coverage; and limit the ability of insurers to exclude coverage of "preexisting conditions."

Probably most important, states can limit the variation in rates that insurers charge. Some states limit the number of price groupings and the range of prices within and among groupings, so that the premium for the highest-cost group is no more than three or four times that of the lowest-cost group. Other states go a step farther, requiring that (except for a few exceptions defined by the state) the same base rate be applied to all groups—a practice known as "modified group rating." Finally, a few states have gone even farther, implementing "pure" community rating laws requiring insurers to apply the same rate to everyone covered under the same plan, regardless of risk factors. By 1994, forty states had adopted some form of pure or modified community rating (Ladenheim & Markus, 1994; Ladenheim et al., 1994).

Evidence on the impact of community rating is still inconclusive. For one thing, the impact of community rating seems to vary depending on the state of the market before the law's enactment, the pace of implementation, and the number of other market reforms that accompany it. In addition, most of the community rating laws are still very new. It is clear, however, that community rating causes an increase in premiums for younger and healthier groups, and a decrease for groups with one or more risk factors or health problems—as intended. Assessments of whether the primary result is to expand coverage or reduce overall costs vary, depending in part on the states studied (Chollet & Paul, 1994; Ladenheim & Markus, 1994), but it is clear that market reforms by themselves cannot make a major inroad into the numbers of uninsured (Markus et al., 1995).

High-risk Pools

Community rating and other market reforms provide one way to extend availability of insurance to individuals in higher-risk groups. An alternative approach is to create an insurance pool for those who would otherwise be denied coverage in the private market because of health status or record of high utilization. Twenty-seven states operate some form of high-risk pool. These pools are generally financed by premium taxes. But because these taxes cannot be levied on self-insured firms because of ERISA restrictions, many states have begun to tap general revenues to help support these pools.

The number of people served by high-risk pools is relatively small—one hundred thousand as of December

1991—and this number has not been growing in recent years ("Evaluation of State Risk Pools," 1995). The primary difficulty with pools is that they tend to be expensive, and therefore they are not affordable unless premiums are very high, subsidies are very high, or both. Once premiums get too high, lower-risk individuals within the pool tend to disenroll, thereby causing a further increase in premiums. Maine, for instance, ended its high-risk pool, maintaining that implementation of a pure community rating system makes such a program unnecessary (Ladenheim et al., 1994).

Redefining the Product

A fourth approach states have used to reduce the cost of coverage is to redefine the product, permitting insurers to create and market a less comprehensive policy to selected groups, generally firms of under twenty-five employees who have been uninsured for at least a year. Typically, benefits waived include alcohol and substance abuse treatments, insurance continuation or conversion, and access to some providers such as chiropractors. But these changes in the benefit package generally only reduce costs by about 10 percent, so most programs also increase cost-sharing requirements. Past evaluations suggest that, at least in their initial stages, sales of these special benefit packages are quite small, numbering only in the hundreds (Butler, 1992).

Targeted Programs for the Poor

A fifth approach, which has evolved considerably in recent years, is to create targeted private or public/private insurance programs for the poor, often funded in part through foundation seed money. Beginning in the 1980s, for example, many states created special programs for children or the low-income employed population. Most involved some sort of subsidy. While these programs were popular and filled a need for those who enrolled, it became clear over time that targeted programs for the poor could not make major inroads unless the programs were both well subsidized and well publicized (Fraser & Hooper, 1988), but states had limited funds for filling either condition.

Medicaid Expansion

A final approach many states have taken is to target programs to new groups of the poor by bringing them in under the Medicaid umbrella. For example, many states extended coverage to pregnant women and children above the AFDC level years before they were required to do so under federal mandates. The attractiveness of this approach has been that the federal government pays from 50 percent to 83 percent of the cost of such programs. The problem, until recently, has been that coverage could only be extended to groups explicitly authorized as "optional" coverage groups under federal law.

In recent years, this expanded waiver authority has permitted states to ignore some of these categorical boundaries and offer a highly subsidized (or even totally subsidized) product to new groups of the poor or near-poor, and to use federal Medicaid dollars to cover at least half of the costs. For example, under their 1115 waivers, subsidized Medicaid coverage is available for all uninsured individuals and families with incomes up to 100 percent of the federal poverty level in Kentucky, Ohio, and Oregon, 250 percent of the federal poverty level in Florida, 300 percent of the federal poverty level in Hawaii, and, on a sliding scale basis, all of the uninsured in Tennessee (U.S. General Accounting Office, 1995).

When these waivers are used, none of the former demographic limitations apply, so the potential for extending coverage is vast. One recent study (Holahan et al., 1995) projected that use of 1115 waivers to cover people up to 200 percent of the poverty level could extend Medicaid coverage to up to 21.1 million previously uninsured people. (Depending on how the programs were designed, up to 19.2 million people who currently have employer-sponsored coverage also would be eligible.) On the other hand, the same study showed that states face a variety of fiscal, economic, and political constraints that make it highly unlikely that enrollments would expand to such levels.

Early reports show that use of this waiver authority has brought some successes in terms of new enrollees. Oregon, for example, expanded eligibility to all people with incomes under the federal poverty level, with the result that more than one hundred thousand previously uninsured persons now have health coverage. Although Tennessee got off to a rocky start because its program was implemented quickly and before adequate system capacity had been built, the program reportedly increased the number of insured by 5 percentage points (Prospective Payment Assessment Commission, 1995).

Another attraction of the waiver for states is that it permits them to reimburse hospitals without regard for the Boren amendment. In the case of Oregon, the waiver has also permitted the state to design its own service package, and therefore to exclude some services that are required under federal law.

While states have generally found the waivers to be to their advantage, the waiver application process is lengthy and difficult, and most states would prefer greater flexibility. The federal government, for its part, has seen a continued increase in Medicaid costs. In fact, because of the way "budget neutrality" is calculated under the waiver process, the use of 1115 waivers has provided states a vehicle for drawing down more federal matching dollars, thereby exacerbating the increase in federal spending (Holahan et al., 1995).

Because of the limitations inherent in the Medicaid waiver process as well as the incremental insurance-based approaches, in the early 1990s some states—Washington, Hawaii, Minnesota, and Oregon—designed more comprehensive insurance approaches. But comprehensive approaches such as these require an exemption from ERISA. Their failure to receive such an exemption, coupled with the 1994 Republican and conservative victories in both congressional and state legislative elections, resulted in these programs being scaled back or put on hold.

THE FUTURE

At least for the near future, it would appear that financing and delivery of health care is likely to continue in the pluralist model, with a mix of public and private approaches and a sizable group of uninsured not covered by either. What is likely to change, however, is the configuration and behavior of each of these compo-

nents. We appear to be on the brink of two major social transformations in the health care system: a downsizing and decentralization of public programs such as welfare, food stamps, and Medicaid, and a major restructuring of the private health care market (Gaus, 1995). Both sectors are evolving quickly and unpredictably, and their interplay is likely to have a profound effect on access. While accurate predictions are difficult, the following is a sketch of a few of the forces affecting access we are likely to see in some form.

Medicaid

The continuing federal imperative to control costs has precipitated recent congressional proposals to eliminate Medicaid as a federal–state entitlement program, converting it instead to a program of block grants to the states, with a cap on the amount of federal contributions to the states. Other proposals would retain Medicaid as a federal–state entitlement program, but still cap the federal contribution. Under any of these scenarios, states are likely to have far greater flexibility in deciding both how to spend their money and how much money to spend, though there may be some maintenance of effort requirements. On the other hand, most states will also find a reduction of federal funds compared with what they would have received under the old system. As one recent analysis (Tallon & Rowland, 1995) noted, a federally capped block grant for Medicaid "passes the buck without the bucks."

Especially if done through a block grant approach, this combination of reduced funding and added flexibility is likely to present states with some tough choices, all of which will have an important impact on access for one or more groups. Following are five brief examples.

How (and If) to Replace Lost Funding

Will the states not only maintain their level of effort but also replace lost federal funds? None of the options for increasing revenues is very attractive politically. Raising taxes is a political "no-no" in most states, although an increase in provider taxes might be an option. States could follow the model currently used in

New York State, raising money through an add-on to private payer hospital rates, though such an approach would run counter to the deregulation trend most regions, including New York, are following. Finally, depending on how federal legislation is worded, states could require local government to pay a share, but this approach also presents formidable political difficulties.

Dividing the State Budget Pie

A second related issue is how to divide the state budget pie between health care and other budget lines. Does the state take from other programs in order to be able to maintain its efforts in health? If so, where does it look for dollars? Ironically, the programs most likely to be tapped, such as education or social services, may have a greater impact on health than the Medicaid program.

Limiting Medicaid Costs

If, on the other hand, the state opts not to replace lost federal funding, it will then have to decide how to do more with less. The hope is that some of the shortfall can be made up through increased efficiency, and in particular through the economic discipline imposed by managed care. But most state managed care programs apply only to the maternal and child health population, and this group only accounts for about a quarter of all expenditures. So even if managed care could produce the 5 percent to 15 percent cost reductions some studies have found, the total program savings would amount to only about 2 percent, according to the Kaiser Commission on the Future of Medicaid (cited in Koppelman, 1995). So most states will have to look in addition to the traditional methods for limiting costs: limiting eligibility, slowing enrollment, limiting services, increasing out-of-pocket expenditures, and reducing payments to providers.

Allocating Dollars among Eligibility Groups

Regardless of its choices on the above questions, severe budget constraints are likely to precipitate some nasty political battles over how to allocate Medicaid dollars among three eligibility groups: pregnant women and children, the elderly, and the disabled. Federal law may provide some guidance to limit these choices, but we are likely to see fierce state-level competition over how to slice up the shrinking health care pie among a growing number of needy and deserving groups.

Restructuring Medicaid Delivery

Another set of issues for states will be how to restructure the delivery system for the Medicaid population. The trend toward managed care is expected to continue almost everywhere, but with a tremendous amount of state variation. Will managed care be voluntary or mandatory? Just for pregnant women and children, or for the elderly and disabled as well? Will mental health services be folded into the capitated rate or not? What will the state look for in selecting plans and providers?

Increase in Managed Care

A second clear trend in the private sector as well as in the Medicaid program is an increased enrollment in health maintenance organizations, preferred provider arrangements, and other forms of managed care. While this movement has many sources, the major driving force is the desire to limit overutilization of services and reduce costs. Although it is clear that this movement will have a profound effect on how care is delivered and received, the impact on access is still not clear.

Depending on how it is done, managed care can create new threats to access. First, capitated programs produce an incentive to underserve, just as fee-for-service creates an incentive to overserve. Some fear that the use of managed care in an already underserved population could produce some real problems, though so far there is little evidence to suggest that Medicaid managed care does a worse job than Medicaid fee-for-service. A second potential access problem takes the form of discontinuities in care, which occur each time a purchaser (either the Medicaid program or an employer) changes health care plans. A third potential access problem for the poor in particular is that community health centers, public hospitals, local Health Departments, and other traditional providers of care to the poor may be excluded from the new managed care networks, thereby depriving them of the revenue they need to stay in business and serve the uninsured.

On the other hand, strong managed care programs—capitated programs in particular—have the potential to improve access, at least for those with public or private coverage. First, capitated plans will have a financial incentive to provide preventive services and to preserve wellness, even if this means expanding the benefit package to include nonmedical services needed by poor and vulnerable populations. Second, the introduction of managed care also has spurred efforts to monitor quality and performance, in part because of the fear of underservice. Third, for the Medicaid population, managed care can mean the difference between theoretical and actual access. Under the old system, possession of a Medicaid card simply gave recipients the right to shop for services; it did not guarantee that a physician would in fact be willing to serve them at the Medicaid rate. Under managed care, possession of a card means that a particular plan is obliged to see them, and a good managed care contract even spells out such things as scheduling and maximum waiting times. Finally, to the extent that managed care does succeed in controlling cost, there is at least some possibility that part of the savings could be used to expand access.

Greater Power of Purchasers

A third important trend with some potential to affect access is the growing power and involvement of purchasers in health care decision making. Driven initially by concern with the rising cost of health care, large employers and business coalitions have for some years been using their purchasing power to exact discounted health care services, both within and outside managed care. In some cases, as in the Minneapolis–St. Paul area, they are moving to direct contracting arrangements with providers in order to have greater control over the cost and content of care. Finally, some of the larger purchasers and business coalitions are becoming increasingly involved in measuring and moni-

toring quality and performance. Some states also are moving in the same directions, using their power as purchasers (of care for Medicaid enrollees, state employees, and others) to both reduce costs and improve quality.

Again, it is still unclear how these trends will affect access. To the extent that purchaser involvement yields improvements in clinical practice, it could improve the quality of access once one enters the system. On the other hand, at least in the short term, the prevalence of deep discounting could have a destabilizing effect on financing for traditional providers of care to the poor by removing hidden subsidies.

The current policy predicament is that, in the face of rapidly rising health care costs, public and private payers are desperately seeking—and, to some extent, finding—ways to contain their expenditures, though so far there has been little success in containing overall system-wide costs. But the traditional "Robin Hood" mechanism for financing care to the uninsured—implicit cost shifts to private payers—presumes a certain level of economic irrationality or financial slippage in the system: that hospitals will be willing to care for people who do not pay, that public and private insurers and other payers will be willing to pay a little extra to help cover the bills of the poor uninsured, and that employees and employers will be willing to pay higher premium costs to help subsidize the care of workers with higher anticipated health care risks or larger families.

Conclusion

Increased competition and cost-consciousness in the health care environment are destroying the traditional financing system, but without creating a new mechanism to assure access and, incidentally, without solving the system-wide cost inflation problem either. Thus far, the response of most major players in the policy arena has been to search for a no-cost solution, when there clearly is not one. One grim scenario that could follow from this constellation of trends could be declining (or at best constant) public coverage, declining private coverage, and a declining provider capacity or willingness to provide free care.

REFERENCES

Acs, Gregory. (1995). Explaining trends in health insurance coverage between 1988 and 1991. *Inquiry, 32* (Spring), 102–110.

American Health Line. (1995).

American Hospital Association. (1993). *Annual survey data.* Chicago, IL: American Hospital Association.

American Medical Association. (1988). Unpublished data from the socioeconomic monitoring system survey. Chicago, IL: American Medical Association.

Bashshur, Rashid L., Rick K. Homan, & Dean G. Smith. (1994). Beyond the uninsured: Problems in access to care. *Medical Care, 32* (May), 409–419.

Berk, Marc L., Claudia L. Schur, & Joel C. Cantor. (1995). Ability to obtain health care: Recent estimates from the Robert Wood Johnson Foundation national access to care survey. *Health Affairs, 14* (Fall), 139–146.

Brown, Sarah S. (Ed.). (1988). *Prenatal care: Reaching mothers, reaching infants.* Washington, D.C.: National Academy Press.

Butler, John A., Judith S. Palfrey, & Deborah K. Walker. (1987). Health insurance coverage and insurance use among children with disabilities: Findings from probability samples in five metropolitan areas. *Pediatrics, 19* (January), 89–98. Cited in John A. Butler, Sara Rosenbaum, & Judith S. Palfrey. (1987). Ensuring access to health care for children with disabilities. *New England Journal of Medicine, 317* (July 16), 162–165.

Butler, Patricia A. (1992). *Flesh or bones? Early experience of state limited benefit health insurance laws.* Portland, ME: National Academy for State Health Policy.

Butler, Patricia A. (1995). *Recent ERISA developments: Implications of the Travelers case for state health policy initiatives.* Washington, D.C.: National Governors Association.

Butler, Patricia, Robert L. Mollica, & Trish Riley. (1993). *Children's health plans.* Portland, ME: National Academy for State Health Policy.

Campbell, Ellen. (1992). Unpaid hospital bills: Evidence from Florida. *Inquiry, 29* (Spring), 92–98.

Cantor, Joel, Stephen Long, & Susan Marquis. (1995). Private employment-based health insurance in ten states. *Health Affairs, 14* (Summer), 199–211.

Chollet, Deborah J., & Rebecca R. Paul. (1994). *Community rating: Issues and experience.* Washington, D.C.: Alpha Center.

Cooper, Philip F., & Alan C. Monheit. (1993). Does employment-related health insurance inhibit job mobility? *Inquiry, 30* (Winter), 400–416.

Davis, Karen, Diane Rowland, Drew Altman, Karen Scott Collins, & Cynthia Morris. (1995). Health insurance: The size and shape of the problem. *Inquiry, 32* (Summer), 196–203.

District of Columbia Hospital Association. (1988). *Prospective uninsured patient survey conducted by Lewin/ICF.* Washington, D.C.: D.C. Hospital Association.

Duke University. (1986). *Health care for the medically indigent: Payment and responsibility for indigent health care.* Raleigh, NC: Center for Health Policy Research and Education.

Duncan, R. Paul, Jan L. Colbert, & Jane F. Pendergast. (1986). *State university study of indigent care.* Volume 2: *The analytic report.* Gainesville, FL: Center for Health Policy Research, University of Florida Health Center.

Dunham, Nancy Cross, et al. (1991). Uncompensated and discounted Medicaid care provided by physician group practices in Wisconsin. *Journal of the American Medical Association, 265* (June), 2982–2986.

Employee Benefits Research Institute. (1995a). *Sources of health insurance and characteristics of the uninsured: Analysis of the March 1994 Current Population Survey.* Washington, D.C.: Employee Benefits Research Institute.

Employee Benefits Research Institute. (1995b). Children without health insurance. *EBRI Newsletter, 16,* 4–7.

Evaluation of state risk pools: The current and potential experience. (1995). *Health Care Financing and Organization News and Progress* (July), 3–4.

Fraser, Irene. (1995). Rate regulation as a policy tool: Lessons from New York State. *Health Care Financing Review, 16* (Spring), 151–175.

Fraser, Irene, Eileen Collins, Lawrence Hughes, & Margaret McNamara. (1990). *Direct financing of uncompensated care: Critical questions in the use and evaluation of uncompensated care pools and other provider-focused approaches.* Chicago, IL: American Hospital Association.

Fraser, Irene, & Cathy Hooper. (1988). *Promoting health insurance in the workplace: State and local initiatives to increase private coverage.* Chicago, IL: American Hospital Association.

Freeman, Howard E., Linda H. Aiken, Robert J. Blendon, et al. (1990). Uninsured working-age adults: Characteristics and consequences. *Health Services Research, 24* (February), 811–823.

Freeman, Howard E., Robert J. Blendon, Linda H. Aiken, et al. (1987). Americans report on their access to health care. *Health Affairs, 6* (Spring), 6–8.

Gaus, Clifton E. (1995). *From innovation to evaluation: Can we meet the evaluation challenge?* Paper presented to Grantmakers in Health and the Robert Wood Johnson Foundation, Princeton NJ, October 13.

Hahn, Beth, & Ann Barry Flood. (1995). No insurance, public insurance, and private insurance: Do these options contribute to differences in general health? *Journal of Health Care for the Poor and Underserved, 6* (1), 41–59.

Health Care Financing Administration. (1995). An overview of OSHRD's staff and responsibilities, Office of Health Reform Demonstrations. December 1 mailing from Lu Zawistowich.

Helms, W. David, Anne K. Gauthier, & Daniel M. Campion. (1992). Mending the flaws in the small group market. *Health Affairs, 11* (Summer), 7–27.

Hendershot, G. E. (1988). Health status and medical care utilization. *Health Affairs, 7* (Spring), 114–121.

Hill, Ian. (1988). *Reaching women who need prenatal care.* Washington, D.C.: National Governors Association.

Holahan, John, Teresa Coughlin, Leighton Ku, Debra J. Lipson, & Shruti Rajan. (1995). *Increasing insurance coverage through Medicaid waiver programs.* Washington, D.C.: Urban Institute.

Jacobson, Peter D., Richard Merritt, Lawrence Bartlett, et al. (1994). *California health care delivery: A competitive model? State health care reform initiatives: Progress and promise.* Baltimore, MD: Health Care Financing Administration.

Kilbane, Kathleen, & Beth Blacksin. (1988). The demise of free care: The visiting nurse association of Chicago. *Nursing Clinics of North America, 23* (June), 2708–2713.

Koppelman, Jane. (1995). *Exploring the impact of Medicaid block grants and spending caps* (Issue Brief). Washington, D.C.: National Health Policy Forum.

Ku, Leighton, & Teresa A. Coughlin. (1995). Medicaid disproportionate share and other special financing programs. *Health Care Financing Review, 16* (Spring), 27–54.

Ladenheim, Kala, Linda Lipson, & Anne Markus. (1994). *Health care reform: 50 state profiles.* Washington, D.C.: Intergovernmental Health Policy Project, George Washington University.

Ladenheim, Kala, & Anne R. Markus. (1994). *Community rating: States' experience.* Special report submitted to The Commonwealth Fund. Washington, D.C.: Intergovernmental Health Policy Project, George Washington University.

Long, Stephen H., & M. Susan Marquis. (1994). The uninsured "access gap" and the cost of universal coverage. *Health Affairs, 13* (Spring), 211–220.

Long, Stephen H., & Jack Rodgers. (1995). Do shifts toward service industries, part-time work and self-employment explain the rising uninsured rate? *Inquiry, 32* (Spring), 111–116.

Markus, Anne, Kala Ladenheim, & Lisa Atchison. (1995). *Small group market reforms: A snapshot of states' experiences.* Report to the Commonwealth Fund. Washington, D.C.: George Washington University, Intergovernmental Health Policy Project.

McDonough, John E. (1995). *The decline of state-based hospital rate setting: Findings and implications.* Portland, ME: National Academy for State Health Policy.

McLaughlin, Catherine G., & Wendy Zellers. (1994). *Small business and health care reform: Understanding the barriers to employee coverage and implications for workable solutions.* Ann Arbor: University of Michigan School of Public Health.

Newacheck, Paul W. (1988). Access to ambulatory care for poor persons. *Health Services Research, 23* (August), 401–419.

New York may abandon rate setting: State eyes market-driven system. (1995). *State Initiatives in Health Care Reform* (September/October), 10, 12.

Nolan, Lisa, Trish Riley, & Jane Horvath. (1995). *Less federal funding for Medicaid: Is state flexibility the answer?* Portland, ME: National Academy for State Health Policy.

Perez-Stable, E. J., G. Marin, & B. VanOss Marin. (1994). Behavioral risk factors: A comparison of Latinos and Non-Latino whites in San Francisco. *American Journal of Public Health, 84* (June), 971–976.

Polzer, Karl. (1995). *Health systems financing after the Travelers case* (Issue Brief). Washington, D.C.: National Health Policy Forum.

Prospective Payment Assessment Commission. (1995). *Medicare and the American health care system.* Report to Congress. Washington, D.C.: Prospective Payment Assessment Commission.

Rowland, Diane. (1995a). *Medicaid: The health and long-term care safety net.* Testimony before the Committee on Finance, U.S. Senate.

Rowland, Diane. (1995b). *Medicaid: A program in transition—the federal–state partnership for state health reform: The role of 1115 demonstration waivers.* Washington, D.C.: Kaiser Commission on the Future of Medicaid.

Rymer, Marilyn. (1984). *Short-term evaluation of Medicaid: Selected issues.* Baltimore, MD: U.S. Department of Health and Human Services, Health Care Financing Administration.

Short, Pamela Farley, & Jessica S. Banthin. (1995). New estimates of the underinsured younger than 65 years. *Journal of the American Medical Association, 274* (October 25), 1302–1306.

Shuptrine, Sarah C., & Vickie C. Grant. (1988). *The relationship of the reasons for denial of AFDC/Medicaid benefits to the uninsured in the U.S.* Columbia, SC: Sarah Shuptrine and Associates.

Tallon, James R., & Diane Rowland. (1995). Federal dollars and state flexibility: The debate over Medicaid's future. *Inquiry, 21* (Fall), 335–340.

U.S. General Accounting Office. (1994). *Access to health insurance: Public and private employers' experience with purchasing cooperatives* (GAO/HEHS-94-142). Washington, D.C.: U.S. General Accounting Office.

U.S. General Accounting Office. (1995). *Medicaid: Spending pressures drive states toward program reinvention* (GAO/HEHS-95-122). Washington, D.C.: U.S. General Accounting Office.

Winterbottom, Colin, David W. Liska, & Karen M. Obermaier. (1995). *State-level databook on health care access and financing* (2nd ed.). Washington, D.C.: Urban Institute.

Zollinger, Terrell W. (1991). Uncompensated hospital care for pregnancy and childbirth cases. *American Journal of Public Health, 81* (August), 1017–1022.

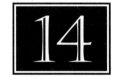

The Politics of Universal
Health Insurance:
Lessons for and from the 1990s

Theodore R. Marmor and Morris L. Barer

For a brief period in the early 1990s (from roughly 1991 to early 1993), the enactment of national health insurance once again appeared imminent in American politics. Public opinion seemed supportive, a new president had campaigned on the promise, and interest groups of all stripes claimed that the medical status quo was unsustainable. To understand how fundamental reform rose to the top of the public agenda and almost as quickly disappeared is the major topic of this chapter. To do so it helps to understand not only the behavior of the Clinton administration but the history of comparable reform efforts in twentieth-century American politics. That background makes possible educated projections of what will happen to medical care issues in the politics of the next decade and beyond.

In 1990, national health insurance was hardly mentioned by pundits, politicians, or the press. The November 1991 election of the largely unknown Democrat Harris Wofford to fill the senatorial seat opened by the unexpected death of Republican Senator John Heinz in Pennsylvania changed all that. In an instant, Wofford's upset victory, widely attributed to his advo-

This commentary expresses some views published elsewhere. See especially Marmor (1994b). Some of the historical commentary appeared in the introductory chapter of Marmor (1994a) and is reprinted here by permission of Yale University Press. The analysis of the failure of the Clinton health plan was previously published by Barer with Marmor and Morrison (1995).

Reprinted from *Social Science and Medicine*, Vol. 41, Morris L. Barer (with T. R. Marmor and F. M. Morrison), "Health Care Reform in the United States: On the Road to Nowhere Again?" pp. 453–460, copyright 1995, with kind permission from Elsevier Science Ltd., The Boulevard, Langford Lane, Kidlington 0X5 1GB, UK.

cacy of national health insurance, suddenly and dramatically turned the attention of the nation's political commentators to the troubled state of American medicine.[1] Yet the very fact of Wofford's groundswell indicated how misleading conventional wisdom's earlier dismissal of national health insurance had been.

The nation's reporters—and many of its politicians—discovered what students of American politics had known for a decade or more. A remarkable consensus had emerged over the 1980s that American medical care, particularly its financing and insurance coverage, needed a major overhaul.

The critical unanimity on this point—what political sociologist Paul Starr rightly termed a "negative consensus"—bridged almost all the usual cleavages in American politics, between old and young, Democrats and Republicans, management and labor, the well-paid and the low-paid. Americans had come to spend more on and feel worse about medical care than our economic competitors, with nine out of ten (including Fortune 500 executives) telling pollsters that American medical care required substantial change. That was the good news for medical reformers, whether in Congress, among interest groups, or in what would become the Clinton administration.

The bad news for reformers was, as had been the case in earlier decades, a bitter truth. A consensus on the seriousness of American medical care problems did not signify agreement on the shape, magnitude, or priority of those problems. Nor did a negative consensus bring with it agreement on remedies. For a variety of ideological and institutional reasons, American politics makes it very difficult to coalesce around any acceptable policy solution. And this applies all the more particularly to a policy that would satisfy the requirements for a stable and workable system of financing and delivering modern medical care. No one has assurance that agreement on the seriousness of the nation's medical ills can generate the legislative support required for a substantively adequate and administratively workable program of reform. That understanding, however, was not

apparent to the enthusiasts President Clinton brought to the White House in January 1993.

The precise shape of the plan President Clinton proposed in October 1993 could not have been anticipated from his campaign promises. As a campaigner, he had understandably avoided the details of health reform or its implementation. As president, he had different obligations, opportunities, and risks. The product of his unprecedented Health Task Force was but the beginning of a furious debate that concentrated more on ideological name calling and mind-numbing claims than clarification of the substantive policy and political choices. Whether the president's plan, or adjustments to it, could have commanded a majority of Congress was made moot by the proposal's slow death in September 1994. This humiliating policy defeat has prompted a furious and continuing round of blaming, exculpatory rhetoric, and scholarly inquiry (including Fallows, 1995; Hacker, 1996; Mashaw & Marmor, 1996; Starr, 1995; Steinmo & Watts, 1995; White, 1995; Yankelovich, 1995). What is far less clear is the meaning of this defeat for the future of American health policy.

HISTORY: LESSON OR LAMENTATION?

The task of substantially changing the rules of American medical care is one of the most difficult any set of reformers faces. At four other moments in twentieth-century American politics, advocates of national health insurance and their presidential backers tried. In the Progressive era, during the New Deal, under President Truman, and during the early 1970s, many advocates thought universal health insurance was imminent only to be ultimately disappointed. In the 1990s, as earlier, entrenched interests helped block national health insurance by skillfully manipulating Americans' deepest fears to protect what they regarded as their interests. In 1993, to be sure, those interest groups seemed to be on the defensive; the time for sweeping reform appeared to have arrived. The president's speech of September 22, 1993, put the issue squarely on the legislative agenda and the initial public response to the call for "comprehensive" reform was favorable. But before the Clinton

---

[1]The details of how the Wofford election affected the coverage of national health insurance are provided and analyzed in Hacker (1996, Chapter 1).

administration and Congress could meet the challenges of workable reform, they had to resolve—or at least cope with—some of the nastiest ideological and budgetary conflicts available in American politics. And that proved impossible.

What might be learned by reviewing this and earlier efforts by presidents committed to reform, but faced with seemingly intractable problems of substance, symbol, and support? Those who do not learn the lessons of history, academics regularly say, are doomed to repeat past mistakes.

Progressive Frustration (1912–20)

Early in this century, reformers of the Progressive era were convinced that broadened medical insurance, financed and administered as social insurance, held the key to improved health, medical, and economic security. But theirs was an elite consensus, helped in the pre–World War I period by the apparent, but momentary, acquiescence of the American Medical Association. Yet, it turned out, there was nothing like a massive popular consensus on the need for change and, when the AMA turned against the idea, the reform movement withered. The transition during this period—from academic reform plans to Progressive state plans to political oblivion—was, as a number of historians[2] have made plain, bitterly disappointing to the reformers. A negative consensus on the need for change may be necessary in American politics. But it has not been a sufficient condition for the enactment of major reform programs in medical care or most other areas of American politics and policy.

The Lost Reform: Compulsory Health Insurance in the New Deal

The agony of the Great Depression opened up enormous opportunities for change in American domestic politics. President Franklin D. Roosevelt led the way,

commissioning expert group after expert group to take up reforms proposed for welfare, unemployment, agricultural failure, banking collapse, and the institutions of economic security more generally.

The opening for universal health insurance came in 1935 with the famous Committee on Economic Security (CES). A cabinet-level special committee, the CES took a year to review the circumstances of welfare, unemployment, child health, and old-age poverty and to arrive at a package of programmatic suggestions. They did their work with admirable skill and timeliness, fashioning workable ideas from a far-flung research investigation of various methods to resolve these difficult problems. Unemployment and welfare were the most pressing and obvious problems. Retirement benefits, though they have loomed much larger in subsequent decades, did not dominate their deliberations. With compulsory health insurance, President Roosevelt hesitated, worried that the presumed opposition of the American Medical Association and their ideological allies might jeopardize the success of the bulk of his social insurance reform package. So it was that the committee refrained from even formally studying health insurance reform, leaving that to congressional advocates. Over the next decade, those advocates, under the banner of successive Wagner-Murray-Dingell bills, would repeatedly but unsuccessfully attempt to generate majority support in Congress for national health insurance.[3]

From NHI to Medicare: The Dogged Retreat

President Truman's experience with national health insurance was no less frustrating. He fought the election battle of 1948 with national health insurance prominent among his proposals for a Fair Deal. But he faced, during the election and after, a barrage of ideological criticism that demonized national health insurance by linking it with socialism, communism, and the Soviet Union. After years of facing certain defeat in Congress, Truman turned his executive advisers to a

---

[2]For a summary of the debate over government health insurance from 1912 to 1920, see Burrow (1977). For an analysis of how organized medicine first embraced and then turned against compulsory health insurance, see Numbers (1978).

[3]The most comprehensive history of this phase of the American debate over compulsory health insurance is Hirshfield (1970).

more modest goal: a health insurance program for Social Security recipients that would in time (fourteen years) become the Medicare program of 1965. During Truman's presidency, the general public was, according to the polls, always supportive of government health insurance. But this support was neither deep nor informed; socialized medicine was a tag that scared many, enough so that no amount of presidential enthusiasm seemed adequate to generate majority support in Congress. Opposition from the conservative coalition of powerful southern Democrats and their ideological counterparts among the Republicans was enough to defeat every attempt at universal coverage—whether for all Americans or just those sixty-five and over.[4]

The fight over Medicare illustrates the conditions required for successful reform, even partial reform. Before the election of 1964, the conservative coalition remained formidable. The Democratic landslide of that year, however, swept away their key institutional bases of power: dilatory tactics symbolically represented by the Rules Committee, control of other key committees without threat from the Democratic caucus, and an ideological balance in Congress as a whole less liberal than Presidents Kennedy or Johnson. But the massive electoral shift of 1964 held a lesson for future reformers. A sufficient condition for reform proved to be the two-to-one Democratic majority in the House of Representatives. This was a margin large enough to contain within it an issue majority on Medicare. In retrospect, a Medicare majority might well have emerged incrementally from the narrow defeats of the early 1960s. The election of 1964 prevents us from ever knowing for sure whether such a development might have taken place at some later date.

The Nixon Years: Seeming Consensus, Undeniable Disappointment

By 1970, the controversial topic of health reform had shifted back from Medicare to national health insurance once again. Though it is difficult for many to remember, the striking feature of the 1970–74 period was the intense competition among proponents of different forms of universal health insurance. There was the catastrophic coverage proposal Senators Russell Long (D-LA) and Abraham Ribicoff (D-CT) advocated, the Kennedy–Corman bill that closely resembled Canada's universal health insurance program, and the Nixon administration's plan for mandated health insurance for employed Americans, known then as the Comprehensive Health Insurance Plan (CHIP).[5]

The lessons of this period were surely relevant to American circumstances in the early 1990s. There was stalemate over the reform proposals of the 1970s because shifting coalitions defeated every attempt at compromise—cycling negative majorities, we might say in political science. The majority that agreed on the need for reform consisted of factions committed to different proposals. The more modest proposals, like the Long–Ribicoff bill, seemed too limited to those who wanted to translate the negative consensus into universal, broad coverage. The proposal for employer-mandated insurance—similar in financing to what President Clinton in fact proposed later—seemed too indirect, incomplete, and incapable of cost control to those favoring more straightforward forms of national health insurance. Even Senator Kennedy, who moved away from his more ambitious version of national health insurance (the Kennedy–Corman bill) to a compromise plan that he and the powerful Ways and Means Committee Chairman Wilbur Mills could accept, was incapable of generating majority support among a coalition of liberal and conservative Democrats.

It is no wonder that many congressional figures from the 1970s were anxious to act once Clinton became president. They had come so close once—and with a Republican president (Nixon) in the White House. However, the cautionary point here is that the lessons of the 1970s are multiple and complicated, not single and simple. What might well have made sense then—namely, mandated, employment-based coverage—need not define the limit of what would be possible twenty years later. Indeed, sensibly sorting out the implications

---

[4]This is the story, told in considerable detail, in Marmor (1973).

[5]These plans were the subject of enormous journalistic and scholarly scrutiny; see Feder, Holohan, and Marmor (1980).

of more than two decades of frustration with partial reform was a major task facing advocates of universal health insurance in the early 1990s.

The Reform Task in 1992–94: Daunting But Do-able?

The lessons of history are never simple. What worked once may not, in changed circumstances, work again. What failed earlier may succeed later. And some constants in American politics are always relevant to lesson drawing. Consider the following regularities.

First, compulsory health insurance, whatever the details, is an ideologically controversial proposal that involves enormous symbolic, financial, and professional stakes. Such legislation does not emerge quietly or with broad bipartisan support, either here or elsewhere. Legislative success requires active presidential leadership, the commitment of an administration's political capital, and the exercise of all manner of persuasion and arm twisting. This President Roosevelt was unwilling to do in the New Deal and President Nixon refrained from doing in the early 1970s. President Johnson was fully willing to use all his legendary legislative energy in 1965, but the composition of Congress then hardly made it necessary. Giving priority to the Medicare bill (with H.R.1 and S.1 as the numerical symbols) represented President Johnson's determination as well as his concentration on Medicare as the legislative centerpiece of his administration's first year.

Second, the limits of political feasibility are far less distinct than Beltway commentators seem to recognize. Political constraints are real, but they do not submit to estimates as precise as the budgetary work of the Congressional Budget Office. For example, the Johnson administration, anxious to make sure its first step would be overwhelmingly acceptable in 1965, requested hospital benefits under Medicare only. But the oddest thing happened. A combination of liberals anxious to make the Medicare program broader and conservative Democrats wishing to head off step-by-step expansion later produced a wider reform than Johnson requested. Not only was physician insurance (what is now known as Part B) added to Medicare by the Ways and Means

Committee, but Medicaid emerged as part of an unexpected "three-layer cake." Accordingly, no one should assume that the substantive and ideological packages sent to Congress as health reform are fixed in stone. And no one should treat legislative outcomes, whether enactment or stalemate, as the purposeful achievements of skillful entrepreneurs. Such outcomes—or resultants—emerge from very complicated bargaining and are a challenge to explain or predict. The lesson is not that anything is possible, but rather that feasibility estimates must acknowledge considerable uncertainty (see Marmor, 1973, Chapter 6).

Third, the role of language and emotive symbols in this policy world cannot be overestimated. How a president reaches out to the public, what counts in the evening news and the morning newspapers as the central reform (or anti-reform) themes, and whether Congress faces a determined grassroots movement—all shape the legislative outcome and, even more important, whether the resultant is sufficiently coherent and implementable to satisfy the expectations for reform. Pressure groups that can prevail in quiet politics are far weaker in contexts of mass attention, as the American Medical Association learned to its regret in the Medicare battle of 1965.

But the central lesson of the past—of both defeats and victories like Medicare—is cautionary in a different sense. It is wise to wait if what is acceptable is not workable. It is foolish to hesitate if what is workable can be made acceptable. If the central elements of a workable plan are acceptable, the pace of implementation can be staggered. But American political history in this area shows that the opportunities for substantial reform are few and far between, precious enough to make their squandering close to a sin.

THE CLINTON REFORM EFFORT REVISITED

It all began with such marvelous intentions, back in the late 1992 U.S. postelection victory glow of the Clinton administration's agenda for the first ninety days. A federally crafted health care reform was finally going to lay to rest the ghosts of health-care-reform-efforts-past, along with the dual bugaboos of out-of-control costs and a large, growing, and embarrassing un- and under-insured population.

But as everyone who cares to know now knows, this road to reform was filled with potholes and poorly concealed land mines as in all efforts past; in September 1994, those traveling along it came to the precipice and turned back (Clymer, 1994). What went wrong, and what is likely to happen next?

To understand the failure of this particular initiative, one must first recall its origins and objectives. Two political imperatives justified the Clinton campaign's promise of reform and the White House mounting a serious effort to deliver it. The first was that the nation's health care costs were predicted, prior to Clinton's election, to reach 18 percent of GDP by the turn of the century (Burner et al., 1992). With the United States already spending far more than all the other advanced industrialized countries (Schieber et al., 1993), and the gap between it and the rest of its economic competitors getting larger, there was increasing concern about the (economic or opportunity) cost of health care costs. Additional resources going into health care meant less competitive American goods and services, lower exchange rates and more expensive imports, or lower American worker wages (Reinhardt, 1989; U.S. Congressional Budget Office, 1992). Health care had become, or at least seemed to be, a burden on general economic growth and prosperity.

The second imperative was the growing insecurity of middle-class America about the adequacy and stability of their health insurance. At any given point in time, approximately 15 percent of the population is without health insurance coverage (with many more having inadequate coverage) (Employee Benefits Research Institute, 1993). But that is a static and incomplete view of the extent of the predicament. Over any recent two-year period, as many as 50 million to 60 million Americans will have had the pleasure of experiencing life without health care coverage.

It was those *with* coverage, who wanted some assurance that they would be able to keep it and that it would be there when they needed it, who represented the potent political force. As the costs of coverage rose, more and more employers were eliminating or modifying the options they offered to their employees, and the private insurance sector was becoming increasingly adept at risk selecting and payment avoidance (Light, 1992). Not only could middle-class working families not be sure that their current coverage would still be there next year, or even next week, but they could be relatively sure that, if they had any health problems, switching jobs was likely to be a costly venture (insurance coverage is rarely, if ever, portable across carriers in the United States).

With these problems widely (if superficially) understood, Clinton's vision of reform expressed two key initial objectives: cost control and "health security" (or guaranteed lifetime insurance coverage for all Americans). The details of Clinton's strategy for achieving these objectives are now well known, and will not be repeated here. There has also been no shortage of blow-by-blow descriptions of the demise of this reform initiative. But there have been few attempts to date to sift the sense from the nonsense, the plausible from the improbable in those many pages of hand wringing and second-guessing that have fed the "Theory of the Month" club (*New York Times*, 1994). It is surely worth considering the claims and counterclaims about the size and placement of the most critical potholes, because such reflection holds the key to understanding what is likely to come next in the U.S. health reform soap opera.

One can usefully group the proffered reasons for failure into six categories: external events; timing; the policy itself; politics; communication/media coverage; and interests. These are not independent, as we will see. But in considering each, it is important to ask ourselves, "Absent this reason, or category of reasons, would we have new federal health care legislation in place today in the United States?" If the answer is "No," or "Probably not," then such individual elements may have been interesting sideshows, *but on their own* they were clearly not decisive. Of course, it is possible that a *collection* of individually unimportant reasons could, nevertheless, be critical. In the analysis that follows, we attempt to do some grouping of elements that appear to be intertwined in this way.

External Events

Closely tied to the "timing" reason is the argument that events beyond control of the Clinton administration (e.g., the fiasco in Somalia, the ongoing distraction of Bosnia) intervened at politically inopportune moments to suck the administration's (and the American public's) energy and attention from the health care reform effort.

Timing

There are two quite separate components to this argument—external and internal. The external version is simply that the recession (and the public concern about jobs, incomes, and employment-related health insurance) ended too soon. This in turn undermined a key source of reform pressure. It was this "premature" recovery that underpinned the Republican challenge to the very need for comprehensive reform. The "What Crisis?" campaign by the Republican leadership, on this view, cast doubt on the case for system overhaul at a critical juncture.

The internal version has to do with the policy development process itself. This argument has included many subthemes. But the dominant version characterizes the administration as squandering its "window of opportunity" by becoming mired in a complex, consultative, time-consuming development process. Why should careful policy development work against the chances of enactment? It is because such policy development takes time, thus giving opponents plenty of opportunity to mobilize their constituencies, refine their rebuttals, and search for allies.

The Policy Itself and the Legislative Process

The Health Security Act, 1,342 pages long, was arguably too complex and bureaucratically cumbersome to have any hope of being understood, let alone embraced by the general public. The proposal tried to find some middle ground that would satisfy both those who would have preferred a single-payer model of national health insurance with no role for the private insurance sector, and those who would have preferred nothing more than "life insurance reform." This strategy satisfied neither group and so, on this argument, was doomed to failure.

In the many arcane details of the American political process, the one legislative feature that some have presented as the key determinant of stalemate over reform is the necessity to obtain at least sixty votes in the Senate in order to overcome a possible filibuster. Had the health reform initiative been piggybacked onto the budget reconciliation bill, it would have required only a simple majority vote for passage. But the administration was unable to get the political support for this approach because of the opposition of a few key members of the Senate.

Electoral Politics

With Clinton's victory in 1992, and Democratic Party control of Congress, was supposed to come the end of policy gridlock in Washington (looking back, one might be excused for not having noticed any difference). The early version of this position was straightforward: the party seen as blocking health care reform would be doomed at the midterm (fall 1994) elections. However, as the process dragged on, as the Democrats failed to reach consensus on their own reform proposal (Rosenthal, 1994), and as the special interests made their influence felt on Congress and public opinion, the Republicans realized they could afford to drag their heels. By the summer of 1994, the official unofficial Republican Party position was that *no* Democratic proposal would see the light of day. And the Republicans had the votes to ensure that this was the case.

To be fair, the Republicans could not have carried out their agenda had it not been for divisions within the Democratic Party. One of the structural realities of American politics is that a partisan majority does not guarantee a *policy* majority. Democrats in Congress rarely stand united on a key policy issue, and this was particularly true during the health care reform debate. Policy solidarity takes a back seat in this process.

Communications/Media Coverage

There are two arguments here that initially appear to be in conflict. One is that the media did an abysmal job of providing informed, balanced analysis of the implications of the administration's plan to the public. Instead, the media treated the reform process as political theater in which who said what today was more important than a careful determination of the likely effects of the reforms on different subsets of real American people (Hamburger et al., 1994).

The second view is that the administration failed to recognize the critical importance of communication in "selling" its policy, and so gave short shrift to involving the press, particularly its Washington corps, in getting the message out. There was no "elevator speech" that could be delivered during the trip up to the fifth floor, and which captured the essence of the plan in a way easily understandable, and attractive, to the (wo)man on the street.

There is the temptation to argue that these cannot possibly both be true. After all, if the administration was unwilling to involve the press in the early stages of policy evolution, how could the press be taken to task for simply reporting on the congressional and committee mudslinging? Or, turning it around, if the administration knew how the media was likely to report on health care reform, how could it possibly entrust the same media with the inner details of the plan's logic and analysis?

In fact, our view is that both are to a large measure correct and that both could (and did) exist. The administration did make some early strategic errors in its failure to hone an "elevator speech" and in its interaction with the Washington press in particular (Fallows, 1995). But once details of the plan were public, there was in fact a dearth of informative reporting and analysis by the media. It is likely that the latter was a more critical determinant of the outcome.

Interests

While the media may not have done its job in sorting out for the public who would gain and who would lose as a result of the Clinton reform plan, those in the latter category were quick to recognize themselves and to mobilize. And the Clinton administration appears to have made some rather egregious errors in sizing up which interests could be counted on as allies, and which were likely to be opposed (Silver, 1995). What resulted may, in retrospect, turn out to have been one of the most effective public influence campaigns ever waged, even in America. It was clear from the outset who the winners and losers were likely to be. The uninsured and underinsured would be better off, at least in terms of insurance security, but also likely in terms of overall cost per family.

Despite the fact that the administration's plan left private insurance as the central player in providing coverage, it was likely that many smaller insurance companies (and those insurers unable to make the transition from fee-for-service to managed care) would have been shaken out of the market. Managed care was likely to take a big bite out of pharmaceutical company bottom lines, and to put downward pressure on (at least specialist) physician incomes. And malpractice reform would be a direct hit on the bottom line of many of the country's trial lawyers.

It was no surprise, then, that the Health Insurance Association of America (HIAA), the American Medical Association, and the Pharmaceutical Manufacturers Association jumped into the fray, early and often, and that, behind the scenes, lobbyists for associations such as the Trial Lawyers of America, the Life Underwriters, and the Health Underwriters were hard at work doing what they do best (and succeeding) (Franklin, 1995). The overall strategy appears to have been best captured by a line in the famous "Harry and Louise" ads sponsored by the HIAA. After anguished discussion about how the plan was going to remove their choice of physician and benefits, they conclude that "There has to be a better way." If the objective of the campaigns, littered in inaccuracies and half truths (*Consumer Reports*, 1994), was to sow seeds of doubt in the minds of the public, then it was wildly successful. And doubt was really all that was needed to scuttle the plan, because there was a dearth of easily digestible, and personally relevant, information being provided by the administration

(Lefebvre, 1994). This made it relatively easy for powerful congressional factions to succumb to the pressures of the lobbyists, knowing full well that doing so would not alienate their increasingly doubtful constituencies. There was also a ready political ear for those targeted campaigns. What the Republicans did not want, most of all, was a made-in-Democrat-country health reform bill (see "Politics," above).

Of course the media was largely complicitous because of the virtual absence of balanced, critical discussion, both of the issues and of the claims (see, e.g., Silver, 1995). In stark contrast to the media coverage of the O. J. Simpson murder case, the media (with few exceptions) did nothing to clear up the confusion created by the paid advertisements (Marmor, 1995).

THE CRITICAL FACTORS OF DEMISE

As we noted above, it is helpful in sifting through the various claims about the reasons for the failure of the Clinton plan (or even of any of the alternatives that came with a rush toward the end), to ask ourselves whether the absence of a particular reason would have meant a different outcome. In some cases, the answer seems relatively simple. For example, we believe that the first three categories—external events, the policy itself, and timing—were secondary at best. If there had not been these particular external events, there would have been others. The nature of politics (as with life itself) is that one never has the luxury of focusing on only one thing, and it would be naive of anyone to believe that the Clintons thought this would be possible or desirable.

As for the policy and the legislative process, despite its length and apparent complexity, one must recall that the details of the act were never meant for public consumption. The details of the American Social Security Act or the Environmental Protection Act are no less complex—little more than the titles are understood by the public—yet they became law. More important by far was the failure to communicate the key features (see below) and to effectively counter the vested interests' clever use of the media.

To sustain the external timing argument, one would have to believe that, had the United States remained in a recession, the plan, or a modification, would by now have been passed into law. There is no evidence of which we are aware that would support such a view. The internal timing arguments are equally difficult to support, requiring that quicker introduction, or introduction as part of the budget bill, would have resulted in passage. In this case that was possible, but unlikely.

But why unlikely? Because of the three other categories—politics, communication/media coverage, and interests. The American constitutional dispersion of power and authority, and the resulting labyrinthian political process, makes passage of much less complex and far-reaching initiatives exceedingly difficult. It is no surprise that American policy is shaped by incrementalism (Morone, 1986). Desperate times may call for desperate measures, but if such are not possible, well, maybe the times are not quite that desperate after all.

It may be, however, that the greatest single impediment to passage of this, or any other significant reform proposal, is the insidious interplay among the special interests, the public, and their elected politicians, through the media. Any major reform involves intent to change the distribution of costs and benefits; if it did not, it would not be reform. In health care, change invariably involves diffuse benefits and concentrated costs—a bit better insurance coverage for a whole lot of people, at the expense of lost or reduced incomes for those involved in the health insurance business; more integrated patient care (and perhaps even better patient outcomes) through managed care, at the expense of reduced pharmaceutical company revenues, fewer (and lower) specialist physician incomes, and fewer hospital-based incomes; less unnecessary defensive medicine and lower medical and legal costs, at the expense of the incomes of malpractice lawyers; and so on.

Those concentrated interests with the most to lose have far more powerful incentives to get their case across than does anyone to make the case for the effect of reform on the average American. And the calamities that are just around the corner if reform X is passed tend to fit much more closely with the sort of story that every editor of every daily newspaper or television news magazine admonishes his or her staff to seek out, than do careful analyses or dull interviews with pointy-headed experts. Most of the latter have already been done, at least once. They are no longer "fresh material," even if they are no less true today than when first run.

Furthermore, the vested interests have at their disposal resources that far outstrip the resources available to (or likely to be committed to) a "voice on the other side." Not only do those interests represent important sources of campaign funding in an environment where election (and reelection) is prohibitively costly (Silver, 1995), but they are also able to support academics promoting "friendly" proposals (*The Lancet*, 1993) and to engage high-priced and obviously quite effective help in the media influence game.

In sum, from where we sit, it appears that politics, media coverage, and interests were the critical factors in undermining this particular effort at significant reform, but these are not separable elements, and it is their interaction that produced the mix of discourse to which the American public was subjected. By November 1994, the American public, which had earlier been so supportive of health care system reform, was now "rejecting a major overhaul of the system" (Henry J. Kaiser Family Foundation, 1994). In the final analysis, disinformation and the spin-doctors won out again.

WOULD IT HAVE MATTERED ANYWAY?

We lose ourselves in such debates over the key reasons for policy development failure at our peril, for there is something more fundamental of which we should not lose sight. As we noted at the outset, two political imperatives drove the Clinton reform initiative—cost control and security of benefits—which leads us to a fundamental question: Would any plan passed in this latest round of health care reform frenzy have achieved either or both of these overarching objectives?

The administration understood that leaving the cost control piece to market forces, whether through managed competition or other mechanisms, was likely to fail (Aaron and Schwartz, 1993). That is why they built limits on premium increases into their proposal, as an explicit attempt to limit the rate of growth of funding, and thus expenditures. Yet very early in the debate, the interest in cost control simply disappeared. The "untouchable" piece of the Clinton plan was universal and lifelong coverage for some basic package of health care benefits; everything else was on the table.

And then even the untouchable became vulnerable. By the summer of 1994, universal coverage had given way to a willingness to accept coverage for 95 percent of Americans as "universal" (Goldberg et al., 1994). By early September, that number had slipped even farther, until it looked not a whole lot different from the unsatisfactory status quo (about 85 percent of the population covered) (Starr, 1994).

And therein lies a continuing and fundamental dilemma for U.S. health reform. The rest of the developed world figured out some time ago that providing universal coverage did not have to mean uncontrolled costs, and that controlling costs did not have to mean foregoing universal coverage. Those simple facts are still largely seen (or at least promoted) within U.S. health policy circles as fundamental contradictions, and for good reason. Those with the most to lose (see above) have compelling reasons (controlled costs = fewer/controlled incomes) to keep the confusion levels high.

In fact, there are a small number of beliefs, promoted by a small number of powerful special interests and embraced for political/ideological reasons by key members of Congress and the Senate, which seem to us to stand in the way of any health reform initiative that is likely to achieve cost control and universal coverage in the United States (Barer, 1995). The first of these, as noted above, is the firmly held belief that universal coverage will require additional revenue. There are good reasons to question this belief (Barer et al., 1994; Wolfe, 1993). The international evidence provides striking proof that the opposite can be true. Where the "made in America" analyses fall down is in their failure to take a population-based approach to estimating the impact of extending coverage to those presently without it.[6]

---

[6]In this, they succumb to the so-called Rand Experiment fallacy. A major finding of the Rand health insurance experiment was that those *in the sample* faced with user fees used less care than those having to pay no user fees, and that the higher the user fee, the less care was sought. Despite the fact

A second fundamental, perhaps even more deeply held, belief that stands as an impediment to successful reform is the notion that "big government" will mishandle it, or, taken the other way, that the private sector is more efficient at providing health insurance coverage than the public sector. This view continues to be promoted heavily by the private insurance sector, for obvious reasons. But that promotion is given weight by many American health economists, who seem (have) to believe fervently that private markets (the invisible guiding hand) must (by assumption) be able to respond to the preferences of a population far better than any government or public-sector structures.

Of course this view conveniently ignores the litany of evidence to the contrary (Friedman, 1991; Light, 1994), largely on the grounds that some additional private market reforms are all that stand between the current problems and health insurance nirvana. Yet it seems obvious to most interested observers outside the United States that much of the activity in which the U.S. private insurance sector engages is little more than waste motion—necessary only because of the peculiar ideological need (powerfully promoted, of course) to cling to the private market and support many corporate players. Risk pooling and community rating would eliminate the need for much of this busy work, but would, by definition, also eliminate many jobs and a lot of insurance company black ink.

Add to these the strong and enduring beliefs in the need to incorporate significant user fees in any reform package (presumably to control costs, but again in the face of compelling evidence to the contrary) and to hitch the funding of the system to place of employment (despite the complications and additional opposition

---

that the experiment precluded, by design, the extrapolation of such results to entire populations, generalizations have nevertheless become commonplace. The results of the experiment have been used to conclude that user fees can control costs, in spite of contrary population-based evidence from Canada, and the fundamental lack of logic in a conclusion that focuses exclusively on the demand side of this market.

Analyses of the effects of extending coverage in the United States have fallen into the same analytical quicksand: differences in service used by subpopulations with different degrees of insurance coverage have been extrapolated to estimate the global, population-based implications of extending coverage to all.

from the small business community so created), and one has a formidable set of structural impediments to any attempt at health care system reform. In the face of such a collection of strongly held beliefs, there seems to us to be little prospect of seeing either universal coverage or, even less likely, cost control in the United States any decade soon.

SO, WHAT WILL HAPPEN NEXT?

In keeping with the American approach to reform, there is a lot of incremental reform activity either in place or being actively considered. This is of three types: federal, state-initiated, or self-propelled (e.g., reform initiated by payers and providers).

Federal Activity

With the 1994 midterm elections, the Republican agenda came to the fore. The Republicans have all along had far less interest in extending coverage, and have argued (even if rhetorically, at times) that costs were not really a problem. Their major thrust in their first few months was to develop an agenda structured around downsizing the role of government. Given the prominence of government programs such as Social Security, Medicare, and Medicaid, we are far more likely to see efforts to shrink coverage (or at least the depth and breadth of benefits) than to expand those programs or create new ones (Iglehart, 1995).

With Clinton's reelection, he might be or may be expected to do what he has done throughout his political career—learn from his mistakes. He has invested considerable political capital in the health care reform effort; it seems unlikely that he would simply turn his back on that. However, any new Clinton-initiated federal reform plan probably would be far more incremental than the Health Security Act, and would involve key concessions to the major players noted above. In the end, any reform that can be supported by all the key interest groups is likely to be tepid at best, with its publicity value far exceeding any real benefits to the average American and most likely leaving the original two driving forces—rising costs and spotty and unreliable coverage—largely intact. For as Steinmo and Watts (1995) have noted, "America cannot pass major comprehensive health care reform that will control costs and offer complete coverage to all Americans because here political institutions are designed to prevent this kind of reform." (For a somewhat less pessimistic emphasis on the same structural barriers to action, see Mashaw and Marmor, 1996.)

State Reform: Spinning Gold from Straw?

Many political observers in the United States now feel that the best hope for significant reform lies at the state level, and that a few successes there will motivate a bandwagon effect. More than twenty years ago, Hawaii went out on a limb and implemented an employment-based health care system built around an employer mandate. Since then, many of the coverage gaps have been filled by supplemental programs, so that virtually all Hawaiians have health care coverage, and at a cost lower than, or comparable to, states with far less extensive coverage.

More recently, a few states have passed legislation that promises to increase coverage and control costs. However, these states, and any that follow in their path, face formidable obstacles (Mashaw & Marmor, 1996), of which the following are but a few:

(a) ERISA exemption: any state wishing to mandate all employers to provide health insurance to their employees requires a federal exemption from the Employment Retirement Income Security Act (ERISA) of 1974. No state has been granted an exemption in the past twenty years, and multistate businesses stand firmly behind ERISA because it allows self-insured employers freedom from state mandates.

(b) fiscal reality: state coffers are notoriously the first to feel the effects of a recession and the last to recover from one. Only now are they beginning to recover from the 1991 recession; in the meantime, the costs of education, justice, and Medicaid, which provides health care coverage for America's most indigent, have all continued to expand. Because of the widespread perception that further health care coverage extension will increase costs (see earlier discussion), this will be an extremely hard sell.

(c) interest group reality: all of the pressures to retain the status quo at the federal level also reside in the states, albeit unevenly distributed. New Jersey, for example, has a high concentration of pharmaceutical companies; Massachusetts and Texas are homes to major academic medical center complexes; Illinois is home to the American Medical Association, the national Blue Cross and Blue Shield Associations, and several major world-class teaching hospitals; and so on. The accounting reality, that cost control must imply income control or job loss, will be even more difficult to hide at the state than at the federal level.

(d) the limits of state policy: many of the key drivers of health care costs are not likely to come under state jurisdiction any time soon. For example, health care professionals are free to cross state borders, irrespective of where they were trained. Even if California chose to get really serious about cost control, and decided to reduce the intake of medical students to state schools, it would have no control over the size of the schools in Massachusetts or Texas. Similarly, the diffusion of expensive technology into clinical sites within a state are largely beyond the direct control of that state. Yet in the absence of control over those cost drivers, there is little hope for long-term cost control unless states are prepared to preside over forceful price and income control policies.

Market, Heal Thyself: Payers, Providers, and Pipe Dreams

And so we come to the last great hope: market reform through capitated health care, total integration, and cost control. Faithful followers of this approach claim that requiring physicians or physician groups to accept financial risk for their clinical decisions will bring both better quality care and lower costs.

Although it is true that some health maintenance organizations and long-standing large physician group practices have been successful in reducing unnecessary care and hospital utilization rates while increasing access to primary and preventive care services, the potential to replicate these successes tends to be grossly overestimated. The environmental and organizational forces required to extend the reach of such truly integrated health care minisystems quite simply do not exist in much of the United States. Many areas continue to be served by rural, solo, fee-for-service physicians, with no logical reason to change their circumstances, and in no position to be able to take on any significant level of financial risk bearing.

Furthermore, even moderate expansion of the reach of such integrated systems would still leave intact a largely patchwork system of coverage, with many opportunities for cost shifting and cream skimming. Where such opportunities exist, they will be taken. The route from individual mini- or microsystem cost control, to macrosystem-level cost control is neither obvious nor simple. But movements such as this need pay little heed to such mundane matters as aggregation fallacies. Nor is it in the interests of many of their disciples to promote such hidden truths.

At the same time, the insurance sector is becoming more vertically integrated by absorbing the managed care sector; this allows large insurers to be better positioned to benefit from a wider range of possible reform initiatives. This may not, in and of itself, be a bad thing. But will it bring cost control or universal coverage? We think not. What seems far more likely is that an increasing share of a still-increasing health care pot will be channeled to nonclinical activity, and this in a country that is already top-heavy in health care administration costs.

That is not to say that the bottom-up process of reform, which has begun and is gaining speed in some jurisdictions such as California, cannot succeed in achieving coverage extension and cost control. The route from here to there is simply not obvious, at least to these observers. So long as the vested interest groups control the political agenda and can continue so effectively and without opposition to sow the seeds of doubt that sup-

port the status quo, and so long as the "market metaphor" (Annas, 1995) with its "invisible hand" dominates thinking about health care, it will be virtually impossible to mobilize change.

In sum, while there are opportunities for incremental reform within both the public and private health care sectors, there are realistically now no opportunities in sight for major and meaningful advances in providing health care coverage to all Americans, or in reining in their runaway health care costs. Where glimmerings of success appear to emerge—where the market may actually be doing what proponents argue it can do, as exemplified in the recent slowing in pharmaceutical cost escalation relative to other sectors of the health care economy (Levit et al., 1994)—one can expect increasingly intense lobbying intended to undermine free market forces. Advocates of markets will be advocates only so long as the stylized, and often highly regulated markets in which they are accustomed to prospering, continue to serve their bottom lines.

REFORM AND UNDERSTANDING: THE ROLE OF POLITICAL SCIENCE

The role of political scientists (and political science) in the twentieth-century battles over universal health insurance is not a subject to which much attention has been paid. That, of course, is no reason to ignore it.

Until the Truman period, political scientists did not play a prominent intellectual role in the debate over what form, if any, government health insurance should play in the American version of a welfare state. The social insurance reformers of the Progressive era took their cues from Europe, especially Germany, and included in their numbers lawyers, public health figures, insurance experts, and what were then known as political economists. By the time of the New Deal, there were two major streams of intellectual commentary: those like I. S. Falk from public health and those like Witte, Perlman, and Epstein from the specialized arena of social insurance. At that time, many American universities, particularly land-grant ones, had within their economics, sociology, and history departments experts in social insurance. At the University of Wisconsin particularly, this expertise was transferred to state reform action (in unemployment insurance, for example) and to the New Deal reforms, where Witte was the executive director of the Committee on Economic Security.

The persistent clash over the Wagner-Murray-Dingell proposal for national health insurance between 1939 and 1948 brought health politics to country-wide media attention. And, in the wake of that, political scientists concerned with public opinion and the operation of pressure groups in American politics came to address national health insurance more directly. The American Medical Association, then the leading critic of "government medicine," expended considerable resources trying to defeat the Truman reform plan and became a prominent example of interest group exertion of power in America's fragmented political system. Stanley Kelley's *Professional Public Relations and Political Power* (1966) addressed this phenomenon directly, supplementing what had become the conventional explanation by journalists for why the United States, unlike most other industrial democracies, had rejected national health insurance.

Kelley's interest in the battles of the 1940s was supplemented by considerable attention to the long struggle over Medicare. Books by political scientists Eugene Feingold (1966), Judith Feder (1977), and Theodore Marmor (1973) addressed the origins, enactment, and early implementation in this controversial program of the Johnson years. But, for all the attention Medicare's legislative struggle generated, political scientists have largely ignored the administrative experience of that program and left the analysis of subsequent disputes over America's so-called health crisis to other fields. There are exceptions to be sure: Larry Brown's (1983) writing on the politics of the HMO movement, Jim Morone's work on health planning (1990), and Mark Peterson's (1993) focus on the health politics of the 1970s and 1980s, as well as Larry Jacobs' recent book (1993) comparing the political struggle over the NHS and Medicare. But the general point remains.

Economists particularly expanded into the health arena in the 1960s, following not surprisingly the expanded market for research on this growing industry. Whether this market development has illuminated our

policy issues is a controversial matter, but it would be surprising to find an essay, like Daniel Fox's (1979) critique of modern health economics, written on the role of political science in the past twenty years of health policy disputes.

The irony, however, is this. As we try to understand the fate of health reform in the 1990s, assumptions about political feasibility are central to the policymaking arguments made and their fate. Those who most regularly voice opinions about this matter tend not to be professional political scientists. Economists like Henry Aaron, Uwe Reinhardt, and Eli Ginzberg,[7] among many others, claim confidently that they know what American politics will and will not permit.

What is striking about such commentary is the thinness of the evidence on which such judgments are made. None of the economists cited have themselves studied the changing constraints of American politics. None of them have systematically investigated the role of public opinion in policymaking in ways, for example, illustrated by the work of Benjamin Page, Robert Shapiro, or Larry Jacobs. Yet the economist commentators appear to have no doubt that their judgments are more than conventional wisdom applied to an arena of politics that has confused even the most searching of scholars. I leave it to historians to wonder about why this should be the case.

There is, however, another side to the fate of health reform in the 1990s. A number of political scientists joined forces to comment on the claims and counterclaims about reform. Organized in reaction to the Jackson Hole Group and known informally as the "No Holes Group," these policy commentators are in fact largely political scientists. Their names will be familiar to those interested in the place of medical care in American political studies: Larry Brown of Columbia, Tom Oliver of Maryland, Jim Morone of Brown, Mark Peterson of Pittsburgh, Larry Jacobs of Minnesota, Christa Altenstetter of CUNY, David Wilsford of Georgia Tech, Deborah Stone of Brandeis, and myself. This group,

[7]For a specific critique of Ginzberg's reasoning about why national health insurance has failed to be enacted, see our chapter "American Health Politics: 1970–90" in Marmor (1994a).

augmented by a number of other sociologists, economists, and lawyers, represents the culmination of a development dating back to the late 1960s: the initiation of a Committee on Health Politics. From that beginning emerged the *Journal of Health Politics, Policy and Law* and a considerable amount of scholarship. What the No Holes Group illustrates is the movement from academic inquiry to a politically more active role, one illustrated not simply by published work, but congressional testimony, media appearances, and other forms of policy participation. Whether that shift in effort will be influential is something no one can be sure about at the time of this writing (summer 1995).

Conclusion

The American politics of universal health insurance was anomalous from the perspective of industrial democracies in the 1990s. Everywhere, it appeared, health reform, with different priorities, was on the agenda, but nowhere was the question of universal coverage in dispute. Cost control, concern about the quality of care, worry about responsiveness to citizen wishes, and the possibility of more efficient delivery and organization of care—all had the attention of national political elites in Japan, France, Holland, Sweden, Britain, Australia, and elsewhere. Because the entitlement to health insurance coverage had been settled earlier, these political battles differed from what took place in the United States, even though the rhetoric of common problems typically obscured this fact.

National health insurance as the reform objective suffered a crushing defeat in the summer of 1994. A kind of political amnesia came over the reporting of the subject. Where it had been one of the two or three most prominent topics on the Clinton administration's agenda during the 1993 and 1994 legislative sessions, universal health insurance disappeared from the president's messages and, with that, from much Washington commentary. But the reform of American medical care hardly died. Indeed, unprecedented change has taken place in the wake of the president's initial reform efforts and only more so since their demise.

In this respect, the stalemated politics of national health insurance had consequences far wider than those initially expected from the legislative battle. The Clinton administration sought to find common ground between liberal and conservative advocates of health reform. It adopted the language of market reform—"managed competition" was its initial slogan—and explicitly rejected universal health insurance on the model of Canada or as an expansion of Medicare (which was very close to the same thing). Instead, it sought the results of traditional health insurance while extolling the virtues of competitive plans vying for customers and bargaining hard with the providers of care. The result is that we have declining insurance coverage, enormous pressure to reduce costs from payers, and enormous uncertainty about what American medical care—or its public policy—will look like by the end of the twentieth century.

The lessons from this experience go beyond national health insurance, however. American politics are fragmented and the opportunities for substantial change are few and far between. What seems striking about the fate of the Clinton reform effort, in retrospect, was the strategy chosen and its unexpected consequences. The very window of opportunity opened up by the conjunction of presidential leadership, a negative elite and public consensus on the need for change, and the presence of energetic advocates let in surprising changes. In prospect, actors tried to adjust to the presumption that the Clinton plan would pass and did so by trying to adapt to its design features. In the wake of defeat, these very same actors had a headstart on change without an organized opposition. The states that tried to anticipate the Clinton program—like Kentucky, Florida, Minnesota, and Vermont—generated changes in the rules of medical organization and finance, but not the funds for universal coverage. The health insurance industry, particularly its largest firms, accelerated its departure from traditional indemnity plans into the role of "health management" companies. Even drug firms took up the banner of management, touting themselves as in the business of disease management. In this respect, the marketing and managerial ethos that dominated the Clinton administration's approach to selling national health insurance survived as their undeniable commitment to universal coverage collapsed. There have been few more ironic episodes in American politics in this or any other century.

REFERENCES

Aaron, Henry J., & William B. Schwartz. (1993). Managed competition: Little cost containment without budget limits. *Health Affairs, 12* (Suppl.), 204–215.

Annas, George J. (1995). Reframing the debate on health care reform by replacing our metaphors. *New England Journal of Medicine, 332* (March 16), 744.

Barer, Morris L. (1995). So near, and yet so far: A Canadian perspective on U.S. health reform. *Journal of Health Politics, Policy and Law, 20* (Summer), 463–476.

Barer, Morris L., Robert G. Evans, Matthew Holt, & J. Ian Morrison. (1994). It ain't necessarily so: The cost implications of health care reform in the United States. *Health Affairs, 13* (Fall), 88–99.

Barer, Morris L., Theodore R. Marmor, and Ellen M. Morrison. (1995). Health care reform in the United States: On the road to nowhere again? *Social Science and Medicine, 41* (4), 453–460.

Brown, Lawrence D. (1983). *Politics and health care organization: HMOs as federal policy.* Washington, D.C.: The Brookings Institution.

Burner, Sally T., Daniel R. Waldo, & David R. McKusick. (1992). National health expenditures projections through 2030. *Health Care Financing Review, 14* (Fall), 1–30.

Burrow, James. (1977). *Organized medicine in the Progressive Era: The move toward monopoly.* Baltimore, MD: Johns Hopkins University Press.

Clymer, Adam. (1994). National health program, president's greatest goal, declared dead in Congress. *New York Times* (September 27), A1.

Consumer Reports. (1994). Health-care hucksters: What their ads say—and don't say (February), 116.

Employee Benefits Research Institute. (1993). *Source of health insurance and characteristics of the uninsured* (Issue Brief No. 133). Washington, D.C.: Employee Benefits Research Institute.

Fallows, J. (1995). A triumph at misinformation. *Atlantic Monthly* (January 26).

Feder, Judith M. (1977). *Medicare: The politics of federal hospital insurance.* Lexington, MA: Lexington Books.

Feder, Judith, John Holahan, & Theodore R. Marmor. (Eds.). (1980). *National Health Insurance: Conflicting goals and policy choices.* Washington, D.C.: Urban Institute.

Feingold, Eugene. (1966). *Medicare: Policy and politics.* San Francisco: Chandler Publishing Co.

Feingold, Eugene. (1993). *The health of nations: Public opinion and the making of American and British health policy.* Ithaca, NY: Cornell University Press.

Fox, Daniel M. (1979). From reform to relativism: A history of economics and health care. *Milbank Memorial Fund Quarterly/Health and Society, 57* (3), 297–336.

Franklin, J. D. (1995). Tommy Boggs and the death of health care reform. *Washington Monthly* (April 31).

Friedman, Emily. (1991). Insurers under fire. *Health Management Quarterly, 13* (3), 23–27.

Goldberg, M., T. Marmor, & J. Mashaw. (1994). The odd jargon of the 95% promise. *Los Angeles Times* (Washington Edition) (August 4).

Hacker, Jacob. (1996). *The road to nowhere: The genesis of President Clinton's plan for national health insurance.* Princeton, NJ: Princeton University Press.

Hamburger, T., T. Marmor, & J. Meacham. (1994). What the death of health reform teaches us about the press. *Washington Monthly* (November).

Henry J. Kaiser Family Foundation. (1994). News release (November 15), 1.

Hirshfield, Daniel S. (1970). *The lost reform: The campaign for compulsory health insurance in the United States from 1932 to 1943.* Cambridge, MA: Harvard University Press.

Iglehart, John K. (1995). Republicans and the new politics of health care. *New England Journal of Medicine, 332* (April 6), 972–975.

Jacobs, Lawrence. (1993). *The health of nations: Public opinion and the making of American and British health policy.* Ithaca, NY: Cornell University Press.

Kelley, Stanley. (1966). *Professional public relations and political power.* Baltimore, MD: Johns Hopkins University Press.

Lancet, The. (1993). Editorial: U.S. health reforms: Clichés, cost and Mrs. C. *341* (March 27), 791–792.

Lefebvre, R. C. (1994). Health reform in the United States: A social marketing perspective. *Journal of Public Policy Marketing, 13,* 319.

Levit, Katherine R., Cathy A. Cowan, Helen C. Lazenby, Patricia A. McDonnell, Arthur L. Sensenig, Jean M. Stiller, & Darleen K. Won. (1994). National health spending trends, 1960–1993. *Health Affairs, 13* (Winter), 14–31.

Light, Donald W. (1992). The practice and ethics of risk-related health insurance. *Journal of the American Medical Association, 267* (May 13), 2503–2508.

Light, Donald W. (1994). Life, death and the insurance companies. *New England Journal of Medicine, 330* (February 17), 498–499.

Marmor, Theodore R. (1973). *The politics of Medicare.* Chicago: Aldine Publishing Company.

Marmor, Theodore R. (1994a). *Understanding health care reform.* New Haven: Yale University Press.

Marmor, Theodore R. (1994b). The politics of universal health insurance: Lessons from past administrations? (Symposium on national health insurance). *PS* (June), 194–198.

Marmor, Theodore R. (1995). Murder, mayhem and medical care reform. *Journal of Health Politics, Policy and Law, 20* (Summer), 817–819.

Mashaw, Jerry L., & Theodore R. Marmor. (1996). Can the American state guarantee access to health care? In Patricia Day, Daniel M. Fox, Robert Maxwell, & Ellie Scrivens (Eds.), *The state, politics and health: Essays for Rudolf Klein* (Chapter 5). Cambridge, MA, & Oxford, UK: Blackwell Publishers.

Morone, James A. (1986). Seven laws of policy analysis. *Journal of Policy Analysis Management, 5* (Summer), 817–819.

Morone, James A. (1990). *The democratic wish.* New York: Basic Books.

New York Times. (1994). Why health care fizzled: Too little time and too much politics (September 27).

Numbers, Ronald. (1978). *Almost persuaded: American physicians and compulsory health insurance, 1912–1920.* Baltimore: Johns Hopkins University Press.

Peterson, Mark A. (1931). Political influence in the 1990s: From iron triangles to policy that works. *Journal of Health Politics, Policy and Law, 18* (Summer), 395–437.

Reinhardt, Uwe E. (1989). Health care spending and American competitiveness. *Health Affairs, 8* (Fall), 5.

Rosenthal, Marilyn M. (1994). Whatever happened to the reform of American health policy? *British Medical Journal, 309* (November 26), 1383.

Schieber, George J., Jean-Pierre Poullier, & Leslie M. Greenwald. (1993). Health spending, delivery, and outcomes in OECD countries. *Health Affairs, 12* (Summer), 120–129.

Silver, George A. (1995). Topics for our times: Clausewitz vs. Sun Tzu—the art of health reform. *American Journal of Public Health, 85* (March), 307–308.

Starr, Paul. (1994). Reform is dead: Long live reform. *New York Times* (September 4), E11.

Starr, Paul. (1995). What happened to health care reform? *American Prospect, 20* (Winter), 20–31.

Steinmo, Sven, & Jon Watts. (1995). It's the institutions, stupid: Why comprehensive health reform always fails in America. *Journal of Health Politics, Policy and Law, 20* (Summer), 329–372.

U.S. Congressional Budget Office. (1992). *Economic implications of rising health care costs.* Washington, D.C.: U.S. Congressional Budget Office.

White, Joseph. (1995). The horses and the jumps: Comments on the health care reform steeplechase. *Journal of Health Politics, Policy and Law, 20* (Summer), 373–384.

Wolfe, Barbara L. (1993). Why changing the U.S. health care system is so difficult. *Social Science and Medicine, 36* (3), iii–vi.

Yankelovich, Daniel. (1995). The debate that wasn't: The public and the Clinton health care plan. In Henry J. Aaron (Ed.), *The problem that won't go away: Reforming U.S. health care financing* (Chapter 4). Washington, D.C.: The Brookings Institution.

CHAPTER

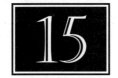

The Elderly and Health Politics: The "Coming of Age" of Aging

William P. Brandon and Dana Burr Bradley

Health politics and policy relating to the elderly involve the biological, social, and economic needs of elderly populations, their specification by the profession of gerontology, and the political expression of those needs.

Health care for the elderly is distinctive in part because aging issues resist narrow definition. In contrast, most other areas of U.S. health politics have historically focused on the provision of acute medical services. What this chapter calls the "aging-support" system incorporates major subdivisions of the health care system.

For example, long-term care and Medicare are leading topics in any review of health care subjects.

Yet the aging-support system also includes many social services that are not usually regarded as health considerations when one thinks about the health care of younger age groups. The principal legislation in the field, the Older Americans Act of 1965, makes coordination of services a primary goal. Although the aging-support system is far from perfect in integrating social and biomedical services, there is growing recognition of the interactions among such problems as social isolation, inadequate nutrition, depression, and failures of "compliance" with medical prescriptions. The emphasis placed on integration and coordination in the aging-support system contrasts with the failure to address the interconnections among problems and among health

The authors wish to thank the Metolina Medical Foundation for establishing the research fund that supported this research; Karen F. Honess, who served as our graduate research assistant; Dr. Gary R. Rassel of the UNCC department of political science, who provided important technical advice; and Dr. Leonard D. Ferenz, who commented on an earlier draft of the manuscript.

and social conditions in dealing with such issues as homelessness, drug addiction, and child abuse.

Finally, it is important to emphasize the great extent to which the elderly rely on family and on formal and informal social institutions with which they interact. It is a mistake to conceive of the aging-support system chiefly as a set of formal programs established by local, state, and national governments. Indeed, one requirement for sound elderly-related public policy is that it should not weaken these nongovernment supports, especially the informal interpersonal ones.

The scope of services and other support for the elderly must be varied because of the remarkable heterogeneity of those who are sixty-five or over (Haber & Gratton, 1994). The simple stereotypes regarding the elderly as poor or near-poor, frail, and bordering on mental incompetence are increasingly inappropriate. Many in this age group still work either for wages or as volunteers. Life expectancy continues to rise, which increases the number of frail elderly, but the average health status at specific ages is also improving. Gerontologists often deal with this diversity by dividing the elderly into subgroups of the young old (65–74), the old (75–84), and the oldest-old (85 and over). Beyond the issue of statistical averages, it is obvious that living longer gives one a chance for greater differentiation and individuation (Moody, 1986). More choices produce a broader array of consequences than those experienced by younger age groups. Therefore, specialists in aging policy emphasize the need for services and programs that recognize the diversity of the target population.

The emerging aging-support system has been generated within this century. For instance, there were no nursing homes, no public pension systems aside from veterans benefits, few private pensions, and little formal retirement as recently as eighty years ago (Haber, 1983; Quadagno, 1988).[1] New structures are arising and ideas of aging are likely to change radically in the first quarter of the next century. In terms of its social definition and institutional evolution, the aging-support system is

roughly where the acute medical care system, which had evolved out of a confused and heterogeneous amalgam of direct and indirect services, was a hundred years ago. Yet the system is changing, especially in the ways in which care is given. The rapid growth in the number of Americans who will be over sixty-five is likely to accelerate change in all aspects of the system.

The politics of aging involves three dimensions: societal understandings, institutional structures, and policy issues. After a brief general explanation of what is meant by societal understandings or meanings, we outline the chief institutional structures that determine public policy related to the elderly. An overview of salient policy issues follows. The conclusion compares aging policy and mainstream health policy.

SOCIETAL UNDERSTANDING

Nothing in biology or in other empirical observations determines the way that we think of life or its phases. At most, physical constraints provide limits for the societal understandings that develop in each culture. These societal understandings give meaning for both the individual and the community. They also structure the details in terms of which we live out our lives. For example, social and political structures like Social Security, private pensions, Medicare, nursing homes, and retirement communities emerged from our particular society's ways of thinking about aging and convictions regarding appropriate or desirable activities and environments for the elderly. Over time, these structures have become givens that guide the evolution of understandings common to our whole society, promote coherence of the values implicit in those understandings, and create an impression of inevitability and legitimacy around the empirical arrangements that they generate. At this level of analysis it is difficult to disentangle "subjective" from "objective," because one reinforces the other and changes in objective social institutions lead or follow changes in

---

[1] In 1910, only forty-nine private companies had pension plans; in 1925, the number had risen to 370. Military pensions, which only became common after the Civil War, were awarded to alleviate particular hardship and were not intended to be a general entitlement. President Theodore Roosevelt pro-

mulgated an executive order that defined age as a disability in 1904, thereby automatically making sixty-two-year-olds eligible for half disability; those sixty-five, for two-thirds disability; and those seventy, for full benefits (Haber, 1983, pp. 108–115).

subjective understandings (Winch, 1958, 1970; Brandon, 1982).

Several brief examples will help clarify the thesis that how we think of aging—and, therefore, the empirical reality that we also "objectively" experience—is a social creation (Estes, 1983). Perhaps the clearest example is the understanding of retirement as a natural phase of life. The idea of crossing a line in time or chronological age at which one stopped productive work altogether was not widely accepted in North America and England during much of the nineteenth century, although the nature of the work undertaken by elderly people might change as their physical powers waned (Quadagno, 1984, pp. 422–424, 436). Formal retirement depended upon the availability of pension schemes. Private pensions could become common only with the concentration of capital and profit produced by large-scale industrial enterprises. Industrialization reduced the heterogeneity of work that had allowed responsibilities in agriculture or traditional hand manufacturing to be altered to accommodate failing physical strength, eyesight, or mental ability (Kreps, 1971, pp. 40, 44; but see Quadagno, 1988, pp. 3–5). As late as 1940, when Social Security began paying benefits, about 40 percent of those sixty-five and over were "retired." By 1984, about 90 percent were "retired" (U.S. Bureau of the Census, 1942, 1986).[2]

Another example of the relation between social meanings and institutional structures is the nursing home, a physical dwelling associated with a way of life. It is easy to forget that the Kerr–Mills Act of 1960 and Medicaid (1965) virtually created the nursing home industry in this country (Brasfield, 1987). In contrast, some social welfare states like Sweden and the United Kingdom strive to keep elderly persons living in their own homes by providing home care and other services and by deemphasizing skilled nursing facilities (Zappolo & Sundstrom, 1989; Johnson, 1989; Jazwiecki & Schwab, 1989). Consequently, individuals in those societies may not experience the same feelings of guilt or failure or run the risks of financial ruin that often attend decisions in the United States regarding the entry of an elderly person into long-term care institutions. In recent years advocates for the elderly and policymakers in the United States have increased the scope, quality, and accessibility of community-based services to enhance the quality of life of the noninstitutionalized elderly and to help them continue living in the community.

The plasticity that makes it possible for different societies to evolve different patterns of living for their elderly is also illustrated by the formation in this country of powerful groups that articulate the political interests of the elderly. The United States began its universal social health insurance program,[3] Medicare, by covering the elderly who receive Social Security. In contrast, other industrial nations began government health coverage for workers and expanded it to the rest of society. During the fifteen years that it took to enact Medicare, proponents had to conceptualize retirees as a group who were uniquely needy, at least in regard to obtaining and paying for health care (Marmor, 1973).[4] This campaign eventually established the legitimacy of demands that society be responsible for providing health care for the elderly, although important insurgent voices have recently begun to question whether the affluent aged should pay more or receive fewer benefits. As we shall see in the section dealing with social structures, the effort to enact Medicare generated or strengthened many of the interest groups that have institutionalized a view of politics based on age cohorts in the United States. The age group to which an American belongs has now become a salient political cleavage, to use the language of political science.

---

[2]These statistics are based on the assumption that data about labor force activity for those sixty-five and over can be used to infer retirement patterns. Respondents, mostly women, who reported in the 1940 survey that they were "engaged in home housework" were considered to be retired. This interpretation is necessary to be consistent with the 1984 data. Males sixty-five and over had a retirement rate of 16 percent in 1940.

[3]Social insurance, which is contrasted with means-tested welfare programs, involves universal entitlement of some easily recognized group (see Brandon, 1992).

[4]The image of the elderly as poor and frail, if not actually sick, may still be the predominant image of the aged in America. Even professionals dealing with the elderly commonly intone the phrase "the elderly living on fixed incomes," despite the fact that the indexing of Social Security to the cost of living in 1972 made the elderly the largest class of Americans to have a major portion of their incomes protected against the ravages of inflation. But Haber and Gratton (1994, Chapter 5) suggest that the stereotypes are changing.

Because the parameters of health insurance were fixed by its initial circumstances, expansions of Medicare have mainly involved providing better protection for current beneficiaries rather than extending coverage to additional population groups. Even organizations like the Gray Panthers and Families U.S.A., which favor universal entitlement and explicitly reject the struggle of one age group against others, probably reinforce our society's tendency to organize around age-defined cohorts. Although the Gray Panthers eschews "ageist" principles (Kuhn, 1988; Gray Panthers, 1987, 13; Friedan, 1993, pp. 632–636), those who respond to its call for "empowerment" are preponderantly over sixty or retirees. This fact suggests that in reality it mobilizes subgroups of older Americans who otherwise might not become active on issues of aging support. In contrast, the elderly in other industrial nations are not organized as political or social pressure groups to such a great extent. Instead, the elderly in many European countries are incorporated into broad-based and socially active labor and political structures.

The fact of social plasticity makes us at least collectively responsible for the condition of the elderly in our society. This consideration is especially important in regard to the future of aging in America. The baby boomers (conventionally, those born from 1945 to 1960) have focused attention on, and often altered social values when they were young. Therefore, we should not expect them to fall passively into accepted twentieth-century patterns when they become old in the next century. The elderly will be far more numerous after 2015 than at any other time in U.S. history. Some research suggests that they may be healthier (Fries, 1980, 1983; Manton, 1982). As the first generation without any experience of the Depression and as the beneficiaries of private pensions and Social Security that increase with the cost of living,[5] as a group the baby boomers may be the most affluent cohort of elderly who have ever

lived. Of course, if they fail to save for retirement, or if significant inflation should occur, or if Social Security is altered, their economic future will be imperiled.

In his seminal *Centuries of Childhood*, the French historian Philippe Aries (1962, p. 22) wrote:

> It is as if, to every period of history, there corresponded a privileged age and a particular division of human life: "youth" is the privileged age of the seventeenth century, childhood of the nineteenth, adolescence of the twentieth.
>
> The variations from one century to another bear witness to the naive interpretation which public opinion has given, in each and every period, of its demographic structure, when it could not always form an objective idea of it.

It is not far-fetched to suggest that the twenty-first century may well be the century of old age and that our generation will be privileged simultaneously to explore and to invent a new kind of human experience. In other words, the new century may see the "coming of age" of aging.

INSTITUTIONAL STRUCTURES

Much of what government does that affects the elderly is conducted by parts of the federal government that are not organized specifically to deal with the needs of the elderly. In these arenas advocates of the aging clash, bargain, or cooperate with other groups representing a multitude of interests in society. Here, for example, aging interest groups encounter the significant substantive lobbying efforts of the American Medical Association, hospital interests, employers concerned about the costs of retirement benefits, and unions. For the next decade, the crucial issue of what kinds of support our society is willing and can afford to give the elderly who lack the personal finances to pay for themselves will be fought out in the generalist government bodies. Over the long term the relative power of the elderly and their advocates in relation to other interests will depend on the ability of the elderly, their families, and professionals working with the elderly to mobilize and to work together.

Yet a policy system that is entirely focused on the elderly has recently been created. In part, the system's components that are dedicated to elderly issues serve largely symbolic purposes; in part, they constitute ad-

---

[5]Recent research on inheritance in the United States also shows that the baby boomers will be the recipients of legacies estimated to be $10.4 trillion in total. This total will constitute the largest intergenerational transfer in U.S. history in nominal dollars. As a proportion of current income, however, the average of about $90,000 per recipient is 12 percent less than the proportion of income received by the boomers' parents (Avery & Renal, 1993a, 1993b; *Journal of Accounting*, 1994).

ministrative routines that are capable of reaching the elderly. The government structures established by Congress to respond to the needs of the elderly are a creation of the 1960s and early 1970s. The first Commissioner of Aging was not appointed until 1965. The first White House Conference on Aging was convened by the Kennedy administration in 1961. There have been three subsequent White House Conferences on Aging.[6] These conferences put issues relating to the elderly and aging in the media limelight and advance the political agenda of the elderly. The most recent White House Conference, which was the culmination of more than a year of grassroots town meetings and organizational preparation, was in 1995.

Interest groups representing the elderly were relatively weak as late as the first half of the 1970s (Pratt, 1976). By 1980, however, voices were beginning to be raised expressing concern that the elderly might become an organized political force of staggering proportions (Samuelson, 1978a, 1978b; Ossofsky, 1978). Their power was demonstrated when grassroots pressure by the elderly forced the repeal of the Medicare Catastrophic Coverage Act of 1988, the first rollback of a major social welfare program in American history (Brandon, 1991a, pp. 345–346; Thompson, 1990). Some voices from younger generations (Third Millennium, 1993) have suggested that chronological age might become a major division in U.S. politics, and the issue may grow under the pressures of fiscal constraints in the latter part of the 1990s. However, at mid-decade neither the elderly nor any anti-elderly groups had coalesced. Whether age will become a fundamental political demarcation or "cleavage" is an important subject that will be discussed later in this section.

The chief institutional features of the political landscape can usefully be divided into three categories: government entities, interest groups, and private service institutions. Government entities, the public sector, include government agencies like the Administration on Aging (AoA), congressional committees and subcommittees, and programs. Each state has its own structures. Programs like Social Security require bureaucratic structures—the Social Security Administra-

tion—to administer them and promote debate about related issues. For example, by the time Medicare was passed in 1965 after a fifteen-year effort, the Social Security Administration had produced a great deal of information supporting the need for government-financed medical care for the elderly. As activities, programs can also be the focus of political disagreements and controversy. For example, the new Republican congressional majority made Medicare funding a major issue in 1995.

Despite the existence of mammoth national programs like Social Security and Medicare, the states and localities are especially important in regard to policy and programs that affect the lives of elderly citizens (Bloksberg, 1989; Liebig, 1992). In the policymaking climate of the late 1970s and early 1980s, which emphasized decentralization and devolution, new state programs such as case management, tax incentives for caregivers, pharmaceutical assistance, and long-term care insurance regulation were created to benefit the elderly. Local governments, often with financial incentives from the state, also undertook new programs. The creation of new programs and services for the elderly cannot be attributed to the efforts of aging organizations or their memberships (Lammers & Liebig, 1990). Much of this service innovation was initiated because state-level policymakers were willing to raise taxes or find alternative sources of revenue.

Interest groups, which are often constituted as voluntary, not-for-profit corporations, are institutions that try to influence public entities. Like private institutions they also often provide significant services to their members. For many years the largest and therefore potentially the most powerful interest group—the American Association of Retired Persons (AARP)—served the information and insurance needs of a growing membership, but was not very active in influencing federal or state government. It did not even work actively for Medicare in 1965 (Pratt, 1976, pp. 90–91).

Finally, private institutions are those nonprofit nongovernmental or for-profit institutions that provide services to the elderly. They range from nursing homes and home health agencies and adult day care centers to more informal social groups that are composed mainly of the elderly. Many of the interactions between private

---

[6]President Bush declined to call one in 1991.

institutions and government involve government efforts to regulate the private sector. Consequently, private institutions commonly form interest groups designed to protect their interests. Examples are the American Association of Homes and Services for the Aging, the trade association representing the interests of approximately four thousand not-for-profit nursing homes, housing retirement communities, and health-related facilities, and the National Association for Home Care, a trade association of more than six thousand home health agencies, hospice, and home care aide businesses.

The pragmatic distinctions among governmental entities, interest groups, and private institutions are useful in ordering the discussion that follows, but should not be pressed too far. Private institutions often attempt to influence government actions, and interest groups receive significant revenue from the sale of services. Government entities are far from shy about trying to influence other government institutions or interest groups. Moreover, because institutional structures may change as the evolution of AARP mentioned above demonstrates, reclassification may sometimes be necessary.

Although our consideration of policymaking in the field of aging must begin by describing structures for making policy, the discussion is infused with the idea that policy usually results from many interactions along issues networks (Heclo, 1978). The understanding of policymaking as involving multiple issues networks contrasts with the conceptualization that policy is determined by a decision of a single powerful decision maker or by bargains made by bureaucrats in the executive branch who are charged with formulating and implementing policy in a particular policy domain, the congressional subcommittees that exercise legislative, budgetary, and oversight jurisdiction over it, and relevant interest groups (so-called subgovernments or iron triangles).[7] The issues networks model for understanding policy is more complex and fluid than other conceptions of policymaking.

Issues networks will vary from one specific issue or time period to another and therefore analysis must be more dependent on context. The networks are composed of individuals whose significance is often dependent on their institutional connections. Part of the evolution in Washington that has produced policy issues networks is the increasing numbers and influence of congressional staff and analysts in executive departments and nonprofit think tanks who communicate with each other and the media. The role of ideas is also important, for the growing acceptance of policy analysis as a rational approach to policymaking has at the very least forced traditional political bargaining to adopt a new vocabulary.

Yet issues networks are still grounded in the institutions that Americans have established to conduct their public and private business. Thus, any exploration of policymaking in regard to issues relating to aging and the elderly needs to begin with a discussion of the institutional matrix within which the policy networks function.

Government Entities

In the executive branch responsibility for government programs to aid the elderly is diffuse. Using 1978 data, Carroll Estes counted at least eighty different federal programs benefiting the elderly directly or indirectly through cash assistance, in-kind transfers, or direct provision of goods and services (Estes, 1983, pp. 77–82). These programs are scattered among six cabinet departments and seven independent agencies. Tax, regulatory, or employment policies would add to the number of programs benefiting the elderly. These programs affect those who give care to the elderly as well as the senior citizens who benefit. Thus, many of them have large constituencies.

In 1978, an outspoken advocate for the elderly, the late Representative Claude Pepper (1900–1989) (D-FL), who chaired the House Select Committee on the Aging (which was abolished in 1993), and a correspondent for the *National Journal* debated both the number and the value of programs that could be regarded as

---

[7]This traditional model of how policy is made in the United States by the stable interactions of congressional subcommittees, executive agency bureaucrats, and narrow interest groups is called a "subgovernment" to indicate its relative autonomy over a defined policy area, as if it were a government over a small stretch of the political landscape. Sometimes it is also called an "iron-triangle" to denote the stability and simplicity of the arrangements over time.

benefiting the elderly (Samuelson, 1978a, 1978b; Ossofsky, 1978). Their dispute vividly demonstrates the difficulty even in defining what programs belong to the aging-support system. It also focused on the question whether the elderly receive a disproportionate share of the gross domestic product in relation to their numbers or average economic status.

The confusion in determining the extent of federal aid to the elderly arises in part from the fact that the federal government is largely organized by function rather than according to beneficiaries or "clientele" groups.[8] Income security and health programs are examples of functional organization. Thus, the Social Security Administration handles old age, survivor, and disability insurance (OASDI) and the Supplemental Security Income program (SSI), which is a national means-tested program for low-income elderly, blind, and the totally disabled. The Health Care Financing Administration (HCFA) is responsible for Medicare, which is an entitlement of the eligible elderly, the disabled on Social Security, and renal dialysis patients, and for Medicaid, the means-tested federal–state program to provide health care to qualifying poor persons without regard to age. Medicaid has been particularly important for the elderly, their families, and their advocates, because it functions as the only significant government program to provide nursing home care. In 1993, for example, Medicaid paid for 52 percent of all nursing home care in the United States (Levit et al., 1994).

The Administration on Aging, which was established under the Older Americans Act of 1965 (PL 89-73), is more important as a symbol of national commitment than for its power as measured in money or staff. It is the apex of a decentralized network of agencies. Amendments to the OAA in 1973 helped codify an existing informal aging services delivery network by requiring states to establish planning and services areas to ensure that OAA funding would be funneled to strengthen local providers (Bradley, 1994, pp. 112–117, 214–217). The 1973 legislation also expanded the

scope of activities that can be undertaken by the aging network, which is composed of the AoA, State Agencies on Aging, the Area Agencies on Aging (AAAs), and other local agencies that receive OAA funding. Over 97 percent of the appropriated moneys are passed to other organizations and governments (U.S. Office of Management and Budget, 1994, 1995, 1996).

The Older Americans Act and its amendments have created a somewhat unusual intergovernment network of agencies, which are supported through a hybrid type of funding. It can be characterized as a prototypical New Federalism program in which the federal government provides funds in broadly defined block grants. It also resembles a categorical grant program due to the large number of detailed program requirements that restrict the actions of both state and area agencies on aging. Although permitted to deliver services themselves, state and area aging agencies are primarily designed to promote and coordinate services delivered by private institutions and other government entities. Overall, the increases in authorized funding for programs administered by the AoA have been modest and have never kept pace with the growth in responsibilities for the state and area agencies on aging (Chemlimsky, 1991). Even more striking is how inflation-adjusted expenditures have not kept up with price inflation (Figure 15-1).

Interest Groups

The administration, Congress, and organized groups representing interested parties largely determine federal policies relating to the aged. A quarter century ago Theodore Lowi could characterize the elderly as unorganized and apathetic and therefore powerless in the struggle to achieve Medicare (Lowi, 1969, p. 64). Nowadays, no one would describe the elderly in these terms. They successfully opposed administration proposals to cut Social Security benefits early in the Reagan presidency, influenced the great Social Security compromise of 1983, and forced the repeal of the 1988 expansion of Medicare that would have covered beneficiaries' catastrophic medical and drug expenses.

A brief survey of the principal organizations making up the nonprofit side of aging-related issues networks is necessary. Yet it should not be assumed that a large array

---

[8]The Departments of Agriculture, Commerce, Labor, and Veterans Affairs constitute exceptions to the generalization that federal programs are organized with reference to function rather than client group. After Republicans won control of Congress in November 1994, the House tried to abolish the Commerce Department.

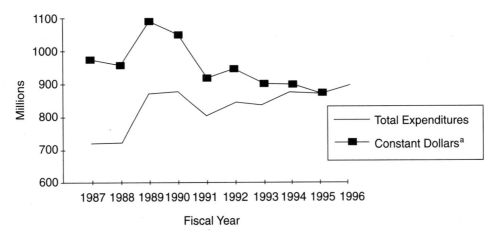

Figure 15–1 Administration on Aging Expenditures, 1987–96

SOURCE: U.S. Office of Management and Budget, Appendices to the Budget, 1987–96

[a]Adjusted to 1995 dollars using Implicit Price Deflator.

of groups organized around some issue means that they control policy relevant to the issue. Recent research (Salisbury, 1990) indicates that when there are many interest groups, they may to some extent cancel each other out, thereby leaving some space for the legislator or policymaker in the executive branch to exercise at least limited autonomy. There is also the possibility of a political backlash against the perceived success of interest groups in frustrating legislative reform. The 1994 Republican election victory, which resulted in the Democratic loss of control of both House and Senate, is attributed in part to voter disgust with "business as usual" in the capital. The charge that interest groups had too much influence over congressional Democrats was prominent in the election rhetoric.

At the national level, a Congress under Republican leadership for the first time in decades began to reconsider the major programs for the elderly and the liberal welfare state philosophy that underlies them. Many members wanted to reform national policy on aging to make it conform more closely to the budgetary and ideological priorities of Republican conservatives. The traditional aging-related interest groups, whether Republican or Democratic leaning, are unlikely to play a decisive role in the fundamental political reordering that is predicted to occur during the last years of the

1990s. The problems of funding entitlement programs for the elderly can no longer be viewed as separate from such national economic issues as balancing the budget, reducing the federal deficit, and capital investment to insure economic growth. In light of these changes, both liberal and conservative interest groups will fight for their constituents and will be influential, but not determinative, in any efforts to resolve elderly-related policy issues.

Mass Membership Organizations

Three membership organizations with more than a million members focus on advancing the interests of the elderly: the American Association of Retired Persons (AARP), with 33.6 million members in 1994–95; the National Committee to Preserve Social Security and Medicare (NCPSSM), which claimed to have 6 million members; and the National Council of Senior Citizens (NCSC), with 5 million members (Table 15-1).

The *American Association of Retired Persons (AARP)* was founded as a retired teachers' association in 1947 and prospered from the sale of life and health insurance to the elderly. It only began vigorously to try to exercise political influence in 1970 over the issue of control of the 1971 White House Conference on Aging (Pratt,

1976, pp. 145–153). Because it is the largest organization and is well funded from the sale of insurance and other services and government grants, it now sponsors a great deal of policy research and employs many lobbyists and policy analysts. It tends to work with Washington insiders in support of programs for the elderly. Although the membership is still slanted toward the middle and upper middle classes, many of its policy positions would benefit low-income elderly if enacted (Day, 1990, pp. 101, 122). Consequently, AARP was the chief target of the insurgent NCPSSM when AARP supported the Medicare catastrophic health insurance proposal in 1988. More recently, efforts were made by conservative Republicans in the 104th Congress to curtail AARP's eligibility to receive federal grants and to lobby (Stehle, 1995). In addition, its tax-exempt status has also been questioned. (NCSC has also been a target.) It should, however, be emphasized that unlike NCPSSM, NCSC, and the smaller ideological groups, AARP is nonpartisan and therefore does not make political contributions. AARP has incorporated the AARP Andrus Foundation, a 401(c)3 foundation that accepts gifts and bequests and uses them to fund research in aging policy and gerontology (Table 15-1). In 1993, it committed $1.7 million to academic research and "action demonstration projects" (American Association of Retired Persons Andrus Foundation, 1994).

The *National Committee to Preserve Social Security and Medicare (NCPSSM)* was founded in 1982 by James Roosevelt (1907–91), former congressman (D-CA) and son of President Franklin Delano Roosevelt. It originally seemed to be little more than a fundraising effort that scared senior citizens with misleading letters about threats to Social Security and Medicare to attract members and donations. The organization became a major irritant to AARP and the congressional elites responsible for passing the Medicare catastrophic legislation in 1988, when NCPSSM became the principal vehicle for

TABLE 15–1 Characteristics of Selected Elderly-Focused Nonprofit Interest Groups

Interest Group[a]	Year Founded	Membership 1994–95	Employees Spring 1995[b]	Revenue (Millions) 1994
American Association of Retired Persons	1958	33,600,000	1,200	469.0
American Society on Aging[c]	1954	10,000	28	2.9
Andrus Foundation	1968	N.R.	9	4.5[e]
Gerontological Society of America	1945	5,900	16	2.2
Gray Panthers	1970	40,000	5	0.31[e]
National Alliance of Senior Citizens	1974	100,000	3	2.0
National Association of Retired Federal Employees	1921	454,178	75	7.2
National Committee to Preserve Social Security and Medicare[f]	1982	6,000,000	75	38.9
National Council of Senior Citizens[g]	1961	5,000,000	140	86.2
National Council on Aging[c]	1950	7,000	105	42.0
Older Women's League	1980	20,000	14	1.5
Third Millennium[g]	1993	1,400	2	0.035
United Seniors Association	1991	400,000	N.A.	5.1[d]

SOURCES: Personal Communications from Diane Welsh (AARP), Marcia Freedman (ASA), Michael Berens (Andrus Foundation), Pam Dawson (GSA), Paula McKenzie (Gray Panthers), Peter Luciano (NASC), Imelda Clark (NARFE), Kristen Brennan (NCPSSM), Dan Schulder (NCSC), Louise Cleveland (NCOA), Vicki O'Reilly (OWL), Richard Thau (Third Millennium). Published materials: 1993 annual reports: Andrus Foundation, Gray Panthers, USA; 1994 annual reports: AARP, NARFE, NCOA, NCPSSM, NCSC; Brandon 1991, p. 341.

[a]Fiscal Year (FY) 1/1–12/31 except as noted.
[b]Full-time equivalent employees.
[c]FY 10/1–9/30.
[d]N.A. = not available, N.R. = not relevant.
[e]Data from 1993 annual report.
[f]FY 4/1–3/31.
[g]FY 7/1–6/30.

mobilizing seniors' discontent against the act. Since the act's repeal, the NCPSSM leadership and fundraising practices have changed in ways that make it somewhat less threatening to Washington insiders and more effective in lobbying. Its professional staff are increasingly part of the aging issues networks that determine policy in Washington as demonstrated by its admission in 1995 to membership in the Leadership Council of Aging Organizations, an umbrella group for centrist and liberal aging advocacy groups (Day, 1995). NCPSSM does not provide the level of member or community services that AARP or NCSC renders. Yet the costs of fundraising and administration amounted to one-third of its 1993–94 revenues. Its annual report (1994) claimed 6 million members, which should give it substantial political clout. However, that figure included many "supporters and spouses" since its $10 membership fee raised barely half of the income that would come from 6 million members (Brennan, 1995). NCPSSM has a political action committee (PAC), which spent over $1 million during an election cycle, with Democrats the primary beneficiaries (National Committee to Preserve Social Security and Medicare, n.d.; Oberlander, 1995).

The *National Council of Senior Citizens (NCSC)* began as Senior Citizens for Kennedy in 1960 under union aegis (Table 15-1). With additional aid from the Democratic National Committee the organization began to grow by developing local senior citizens clubs across the country. NCSC, as it became in 1961, focused almost entirely on Medicare until that legislation was enacted (Pratt, 1976, pp. 88–89). It still focuses on income security and health issues. Its unity of purpose, grassroots foundations in about 4,800 affiliated local clubs, access to AFL-CIO lobbying resources, and experience of coalition building made it a potent force in the debates about Social Security in the early 1980s.

In 1995, its annual report promised,

> NCSC can be counted on to work shoulder-to-shoulder with the AFL-CIO and its affiliated unions on a number of shared goals, chief among them being the protection of "entitlements," principally Social Security, Medicare and Medicaid. And, once again, we will join forces to oppose

the Balanced Budget Amendment, the lowering of the capital gains tax rates—which is nothing more than massive new tax cuts for the wealthy—and increased military spending (National Council of Senior Citizens, 1995).

It fulfilled these promises by organizing protests in hearings and outside the Capitol in 1995 when House Republicans tried to enact legislation to cut $270 billion from the Medicare program.

One the other hand, in its 1993–94 budget, over $81 million of its $86.2 million in revenues came from "grants and contracts from government agencies," which suggests the magnitude of the housing programs, employment programs for seniors in social and environmental services, and other programs that it provides. These funded activities make NCSC vulnerable to Republican efforts to attack the tax-exempt status and federal funding of organizations that use their non-government funds to advocate on behalf of their members and constituents. It also has a PAC (whose funds are raised from member contributions and are not included in its $86 million revenues), which gave contributions of $100,000 to $400,000 to support specific political candidates (almost all of whom were Democrats) and causes in election cycles during the first half of the 1990s.

Ideological Advocacy Groups

Among the organizations that are more interesting for their ideas than for the size of their memberships are the Gray Panthers, the Older Women' League (OWL), the National Alliance of Senior Citizens (NASC), and the United Seniors Association (USA). Whereas the first three were founded between 1970 and 1980, USA began in 1991. It is the clearest example of the new phenomenon of organizations established by Washington insiders using the latest high-tech direct mail marketing techniques to generate a high volume of contributions while building an advocacy organization from the top down (Nielsen, 1985, Chapter 3). Day (1990, pp. 78–79) claims that NASC and NCPSSM are also the creation of "direct mail political operations."

The *Gray Panthers* was founded in 1970 by six professional women facing forced retirement by their employers—nonprofit charitable, religious organizations and the United Nations (Kuhn, 1991, pp. 128–132). At the time, both custom and considerable legal sanction endorsed retirement at the arbitrary age of sixty-five. However, instead of accepting retirement, these six friends decided to change a system that in their view was unjust. By the end of the 1970s, the Gray Panthers had achieved considerable success in repealing retirement policies defined by chronological age (Long, n.d.). It continues to have a broad social justice agenda that transcends issues benefiting only the elderly and describes itself as an intergenerational group. In a signed editorial in its official newspaper *Network*, charismatic founder Maggie Kuhn (1988) proposed that the Gray Panthers should concentrate on organizing college campuses and urged local networks to have members of diverse ages. Yet despite this aspiration, the Gray Panthers focuses on the tasks of consciousness raising, empowering, and organizing the elderly. The organization has approximately forty thousand members and fifty chapters that are active in local grassroots networks (Table 15-1). Revenues in 1995 were a quarter of a million dollars, excluding some restricted endowment income. In the past, imaginative lobbying, protest activities, and network membership magnified its effectiveness beyond its numbers and its leadership sought to build coalitions with larger organizations. Its membership, however, fell by a third between 1989 and 1995 and revenues fell by two-thirds. The death of its founder in 1995 at the age of eighty-nine (Thomas, 1995) is likely to lead to problems and further change for the organization (see Kuhn, 1991, pp. 221-224).

The *Older Women's League (OWL)* is similar in many respects to the Gray Panthers. Founded ten years later, it had only twenty thousand members and claimed to have revenues of $1.5 million in 1994 (Table 15-1). Like the Gray Panthers, it has a broad-ranging liberal agenda focused on economic security (maintaining a non-means-tested Social Security indexed to the cost of living), a single-payer national universal health care system, housing, and antiviolence and antidiscrimina-

tion positions. As its name suggests, its special role is to advocate for the interests of middle-aged and older women. OWL is particularly sensitive to the need for more recognition and support for unpaid caregivers, a role that most often falls on middle-aged and older women.

The *National Alliance of Senior Citizens (NASC)* and the *United Senior Association (USA)* work for conservative political positions. Both opposed the Clinton health reform proposal, although it is impossible to judge the significance or vigor of their opposition. NASC, with one hundred thousand members but only three staff in 1995, appears to be the more established of the two (Table 15-1). It is in competition with AARP in selling insurance and other services to its members (National Alliance of Senior Citizens, 1994). USA, which was founded by the late Hollywood actor and former conservative Republican senator from California, George Murphy (1902–92), and conservative direct-mail guru Richard Viguerie, claimed to have four hundred thousand members and revenues of $5.1 million in 1993. In light of the large cost of direct-mail fundraising, some have dismissed the organization as the latest vehicle to enrich Viguerie's for-profit corporations (Hutcheson, 1995). Its staff is larger then that of NASC, but it does not attempt to provide insurance and other benefits for members. It seems, however, to be making something of an impression on the media. Its staffers appear to participate in the issues networks developed by the political right (United Seniors Association, n.d.; Day, 1995), which may make it influential in coming years.

The political orientation of the membership organizations is affected by their origins. Retirees from the professions, who often held conservative views, made up the bulk of AARP membership in its early years. It now has a broader membership and is more middle-of-the-road. Yet it must be careful about offending members, many of whom are more attracted to the services and information that it offers than to its ideological commitment. Thus, when its policy analysts at the center of the issues networks in Washington, D.C., get too far in front of its membership—as happened with the Medicare catastrophic health insurance act—the organization will suffer. In contrast to AARP, NCSC reflects the mainstream liberal outlook of the large proportion of its members, who are former union members, and of its leadership, which is predominantly composed of retired labor leaders. The Gray Panthers champions both the causes and methods of the 1960s. Thus, its newspaper agitates for racial equality, anti-ageism, peace, and universal health care through a national health service (or "socialized medicine"). OWL supports many of the same issues as the Gray Panthers, but with a greater feminist emphasis. Another large membership organization, the National Association of Retired Federal Employees, aggressively pursues the narrow self-interest of its approximately half million members on issues relating to federal retirement benefits without regard to political orientation. It lacks a broad agenda and is politically important only when federal benefits are threatened.

Although the political climate in America has become more conservative since the 1994 election, it is not certain that NASC or USA will become more influential. While some of the ideas that they espouse are currently popular in right-wing circles, there is little evidence that these organizations are opinion leaders. In the field of aging policy there is as yet no equivalent to the role that Ralph Reed and his Christian Coalition play in advancing the family values agenda.

Professional Associations and Resources

In addition to the elderly mass membership groups and the ideological advocacy groups, three other organizations provide the professional infrastructure that helps define aging and gerontology as a distinctive field. The Gerontological Society of America (GSA), the American Society on Aging (ASA), and the National Council on Aging (NCOA), the major professional and resource organizations in the United States, reflect the liberal mainstream views of the engaged professional social services and health workers. Each was founded between 1945 and 1954 and now has between five thousand and ten thousand members.

The *Gerontological Society of America (GSA)*, which publishes the *Gerontologist* and the *Journal of Gerontology*, is the main forum for academics who specialize in aging.[9] GSA's mission is "to promote the scientific study of aging, to encourage exchanges among researchers and practitioners . . . and to foster the use of gerontological research in forming public policy" (Gerontological Society of America, 1987). As the focus of mainstream professional and academic experience and an important element sustaining issues networks dealing with the elderly, it engages in research projects and "education" to inform government officials and interest groups about gerontological issues (Gerontological Society of America, 1987, pp. 1, 2). It also sponsors the most important annual meeting that brings together experts on aging issues. Its membership has decreased by about one thousand in the past six years after tripling between the mid-1970s and 1989 (Pratt, 1976, p. 87; Brandon, 1991; Rayazuddin, 1995) (Table 15-1).

The *American Society on Aging (ASA)*, in contrast, has experienced rapid growth to about ten thousand members during the first half of the 1990s (Table 15-1). The focus of ASA is on professional practitioners and advocates for the elderly, rather than on researchers and university-based teachers. It provides much of the professional education for practitioners and is active in providing public information on the aged, including its well-respected and readable quarterly journal, *Generations*. ASA leadership believes that recent membership growth is due to efforts to reach new and lower-income professionals in the field. ASA has also developed targeted sections within the organization that can function as specialty organizations.

The *National Council on Aging (NCOA)* is the nation's leading resource center in the field of aging. Its organizational and individual members are involved in all

---

[9]However, physicians who specialize in the medical field of geriatrics, the branch of medicine dealing with the pathology and physiology of aged patients, are likely to belong to the American Geriatrics Society (AGS). AGS, which was founded in 1942 and now has about six thousand members, publishes the *Journal of the American Geriatrics Society*. It is not a politically important interest group except in matters of relating to the medical field of geriatrics.

facets of aging issues networks. It engages in advocacy on national and state levels and also tries out new programs. For example, NCOA takes credit for developing Meals on Wheels into a national program. Its extensive programs require it to have a large annual budget, which amounted to $42 million in 1994, with almost $40 million in government grants and contracts (National Council on Aging, 1994) (Table 15-1). Many senior centers are affiliated with NCOA and provide some of its membership, but professionals and organizations that provide services to the elderly constitute much of its constituency.

Summary Discussion

This section has developed several themes. The emergence of an increasingly distinct aging-support system began with the development of government civil service pensions and Social Security. It became increasingly differentiated from other medical and social service programs during the fifteen-year campaign that followed the decision in 1951 to pursue social health insurance only for the elderly (Marmor, 1973, pp. 13–15). Nonetheless, federal agencies and congressional committees charged with the most important substantive decision making generally combine responsibility for aging-support issues with other domestic policy issues. In the aftermath of the 1994 congressional elections, the generalist structures of the federal government are especially important, because they alone must sort out the fundamental issues of what programs and beneficiaries will suffer the largest funding cuts and who benefits when new resources are parceled out. The interest groups that focus on the elderly have become increasingly strong in the past quarter century. They span a wide range of political outlooks and use diverse methods.

As the numbers of elderly grow, writers such as Phillip Longman (1987) have expressed fear that the elderly will become politically invincible. (See also Feldstein, 1988, pp. 199–204; Day, 1990, p. 35.) More recently, Third Millennium (1993), an advocacy and educational association representing Americans born after 1960, published a manifesto that, while explicitly eschewing generational war, calls for an end to short-sighted political decisions that mortgage their constituents' futures and the futures of *their* children in the next millennium. Increasing government debt and the growing costs of Social Security and Medicare are the principal issues that Third Millennium has targeted.

It is not clear how effective the elderly will be in protecting the entitlements that they have gained and in achieving further advantages from the political system. The elderly do vote in much greater percentages than other age groups. (In the 1994 House elections, voters sixty and over cast a quarter of the votes; *New York Times*, 1994.) Yet gerontologist Robert H. Binstock (1989) argues that the very diversity of the elderly keeps them from forming an effective voting bloc: "A person who celebrates an older birthday does not suddenly change a lifetime of political attachment, self-and group-identities and specific economic and social interests." Data from public opinion polls indicate that the political attitudes of the elderly are not noticeably different from those of other age groups (Day, 1990, pp. 36–62).

Diversity in the views of the elderly is increasingly registered by the proliferation of interest groups that purport to represent the elderly and increasing ideological disagreement among them. Yet, as noted earlier by Salisbury (1990), there is a "paradox" of interest groups: as more and more groups develop, they become increasingly ineffective. In part, their conflicting voices drown each other out. But when a plethora of interest groups contend against each other, the bureaucrat or politician is also left with a "political space" in which there is some freedom to maneuver and to make policy decisions that accord with considerations that government decision makers deem important.

This view of interest groups, which questions their power as organizations to determine the outcome of political issues, is consonant with the new emphasis on issues networks in understanding American political phenomena (Heclo, 1978; Day, 1990, pp. 97–98). When the organization's power as one side of the "iron triangle" of government bureaucrat, interest group, and congressional committee is undermined, individuals talking across these government institutions and other structures become important. Position papers and analytic studies by interest groups, along with the more important government reports and congressional hearings, are ways to legitimate ideas. In such a policy environment consensus about policies is built on conventional wisdom resulting from shared assumptions and the ideas of policy analysts. Machiavellian political manipulation and the threat or exercise of bald political power are less important in understanding how policy is made (Day, 1990, pp. 101–102). Thus, explanatory models based on bargaining from positions of political power, which characterized the iron triangle as a relatively definable and stable structure that is rooted in continuing realities of power, are generally considered to be less useful for understanding contemporary policymaking than the modern information model. Information models, however, are notoriously slippery, because they tend to dissolve distinctions between structure and process and to make each very context-dependent.

With this background we move to an examination of several important aging issues. In so doing, we use the framework of issue networks, government structures, interest groups, and private institutions to examine the security of retirement income, financing acute medical care, and the provision of long-term care.

POLICY ISSUES

Sometimes political elites and the average voter fail to discern the same broad fundamental issues. In the arena of aging policy, however, they currently identify the same issues. A Gallup poll of voters of all ages in June 1988 showed that "health care, retirement and long term care" were the most important family policy issues in that year's presidential campaign (Brandon, 1991). These issues remain salient. Over half of American workers express concern that they will not be able to afford retirement according to a 1993 Gallup Poll, with younger workers (18–49) voicing the most apprehension. Access to affordable health care and rising long-term care costs continue to concern Americans of all ages (Williams, 1994; Gallup & Saad, 1993).

Income Security

For most Americans, enjoying a comfortable retirement depends on the adequacy of a "three-legged stool," comprised of income from employer-sponsored retirement plans, personal savings, and Social Security. The Employee Retirement Income Security Act of 1974 (ERISA), which governs pensions and other benefits of employment in the private sector, requires vesting after five years and guarantees the financial security of private pension funds. The third stool, private savings amassed during prime working years, has long concerned economists, who point out that the average American has a very low rate of personal savings when compared to citizens of other advanced industrial states (Moynihan, 1988). Despite recent rhetoric from conservatives about the importance of personal rather than social responsibility and the development of such instruments as 401(k) plans that reward savings with tax benefits, it remains to be seen whether Americans will allot more of their discretionary incomes to savings and less to current consumption.

Social Security, which is the largest domestic government program in the United States, covers 90 percent of those sixty-five and over.[10] For most beneficiaries, it is their single largest source of income. Unlike most company pensions and personal savings, Social Security has been indexed since 1972 so that payments increase as the cost of living rises. The large reduction in poverty rates among older Americans since the 1960s is mainly due to increases in Social Security. In fact, eight out of ten older families would have fallen below the poverty line if Social Security were not indexed (U.S. Bureau of the Census, 1990). Thus, the long-term economic stability of Social Security is crucial, because it is the principal financial source of well-being for seniors and their families.

---

[10]Of course, many beneficiaries of Social Security are younger than sixty-five, since the law provides for early retirement with lower income and the provisions relating to survivors provide young dependents of a deceased eligible worker or retiree with an inflation-adjusted income until they are old enough to work or have begun college. Recipients of disability income may be of any age so long as they have worked long enough to qualify for Social Security and have met the two-year waiting period.

One of the major achievements of the 1980s was the eleventh-hour cooperation among Congress, the president, and major private interests that corrected a significant imbalance between revenues and expenditures in the Social Security trust funds. The agreement was reached by an important process. It involved establishing a bipartisan National Commission on Social Security Reform (which was also known as the Greenspan Commission after its chairman, Alan Greenspan). Like other commissions organized during the Reagan administration to work out compromises between apparently implacable opponents, this bipartisan commission allowed the president to back away from his seemingly intransigent public opposition to the Democratic Congress without angering supporters on the political right. The political cover was also important to members of Congress. The commission's proposed compromise shielded them from Social Security beneficiaries who were upset about the one-time postponement of a cost-of-living allowance (COLA), from federal employees and retirees who were angry that new civil servants would have to enroll in Social Security, from taxpayers who would have to pay more in payroll taxes, and from other disgruntled interests such as AARP (Light, 1985, pp. 198–203). Although the National Commission on Social Security Reform (1983) played a prominent role, it was behind-the-scenes negotiations between David Stockman (President Reagan's director of the Office of Management and Budget) and Robert M. Ball (a mainstream liberal who had served as commissioner of Social Security from 1962 to 1973) that forged the final bipartisan, intergenerational compromise (Achenbaum, 1986, p. 86; Moynihan, 1988).

The compromise, which was enacted as the Social Security Amendments of 1983 by a vote of 282–148 in the House of Representatives and 88–11 in the Senate, was designed to create a $5.5 trillion reserve fund by the year 2025 that will make Social Security financially sound well into the next century.

However, the existence of burgeoning reserves in the Social Security trust funds since 1983 instead of the rapid decline experienced in the earlier decade has generated its own political controversy. The issue is whether the growing Social Security trust funds should be regarded as part of the annual federal budget or separate (Dattalo, 1992, pp. 377–379). If the budget includes the revenue of the Social Security trust funds, the federal deficit appears smaller. Yet to exclude this major revenue source gives an inappropriate picture of the proportion of the national wealth that is going to government and makes the deficit appear to be worse than it actually is. Senator Daniel Moynihan (D-NY) has been particularly strong in rejecting the use of the Social Security trust funds to mask current federal revenue shortfalls, which he charges violates the program's integrity (Moynihan, 1990, p. 13).

When the baby boomers retire (from about 2010 to 2030), their Social Security benefits will be supported by a relatively smaller workforce paying payroll taxes. A prefunded surplus allows the Social Security system to shift some of the retirement burden from future workers to the current generation of workers (National Academy on Aging, 1995). Recent analysis indicates that the Old Age and Survivor Insurance Trust Fund (OASI) can pay benefits until 2030 without expenditures exceeding revenues, whereas the Disability Insurance (DI) fund will be in a deficit situation by about 2016 (Federal Old Age and Survivor Insurance Trust Fund and Disability Insurance Trust Fund Board of Trustees, 1995, pp. 27–28).

One simple way to strengthen the balances in all the trust funds is to again raise the age at which retirees will receive full benefits. Increasing the accepted retirement age will keep people working and contributing payroll taxes longer and reduce the period during which they will receive benefits. However, raising the normal retirement age has the potential disadvantage of producing greater alienation among younger workers, many of whom are already skeptical about ever receiving any return from the contributions that they are forced to pay to Social Security (Bernstein, 1995; Third Millennium, 1993).

Acute Health Care

To the surprise of many observers, acute medical care for the elderly became a vexed issue in the mid-1990s. As recently as five years ago, the principle of federal responsibility to provide health care and the necessity of federal oversight of programs to insure that health care reached the elderly seemed beyond question. Indeed, according to the Washington cliché, Medicare was the third rail of politics—"touch it and you die." The similarity between Medicare and the electrified middle rail of a New York subway was dramatized for Congress by the backlash generated when it enacted the Medicare catastrophic coverage health insurance act in 1988. Had the act not been repealed, it would have greatly improved Medicare coverage but would have required that the elderly, especially the affluent elderly, pay for the sickness benefits.[11]

Ostensibly, reform of Medicare and Medicaid moved onto the congressional agenda in 1995 as part of the effort to balance the federal budget and reduce the public deficit. These were important provisions in the Republican's "Contract with America," a campaign document developed by Congressman Newt Gingrich (R-GA) that defined the policy goals and ideology of many Republican members of Congress during the elections of 1994. Many of these conservatives, however, wanted to use budget issues to alter the fundamental relationship between the federal government and the states. Specifically, some saw the nation's budget difficulties, which were certainly exacerbated but not necessarily caused by the health care programs, as an opportunity to attack so-called entitlements.

Entitlements have come to mean the nationally mandated programs that individuals must be given if they meet eligibility qualifications. Thus, an entitlement in this context is a legally enforceable right. While some other countries do guarantee their populations broad social rights as a fundamental right of citizenship, there is no blanket constitutional right to health care in the United States as there is a legal right to freedom of speech, religion, and the other civil rights. A number of statutes, however, have given guarantees that particular groups of Americans will enjoy what are sometimes called "social rights," such as health care or retirement pensions.

In complex democratic industrial and postindustrial societies the overall structure of social programs that insure a minimal level of material support for everyone is commonly called the "welfare state." For example, some U.S. programs reaching a broad spectrum of the population, such as Social Security and Medicare, are part of the modern welfare state. The United States began to create a welfare state with FDR's New Deal. Yet the United States never really became a full-fledged welfare state, as demonstrated most recently by the defeat of President Clinton's effort to secure the full benefits of access to modern health care for all citizens.[12] The initial attack on entitlements has concentrated on Medicare and Medicaid rather than on the pension funds. These smaller programs may be more vulnerable than the giant Social Security program, because they are newer and have had greater financial difficulties in recent years. This attack on existing, limited entitlements to health care, then, may portend only the opening battle against those who want the United States to achieve a more complete welfare state or at least to maintain the admittedly imperfect social welfare institutions that are already in place.

Medicare

The immediate occasion for attention to Medicare was the report of the board of trustees of the Federal Hospital Insurance Trust Fund (1995), which predicted bankruptcy by 2002, with high- and low-cost estimates projecting bankruptcy in 2001 and 2006, respectively, if nothing more was done to alter revenues or spending. While Part B, which pays for doctors' fees and is financed from general federal revenues and a premium paid by beneficiaries, also experienced sharply rising costs during the first half of the decade, its sources of financing cannot become bankrupt. Over the years each annual report of the trustees has predicted the impending exhaustion of the hospital insurance trust

---

[11]For additional discussion on the Medicare Catastrophic Coverage Act of 1988 and its aftermath, see Brandon (1991, pp. 344–347).

[12]Although the typical array of U.S. programs and entitlements provide cash and other benefits for low-income individuals, the general notion of the "welfare state" is much more comprehensive than the narrow American use of "welfare" to mean the often punitive means-tested income and health care programs for limited numbers of the poor.

fund. For example, as late as the mid-1980s, deficits in the Part A trust fund were expected early in the 1990s (Board of Trustees, Federal Hospital Insurance Trust Fund, 1988; Brandon, 1991, p. 344). Thus, it should not have been startling news when the trustees repeated earlier warnings of impending financial problems.

Medicare Part A bankruptcy kept retreating into the future partly due to the considerable success of efforts initiated in the 1980s to reduce the rate of increase in Medicare costs. Implementation of the prospective payment system (PPS), which uses diagnosis-related groups (DRGs) to pay hospitals a flat fee depending on a patient's diagnosis, reduced Medicare costs and permitted efficiencies in hospital management (Russell, 1989). After establishing long-term programs to bring hospital payments under control, Congress focused on Medicare Part B payments to doctors. In the late 1980s, HCFA supported the development of the resource-based relative value system, a fee schedule designed to shift incentives toward primary care rather than specialty care and reward cognitive activities by providers over procedures (e.g., more X-rays, tests, etc.).

These changes in paying hospitals and doctors essentially nationalized health care finance in America, whereas previously each locality had its own cost structures that had been carefully preserved by Medicare. In consequence, the administration and Congress created a ready handle that allowed them to control federal Medicare payments throughout the country. These payment mechanisms have made it much easier for the Republican-dominated Congress to implement cuts in Medicare. Ironically, both of these centralizing reimbursement reforms were inaugurated and implementation at least begun with the support of Republican administrations whose rhetoric favored decreasing federal power and increasing state and local responsibility over government programs.

Proposals to improve Medicare's balance sheets include expanding revenue (by increasing Medicare Part B premiums, with wealthier beneficiaries paying more), reducing expenditures by cutting provider reimbursement, fostering membership in managed care programs, and creation of "medical savings accounts" (Rubin, 1995; Fraley, 1995a). The latter would allow elderly in-

dividuals to receive a lump sum for Medicare that would be used to purchase a catastrophic insurance or HMO membership and pay for co-payments, deductibles, and other health care expenses. Any surplus at the end of the year could be kept for future health care expenses or used by the elderly for other purposes.

Of particular concern to those who wish to insure that the elderly poor continue to receive health care have been congressional efforts to end the federal requirement that state Medicaid programs pay co-insurance, deductibles, and Part B premiums for low-income elderly. Linking Medicare and Medicaid in this manner has enabled low-income elderly to use the same doctors and other health care providers that serve middle-income elderly (Fraley, 1995b, p. 3540).

The principal purpose of these proposed changes is to wring very large savings out of federal payments for health care. However, the elimination of the Medicaid–Medicare dual eligibility entitlement and the creation of alternative arrangements would make fundamental changes in the traditional Medicare indemnity program as it has existed for the past thirty years. Creating medical savings accounts and more attractive managed care options may result in separating low-risk individuals from older, sick, and higher-risk elderly who are unable or unwilling to leave established relationships with health care providers. It may also lead to the development of delivery networks that cater to the elderly who wish to purchase more care than the basic Medicare program allows. If different levels of risk begin to separate out—and especially if individuals with lower risks or their insurers are rewarded by receiving some part of what Medicare does not have to spend on them—total Medicare costs could actually rise. This seemingly counterintuitive result is likely to occur because what Medicare currently spends on low users helps cover those with large medical expenses (since in most places full-fledged managed care is not yet a significant factor in covering the Medicare population). If significant financial incentives are returned to the low utilizers and their insurers, there will be less left to cover those needing more medical care. Moreover, Republicans in the 104th Congress proposed a fail-safe budget mechanism that would reduce payments to physicians who treat patients in traditional Medicare, if budget reduction targets were not met. With such changes, it is possible that managed care and medical savings accounts would provide care for the relatively healthy and affluent and that a residual health care system composed of more marginal providers, hospital outpatient clinics, and emergency rooms would provide a different type of medicine to sicker, elderly, and less affluent patients.

Despite all the proposed changes that have a fair measure of support in Congress, Medicare is certain to continue to exist as a national program with many elements of the traditional Medicare program. Continuity and some level of stability seem assured, because Medicare serves a broad cross-section of elderly Americans and is one of the principal programs that many of the elderly interest groups discussed in the previous section have vowed to defend. Medicaid, however, is quite a different story.

Medicaid

Medicaid has been a joint federal–state program for which Washington pays 50 percent or more of the program costs and stipulates federal regulations that specify core eligibility and basic benefits that ensure a basic uniformity throughout the United States. The states are charged with administering Medicaid, so each state program is different. States also have the option of including additional categories of recipients and may choose to cover additional services; these expanded Medicaid programs receive the same proportion of federal cost sharing.

There are significant disparities between the reality of Medicaid and the popular perception of it. The perception that Medicaid is a program for single mothers on welfare and their children ignores the fact that almost 70 percent of Medicaid spending is for care of senior citizens and the disabled. (It is, however, true that more than 70 percent of *individuals* who are beneficiaries are under sixty-five years old.) The somewhat more sophisticated understanding that Medicaid is important for the elderly because it provides the bulk of long-term care is true, but it overlooks the fact that *half* of Medicaid payments for care of elderly and disabled pa-

tients are spent for *acute health care services*. HCFA Administrator Bruce C. Vladeck dramatizes this reality with the slogan "Medicaid serves . . . as Medicare's safety net" (Vladeck & Davenport, 1995).

As part of the attack on entitlements, conservative congressional sentiment in the 104th Congress favored giving the states the power to determine what kind of Medicaid programs to provide. Federal payments would continue, but would be converted to a block grant, capped at a fixed dollar amount calculated according to funding formulas,[13] in place of the current open-ended promise to pay a given percentage of state costs. While some members of Congress wanted to end federal mandates entirely, at least in the crucial area of nursing home regulation, the federal government remains responsible for specifying detailed standards that require nursing homes to provide decent quality of care. States would be required to enforce these standards on the nursing homes within their jurisdiction as a condition of receiving federal Medicaid funds, although it is possible that Congress will leave the formal standards in place without requiring enforcement mechanisms (Rovner, 1995; Cotton, 1995; Rubin, 1995; Fraley, 1995b).

In addition to paying co-payments, deductibles, and Medicare Part B premiums for low-income elderly (discussed in the Medicare section above), Medicaid picks up the cost of eyeglasses, hearing aids, and prescription drugs for low-income seniors. Without access to drugs, glasses, and hearing aids, much of the medical care reimbursed by Medicare will do the patient little good. Many of the more affluent elderly have "medigap" health policies—private insurance that picks up the costs of health care and health-related services that Medicare does not cover. However, such medigap policies are unaffordable for the typical low-income retiree, for whom Social Security is the chief source of income. For example, the most generous medigap insurance in Ohio cost $1,122 in the mid-1990s and yet provided less complete coverage than Medicaid (Vladeck & Davenport, 1995).

Policy analysts and legislators should not be fooled by the fact that as an age cohort the economic status of

---

[13]States would be allowed to choose between two formulas.

the elderly has improved greatly since the middle of the century. Social Security and Medicare have performed magnificently in raising many poor elderly to a point above privation, but the consequence is that many live only slightly above the federal poverty level. Almost a quarter of Americans over sixty-five survive on incomes below 125 percent of the poverty line and 15 percent are still below that level. Women without partners and older seniors are especially prone to fall below the poverty level (Vladeck & Davenport, 1995). This age group is also especially likely to have cascading medical problems, which are exacerbated by social isolation. Those wishing to reduce Medicaid spending and re-structure Medicare for budgetary reasons may, perhaps inadvertently, destroy the Medicaid safety net that sup-ports the basic health benefits of Medicare for these needy and deserving beneficiaries.

Summary Discussion

Will conservatives dismantle the half-completed ef-forts to insure that society provides all Americans with a modicum of social welfare? Or has the high tide of conservative reform been recorded at mid-decade? The rate of increase in federal health expenditures will surely be cut, but will the basic federal responsibility for most health programs continue? Although it is impossible to answer these questions definitively, there is a useful his-torical parallel that may provide insight into develop-ments later in the decade.

The first budget prepared by the Reagan adminis-tration in 1981 embodied the principal elements of the "Reagan revolution"—returning power to the states by substituting block grants to the states for categorical grants, cutting federal taxes, and reducing federal ex-penditures. Income taxes were reduced; many federal mandates were eliminated or reduced; a number of cat-egorical programs were shifted to block grants; and fed-eral spending for most domestic programs was cut, al-though not by the amounts that fiscal conservatives in the administration desired (Stockman, 1986, pp. 135–158, et seq.). However, the Reagan administration failed to achieve its goals in one area: the health-related pro-grams. A young congressman, Henry Waxman (D-CA),

frustrated the administration's effort to shift much of the responsibility for health to the states. In order to maintain the principle of federal responsibility he had to accept cuts in federal expenditures for health care programs. However, as congressional elections loomed and the Democrats regained control of the Senate, spending began to creep up again in the areas where fed-eral responsibility for programs had been maintained (Stockman, 1986; Brandon, 1991b). By some mea-sures, health spending increased as a proportion of fed-eral domestic spending, because the programs remained in place (Salamon, 1987).

History does not repeat itself, of course, but the Rea-gan era budget battles have implications that are rele-vant to the current controversies over budget and gov-ernment responsibility for domestic social programs.

- The underlying program structures and the govern-ment level that is responsible for a program are cru-cially important.
- Struggles over increases or decreases in dollars appro-priated for programs are less important over the long run. Changing economic conditions, demands for services, technologies, and so on, will alter the level of future expenditures if institutional mechanisms that keep the program or spending category on the government's agenda are retained.
- Shifting program responsibility to the states under the guise of capping budget increases in the near and intermediate terms is an effective way to attack enti-tlements of citizens to (relatively) uniform national social welfare programs.

Long-term Care

Although political elites in Washington worry about the future of Social Security and Medicare, the most vexing health problem for many of the elderly and their families is long-term care. Long-term care (LTC) is the generic term for the help needed by an older adult or his or her family when physical or mental disabilities impair his or her capacity to perform the basic tasks of everyday life, such as eating, bathing, dressing, and housekeeping. LTC includes preventive, supportive, diagnostic, maintenance, and rehabilitative services in a variety of settings appropriate to individual needs (Crogan, 1993). It is a political and budgetary problem with great salience for both elites and many voters.

There are many dimensions to this problem:

- Older Americans are expected to make up a fifth of the population by 2035 (Schulz, 1995).
- Increasing longevity in the United States means that there will be more of the "oldest-old," who generate the greatest individual need for LTC.
- Families are the predominant provider of care for seniors (Cantor, 1980; Stone et al., 1987).
- Individuals find that the most difficult problem of health care financing is to pay out of pocket for LTC or to purchase adequate LTC insurance.
- Household out-of-pocket health expenditures, including health insurance premiums, will continue to increase substantially (Rubin et al., 1995).
- LTC commonly requires both social services and health care, which have traditionally been separated in the United States to the detriment of each and the frustration of those assigned to coordinate them.

The Anatomy of Long-term Care Problems

The politicization of long-term care is resulting in an overly narrow focus on finance. Many of the underlying problems faced by the elderly and their families are not fundamentally financing issues, but instead are questions regarding the organization and delivery of care. The consequence of the disjunction between private problems and public issues is that the political resolutions of public issues, when finally generated, are likely to leave many citizens dissatisfied. Some of the problems of organizing and delivering long-term care are even likely to be exacerbated by attempts to force misguided solutions.

The problem of LTC is framed mainly in terms of the strict dichotomy between skilled nursing care and home- or community-based care. Most private health insurance policies do not cover LTC: only about one percent of total LTC expenditures are paid by private insurance. Public LTC expenditures are overwhelmingly for nursing home rather than home care. Medicare covers short stays in skilled nursing facilities, but Medicare spending amounted to less than 5 percent of nursing home expenditures in 1991. This leaves Medicaid as the dominant source of public funding for LTC (Wiener et al., 1994, pp. 6–12). Because the cost of LTC often exceeds the personal financial resources of many elderly, many become poor by depleting their income and assets paying for care, a process known as "spending down" (Adams et al., 1993). By spending down, elderly individuals or couples gain access to Medicaid funding.

Difficulties both in defining the problem and in finding appropriate political solutions for a heterogeneous population with a wide range of specific sorts of problems are notable. An example of the difficulties in reaching agreement about seemingly simple issues is provided by the shifting conceptions of "home" found in various LTC contexts. Under Medicaid waiver programs, state policymakers have some leeway in determining coverage for services outside a skilled nursing facility. Some states have defined a home by the presence of attendant cooking facilities and a bathroom within a housing unit. Others define home to include any residential setting in which formal medical services are not provided (Benjamin, 1992, p. 13). In some states home care agencies provide services to people living in group residential settings as diverse as board and care homes (Hawes et al., 1993) and adult foster homes (Kane et al., 1991).

The most common attempt to resolve LTC issues involves comparing institutional costs with the cost of those home expenses that are reasonable candidates for reimbursement. The problem is operationalized by asking whether institutional care (e.g., in skilled nursing facilities) or home- or community-based LTC is less costly. The conventional wisdom had been that it was cheaper to care for all but the most impaired elderly in their homes. However, a number of careful studies using control groups, often along with random assignment and multivariate statistical techniques, showed that the home- and community-based care provided in such settings did not save money that would otherwise have been spent for institutional care (Weissert et al., 1988; Rivlin & Wiener, 1988, pp. 190–202).

In contrast to the political issues of financing LTC, the chief delivery question is whether a patient's health status, quality of life, or subjective satisfaction is typically greater when home- or community-based care permits patients to reside outside a skilled nursing facility. Evidence in thirty-one studies suggested that mortality is little affected and indices of physical functioning registered mixed results but nothing startling. "Increased life satisfaction appears to be a relatively consistent benefit of community care. Caregivers and patients who use community care are more satisfied" (Weissert et al., 1988, pp. 347–366). Seniors express a strong desire to remain in their own homes for as long as possible (Straw, 1991). Clearly someone is listening. Home care is the fastest-growing component of personal health care expenditures. Home care was a $20 billion industry in 1993 (Levit et al., 1994) and is expected to reach $40 billion in 2018 (Wiener et al., 1994). The expanding role of home care and assisted living providers adds to the complexity of organizing and delivering LTC for seniors, their families, and health policy analysts (Kane, 1995).

The rapidly increasing need for long-term care on the one hand and, on the other hand, decreasing fertility rates, increased labor force participation by women, and increasing marital disruption within our society threaten the availability of family caregivers. Quiet concern has also been raised about the possibility that providing long-term home care will inadvertently *monitize* home care; that is, that paid care will slowly drive out unpaid care. Paying for services that family and friends have been supplying outside market arrangements inevitably leads to increasing dependence on paid care and rising public and private costs. Moreover, as Titmus's classic *Gift Relationship* (1971) suggests, quality may be lower when services are bought and sold rather than freely given. The research to date suggests that families continue to provide the majority of LTC to frail elders even when formal services are used (Branch et al., 1988; Tennstedt & McKinley, 1989). Several longitu-

dinal studies have also concluded that informal caregivers do not relinquish their caregiving roles to the formal network (Jette et al., 1992).

Gerontologists and health services researchers who focus on LTC for the elderly must deal with many unresolved problems and unanswered questions, which are compounded by the heterogeneity of the aging population. For example, there are problems faced by physically or mentally impaired elderly living alone, including the likelihood of social isolation and difficulties in securing adequate nourishment and compliance with medication schedules. These problems must be balanced against the loss of self-esteem or even clinical depression that may result from the loss of independence when a senior leaves his or her long-time personal residence. Such decisions have to be made for each case in light of personal characteristics and the availability—or, too often, the lack of availability—of home and community services in a specific patient's community.

This broad-scale characterization of the kinds of problems facing service providers suggests the countless issues that confront professionals in the aging-support system. Because this chapter is an essay on the politics of aging, it can only nod at the range of problems that are difficult to translate adequately into political discourse. The common ground on which the problem definitions discerned by long-term health care workers and the formulation of public issues should focus is the organization and delivery of care. Both concerned caregivers and public servants want elderly citizens and their families to have whatever arrangements make them happy so long as public costs and low quality (as measured by elder abuse and other indicators) are minimized. Although costs must be considered, they should not be the only criterion in determining public policy. The reality, however, is that so long as budget problems are the principal focus in Washington and the state capitals, it will be difficult for politicians to define LTC needs as more than problems in health care finance.

The emerging models of LTC service delivery increasingly emphasize (1) greater reliance on home- and community-based services, (2) consolidation and decentralization of administrative responsibility for LTC, and (3) limits on the supply of institutional care. Together these changes constitute a paradigm shift away from care provided solely in an institutional setting.

It is unclear how these conceptual changes and their attendant costs will be handled by emerging issues networks. Thus, it is necessary to conclude this section by examining the options that face both federal and state governments as they come under increasing pressure to take some action to increase their financing of LTC.

Four Options for Long-term Care

There are four broad options for financing LTC services. While each comes with implications for the organization of care and therefore the delivery of services, our discussion is restricted chiefly to the financial implications of each alternative.

Medicaid as national LTC insurance. Continuing the current system in which Medicaid pays for more than 40 percent of the cost of nursing home care is always possible. Since relatively few elderly qualify as "poor" by official income criteria, most of those for whom government ultimately pays have exhausted their private resources by "spending down" to receive Medicaid assistance (Adams et al., 1993; Vladeck & Davenport, 1995). Although the Catastrophic Coverage Act had sought to ease some of the rules that forced "spousal impoverishment" (Iglehart, 1989; Rovner, 1988), elderly individuals and couples who live independent and economically productive lives still often have to turn to means-tested welfare to pay for long-term care in their final years. Medicaid, which was initially regarded as serving mothers and children receiving Aid to Families with Dependent Children (AFDC), has developed into a perverse kind of national LTC insurance program that covers elderly Americans after they pay a gigantic and variable deductible that amounts to their entire life savings.

While the bulk of public LTC funding is from federal sources, state governments have taken the lead in developing and administering public LTC programs. Medicaid costs now rank third in aggregate state expenditures, behind public schools and higher education

(Gold, 1993). Some of the state innovations were pioneered under the Medicaid waiver program.[14] Since 1981, states have had the option of applying for Medicaid waivers to fund home- and community-based services for people who meet Medicaid eligibility requirements and would otherwise require expensive institutional care. All states now provide some home- and community-based services in their Medicaid programs. The experience of three states with long-standing Medicaid waiver programs—Oregon, Washington, and Wisconsin—is worth noting. Through restrictions involving financial eligibility criteria, functional eligibility criteria, and a variety of program management techniques, these states were able to provide services to more people with available funds (U.S. Government Accounting Office, 1994). Some state officials believe that the ability to provide home- and community-based care through state-funded and Medicaid waiver programs has allowed states to successfully contain growth in overall state spending. Controls on program growth, however, have at times resulted in waiting lists for some programs (U.S. General Accounting Office, 1995).

There are some other steps that could be taken to ameliorate the current system. An obvious development is to liberalize the qualifications necessary for the elderly to receive Medicaid (Wiener et al., 1994, pp. 124–130). Another suggestion is the reverse annuity mortgage, a form of home equity conversion that allows an elderly homeowner to tap the heretofore nonliquid assets represented by the family home. The best evidence is that making available assets that are currently nonliquid can help some individuals cope with long-term care costs, but does not constitute a systemic solution (Rivlin & Wiener, 1988, pp. 123–145).

Private long-term care insurance. Private insurance is now sold to protect individuals against the financial consequences of extended need for long-term care. Al-

---

[14]The changes made by the Omnibus Budget Reconciliation Act of 1981 (PL 97-35) authorized the secretary of HHS through HCFA, the federal agency in charge of Medicaid, to approve exceptions or waivers to Medicaid program rules. These waivers allow the states to offer packages of services, including nonmedical services, which may not be covered by the states' regular Medicaid programs.

though this product did not exist before the mid-1980s, the market is growing rapidly. According to surveys conducted by the Health Insurance Association of America (HIAA), the number of policies sold increased from 815,000 in December 1987 to more than 2.9 million in December 1992 (Wiener et al., 1994, p. 50). These numbers obscure the fact that relatively few policies are in force at any one time and only a minuscule portion of the more than 31 million who are sixty-five and older are covered (Temkin-Greener & Meiners, 1995, p. 196). Unless one begins to pay for insurance well before retirement, when the possibility of needing expensive LTC becomes apparent, premiums are usually too expensive for most individuals to purchase. Private insurance companies are also not eager to promise service benefits or indemnity benefits that are indexed to inflation, because the future incidence and costs of long-term care defy accurate prediction. Private insurance companies, of course, are required to have reserves set aside against future claims.

Under current practices, where private LTC insurance is aimed primarily at the elderly population, Wiener, Illston, and Hanley (1994, p. 79) estimate that only a minority are likely to have such coverage in 2018. The percentages would, however, be significantly higher if employers could be persuaded to offer private LTC insurance to their younger employees and if workers would willingly purchase the product. Private LTC policies can be affordable only if it is possible to convince people to buy policies at a younger age.

Social insurance. Social insurance would provide a way to avoid the problems of predicting future demand and costs and determining adequate reserve requirements. Social Security and Medicare Part A are examples of social insurance. The difficulty of calculating reserves and predicting future costs and demand are not relevant, because social insurance can use each year's income to pay obligations as they arise. Federal taxing power guarantees that government promises will be kept. Universal compulsory public LTC insurance would also avoid the problem of adverse selection, since everyone within a given group would have to participate (Brandon, 1989, 1992).

Both social insurance and private insurance might lead to an expansion of demand and price increases. Even public comprehensive coverage of long-term institutional care at its current costs would strain the federal budget. The failure of the Clinton administration's 1993 Health Security Act and the criticism that it generated reduce the chances that a social insurance model for long-term care will be politically feasible in the future.

Public–private partnerships. Given the inadequacies of both private LTC insurance and public insurance, a new hybrid option is developing in some states. This approach permits purchasers of state-approved private LTC insurance to use Medicaid as catastrophic coverage without pauperizing themselves. This public–private partnership is being tested in California, Connecticut, Indiana, Iowa, and New York with grant support from the Robert Wood Johnson Foundation. Although the state programs differ in details, they generally feature a model that promotes a partnership between state Medicaid agencies and private LTC insurers. Purchase of a policy entitles the holder to private LTC coverage and, when those benefits are exhausted, to skilled nursing benefits under Medicaid without spending his or her financial assets. This alternative allows the insured to obtain significant asset protection (Wiener et al., 1994, p. 16). By linking private insurance with improvements in Medicaid, this approach might offer a positive model for financing and delivering LTC that can be replicated in all fifty states (Meiners & McKay, 1990).

Summary Discussion

The current narrow focus on balancing the federal budget is incompatible with any systematic enlargement of the government's responsibility for the aging-support system. Services cannot be significantly expanded and access increased without increasing expenditures. Thus, the future of at least the long-term care portion of the aging-support system may be decided in part by the ability of the U.S. economy to continue to create abundant wealth. If we are to develop a rational, comprehensive, government-funded and -monitored system that does not permit the existence of two classes of care to continue, we must develop some way to see around the budget deficit blinders that currently preclude significant innovation in domestic public policy. We should remember that we are an *aging society*, in which everyone—young and old alike—participates. The interdependence of the generations is receiving strong emphasis across the entire spectrum of aging-support issues. For example, the 1995 White House Conference on Aging emphasized the intergenerational perspective when it examined issues relating to older adults and their families. It will be easier to promote planned change for citizens of all ages before great vested interests like insurance companies achieve a position in the long-term care field that enables them to force government to share power with corporate interests.

This overview of the acute medical system and LTC and their implications for the aging-support system suggest the continuing validity of Saward's law that "if form follows function, function follows funding." When the late Ernest Saward enunciated his half-facetious "law," government was still able to direct significant amounts of money to projects to effect ends that it chose. It had the confidence and political support necessary to plan and implement government programs with a view to improving the organization and delivery of services. Yet function still follows funding when government devotes its energies to reducing the cost of its purchases from the private sector or to avoiding what had been regarded as established public obligations. This truth is demonstrated by cost shifting on the part of providers and the rush to managed care by both the private and public sectors in the wake of the defeat of Clinton's health reform.

Major changes, either in resources or in the locus of administrative responsibility, change programs. It is possible to think in advance about these changes—a practice that used to be dignified by the name "planning." Alternatively, one may let events happen and feign surprise. The move to give states the primary responsibility for setting standards for Medicaid, if it is fully implemented, exemplifies the second alternative. Sometimes it is easier to obtain desired political and ideological goals if one does not think very carefully about their practical consequences.

Conclusion

This chapter has emphasized the relatively recent emergence of a definable aging-support system providing income, social services (including transportation), and health care. In keeping with the political focus of this book, the chapter provided considerable detail about the relevant public structures and those private interests that have developed to support and influence them. It is now time to address the potential for fundamental political change and the impact of such change on an aging population and the support system that helps the elderly and their families cope with infirmity and difficult living situations.

According to congressional Republicans, the 1994 elections initiated a political revolution that will see the federal government disengage from efforts to help its citizens cope with life's everyday problems. Indeed, many of the newly elected members of the House of Representatives, who claim to represent the true political beliefs of their constituents, express their intention to reduce the power and influence of the national government as such. If they only accomplish their budgetary aims, a major change will occur in the organization of services in the United States. But their larger political and constitutional aims are profoundly revolutionary.

The conservative Republican administrations of Ronald Reagan and George Bush were still committed to helping citizens cope with health and social problems that they faced. A major accomplishment of their administrations was to strengthen Medicare and Medicaid by developing new ways to control health care costs. Although it is rarely made explicit, the breathtaking achievement in health care of twelve years of Republican administrations (1981–93) was the nationalization of health care finance. The prospective payment system (PPS), which uses diagnosis-related groups to reimburse hospitals and the resource-based relative value scale (RBRVS) for physician payment, replaced the diversity of local charges and cost-based reimbursement with a national system that only allows for minor variation in local labor and practice costs.

Ironically, these assertions of national power could hardly be described as "bold," because virtually no one even asked whether federal power should be asserted over the remaining vestiges of localism in the health care system. Political questions about the wisdom of asserting federal dominance over this aspect of social interaction were largely left unasked. Instead, debate was mainly left to policy analysts and other specialists who focused on technical issues about the ability of the system to function as intended and the potential that consequences might be detrimental or unfair to some providers or patients.

In contrast, the outcome of the congressional elections of 1994, which were fought by the Republicans under the banner of the "Contract with America," has legitimized talk among conservatives about a significant reduction in the power of the federal government. Thus, for example, instead of the technical issues of effectiveness and unanticipated consequences that were raised in regard to PPS and RBRVS in the 1980s, recent debates about welfare turned on conflicts over the power and appropriateness of action by the national government. For example, some of the new "antifederalists" in the 104th Congress anguished over the conflict between their conviction that the federal government should leave to the states any attempt to influence how citizens live and their strong desire to attack illegitimacy by passing national mandates that prohibit welfare payments to teenage mothers or increases in payments for children born to mothers who already received welfare for older children. It was probably only a matter of time before similar issues about the fundamental role of government arise in regard to the health care agenda.

Changes in the Medicare program were made by Congress in the mid-1990s. The ostensible issue on the agenda was how to control costs and reduce the federal budget deficit. But the most committed proponents on both sides saw the controversy as much more fundamental: at issue was the role of the federal government in securing health care for the elderly.

The Medicare debate about savings and alternative ways to organize and deliver care was important in its own right, but it was also a preliminary event before insurgent conservatives put Social Security on the action agenda. Social Security, the paradigmatic New Deal program, is fraught with symbolic importance for the role of government in our polity. The political significance of the coming battles over Social Security does not, however, gainsay its practical importance for tens of millions of citizens who are counting on Social Security to provide a comfortable retirement.

The contrast with earlier debates is again instructive. As explained in the section on income security, the deliberations about Social Security a decade and a half ago involved Democrats and Republicans who worked together on technical issues. They aimed to restore Social Security to fiscal health and to deal with a considerable portion of the projected shortfall that will occur in the second quarter of the next century, when the baby boomers are all receiving Social Security checks. This collaborative purpose and the format of an independent bipartisan commission allowed them to achieve most of their goals, although the process involved much hard bargaining. The character of debate about ways to resolve the Social Security crisis of the 1980s was fundamentally different from the debate that would be held if the same crisis emerged in the 1990s. The debate in the 1980s did not question the legitimacy of Social Security or the principle of social insurance. Concerns about both are certain to be raised later this decade when Congress turns to Social Security, for Social Security represents the "mother" of social insurance or "entitlement" programs in America.

If Medicare and Social Security are both on the agenda in the 1990s in a manner that is unprecedented since the 1930s, the third aspect of the aging-support system to be addressed in this chapter—long-term care—appears to have largely dropped off the national agenda. In part, its disappearance may be due to increasing awareness that many of the issues of LTC are individual problems that must be negotiated between the elderly and their families. It is also likely that this field will see ever more experimentation by states, if the devolution of federal power and resources proceeds as promised.

Yet, given the history of demands by the American public for government help in solving private problems, it is hard to believe that LTC will be permanently off the public agenda. Moreover, the logic of attempts to reform the cash payment portion of welfare would seem to lead ineluctably to reform of the health care that comes with monetary Aid to Families with Dependent Children (AFDC). As part of such reform, legislators should deal with the artificial and illogical combination in a single program of a LTC program for the middle class in nursing homes and an acute care program for single poor mothers and their children.

Of course skeptics may be justified in refusing to underestimate the willingness of Congress to ignore the "logic" of reform. The views of such pessimists seem more compelling when a substantial number of the majority in Congress claim to believe that such social and health programs are not really the business of the national government in the first place.

REFERENCES

Achenbaum, W. Andrew. (1986). *Social Security: Visions and revisions.* Cambridge: Cambridge University Press.

Adams, E. Kathleen, Mark R. Meiners, & Brian Burwell. (1993). Asset spend-down in nursing homes: Methods and insights. *Medical Care, 31* (January), 1–23.

American Association of Retired Persons, Andrus Foundation. (1994). *1993 annual report.* Washington, D.C.: American Association of Retired Persons, Andrus Foundation.

Aries, Philippe. (1962). *Centuries of childhood: A social history of family life.* Trans. Robert Baldick. New York: Alfred A. Knopf.

Avery, Robert B., & Michael S. Rendall. (1993a). Estimating the size and distribution of baby boomers' prospective inheritances. *Proceedings of the Annual Meeting of the American Statistical Association, Social Statistics Section.* Alexandria, VA: American Statistical Association.

Avery, Robert B., & Michael S. Rendall. (1993b). *Inheritance and wealth.* Paper presented to the Philanthropy Roundtable, November 11.

Benjamin, A. E. (1992). In-home health and supportive services. In M. G. Ory & A. P. Duncker (Eds.), *In-home care for older people: Health and supportive services.* Newbury Park, CA: Sage.

Bernstein, Merton C. (1995). Social Security's most likely change—and least understood. *Aging Today, 16* (July/August), 3–4.

Binstock, Robert H. (1989). The phantom old age vote. *New York Times* (January 2), 23.

Bloksberg, Leonard M. (1989). Intergovernmental relations: Change and continuity. *Journal of Aging and Social Policy, 1* (3/4), 11–36.

Board of Trustees, Federal Hospital Insurance Fund. (1988). *The 1988 annual report,* H.R. Doc. 100-193, 100th Congress, 1st session. Washington, D.C.: U.S. Government Printing Office.

Board of Trustees, Federal Hospital Insurance Fund. (1995). *The 1995 annual report,* H.R. Doc. 104-56. 104th Congress, 1st session. Washington, D.C.: U.S. Government Printing Office.

Bradley, Dana Burr. (1994). *Constructing state old-age policy: A Pennsylvania perspective.* Unpublished Ph.D. diss., Carnegie-Mellon University, Pittsburgh, PA.

Branch, Laurence G., et al. (1988). A prospective study of incident comprehensive medical home care use among the elderly. *American Journal of Public Health, 78* (3), 255–259.

Brandon, William. P. (1977). Politics, administration and conflict in neighborhood health centers. *Journal of Health Politics, Policy and Law, 2* (Spring), 79–99.

Brandon, William P. (1982). "Fact" and "value" in the thought of Peter Winch: Linguistic analysis broaches metaphysical questions. *Political Theory, 10,* 215–244.

Brandon, William P. (1989). Cut off at the impasse without real catastrophic health insurance: Three approaches to financing long term care. *Policy Studies Review, 8.*

Brandon, William P. (1991a). Politics, health and the elderly: Inventing the next century—the age of aging. In Theodor J. Litman & Leonard S. Robins (Eds.), *Health politics and policy* (2nd ed.). Albany, NY: Delmar.

Brandon, William P. (1991b). Two kinds of conservatism in U.S. health policy: The Reagan record. In Christina Altenstetter & Stuart C. Itaywood (Eds.), *Comparative health policy and its new right: From rhetoric to reality.* Houndsmills, Basingstoke, UK: Macmillan.

Brandon, William P. (1992). The promise of Medicare. In Miriam K. Mills & Robert H. Blank (Eds.), *Health insurance and public policies: Risks, allocations and equity.* Westport, CT: Greenwood Press.

Brasfield, James M. (1987). *The management of invisible policies: Medicaid and long term care.* Paper presented at the meeting of the Southwestern Social Science Association, Dallas, TX, March 18–21.

Brennan, Kristen (Public Affairs Representative, National Committee to Preserve Social Security and Medicare). (1995). Telephone conversation with Karen Honess (July 26).

Cantor, Marjorie. (1980). The informal support system: Its relevance in the lives of the elderly. In Elizabeth Borgotta & Neil McClusky (Eds.), *Aging and society.* Beverly Hills, CA: Sage.

Chelimsky, E. (1991). *The administration on aging: Harmonizing growing demands and shrinking resources* (GAO/T-PEMD-91-9). Washington, D.C.: U.S. General Accounting Office.

Cotton, Paul. (Ed.). (1995). Moderate Republicans join attack on nursing home regulations rollback. *Medicine and Health, 49* (December 11), 2.

Crogan, Neva. (1993). Choices in the long-term care continuum. *Geriatric Nursing, 14*, 323–326.

Dattalo, Patrick. (1992). Social Security's surpluses. *Social Work, 37* (July), 377–379.

Day, Christine L. (1990). *What older Americans think: Interest groups and aging policy.* Princeton, NJ: Princeton University Press.

Day, Christine L. (1995). *Old-age interest groups in the 1990's: Coalition, competition, and strategy.* Paper presented at the annual meeting of the American Political Science Association, Chicago, IL, August 3–September 30.

Donabedian, Avedis, et al. (1986). *Medical care chartbook* (8th ed.). Ann Arbor, MI: Health Administration Press.

Estes, Carroll L. (1983). *The aging enterprise: A critical examination of social policies and services for the aged.* San Francisco: Jossey-Bass.

Federal Old-Age and Survivors Insurance and Disability Insurance Trust Fund Board of Trustees. (1995). *The 1995 annual report.* H.R. Doc. 104-57. 104th Congress, 1st session. Washington, D.C.: U.S. Government Printing Office.

Feldstein, Paul J. (1988). *The politics of health legislation: An economic perspective.* Ann Arbor, MI: Health Administration Press.

Fraley, Colette. (1995a). Health: GOP scores on Medicare. But foes aren't done. *Congressional Quarterly* (November 8), 3535–3538.

Fraley, Colette. (1995b). Reconciliation: Scaled-back Medicaid savings plan emerges from conference. *Congressional Quarterly* (November 18), 3539–3540.

Friedan, Betty. (1993). *The fountain of age.* New York: Simon & Schuster.

Fries, James F. (1980). Aging, natural death, and the compression of morbidity. *New England Journal of Medicine, 303,* 130–135.

Fries, James F. (1983). The compression of morbidity. *Milbank Memorial Fund Quarterly, 61* (Summer), 397–419.

Gallup, Alec, & Lydia Saad. (1993). America's top health care concerns. *Gallup Poll Monthly* (June), 2–5.

Gerontological Society of America. (1987). *To meet the challenge of aging: Annual report 1987.* Washington, D.C.: Gerontological Society of America.

Gold, S. D. (1993). Cadillac or Yugo? *State Legislatures, 19* (6), 32–36.

Gray Panthers. (1987). *Disability Task Force Newsletter: Age and Youth in Action, 3* (March).

Haber, Carole. (1983). *Beyond sixty-five: The dilemma of old age in America's past.* Cambridge: Cambridge University Press.

Haber, Carole, & Brian Gratton. (1994). *Old age and the search for security: An American social history.* Bloomington: Indiana University Press.

Hawes, C., J. B. Wildfire, & L. J. Lux. (1993). *Regulation of board and care homes: National summary.* Washington, D.C.: American Association of Retired Persons.

Heclo, Hugh. (1978). Issue networks and the executive establishment. In Anthony King (Ed.), *The new American political system* (1st ed., pp. 87–124). Washington, D.C.: American Enterprises Institute.

Hutchinson, Ron. (1995). There's a new kid on the senior's block (op-ed.). *Charlotte Observer* (March 1).

Iglehart, John K. (1989). Medicare's new benefits: "Catastrophic" health insurance. *New England Journal of Medicine, 320,* 329–336.

Jazwiecki, Tom, & Teresa Schwab. (1989). Conclusion. In Teresa Schwab (Ed.), *Caring for an aging world: International models for long term care, financing, and delivery* (pp. 366–376). New York: McGraw-Hill.

Jette, Alan M., Sharon L. Tennstedt, & Laurence G. Branch. (1992). Stability of informal long-term care. *Journal of Aging and Health, 4* (May), 198–211.

Johnson, Malcolm. (1989). Long-term care for the elderly in England. In Teresa Schwab (Ed.), *Caring for an aging world: International models for long term care, financing, and delivery* (pp. 162–192). New York: McGraw-Hill.

Journal of Accounting. (1994). *178* (July), 6.

Kane, Rosalie A. (1995). Expanding the home care concept: Blurring distinctions among home care, institutional care, and other long-term-care services. *Milbank Quarterly, 73* (2), 161–186

Kane, Rosalie A., Robert L. Kane, Laurel H. Illston, John A. Nyman, & Michael D. Finch. (1991). Adult foster care for the elderly in Oregon: A mainstream alternative to nursing homes? *American Journal of Public Health, 81* (September), 1113–1120.

Kreps, Juanita M. (1971). *Lifetime allocation of work and income: Essays in the economics of aging.* Durham, NC: Duke University Press.

Kuhn, Maggie. (1988). Editorial. *Network, 17* (November/December), 13.

Kuhn, Maggie. (1991). *No stone unturned: The life and times of Maggie Kuhn.* New York: Ballantine Books.

Lammers, William W., & Phoebe S. Liebig. (1990). State health policies, federalism and the elderly. *Publius, 20* (3), 1331–1348.

Levit, Katharine R., et al. (1994). National health expenditures, 1993. *Health Care Financing Review, 16* (Fall), 247–294.

Liebig, Phoebe S. (1992). Federalism and aging policy in the 1980s: Implications for changing interest group roles in the 1990s. *Journal of Aging &Social Policy, 4* (1/2), 17–33.

Light, Paul. (1985). *Artful work: The politics of Social Security reform.* New York: Random House.

Long, Christina G. (n.d.). *Blueprint for a new age.* Radnor, PA: Gray Panthers. Photocopy.

Longman, Phillip. (1987). *Born to pay: The new politics of aging in America.* Boston: Houghton Mifflin.

Lowi, Theodore J. (1969). *The end of liberalism: Ideology, policy, and the crisis of public authority.* New York: W. W. Norton.

Manton, Kenneth G. (1982). Changing concepts of morbidity and mortality in the elder population. *Milbank Memorial Fund Quarterly, 60* (2), 183–244.

Marmor, Theodore R. (1973). *Politics of Medicare.* Chicago: Aldine.

Meiners, Mark R., & Hunter L. McJay. (1990). Private vs. social LTC insurance: Beware the comparison. *Generations, 14* (2), 32–36.

Moody, Harry R. (1986). The meaning of life and the meaning of old age. In Thomas R. Cole & Sally A. Gadow (Eds.), *What does it mean to grow old?: Reflections from the humanities* (pp. 9–40). Durham, NC: Duke University Press.

Moynihan, Daniel P. (1988). Conspirators, trillions, limos in the night. *New York Times* (May 23), A19.

Moynihan, Daniel P. (1990). Surplus value. *The New Republic, 202* (June 4), 13–16.

National Academy on Aging. (1995). Facts on Social Security: The old age and survivors trust fund. National Committee to Preserve Social Security and Medicare. *1994 annual report (1993–4).* Photocopy. Washington, D.C.: National Committee to Preserve Social Security and Medicare.

National Alliance of Senior Citizens. (1994). *Annual report 1994.* Photocopy.

National Committee to Preserve Social Security and Medicare. (n.d.). What is the National Committee? Washington, D.C.: National Committee to Preserve Social Security and Medicare.

National Council on the Aging, Inc. (1994). *Annual report 1994.* Washington, D.C.: National Council on the Aging, Inc.

National Council of Senior Citizens. (1995). Progress report, *NCSC Annual Report.* Washington, D.C., January.

New York Times. (1994) The 1994 election: Tracking shifts over eight elections (November 13), 24.

Nielsen, Waldemar A. (1985). *The golden donors.* New York: E. P. Dutton.

Oberlander, Jon. (1995). National Committee to Preserve Social Security and Medicare (NCPSSM). In Craig Ramsay (Ed.), *U.S. health policy groups: Institutional profiles* (pp. 314–317). Westport, CT: Greenwood Press.

Ossofsky, Jack. (1978). Correspondence. *National Journal, 18* (March 11), 408–409.

Pratt, Henry J. (1976). *The gray lobby.* Chicago: University of Chicago Press.

Quadagno, Jill S. (1984). From poor laws to pensions: The evolution of economic support for the aged in England and America. *Milbank Memorial Fund Quarterly, 62* (Summer), 417–446.

Quadagno, Jill S. (1988). *The transformation of old age security: Class and politics in the American welfare state.* Chicago: University of Chicago Press.

Rayazuddin, Mohammed. (1995). (Director of information, Gerontological Society of America). Telephone conversation with Karen Honess. (March).

Rivlin, Alice M., & Joshua M. Wiener. (1988). *Caring for the disabled elderly: Who will pay?* Washington, D.C.: The Brookings Institution.

Rovner, Julie. (1988). Catastrophic-costs measure ready for final Hill approval. *Congressional Quarterly Weekly Report, 46* (June 4), 1494–1495.

Rovner, Julie. (1995). Nursing home standards: Flashpoint for federalism. *Medicine and Health Perspectives, 49* (October 23).

Rubin, Alissa J. (1995). Reconciliation: Highlights of conference report. *Congressional Quarterly* (November 18), 3513–3515.

Rubin, Rose M., Kenneth Koelln, & Roger K. Speas. (1995). Out of pocket health expenditures by elderly households: Change over the 1980s. *Journal of Gerontology: Social Sciences, 50B* (5), S291–S300.

Russell, Louise B. (1989). *Medicare's new hospital payment system.* Washington, D.C.: The Brookings Institution.

Salamon, Lester M. (1987). Partners in public service: The scope and theory of government–nonprofit relations. In Walter W. Powell (Ed.), *The nonprofit sector: A research handbook.* New Haven: Yale University Press.

Salisbury, Robert H. (1990). The paradox of interest groups in Washington—more groups, less clout. In Anthony King (Ed.), *The new American political system* (2nd ed., pp. 203–229, 327–330). Washington, D.C.: AEI Press.

Samuelson, Robert J. (1978a). Another look at those figures on the aged. *National Journal, 18* (March), 399.

Samuelson, Robert J. (1978b). Busting the U.S. budget—the costs of an aging America. *National Journal, 18* (February), 256–260.

Schulz, James H. (1995). *The economics of aging* (6th ed.). New York: Auburn House.

Stehle, Vince. (1995). Welfare for lobbyists? *Chronicle of Philanthropy, 7* (July 13), 32–33.

Stockman, David A. (1986). *The triumph of politics: How the Reagan revolution failed.* New York: Harper & Row.

Stone, Robin, Gail Cafferata, & Judith Sangl. (1987). Caregivers of the frail elderly: A national profile. *Gerontologist, 27*, 616–626.

Straw, Margaret K. (1991). *Home care: Attitudes and knowledge of middle aged and older Americans*. Washington, D.C.: American Association of Retired Persons.

Temkin-Greener, Helena, & Mark R. Meiners. (1995). Transitions in long-term care. *Gerontologist, 35* (2), 196–206.

Tennstedt, Sharon, & J. McKinley. (1989). Informal care for frail older persons. In M. Ory & N. Bond (Eds.), *Aging and health care: Social science and policy perspectives*. London: Routledge.

Third Millennium. (1993). *Third Millennium declaration*. New York: Third Millennium.

Thomas, Robert McG., Jr. (1995). Maggie Kuhn, 89, The founder of the Gray Panthers, is dead. *New York Times* (April 23), L47.

Thompson, Carolyn R. (1990). *What happened to Medicare catastrophic care?* Paper presented at the 1990 annual meeting of the American Political Science Association, San Francisco, August 28–September 2.

Titmus, Richard M. (1971). *The gift relationship: From human blood to social policy.* New York: Pantheon Books.

United Seniors Association. (n.d.). *1993 annual report.* Photocopy.

U.S. Bureau of the Census. (1942). *Statistical abstract of the United States 1941* (No. 63). Washington, D.C.: U.S. Government Printing Office.

U.S. Bureau of the Census. (1986). *Economic characteristics of households in the United States: Fourth quarter 1984* (Current Population Reports, Series P 70, No. 6). Household Economic Studies. Washington, D.C.: U.S. Government Printing Office.

U.S. Bureau of the Census. (1990). *Money income and poverty status in the United States: 1989* (Current Population Reports, Series P-60, No. 169). Washington, D.C.: U.S. Government Printing Office.

U.S. General Accounting Office. (1994). *Medicaid long-term care: Successful efforts to expand home services while limiting costs* (GAO/HEHS-94-167). Washington, D.C.: U.S. General Accounting Office.

U.S. General Accounting Office. (1995). Long-term care: Current issues and future directions (Letter Report, 4/13/95, GAO/HEHS-95-109). Washington, D.C.: U.S. General Accounting Office.

U.S. National Commission on Social Security Reform. (1983). *Final report*. Washington, D.C.: U.S. Government Printing Office.

U.S. Office of Management and Budget. *Appendices to the Budget, 1982–1996*. Washington, D.C.

Vladeck, Bruce, & Karen F. Davenport. (1995). Medicaid: A safety net in peril. *NCOA Perspective on Aging, 24* (4), 4–7.

Weissert, William G., C. Matthews Cready, & James E. Pawelak. (1988). The past and future of home and community based long-term care. *Milbank Quarterly, 66* (2), 309–388.

Wiener, Joshua M., Laurel Hixon Illston, & Raymond J. Hanley. (1994). *Sharing the burden: Strategies for public and private long-term care insurance*. Washington, D.C.: The Brookings Institution.

Williams, T. Franklin. (1994). Integrating the needs of older Americans into the goals and structures of health care reform. *Gerontologist, 34* (1), 616–617.

Winch, Peter. (1958). *The idea of a social science and its relation to philosophy*. London: Routledge & Kegan Paul.

Winch, Peter. (1970). Understanding a primitive society. In Bryan R. Wilson (Ed.), *Rationality*. New York: Harper & Row.

Zappolo, Aurora A., & Gerdt Sundstrom. (1989). Long-term care for the elderly in Sweden. In Teresa Schwab (Ed.), *Caring for an aging world: International models for long-term care, financing, and delivery* (pp. 22–57). New York: McGraw-Hill.

CHAPTER

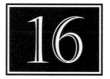

Health Politics and Mental Health Care

David A. Rochefort

Mental illness and its treatment are fundamental to the operation of the health system. Among biomedical researchers today, there is growing appreciation of the role of psychological factors in the development of a host of physical illnesses, ranging from lower back pain, to allergies, to diabetes, to heart attack. And emotional stress is a predictable outcome of the discovery and management of any serious medical problem. At the same time, many (some would say "all") mental illnesses have a well-established biological component to them. From a service perspective, mental health care facilities represent an important element of the nation's health care infrastructure. Many patients also receive treatment for mental disorders in general medical settings.

Reflecting this close interrelationship, mental health policy analysis is, in part, an offshoot of broader health policy studies, and the insights of each field can help advance the other. However, key distinctions between the mental health and health care sectors must also be made

that, taken together, give to mental health policy analysis a unique quality. For much of American history, the bulk of mental health services were provided in public facilities, and public care sources remain crucial to a large number of mentally ill individuals today. Although mainstream health insurance programs supply a portion of mental health funding, it is impossible to understand the evolution or current structure of the U.S. mental health system without reference to income maintenance entitlements, such as Supplemental Security Income. Policy innovations in mental health care have also followed their own rhythm, only sometimes coinciding with general health policymaking. Last but not least, mental illness is associated with a social stigma that finds few parallels among other diseases and conditions.

The purpose of this chapter is to review the politics and policies of mental health care, paying heed to the ways in which mental health care and health care trends both converge and diverge. We begin by surveying the scope of the problem of mental illness and patterns in its treatment. This is followed by a discussion of major influences in mental health policymaking. Next, an analysis of the campaign for national health care reform during the early Clinton administration is provided from a mental health care perspective. Finally, we make note of the driving forces, such as managed care and Medicaid reform, which promise to shape the U.S. mental health system into the twenty-first century.

SIGHTING THE BOUNDARIES OF MENTAL HEALTH CARE

The population afflicted with mental health problems ranges from more to less visible, depending on the type and location of services sought for treatment. How we define what constitutes mental health care also determines what portion of this sector falls within our sight.

One basic measure of mental health care in the United States is provided by activity in the specialty mental health sector. The specialty mental health sector is a construct that has been employed by the National Institute of Mental Health (NIMH), and now the federal Center for Mental Health Services, to guide data collection efforts. A primary focus of the biennial *Mental Health, United States* series, it encompasses those facilities and organizations with a specific, narrow-purpose mission of serving psychiatric patients—for example, public and private psychiatric hospitals, general hospital psychiatric units, and various ambulatory mental health care organizations. According to this conceptualization of the mental health system, and using the latest published data, there were some 5,300 provider organizations in 1990. The number of inpatient admissions, readmissions, returns from leave, and transfers slightly exceeded 2 million; outpatient additions approximated 3 million (Redick et al., 1994).

Yet this specialty mental health sector omits millions of patients who receive psychiatric care in other settings. For example, Kiesler and Sibulkin (1987; see also Kiesler & Simpkins, 1993) have drawn attention to the large volume of services provided to mentally ill persons in general hospitals outside specialized psychiatric units.

In fact, by 1980, the number of such episodes topped one million, exceeding episodes within specialized psychiatric units by a ratio of about 3:2. A more recent analysis of service usage for mental and addictive disorders found that only 40 percent of all persons treated received care from the "specialty mental addictive" sector, compared to 43 percent in the "general medical" sector (Bourdon et al., 1994).

Focusing on outpatient care, Olfson and Pincus (1994) examined three levels of mental health service use: (1) specialty mental health care, in which a patient visited a mental health specialist for a diagnosed mental health condition and was treated with either psychotropic medication or psychotherapy; (2) explicit mental health care, in which a patient visited a provider in the specialty or general medical sectors and was treated with either psychotropic medication or psychotherapy; and (3) broadly defined mental health care, in which a patient either was treated with a psychotropic medication, or visited a practitioner for a mental health condition, or obtained psychotherapy. The number of people falling into these three respective categories was 3.2 million, 6.4 million, and 21.6 million, respectively.

Finally, a still broader perspective on the mental health sector would include those suffering from mental illnesses who do not receive treatment, in addition to those under care. Data compiled as part of the National Comorbidity Survey in 1990–92 supply estimates of lifetime and twelve-month prevalence rates for fourteen major mental disorders among those fifteen to fifty-four years old (Kessler et al., 1994). According to this study, nearly 30 percent of the general population experienced at least one mental disorder during the past year, most of whom did not receive any professional mental health treatment. About 50 percent of the respondents had suffered a mental disorder at some time in their lives.

The fact that the boundaries of the mental health sector can be, and are, visualized so variously has important consequences for the content of mental health policy analysis and for mental health policy development. First, it is obvious that our awareness of the scope of the problem of mental illness hinges on the population group encompassed—users of specialty services, users by diagnosis, or sufferers outside the service system. So, too, does the estimated fiscal impact of mental illness. For example, the Center for Mental Health Services placed total expenditures by specialty mental health organizations at $28.4 billion in 1990. Yet if we look at the total economic costs of mental illness in this same year, including not only direct services but also morbidity and mortality and other indirect costs, the figure reached nearly $148 billion (National Advisory Mental Health Council, 1993).

Not just aggregate figures, but their composition and distribution also reflect how the counting is done. This is so because different components of the mental health sector are used and paid for by different groups in society. As an illustration, the chronically and severely mentally ill are a more central concern in the specialty mental health sector than in general medical settings, and state governments bear a greater share of the financial burden in the former than in the latter.

Second, our conception of boundaries also relates to our understanding of how the mental health sector does and should operate. For example, whether the rate of hospitalization for mental disorder in the United States over the 1960s and 1970s remained stable or climbed sharply depends on whether we count only inpatient episodes in specialty units or all episodes for mental disorder in general hospitals (Kiesler & Simpkins, 1993, p. 3). The large volume of mental health services being delivered in nonspecialized sites, including both general hospitals and physicians' offices, prompts clinical questions about appropriateness of care and the practice of referral between general and specialty sectors. Such normative concerns, in turn, relate to potential policy choices about responsibility for oversight of mental health service delivery and the operational standards that will be applied.

The role of problem definition in public policymaking is well recognized (Rochefort & Cobb, 1994)—whether a given situation ranks as a significant social issue, whom it is seen as affecting, and in what ways these factors influence how public officials will respond. In this way, deciding what qualifies as mental illness and mental health care has real political import for the standing of mental health concerns on the policy agenda. Different perceptions of degrees and types of mental health need also predispose different policy approaches, as in the choice between universal entitlements and more targeted programs, or in the investment of resources in preventive, curative, and long-term care services. Increased sophistication of health services research has contributed substantially to a more complete picture of the mentally ill than ever before, but it remains for policymakers to decide how much of this picture represents legitimate need in light of available resources, social norms, and their own political philosophies.

It is in deliberations over health insurance reform that all these definitional questions come to a focal point, first, in the priority given to coverage of mental illnesses and, second, in the means by which this coverage is arranged. Several analysts (Mechanic, 1993; Rochefort, 1993; Kiesler & Simpkins, 1993) have pointed out that the medically oriented, acute care health system is poorly oriented to the needs of many mentally ill persons who require long-term social support. Further, the cost and quality control instruments that are now spreading rapidly throughout the general health sector, including patient cost sharing, utilization review, and prospective payment, often impact differently on the mentally ill than on other patient groups. Given how deeply interwoven mental health and health care needs can be, as well as the increasing use of general medical services by the mentally ill, a genuine policy dilemma is how to include mental health care in the overall movement for health reform without subjecting the mentally ill to a service model that would be inefficient and ineffective for them.

THE MENTAL HEALTH POLICYMAKING ENVIRONMENT

The roots of U.S. mental health policy development, and the sources of change in this policy, lie in many influences. These influences have combined and conflicted in a variety of ways over time to produce the organization and functioning of the contemporary mental health sector.

Causal Theories

The history of mental health care is marked by the rise and fall of many different theoretical schools on the etiology and treatment of mental illness. As various perspectives have gained and lost ascendancy, major policy shifts have occurred, leading to changes in resource allocation and the locations and forms of treatment.

The initial establishment during the early 1800s of a system of state mental hospitals reflected one such shift in causal thinking. A new philosophy of care known as "moral treatment" asserted the role of environmental and emotional factors in the development of mental illness, supplanting earlier interpretations of insanity as the will of God. These new causes argued for specialized treatment settings that could deliver consistent, controlled, individualized, and humane attention to the residents. More and more, mental illness was viewed as a medical problem requiring a specific form of professional intervention, and numbers of mentally ill persons were removed from the local poorhouses and jails to which they had been consigned.

New ideas about the genetic basis of mental disorder help account for the deterioration of this public mental hospital system in the late 1800s. A belief that little could be done to aid the mentally ill led to custodial confinement on a large scale, including the widespread use of patient restraints. Facilities became badly overcrowded and run-down, as state legislatures kept operating budgets low. Moral treatment gave way to therapeutic pessimism and the decline of active treatment efforts.

The community mental health movement of the 1960s and 1970s offers a more recent example of the power of new theoretical formulations. In this case, it was the traditional medical model that came under attack, as researchers and writers in numerous fields sought to link mental illness to social process and external pressures. A key tenet of the community mental health movement was that patients should be treated in the community, rather than in artificial, "desocializing" hospital environments. Further, new resources were sought to prevent mental illness through public health-style interventions. As a result of this revision in mental health thinking, the federal Community Mental Health Centers Act of 1963 was passed, funding a network of local organizations providing clinical and educational services.

The mental health field is perennially in ferment, as myriad etiological notions centered on biological, emotional, social, genetic, and interpersonal factors vie for legitimacy and financial support. In part, this competition results from the limited success of past treatment efforts, particularly for the most seriously mentally ill. It also speaks to the uncertain knowledge base on which the field of psychiatry rests. Today, the struggle of ideas in mental health care continues over such issues as whether mental disorders are truly medical diseases; the role of drug treatments versus psychotherapy; and the value of contributions by mental health practitioners in rival disciplines (Barbour, 1995).

Intergovernmental Relations

As mental health policy objectives have changed from one period to another, there often have been associated shifts in federal, state, and local responsibilities for mental health care. Indeed, changes in intergovernmental relations have been the primary vehicle for implementing several of these new policies.

During the 1800s, a hospital system run by state authorities marked the turning away from local mental health practices based on poor relief arrangements. Then, after World War II, it took the intervention of the federal government to spur the community mental health movement. In the 1980s, the block grant initiative of the Reagan administration gave state policymakers the means to reorient this community-based system to the needs of severely mentally ill persons. In the current decade, many mental health advocates have seen the watershed creation of some kind of national health insurance program as the most promising route to improve mentally ill persons' access to services.

However, even as different parts of government may come to assume new roles periodically, mental health care in the contemporary United States is unavoidably a multilevel activity, due to the tiered nature of our social service and health programs. The deinstitutionalization program of the 1960s and 1970s led to a massive downsizing of state hospital populations, from 559,000 in 1955 to 110,000 in 1985. One direct effect of this movement was the increased "localization" of the mental health system, placing greater reliance on general hospitals, shelters, and other facilities that are run by municipal and county governments. Meanwhile, the federal government helps finance state and local services through its Medicare, Medicaid, and block grant programs. Effective mental health policy depends on cooperation among all these intergovernmental actors, but what often occurs is a kind of gaming in which the various levels play off against each other in an attempt to avoid unwanted burdens and conserve resources. Populations such as the mentally ill homeless that present complicated service needs expose the gaps in this tangle of relationships and the absence of joint planning.

The United States has a powerful political tradition of decentralization, with the states serving as "laboratories" for testing innovative programs. In some cases, however, national policy standards have been deemed essential, as with civil rights. The balance between variability and consistency is struck by decision makers within each policy area, based on specific historical and ideological factors. In mental health care, this balance customarily has favored state and local autonomy. This country does not have one national mental health system; it has fifty state systems. Quality varies tremendously, and funding levels per capita differ by as much as sevenfold (Arons et al., 1994). Intergovernmental grant transfers are one potential means of equalizing mental health care resources around the nation—and they have been used for this purpose, to a limited extent, in the past. Yet political and need-based considerations inevitably clash in allocation decisions of this kind, as has been seen in the history of the Alcohol, Drug Abuse, and Mental Health block grant (Rochefort, 1993). Moreover, federal cost-sharing initiatives can sometimes have the ironic effect of bolstering already strong state systems that seize the opportunity for program expansion—a trend evident under Medicaid's optional funding of community-based mental health services.

Political Economy

Mental health care delivery reacts to a complex of political and economic incentives. On the one hand, mental health policy enactments provide a blueprint for the desired operation and impacts of the system. On the other hand, that system also depends on market forces and the often unexpected interconnections between mental health care and other public and private programs.

The shaping power of this political economy is seen directly in the movement of patient populations out of state and county mental hospitals during the 1960s and 1970s. Most influential in the timing and state-by-state pattern of patient discharges (far beyond the impact of the federal Community Mental Health Centers program) were the Supplemental Security Income and Medicaid programs. Although neither of these programs had been developed primarily for the mentally ill, they nonetheless provided financial means for supporting the mentally ill in the community, and for relocating mental hospital residents to private health care facilities.

Using a political-economy framework, Brown (1985) has argued that mental health policy "reinforces and replicates" inequalities and power relationships of the social structure. In this light, the transfer of thousands of patients to private living and service settings attests to the dominance of the private enterprise model in the United States, including the willingness to use public funds to subsidize private profit making. This same process can be seen today in the ongoing privatization of mental health services, as states contract with health maintenance organizations and other corporate entities for the care of mentally ill persons.

However much emphasis one places on a transcendent logic of capitalism in mental health policy developments, it is clear that the mental health system is extraordinarily fragmented and pluralistic. This makes it resistant to top-down control, while exposing it to programmatic and economic forces from outside the mental health sphere. So it is that there are really two U.S. mental health systems: a de jure system based on the planned interventions of mental health policymakers, and a de facto system based on the net outcome of all policies and practices bearing on mental health care from the mental health, health, and social welfare fields (Kiesler & Sibulkin, 1987).

Decision-making Structures and Venues

Aiding the passage of federal community mental health legislation in the decades following World War II was a potent informal decision-making structure. A small group of actors in the executive and legislative branches of the federal government joined forces with private advocates to form a classic "iron triangle," characterized by a strong consensus on policy philosophy, exclusion of opposing interests, and an ability to command resources. Owing to its high ideological and organizational cohesion, this alliance had the capacity to overturn the long-established hegemony of state hospital care.

As Baumgartner and Jones (1993) have argued, such "policy monopolies" typically erode in time under the pressure of new ideas, "negative feedback" arising from implementation disappointments, emergence of new interest groups, and shifts in public opinion. By the late 1970s, when President Carter's Mental Health Systems Act was being considered, the equilibrium in national mental health policymaking had given way to a much more open contest involving a greater variety of interest groups who disagreed on future policy directions and the distribution of resources.

Today, the mental health policy environment has grown very fluid and diversified on both the national and state levels, exhibiting many of the qualities of an "issue network" that Peterson (1993) identifies for health care. This puts unprecedented stress on coalition building, both among professional, consumer, family, and organizational interests inside the mental health care arena, and with potential collaborators in the disabilities, public health, and other communities.

In addition to federal and state legislatures, the courts are another decision-making venue of signal importance for mental health policymaking. Although court decisions played a crucial part in defining the right to treatment, the right to refuse treatment, and the right to treatment in the least restrictive setting that contributed to deinstitutionalization, the courts have proved a less effective method of improving the quality of community mental health services. Moreover, strict involuntary commitment procedures based on the criterion of dangerousness delimit contemporary mental health policy strategies by hampering, for example, the kind of "round-up" and hospitalization of the homeless mentally ill that New York City tried in the late 1980s (Rochefort, 1993). In 1990, the enactment of the Americans with Disabilities Act provided new legal grounds for the fight against mental illness-based discrimination in the workplace, thereby guaranteeing the judicial system a central place in the ongoing evolution of the rights of the mentally ill.

Values

The nature and limits of mental health policymaking are partly a function of the same cluster of social values that constrains health care policymaking in general. According to Morone (1990), American political culture has "shaped past policies" and "frames future possibilities" in health care. Among the national traits he cites in this connection are a distrust of social problem solving in the political sphere, the avoidance of systematic priority setting, a devaluation of public administration, uncertain commitment to indigent patients, and antipathy to welfare programs.

In addition to these biases, mental health policymakers must also contend with the heavy social stigma of mental illness, which reflects widespread popular fear, ignorance, and hostility. The motives underlying policy development toward this perceived deviant group have always been decidedly mixed, a strange blend of compassion, medical humanitarianism, control, coercion, isolation, and cost control. In a 1989 national poll commissioned by the Robert Wood Johnson Foundation, 65 percent agreed that a lot of stigma still remains attached to mental illness. Although most respondents recognized the potential value of treatment for serious mental health problems, opinion was very divided on the dangerousness of mentally ill individuals and the comparability between physical and mental illnesses.

The impact of social stigma on mental health care systems is especially evident in programs that bring the severely mentally ill into close proximity with the general community. The Robert Wood Johnson survey found facilities for the mentally ill to be among the least well accepted of a group of possible neighborhood facilities. Such attitudes are consistent with behavior, as community residential facilities throughout the country have met vigorous resistance from local residents and their elected representatives. Supporting this "Not in My Backyard" phenomenon have been a variety of formal and informal methods of exclusion, including municipal ordinances and regulations, bureaucratic obstacles, and public protests.

There is some experience to suggest that local opposition can subside remarkably once community residences are in operation and neighborhood members' worst fears of violence and disruption go unrealized (Winerip, 1994). Nonetheless, the challenge for administrators remains how to launch these programs into welcoming environments. In this sense, cultural attitudes toward the mentally ill are a significant variable in the implementation phase of mental health policymaking, and the ability to achieve social integration is essential to the clinical efficacy of community-based care.

MENTAL HEALTH INSURANCE COVERAGE PROBLEMS

The problems of uninsurance and underinsurance that helped convert health care reform into a major national issue by the early 1990s are found nowhere more clearly than in the mental health care sector.

Whereas 14 percent of the U.S. population lacked insurance coverage in 1990, 18 percent of all persons with mental disorders were without insurance (National Advisory Mental Health Council, 1993). Overall, the mentally ill are much more dependent on government programs to pay for their health services. For instance, it is estimated that 42 percent of health care expenditures for the population as a whole comes from public sources, compared to 54 percent for the mentally ill and 57 percent for the severely mentally ill. Moreover, even though the vast majority of persons with health coverage also have mental health care benefits—an estimated 98 percent of those in private health plans (Carter, 1993)—mental health benefits are almost never provided on a par with those for other illnesses and conditions. Instead, insurers limit coverage through a variety of methods, including fewer allowable days of inpatient care per year, lower annual expense maximums, lower lifetime expense maximums, fewer outpatient visits per year, and higher patient cost sharing. Health maintenance organizations are no exception, often applying benefit restrictions for inpatient days and outpatient visits per year that do not exist for other forms of health care (National Advisory Mental Health Council, 1993).

Public insurance programs also discriminate against the mentally ill. For example, Medicare requires a 50 percent co-payment for outpatient mental health services, compared to 20 percent for other services. Medicaid excludes payments for persons between twenty-two and sixty-four years of age in "institutions for mental disease," that is, facilities in which 50 percent or more of the patients have a primary diagnosis of mental illness. Also uncovered is care in small residential facilities (Taube et al., 1990).

Another mental health insurance problem is lack of comprehensiveness in the services eligible for coverage. One analysis estimated that only 11 percent of all those with health insurance coverage had benefits for "partial hospitalization," a valuable service for mental illness (Carter, 1993). Nor are residential and rehabilitation services or case management typically covered. Somewhere between 60 percent and 65 percent of all mental health expenditures are for institutional care (Arons et al., 1994), despite abundant evidence of the cost-effectiveness of alternative treatments for most psychiatric patients (Kiesler & Sibulkin, 1987).

The problem of health insurers curtailing coverage because of "preexisting conditions" has been widely noted. Such practices may involve exclusions of specific illnesses or sometimes the denial of coverage entirely to an individual with a certain medical history. The risk of falling subject to this insurance cost-containment device is one of the main reasons behind "job lock," wherein an employed person hesitates to change jobs because of the potential impact on coverage status (Starr, 1994). Mental illness is one of the factors commonly used in this process of "medical underwriting." Reportedly, many individuals resort to out-of-pocket payment for mental health care rather than make use of the benefits available to them, simply to avoid the possibility of future coverage denials (Carter, 1993).

A main impetus behind the expansion of insurance coverage during the 1970s and 1980s was the passage of legislation in a majority of states mandating minimum coverage of mental disorders in private health insurance plans. These mandates have failed, however, to expand access to mental health insurance coverage as expected. Many companies avoided mandates through self-insurance, and a number of states passed "bare-bones" legislation to allow the marketing of health insurance policies without mental health and substance abuse benefits. Moreover, the growing size of the uninsured population has blunted the impact of mental health mandates.

All told, in addition to the roughly 40 million Americans who have no insurance coverage, an estimated 15 million to 30 million Americans are without adequate insurance for mental health problems (Sharfstein et al., 1993). Several consequences result, including financial disincentives to seeking mental health treatment on a timely basis; widespread vulnerability in the face of catastrophic mental illnesses; and the necessity of maintaining a residual system of mental health facilities for those unable to pay for care, leading to a two-tiered, public–private mental health care structure (Arons et al., 1994). On a macrolevel, the variety of different payers and coverage gaps produces tremendous disorganization marked by "excess capacity, uncoordinated service use, access problems, and excess costs" (Arons et al., 1994, p. 194; see also Sharfstein et al., 1993).

MENTAL HEALTH CARE REFORM AND THE NATIONAL HEALTH CARE DEBATE: POLITICS AND POLICY ALTERNATIVES

Universal coverage and cost containment were the two dominant aims of the movement for national health care reform. Crucially related to both is the ques-

tion of what services to include in the basic benefit package guaranteed to all of the insured. From the outset, mental health care stood on uncertain ground in this discussion.

For mental health advocates, of course, the inclusion of mental health benefits was essential, a pivotal test of the very concept of reform. Universal basic mental health benefits would move mental health coverage toward parity with other forms of health care. To justify this long-sought objective, the advocates presented several arguments. For example, former First Lady Rosalynn Carter, honorary chairperson of her husband's presidential commission on mental illness, made the following points in testimony before the Senate Labor and Human Resources Committee in March 1994 (Carter, 1994):

1. Mental illness is a "serious and pervasive" social problem.
2. Like physical illnesses, some of the major mental illnesses are related to chemical or structural brain disorders.
3. There is clear evidence of the efficacy of many mental health treatments.
4. Model benefit plans from the private sector demonstrate that comprehensive mental health coverage is a controllable cost that is capable of reducing health costs in general.

Advocates also argued that clear public support exists for expanding mental health benefits. For example, in February 1994, the Judge David L. Bazelon Center for Mental Health Law commissioned a national poll on views toward coverage of mental health care and substance abuse under health care reform. It found that 65 percent of Americans wanted mental health benefits to be covered in the national reform package. Forty-three percent said including these benefits was "one of the most important" or "a very important" component of any new program. Asked whether it was important to cover mental health problems to the same extent as physical health problems, 62 percent answered affirmatively. Most respondents opposed limits on inpatient and outpatient mental health coverage, as well as high co-payments (Bazelon Center, 1994b).

An unprecedented coalition of thirty-three mental health organizations, including advocacy groups, state mental health systems, professional associations, provider agencies, and family and consumer groups, was formed in March 1993 to give input to the president's Task Force on National Health Care Reform (Koyanagi et al., 1993). Hoping to enhance its influence by presenting a unified position, this Mental Health Liaison Group recommended a "broad array of health and mental health treatment, rehabilitation and prevention services, emphasizing treatment in the least restrictive setting consistent with the patient's clinical needs" (Mental Health Liaison Group, 1993, pp. 539–540). It also called for an organized system with capitated premiums, prior authorization, and utilization controls. Variable co-payments were considered to be acceptable for psychotherapy, however, in order to discourage inappropriate utilization. The coalition also underscored maintaining a strong public mental health system to meet any specialized service and financing needs left unaddressed by health reform, as well as bringing these state systems into close linkage with the private care system.

Notwithstanding such an unusual and timely mobilization of mental health interests, including the participation of esteemed public figures like former First Ladies Rosalynn Carter and Betty Ford, the idea of mental health insurance expansion evoked a cautious response among most health planners and policymakers. Within the Clinton administration, the vice president's wife Tipper Gore was a strong and faithful ally. Still, as the formulation of the president's proposal took place between January and September 1993, there were many mixed signals as to how mental health care would be handled. On March 16, 1993, the *New York Times* reported that the administration intended "to guarantee mental health coverage" and "to eliminate what they [administration planners] see as discriminatory treatment of mental illness by insurers" (Pear, 1993a). Yet by June, the *Times* disclosed that "concerns about cost have forced the administration to reconsider its initial plan to provide open-ended, comprehensive" mental health benefits (Pear, 1993b). A growing tension between Mrs. Gore and Mrs. Clinton was attributed to

this issue. In September, shortly before the president's plan was released, administration officials indicated that earlier ambitious plans for mental health care were being scaled back (Pear, 1993c).

Comparing provisions in President Clinton's Health Security Act with other reform initiatives in Congress, it is possible to identify five distinct approaches to mental health care coverage (Hoehn, 1993; Bazelon Center, 1994a).

At one extreme lay a "comprehensive coverage model," exemplified in the American Health Security Act, a single-payer bill sponsored by Senator Paul Wellstone (D-MN) and Representative James McDermott (D-WA). This approach featured no restrictions on the population to receive services, except for "special care coordination," which was reserved for the severely and chronically mentally ill. The spectrum of medical, psychiatric, and social support services encompassed was very extensive, including assessment, diagnosis, and referral; crisis intervention; partial hospitalization; psychosocial rehabilitation; pharmacotherapy; residential treatment; and inpatient care. Cost containment was to be achieved by utilization review, rather than by any patient cost sharing or preset service limitations.

A second "enhanced private insurance model" describes the Clinton proposal (Arons et al., 1994). Included in the basic plan were thirty days of hospitalization (extendable to sixty days in dangerous situations); thirty sessions per year of outpatient psychotherapy (extendable to 120 days with a trade-off against inpatient days); specified intensive nonresidential services, such as partial hospitalization, day treatment, and psychiatric rehabilitation (120 days a year, with a trade-off against inpatient days for the first sixty days and high co-payments for the second sixty days); and unlimited case management on an as-needed basis. Co-payments and deductibles were a function of the cost-sharing options in the overall plan, ranging for outpatient psychotherapy between $25 per visit and 50 percent coinsurance. With no lifetime limits and no exclusions due to preexisting conditions, the plan essentially provided benefits tantamount to the best private mental health care coverage available. A further part of the proposal was "full integration" of the public and private mental health sectors in the year 2001, with the elimination of annual day and visit benefit limits at that time.

A third "restricted private insurance model," embodied in a number of congressional reform plans, took the approach of more modest private mental health plans. A specific illustration was the "Health Access America" proposal of the American Medical Association, which provided for twenty outpatient visits per year, forty-five inpatient days, and deductibles of $350 (individual) and $750 (family) plus co-payments.

A fourth "severe mental illness model," such as in mental health legislation sponsored by Senator Pete Domenici (R-NM), restricted eligibility for services to certain illnesses defined by diagnosis, disability, and duration, with a narrow focus on the most severe and incapacitating disorders like schizophrenia and manic depression. For individuals with these problems, coverage of treatment and cost controls were to be on a par with those for physical illnesses. Senator John Chafee's (R-RI) Health Equity and Access Reform Today Act similarly limited the mental health benefit to services for severe mental illness.

Finally, a "mental health coverage unspecified model" applied to proposals like the Managed Competition Act of 1993 (Cooper [D-TN]/Breaux [D-LA]), the Affordable Health Care Now Act (Michel [R-IL]/Lott [R-MS]), and the Comprehensive Family Health Access and Savings Act (Gramm [R-TX]). These bills contained no unequivocal statement of mental health benefits, leaving these instead to be defined by boards after passage and, in some cases, allowing for the continuation of exclusionary insurance practices. None of these proposals guaranteed universal population coverage.

It was the administration's bill, however, that commanded center stage in legislative deliberations, at least in the early period. The reaction of the mental health community to its provisions was ambivalent, but, in a spirit of compromise, on the whole supportive. The proposal did not give full parity between mental health and health care, as many advocates desired. And social support and rehabilitation services for the chronically and severely mentally ill in the community were restricted. One of the most critical appraisals came from the National Alliance for the Mentally Ill, an organiza-

tion representing mentally ill persons and their families, which characterized the Clinton plan's limitations on mental health benefits as "totally unacceptable" and "federally mandated discrimination against persons with severe mental illness" (*News & Notes*, 1993).

Still, many mental health advocates well realized that the Health Security Act featured better benefits than many of the rival plans in Congress, with the advantage of guaranteed universal coverage. If not ideal in all ways, the administration's bill would translate nonetheless into vastly improved mental health protections for millions of Americans. Although it was but a promise, the vision of mental health and health care integration by 2001 also held strong appeal.

Meanwhile, the legislative process afforded the mental health coalition and its collaborators the chance to work at broadening the mental health component before a final health bill was enacted, and that is exactly what they set about doing. A bipartisan Working Group on Mental Illness and Health Issues, whose members included Representatives James McDermott (D-WA), Ronald Machtley (R-RI), and Eleanor Holmes Norton (D-DC) and Senators Pete Domenici (R-NM), Paul Wellstone (D-MN), and Edward Kennedy (D-MA) spearheaded the cause, with the assistance of the organized mental health interests. A primary thrust of the group was the refutation of claims that expanded mental health coverage necessarily meant excessive utilization and costs. What resulted from this initiative, in the words of one leading national mental health advocate, was dramatic improvement in the mental health benefits of various bills, which became "more comprehensive, more flexible, and even some calling for parity" (Koyanagi, 1995).

By the end of the summer of 1993, there were two main health reform plans from the House and Senate Democratic leaderships. Both included substantial mental health provisions (Gosselin, 1994). Increasingly, however, such details of legislation were being lost in the midst of a bitter ideological battle between Democrats and Republicans over the proper role of government. At one point, Senator Phil Gramm (R-TX) claimed that Senate Majority Leader George Mitchell's (D-ME) bill would pave the way to socialized medicine and a "medical Gestapo knocking on your parents' door" (Toner, 1994). In this heated atmosphere, and with widespread public doubts over a new health program's impact on the economy and existing private health care arrangements, the effort for national health care reform collapsed. With it went the hopes for a federal solution to mental health insurance coverage problems.

AFTER THE FAILURE OF REFORM

The community mental health revolution of the past forty years has wrought profound changes in mental health care across the United States. Public hospital facilities have been massively downsized, alternative inpatient and outpatient treatment settings have proliferated, and there is increasing reliance on drugs and other new therapies. This was anything but a careful public policy experiment, however. In fact, it was hardly planned change at all in certain respects. Instead, the movement was driven by a host of coinciding forces ranging from biomedical advances, to civil liberties struggles, to expanded public and private insurance coverage, to a heightened popular receptivity to psychological concepts, to federal activism. Today the call is heard from some quarters for a return to a mental health system centered around inpatient care in large public institutions. This notion, however, is a clinical and social anachronism. Largely as a result of deinstitutionalization and other transformations of recent decades, progressive mental health care is now viewed in "biopsychosocial" terms, dictating both a balanced and comprehensive service system (Bachrach, 1993). This concept goes far beyond the traditional functions of the state hospital.

Rapid and spontaneous in its spread, contemporary community mental health care is still poorly understood in many ways. Unknown, for example, are the fates of all former long-term hospital patients. It is also unclear which types of patients respond best to particular treatments among the broad spectrum of alternatives currently available. Further, the sources of community reaction to the mentally ill remain largely obscure, a prime obstacle in developing strategies to combat stigma and

rejection. Yet one key fact may be stated with a high degree of certainty: community care can work effectively, even with persons suffering from severely disabling and chronic mental illnesses. Numerous rigorously "controlled" studies have established the superiority of "alternative treatment programs" to hospitalization with regard to a whole array of clinical and social outcome variables (Kiesler & Sibulkin, 1987). As their common elements, such programs include extensive social support and behavioral skill building, as well as practical intervention in patients' social environments.

Yet a central problem of mental health policymaking is that not all mentally ill persons have access to good quality programs possessing these components. Mental health advocates had looked to the passage of federal health reform not only to give mental health coverage to the uninsured, but also to stimulate the reorganization and expansion of the mental health system. Once that legislative effort collapsed, the field was left open for other kinds of influences to define future scenarios in U.S. mental health care.

For one thing, the failed campaign for national health reform meant that the states would be the prime shapers of their own future mental health systems, free to pursue those improvements for which they can muster political and financial support. The states have been working at this task for many years, albeit with widely varying commitment. One basic reform direction that has emerged is the creation of coordinated local service systems in which the resources of diverse public and private agencies are used to create individually tailored frameworks of community support for patients with complex needs. The "Program for Assertive Community Treatment" (PACT) is one such approach. First developed in Wisconsin in the 1970s, it now operates in more than three hundred localities in thirty-four states. At its core, PACT involves "multidisciplinary teams of mental health professionals who share a common and limited caseload and provide comprehensive care in the community for adults with long-term psychotic illnesses" (Deci et al., 1995, p. 676). The Robert Wood Johnson Foundation also launched a multiyear demonstration program in the late 1980s, called the "Program on Chronic Mental Illness," to promote the centralization of administrative, fiscal, and clinical responsibility for long-term mental health care in the hands of single mental health authorities. Selected to participate in the initiative were nine cities that also received special rental subsidies from the U.S. Department of Housing and Urban Development to expand community housing for the program's clientele (Talbott, 1995).

These attempts at subnational mental health system change have not been without their problems. Bureaucracies are prone to resist the new organizational relationships that meaningful coordination of services demands—a classic implementation obstacle. Funding to commence new programs and then to sustain activities at acceptable quality levels has also been difficult to arrange in many places. In these and other ways, the reform process hinges on strong political will matched by effective public leadership—a rare combination. In the case of the more ambitious systemic reorientation represented by the Robert Wood Johnson program, great doubt exists about the impact of structural-level changes on individual patient outcomes (Goldman et al., 1994).

Meanwhile, as the states explore community treatment innovations, the phenomenon of managed care is spreading throughout the mental health sector, and with startling rapidity. Well over 100 million Americans were enrolled in managed mental health and substance abuse programs by 1995 (Law, 1995). In simplest terms, managed mental health care is an administrative process of overseeing the utilization of mental health services. Managed mental health care is associated with multiple objectives (quality improvement, cost control, services integration) and it has been operationalized variously depending on the context (e.g., within conventional insurance plans, health maintenance organizations, or other organized systems of care). Managed mental health is found in both public and private sectors, and it is worth highlighting certain distinctions between these two forms.

Already by 1990, most large firms in the United States were providing health insurance coverage with a managed care feature (Garnick et al., 1994). Four com-

mon types of programs were (1) case management, in which an "ombudsman" service coordinator arranges all care and support services; (2) preadmission certification, in which insurers approve all hospital admissions prospectively; (3) concurrent review, in which a patient's course of inpatient treatment is reviewed as care is delivered, with periodic approvals for continuation; and (4) outpatient review, in which the course of outpatient treatment is reviewed on either a prospective or concurrent basis. Beyond the use of these fundamental mechanisms either singly or in combination, private managed mental health care programs are enormously diverse, relying on different kinds of review personnel, clinical criteria, and penalties.

Even less consensus exists on the meaning of managed mental health care in the public sector. For example, one attempt to formulate a standard definition states: "the organization of an *accessible* and *accountable* service delivery system that is designed to *consolidate* and *flexibly deploy* resources so as to provide *comprehensive*, *continuous*, *cost-effective*, and *effective* mental health services to *targeted* individuals in their *home communities*" (Hoge et al., 1994, p. 1087). Thus do the aims of public-sector managed care extend beyond those of the private version, to include a wholesale organizational remedy for all the problems of "unmanaged" mental health systems. In practice, public-sector managed care often is delivered through a "carve-out" arrangement, wherein a state agency contracts out to a separate private or public entity for the care of a defined population for a set budgetary amount. Several states have already received federal waiver approvals to provide mental health and substance abuse services under Medicaid by this method.

In a cacaphony of voices, payers, providers, consumers, and advocates are now registering competing claims about the efficiency, equity, and cost savings of managed care programs. The result is fast becoming the major controversy of the day in mental health care. In Rhode Island, for example, the Department of Health, prompted by consumer complaints, investigated and found serious deficiencies in the practices of one private managed care company, United Behavioral Systems. As a result, the company was both fined and ordered to revamp its operation. Around the same time, in Massachusetts an investigation was begun to account for a sharply elevated death rate among the clientele of the state Department of Mental Health simultaneous with its shift to a privatized care system (Bass, 1995). It is uncertain how widespread such problems might be across the nation or what the precise reasons are for their occurrence. Nonetheless, they underscore concerns about the financial incentives under managed care to minimize service delivery. Further research is needed, with much more detailed analysis of the organizational auspices and design of managed care instruments as these impact on patient care as well as costs (Garnick et al., 1994).

The potential transformation of Medicaid from an open-ended federal–state matching program with defined standards of eligibility to a fixed block grant lacking entitlement status, as proposed by the Republican Congress in the fall of 1995, riveted the attention of all in the health policy community, stimulating great speculation about the likely consequences for health care for the poor. Less well-examined, however, were the far-reaching effects these changes could have on mental health care in the United States. Historically, Medicaid has played a crucial role in the development of community mental health care. As noted earlier, Medicaid funding of general hospital and nursing home care helped spur the process of deinstitutionalization. More recently, Medicaid also became a prime source of funding for a range of community mental health services under special program options that allow states to leverage federal funds for such activities as case management. Nationwide, Medicaid accounted for 30 percent of all public mental health and substance abuse funding in 1990 (Law, 1995). The program has become one of the most important sources of third-party reimbursement for community mental health agencies in many states.

The conversion of Medicaid to a block grant would result in a reduced level of public financing for mental health services and less opportunity to expand innovative services. While to some extent the states might make up for federal cutbacks, many are already struggling with severe budget problems of their own, and the mentally ill have never wielded much political power in the battle for scarce resources. In any event, state governments around the country are sure to be uneven in their responses to Medicaid shrinkage. Some may even retarget funds away from the mentally ill population to other program constituencies, in the process increasing geographic inequities in the quantity and quality of mental health services.

Thus the challenges of mental health care delivery will continue to evolve, partly as a function of internal issues and the unique history of the mental health sector and partly as a function of broader health system currents. To return to a theme at the opening of this chapter, mental health and health care are two distinct but conjoined fields. Because of this connection, effective policy development in the two areas, as well as sound policy analysis, depends on appreciating the interrelationship.

REFERENCES

Arons, Bernard S., Richard G. Frank, Howard H. Goldman, Thomas G. McGuire, & Sharman Stephens. (1994). Mental health and substance abuse coverage. *Health Affairs, 13* (Spring), 192–205.

Bachrach, Leona L. (1993). The biopsychosocial legacy of deinstitutionalization. *Hospital and Community Psychiatry, 44* (6), 523–524.

Barbour, William. (1995). *Mental illness: Opposing viewpoints.* San Diego: Greenhaven Press.

Bass, Alison. (1995). DMH sees increase in deaths. *Boston Globe* (June 11), 1.

Baumgartner, Frank R., & Bryan D. Jones (1993). *Agendas and instability in American politics.* Chicago: University of Chicago Press.

Bazelon Center for Mental Health Law. (1994a). *Health care reform fact sheets.* Washington, D.C.

Bazelon Center for Mental Health Law. (1994b). *Survey of voters' views on coverage of mental health care and substance abuse treatment under health care reform.* Washington, D.C.

Bourdon, Karen A., Donald S. Rae, William E. Narrow, Ronald W. Manderscheid, & Darrel A. Regier. (1994). National prevalence and treatment of mental and addictive disorders. In Ronald W. Manderscheid & Mary Anne Sonnenschein (Eds.), *Mental health, United States, 1994.* Washington, D.C.: Center for Mental Health Services, Superintendent of Documents, U.S. Government Printing Office.

Brown, Phil. (1985). *The transfer of care: Psychiatric deinstitutionalization and its aftermath.* London: Routledge & Kegan Paul.

Carter, Rosalynn (1993). Mental health policy and health care reform. *National Forum, 73* (Winter), 13–15.

Carter, Rosalynn. (1994). Testimony of former First Lady Rosalynn Carter before the Senate Labor and Human Resources Committee, March 8. Unpublished.

Deci, Paul A., Alberto B. Santos, D. Walter Hiott, Sonja Schoenwald, & James K. Dias. (1995). Dissemination of assertive community treatment programs. *Psychiatric Services, 46* (July), 676–678.

Emery, C. Eugene, Jr. (1995). R.I. fines health insurer $100,000. *Providence Journal-Bulletin* (July 12), 1.

Garnick, Deborah W., Ann M. Hendricks, Jane D. Dulski, Kenneth E. Thorpe, & Constance Horgan. (1994). Characteristics of private-sector managed care for mental health and substance abuse treatment. *Hospital and Community Psychiatry, 45* (December), 1201–1205.

Goldman, Howard H. (1993). Politics of inclusion: Mental health coverage in national health reform. *National Forum, 73* (Winter), 42–43.

Goldman, Howard H., Joseph P. Morrissey, & Susan M. Ridgely. (1994). Evaluating the Robert Wood Johnson Foundation program on chronic mental illness. *Milbank Quarterly, 72* (Winter), 37–48.

Gosselin, Peter G. (1994). Mitchell airs health plan that covers 95%. *Boston Globe* (August 3), 1.

Hoehn, Karen. (1993). *Proposals in the 103rd Congress calling for inclusion of mental health in healthcare reform.* Washington, D.C.: Mental Health Policy Resource Center.

Hoge, Michael A., Larry Davidson, Ezra E. Griffith, William H. Sledge, & Richard A. Howenstine. (1994). Defining managed care in public-sector psychiatry. *Hospital and Community Psychiatry, 45* (November), 1085–1089.

Kessler, Ronald C., et al. (1994). Lifetime and 12-month prevalence of DSM-III-R psychiatric disorders in the United States. *Archives of General Psychiatry, 51* (January), 8–19.

Kiesler, Charles A., & Amy E. Sibulkin. (1987). *Mental hospitalization: Myths and facts about a national crisis.* Newbury Park, CA: Sage.

Kiesler, Charles A., & Celeste G. Simpkins. (1993). *The unnoticed majority in psychiatric inpatient care.* New York: Plenum Press.

Koyanagi, Chris. (1995). Lessons learned—looking ahead: A national advocate's point of view. *Policy in Perspective (Mental Health Policy Resource Center)* (March), 3–5.

Koyanagi, Chris, Joseph Manes, Richard Surles, et al. (1993). On being very smart: The mental health community's response in the health care reform debate. *Hospital and Community Psychiatry, 45* (September), 537–539.

Law, Colleen E. (1995). Database: Mental health and substance abuse managed care statistics. *Policy in Perspective (Mental Health Policy Resource Center)* (September), 5.

Mechanic, David. (1993). Mental health services in the context of health insurance reform. *Milbank Quarterly, 71* (March), 349–364.

Mental Health Liaison Group. (1993). Recommendations for mental health services in health care reform. *Hospital and Community Psychiatry, 44* (June), 539–542.

Morone, James A. (1990). American political culture and the search for lessons abroad. *Journal of Health Politics, Policy and Law, 15* (Spring), 129–143.

National Advisory Mental Health Council. (1993). Health care reform for Americans with severe mental illnesses: Report of the National Advisory Mental Health Council. *American Journal of Psychiatry, 150* (October), 1447–1465.

News & Notes. (1993). Mental health groups seeking equal coverage give Clinton's health care plan mixed reviews. *Hospital and Community Psychiatry, 44* (November), 1112–1113.

Olfson, Mark, & Harold A. Pincus. (1994). Measuring outpatient mental health care in the United States. *Health Affairs, 13* (Winter), 172–180.

Pear, Robert. (1993a). White House plan would cover costs of mental illness. *New York Times* (March 16), A1.

Pear, Robert. (1993b). Administration rethinking mental health coverage. *New York Times* (June 10), A24.

Pear, Robert. (1993c). Clinton cuts aims on mental health and dental costs. *New York Times* (September 3), A1.

Peterson, Mark A. (1993). Political influence in the 1990s: From iron triangles to policy networks. *Journal of Health Politics, Policy and Law, 18* (Summer), 395–438.

Redick, Richard W., Michael J. Witkin, Joanne E. Atay, & Ronald W. Manderscheid. (1994). Highlights of organized mental health services in 1990 and major national and state trends. In Ronald W. Manderscheid & Mary Anne Sonnenschein (Eds.), *Mental health, United States, 1994* (pp. 77–125). Washington, D.C.: Center for Mental Health Services, Superintendent of Documents, U.S. Government Printing Office.

Rice, Dorothy P., Sander Kelman, & Leonard S. Miller. (1992). The economic burden of mental illness. *Hospital and Community Psychiatry, 43* (December), 1227–1232.

Rochefort, David A. (1993). *From poorhouses to homelessness: Policy analysis and mental health care.* Westport, CT: Auburn House.

Rochefort, David A., & Roger W. Cobb. (Eds.). (1994). *The politics of problem definition.* Lawrence: University Press of Kansas.

Sharfstein, Steven S., & Anne M. Stoline. (1992). Reform issues for insuring mental health care. *Health Affairs, 11* (Fall), 84–97.

Sharfstein, Steven S., Anne M. Stoline, & Howard H. Goldman. (1993). Psychiatric care and health insurance reform. *American Journal of Psychiatry, 150* (January), 7–18.

Starr, Paul. (1994). *The logic of health care reform.* New York: Penguin Books.

Talbott, John A. (1995). Evaluating the Johnson Foundation program on chronic mental illness: An interview with Howard Goldman. *Psychiatric Services, 46* (May), 501–503.

Taube, Carl A., Howard H. Goldman, & David Salkever. (1990). Medicaid coverage for mental illness: Balancing access and costs. *Health Affairs, 9* (Spring), 5–18.

Toner, Robin. (1994). Senate G.O.P. heats up attack on health bill. *New York Times* (August 4), A15.

Winerip, Michael. (1994). *9 highland road.* New York: Pantheon.

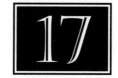
The Health Politics of Disability

Gary L. Albrecht

Health politics in America exemplifies the post-modern struggle over what constitutes core social values, culture, human rights, and the meaning of democracy in our society (Elster, 1992; Wilson, 1993). Political activity occurs around health issues when citizens with divergent opinions or interests engage in a discourse over what policies should be enacted and made binding on the group (Miller, 1991, p. 390). Health symbolizes an individual's quality of life and a society's well-being, for we judge societies in terms of the mortality, morbidity, disability, and health-related quality of life of their citizens. In general, societies are thought to be better places to live if their citizens live long lives, have high-quality, accessible, and affordable medical care, experience little or delayed morbidity, re-port few disability days, and enjoy a high quality of life (Albrecht and Fitzpatrick, 1994). An examination of the heated debate in the United States and many other countries over health care reform reveals that, despite expensive and complex national systems, health is not perceived by many to be distributed justly or econom-ically in society (Batavia, 1993; Feinstein, 1993; Melville, 1994).

Debates rage over prevention versus treatment, access to and costs of care, and what posture to take toward persons who are unborn, disabled, or older. When confronted with agreeing on a core set of values or allocating scarce resources to expensive problems, people's emotions flare and, undeterred by fact or the good of society, they often act according to their own self-interests. This chapter focuses on disability debates as examples of more general health care politics. Analysis of disability politics is important for many reasons. As populations

Work on this chapter was supported by the Award for the Promotion of Human Welfare, 1993; Emory University and the Southern Sociological Society.

age and as technology keeps people alive who previously would have died, more citizens are living with disability. Disability implies the threat of dependence and increased costs to society. In terms of values, humanity and respect in a society can be measured by how government and citizens treat their children, older people, and persons with disabilities. The inclusion of persons with disabilities in society raises issues of human rights and morality. What are the mutual obligations that citizens have to their country and the nation has to its members? What is a just distribution of resources? An analysis of disability politics addresses these timely and fundamental issues.

This chapter reviews current definitions of disability and conceptualizations of the disability process. It highlights the relationship of disability to health and examines the distribution of disability in society. The chapter then analyzes the political economy of disability in the United States and points out the historical evolution of needs-based and entitlement systems to support persons with disabilities. Needs-based benefit systems are predicated on what a person "needs" to live at least a minimum-level quality of life. Entitlement systems are based on laws that distribute benefits according to a person's membership in a group such as those over sixty-five or those with disabilities. Entitlement does not always indicate need and those in need are often not entitled. Next, the chapter describes and analyzes the history of disability legislation and politics in the United States, including the Americans with Disabilities Act and its effect on society. It indicates how disability and chronic illnesses are major problems in health care reform. The chapter concludes with some thoughts on formulating a national disability policy.

WHAT IS DISABILITY?

For years, clinicians, researchers, and government welfare agencies have struggled with disability definitions, their measurement, and their interpretation. Disability is a concept that refers to limitations in an individual's activity and role performance that require adjustments in the regimens of daily life and preestablished social relationships (Albrecht, 1992, p. 17). Peo-

ple who are recognized as having a disability usually are thought to be limited in physical, mental, or emotional function due to some impairment. Impairments refer to anatomical or functional abnormalities, such as the loss of a limb, brain damage, or hormonal imbalances, which exist on the physiological or biochemical level. These impairments are the result of genetic anomalies, accidents, or sequelae of chronic illness. Functional limitations are often operationally defined in terms of difficulties in performing activities of daily living, such as walking, moving up and down stairs, lifting a ten-pound weight, hearing, speaking, functioning cognitively, bathing and toileting, and less frequently in terms of instrumental activities such as preparing meals or taking medications. Taken in concert, impairments, disabilities, and functional limitations are indicators of an individual's dependency in society.

Disability is conceptually related to disease and diagnostic categories and indirectly to health-related quality of life. Researchers have been struggling for years to build these multiple concepts into a coherent conceptual model that has multiple uses in clinical medicine, research, and determining health and welfare benefits. During the 1970s and 1980s, most disability studies relied heavily on the conceptual model developed by Nagi (1965) and the World Health Organization's International Classification of Impairments, Disabilities, and Handicaps (ICIDH) framework (Grimby et al., 1988). These two frameworks adapted from Verbrugge and Jette (1993) are presented in Figure 17-1.

Many researchers continue to build their work on these two models. Verbrugge and Jette (1993), for example, use them to elaborate and explain the process of becoming disabled. They point out that clinicians and survey researchers alike tend to focus on the intrinsic, personal capacities of persons with disabilities without paying sufficient attention to constraints in the external environment, such as steps, transportation, and discrimination in the workplace. Building on the Nagi and ICIDH models, they suggest that disability is a gap between personal capability and environmental demand. This more complete formulation draws needed attention to the ongoing interaction between people and their environments.

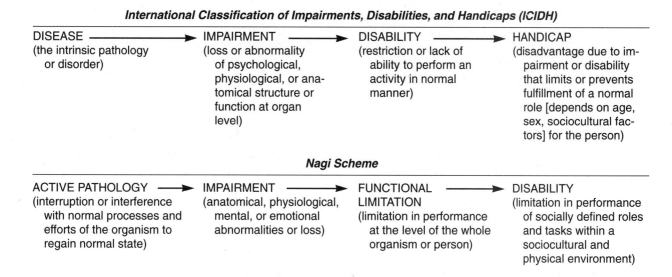

International Classification of Impairments, Disabilities, and Handicaps (ICIDH)

DISEASE ⟶	IMPAIRMENT ⟶	DISABILITY ⟶	HANDICAP
(the intrinsic pathology or disorder)	(loss or abnormality of psychological, physiological, or anatomical structure or function at organ level)	(restriction or lack of ability to perform an activity in normal manner)	(disadvantage due to impairment or disability that limits or prevents fulfillment of a normal role [depends on age, sex, sociocultural factors] for the person)

Nagi Scheme

ACTIVE PATHOLOGY ⟶	IMPAIRMENT ⟶	FUNCTIONAL LIMITATION ⟶	DISABILITY
(interruption or interference with normal processes and efforts of the organism to regain normal state)	(anatomical, physiological, mental, or emotional abnormalities or loss)	(limitation in performance at the level of the whole organism or person)	(limitation in performance of socially defined roles and tasks within a sociocultural and physical environment)

FIGURE 17-1 International Classification of Impairments, Disabilities, and Handicaps (ICIDH) and Nagi Scheme

SOURCE: Reprinted from *Social Science and Medicine, 38,* Lois M. Verbrugge and Alan M. Jette, The disablement process, p. 1, 1993, with kind permission from Elsevier Science Ltd, The Boulevard, Langford Lane, Kidlington 0X5 1GB, UK.

Johnson and Wolinsky (1993) note that while previous work based on the Nagi and ICIDH models has been informative, it does not represent the complexity of the disability process nor the multiple paths to a particular health status. Addressing these issues, Johnson and Wolinsky develop, test, and confirm a multi-equation model of perceived health status (presented in Figure 17-2) that demonstrates the complexity of the relationships among disease, disability, activities of daily living, and perceived health status.

The confirmed model highlights the differences between upper and lower body disability, the different types and levels of activities of daily living, and the direct and indirect effects of sociodemographic variables like age, sex, race, education, and disease on disability, activities of daily living, and perceived health status.

The work of Albrecht and Higgins (1977), Pope (1984) and Verbrugge et al. (1994) emphasizes the importance of considering disability as a dynamic process. People with disabilities, for instance, have "good days and bad days" (Charmaz, 1991), disabling conditions can go into remission and then recur without warning, and the cycle of disability often is experienced as an ebb and flow

even as function gradually deteriorates. This work on elaborated conceptual models and sensitivity to disability as a process is refining our understanding of disability and its relationships to disease and health status.

The analytical work of researchers, however, must be considered in conjunction with the legal definitions of disability to understand how disability policies are implemented in government benefit programs. Government and industry programs, policies, and practices are bound by the most recent federal and local law. The most recent major disability legislation in the United States is the Americans with Disabilities Act of 1990 (ADA), which states that persons have a disability if they meet one or more of the following criteria (LaPlante, 1991):

A. a physical or mental impairment that substantially limits one or more of the major life activities of such individuals
B. a record of such an impairment
C. being regarded as having such an impairment

Section 504 of the Rehabilitation Act of 1973 used Part A as the core working definition of disability, while

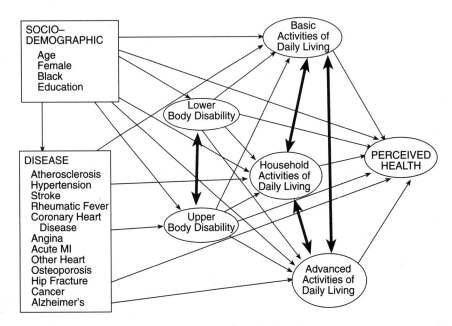

Figure 17-2 Specified Conceptual Model for Composite Scales and Latent Variables of Disease, Disability, Functional Limitation, and Perceived Health

SOURCE: Robert J. Johnson and Frederic D. Wolinsky. (1993). The structure of health status among older adults: Disease, disability, functional limitation, and perceived health. *Journal of Health and Social Behavior, 34,* 114. Used by permission of the American Sociological Association and the author.

the ADA added Parts B and C. Under this expanded definition, persons who consider themselves to be disabled but who are not perceived by others to be so are, nevertheless, implicitly included.

In applying disability definitions to individuals, disagreement has frequently occurred over what is meant by "impairments that substantially limit one or more of the major life activities." The Senate and House reports that accompanied the 1990 ADA legislation attempt to clarify this language:

A physical or mental impairment does not constitute a disability under the first prong (Part A) of the definition for purposes of the ADA unless its severity is such that it results in a "substantial limitation in one or more major life activities." A "major life activity" means functions such as caring for one's self, performing manual tasks, walking, seeing, hearing, speaking, breathing, learning, working, and participating in community activities (U.S. House of Representatives, 1990, p. 51).

Since disability and major life activities are often defined through examples, the congressional reports further addressed the problem of characterizing "substantial limitation" by adding:

A person is considered an individual with a disability for purposes of the first prong (Part A) of the definition when the individual's important life activities are restricted as to the conditions, manner, or duration under which they can be performed in comparison to most people (U.S. House of Representatives, 1990, p. 52).

When all of this material is considered, it is evident that disability determination by government agencies and medical staff remains a "judgment call" subject to interpretation (Albrecht, 1992). The very ambiguity of these legal definitions and interpretations, the economic consequences of inclusion and exclusion criteria, and disagreement over the allocation of scarce resources in society make disability determination a political as well as a medical and social welfare activity.

TABLE 17-1 Conditions with Highest Prevalence of Activity Limitation, All Ages, United States, 1983–85

Main Cause	Prevalence	Percent	All Causes	Prevalence	Percent
All conditions	32,540	100.0	All conditions	52,718	100.0
Orthopedic impairments	5,220	16.0	Orthopedic impairments	6,987	13.3
Arthritis	4,000	12.3	Arthritis	6,130	11.6
Heart disease	3,736	11.5	Heart disease	5,575	10.6
Visual impairments	1,438	4.4	Hypertension	3,506	6.6
Intervertebral disk disorders	1,424	4.4	Visual impairments	2,900	5.6
Asthma	1,411	4.3	Diabetes	2,111	4.0
Nervous disorders	1,289	4.0	Mental disorders	1,837	3.5
Mental disorders	1,284	3.9	Asthma	1,783	3.4
Hypertension	1,239	3.8	Intervertebral disk disorders	1,699	3.2
Mental retardation	947	2.9	Nervous disorders	1,601	3.0
Diabetes	885	2.7	Hearing impairments	1,405	2.6
Hearing impairments	813	2.5	Mental retardation	1,047	2.0
Emphysema	649	2.0	Emphysema	994	1.9
Cerebrovascular disease	610	1.9	Cerebrovascular disease	939	1.8
Osteomyelitis/bone disorders	360	1.1	Abdominal hernia	595	1.1

SOURCE: Mitchell P. LaPlante. (1991). The demographics of disability. *Milbank Quarterly, 69,* 66. Used by permission of the Milbank Memorial Fund.

THE DISTRIBUTION OF DISABILITY IN SOCIETY

While estimates that there are some 43 million persons in this country with disabilities as cited in the ADA legislation seem reasonable according to diverse national surveys (Kraus & Stoddard, 1991; Louis Harris & Associates, 1986, 1994; Social Security Administration, 1994; Bales, 1995), such figures are likely to be understated when the expanded ADA definition is applied to the American public. In addition, the numbers of persons who report activity limitations are gradually increasing due to several other factors. Advances in medical technology have saved the lives of young and middle-aged people who earlier would have died from their health conditions (Levinsky, 1993). Now these individuals survive, but with impairments that cause activity limitations. Likewise, older Americans are living longer but are experiencing more diseases and more of the disabling consequences of old age. Improved personal health, medical technology, and health services explain these trends (Monahan, 1988).

To provide an overview of dependency due to disability in the United States, Table 17-1 portrays those conditions most responsible for activity limitations among all age groups.

The majority of persons with activity limitations experience chronic illnesses, and typical persons in this group have an average of 1.6 conditions that cause them to be limited. Health conditions vary considerably in their likelihood of causing activity limitation. The conditions in Table 17-2 are ranked in terms of their likelihood of causing an activity limitation. The most disabling conditions are often childhood-onset diseases like mental retardation and cerebral palsy. Generally, those diseases that are the most disabling are low in prevalence. The prevalence of disabling conditions is a product of the prevalence of the condition and the likelihood that the condition causes disability. For example, mental retardation is very disabling but not very prevalent so it is not a major cause of disability. Arthritis, on the other hand, although not as disabling, is quite prevalent and therefore is a major cause of disability.

Disability adds burdens to those who are already disadvantaged (Wright & Leung, 1993). People with disabilities are more likely to be in poor general health, over age sixty-five, female, minority group members, poorly educated, and living alone than are individuals

TABLE 17-2 Conditions with Highest Risk of Disability, by Type of Disability, All Ages, United States, 1983–86

Chronic Condition	Number of Conditions	Percent Causing Activity Limitation	Rank	Percent Causing Major Activity Limitation	Rank	Percent Causing Need for Help in Basic Life Activities	Rank
Mental retardation	1,202	84.1	1	80.0	1	19.9	9
Absence of legs(s)	289	83.3	2	73.1	2	39.0	2
Lung or bronchial cancer	200	74.8	3	63.5	3	34.5	4
Multiple sclerosis	171	70.6	4	63.3	4	40.7	1
Cerebral palsy	274	69.7	5	62.2	5	22.8	8
Blind in both eyes	396	64.5	6	58.8	6	38.1	3
Partial paralysis in extremity	578	59.6	7	47.2	7	27.5	5
Other orthopedic impairments	316	58.7	8	46.2	8	14.3	12
Complete paralysis in extremity	617	52.7	9	45.5	9	26.1	6
Rheumatoid arthritis	1,223	51.0	10	39.4	12	14.9	11
Intervertebral disk disorders	3,987	48.7	11	38.2	14	5.3	—
Paralysis in other sites (complete/partial)	247	47.8	12	43.7	10	14.1	13
Other heart disease/disorders	4,708	46.9	13	35.1	15	13.6	14
Cancer of digestive sites	228	45.3	14	40.3	11	15.9	9
Emphysema	2,074	43.6	15	29.8	—	9.6	15
Absence of arm(s) hand(s)	84	43.1	—	39.0	13	4.1	—
Cerebrovascular disease	2,599	38.2	—	33.3	—	22.9	7

SOURCE: Mitchell P. LaPlante. (1991). The demographics of disability. *Milbank Quarterly, 69,* 67. Used by permission of the Milbank Memorial Fund.

in the general population (Mathematica Policy Research, 1989). Among the 35.3 million persons under sixty-five years old who are without health insurance in the United States, 4.1 million are limited in activity, comprising 11.5 percent of all uninsured people (La-Plante, 1991, 1993). About 547,000 children with limitations in school or play (for those under age five) are uninsured (National Council on Disability, 1993). Those children and adults who are uninsured have from 19 percent to 44 percent fewer physician contacts and from 29 percent to 65 percent fewer hospitalizations than similarly disabled individuals with insurance, depending on the level of disability. Persons who are fortunate enough to receive disability benefits are more prone to be hospitalized and visit a physician than are members of the general population; they are also twice as likely to live alone (Pope & Tarlov, 1991). Men with severe disability have more access to Medicare than women, but women have more access to Medicaid, regardless of disability status (LaPlante, 1991). Finally, 51 percent of people who require assistance with activities

of daily living (ADL), such as eating, dressing, and using the toilet, report that they are in poor health (La-Plante, 1993).

The consequences of disability are far-reaching for both individuals and society. Persons with activity limitations have difficulty working and holding a job. More than 39 percent of individuals with substantial activity limitations live below or just slightly above the poverty level. These individuals rely on Social Security benefits, Supplemental Security Income (SSI) programs, and other government programs for over one-third of their income. In 1989, approximately 70 percent of all working-age adults were employed, compared with only 20 percent of those who required assistance with ADL (Monahan, 1991). Nonetheless, work is essential for persons with disabilities because it influences their ability to live by themselves, be financially self-sufficient, have access to health benefits, maintain self-esteem, and be seen as contributing members of society.

Children and adolescents are particularly vulnerable in a disabling environment that discourages persons with disabilities from living independently. Young people with disabilities are often helped for a time and then have to fend for themselves. Each year almost 650,000 students with disabilities graduate from special education programs or are declared ineligible for further services. Of these, 22 percent will become fully employed, 40 percent will be underemployed and live at the poverty level, 27 percent will be unemployed and on welfare, 8 percent will be idle at home, and 3 percent will be institutionalized (Hipplitus, 1985). In spite of extensive public programs, more than two-thirds of young people with disabilities are unemployed or underemployed after they leave school. The consequences of this feeder system are that persons with disabilities who leave school without a job and become dependent on others are likely to remain dependent throughout their adult years (Rusch & Phelps, 1987). These patterns also hold for adults who drop out of the labor force because of a disability. The longer they are away from work, the less likely they are to be able to live independently and return to the labor force.

From a subjective viewpoint, disabilities constrain people's daily activities and social lives. People with disabilities perceive their environments as disabling and often inhospitable. They are afraid that their disabilities will cause them to become sick, be hurt, or be victimized by criminals. Because of architectural barriers, they frequently cannot use their own bathrooms or kitchens without assistance. When they leave home, they confront inaccessible stairs, sidewalks, buildings, and bathrooms. They often do not have access to public transportation, specially equipped vehicles, or people who can drive them to work or to the store. In addition, persons with disabilities meet similar barriers in the workplace; 47 percent report that employers do not recognize that they are capable of doing a full-time job, 40 percent say that they cannot find suitable employment, and 25 percent have encountered job discrimination. Over 50 percent of persons with disabilities find it difficult to locate services that help them (Louis Harris & Associates, Inc., 1986, 1994). On a personal level, such individuals feel stigmatized or negatively marked by their disabilities, and experience isolation and prejudice in their daily lives. Clearly, disability is a social problem when viewed from either an objective or subjective perspective.

THE POLITICAL ECONOMY OF DISABILITY IN THE UNITED STATES

The financial costs of disability are enormous. In 1986, expenditures for persons with disabilities were estimated to be $169.4 billion for the working-age population and are thought to have risen to about $190 billion (Berkowitz & Dean, 1990; Melville, 1994) ten years later. Of these funds, $78 billion financed federal programs such as Social Security Disability Insurance, SSI, Medicare, Medicaid, food stamps, and veterans' compensation for persons with disabilities. The remaining funds were spent by state and local governments, workers' compensation, private insurance, industry, charitable organizations, and private citizens for disability-related expenses. These figures do not include all the programs directed at older Americans or younger people with disabilities. Federal, state, and local governments, for example, spend more than $7 billion annually on individuals with developmental disabilities such as mental illness, epilepsy, and mental retardation.

Government Responses to Disability

Government initially reacted to disability by instituting programs that provided benefits to the workers who were the most valuable to the political economy of the emerging nation. The first national disability-related law was the Pension Act of 1776, which provided compensation for veterans of the Revolutionary War. Soldiers or sailors who lost a limb or became so disabled by a war injury that they could not work received half pay for life or for as long as the disability lasted (Oberman, 1965; Berkowitz, 1987). The second piece of disability legislation was the Act for the Relief of Sick and Disabled Seamen passed by Congress in 1798. These two laws were intended to protect the military and merchant marine, which were vital occupations in the early years of the nation. Similar legislation was passed after the Civil War, the Spanish American War, and the Boxer Rebellion. During the nineteenth century, railroad workers and miners were added to these favored groups.

A disjointed national disability system emerged during the presidency of Theodore Roosevelt (1901–9), based on two separate systems designed to distribute benefits to persons with disabilities. The primary work-based entitlement system allocated benefits on the basis of an individual's place, importance, and work potential in the labor force. A secondary needs-based system was developed to help persons with disabilities who were dependent and unable to work. These two systems based on different and sometimes conflicting values constitute the bedrock of modern welfare in the United States (Coll, 1969; Skocpol, 1992). Workers' compensation laws were passed in most states by 1911 to provide disability benefits to workers who were injured or became ill on the job. The National Rehabilitation (Smith–Fess) Act of 1920 extended vocationally oriented rehabilitation benefits to members of the general public who were physically disabled. A series of permanent Social Security acts were passed by Congress from 1935 to 1972, providing disability benefits to workers and their families (Berkowitz, 1979). While this piecemeal legislation provided income support and disability benefits to many workers and their families, it left huge portions of the population unprotected.

The three most important contemporary laws dealing with disability and rehabilitation are the Rehabilitation Act of 1973, the Education for All Handicapped Children Act of 1975, and the Americans with Disabilities Act of 1990, along with their amendments. The Rehabilitation Act of 1973 and its subsequent amendments established the Rehabilitation Services Administration within the U.S. Department of Health and Human Services, emphasized coordinated services for those with severe disabilities, improved physical access to buildings and transportation, and provided for affirmative action in the employment of persons with disabilities. The Handicapped Children Act of 1975 stressed the idea that education is a right of all children, provided special education programs, and encouraged the mainstreaming of children with disabilities in regular classrooms whenever possible. The Federal Fair Housing Amendment of 1988 included persons with disabilities as a group protected from discrimination in housing. This was the first time that the antidiscrimination principle regarding people with disabilities was extended to the private sector. The broad-based Americans with Disabilities Act of 1990 and its amendments established the rights of and prohibited discrimination against persons with disabilities in employment, transportation, accessibility, and access to services in the private and public sectors. These acts provide income support, rehabilitation opportunities, and "civil rights" for persons with disabilities (Berkowitz, 1989, 1994).

The Rise of a Rehabilitation Industry

Government funds and enabling legislation helped create a gigantic market for disability care and rehabilitation services. This market is shared by three types of organizations: not-for-profit health care institutions, for-profit corporations, and hybrid organizations that exhibit characteristics of both. Health care institutions and rehabilitation facilities are now operated like businesses (Kerr, 1993). Disability or rehabilitation organizations are compelled to break even or show a profit or they will not survive and grow. For similar reasons, public hospitals often have to cut services when they do not have the staff and resources to deliver care.

By all indicators, rehabilitation is a major growth area in health and welfare services. During 1993, over $160 billion in disability claims was paid by government and business to help recipients support themselves, purchase health care, and engage in rehabilitation. Big business has entered this arena. Abbott Laboratories, a multibillion-dollar supplier of medical goods and pharmaceuticals to the rehabilitation marketplace, reported gross profit margins of 50.9 percent in 1986, 51 percent in 1987, and 52.3 percent in 1988 (Teitlebaum, 1989). Although these margins dropped a bit in the late 1980s, they are still remarkable. In 1994, Abbott Laboratories reported a 39.4 percent five-year average return on equity and a profit margin of 16.7 percent compared with a median profit margin of 3 percent to 4 percent for most other businesses (Walsh, 1995). By any measure, the health sector of the economy, while experiencing renewed competition and cost constraint pressures, continues to exhibit noteworthy growth and profitability. In 1994, for example, drug, health care service, medical supply, and biotechnology companies taken together showed a 5.8 percent profit margin while all American industries reported a 4.3 percent profit margin (Walsh, 1995).

Similarly, in hospitals, the number of rehabilitation beds rose 18 percent from 1983 to 1985, and these numbers continue to rise (American Hospital Association, 1989). For-profit companies such as Crawford Rehabilitation Services, Inc., Rehab Services Corp, and Hospital Corporation of America have grown with the market. These corporations make drugs, surgical equipment, wheelchairs, hospital beds, and orthopedic devices and provide services for persons with disabilities. Their profit margins can be up to ten times those of other manufacturing industries.

The nursing home industry has also flourished in an environment where there is a shortage of beds to meet the demand. This is due principally to two factors: (1) the number of older Americans, especially those over eighty-five, is increasing; and (2) nursing home beds are being used as less expensive alternatives to hospital beds (Sirrocco, 1994). In 1990, there were 31.5 million persons over the age of sixty-five; by 2010, these numbers are expected to swell to 45 million. During the same time period the number of those over eighty-five is expected to double. Besides offering custodial care, nursing home companies are directly competing with hospitals for postoperative and subacute patients. This is also an extraordinarily profitable segment of the business. Dean Whitter analysts note that the operating margins for treatment of subacute and rehabilitation care are roughly twice those for custodial geriatric care (Gilpin, 1994, p. F5). As a consequence, large nursing home chains such as Health Care and Retirement Corporation, Beverly Enterprises, Hillhaven Corporation, and Living Centers of America are branching into this burgeoning market. Together these four institutions operate over 1,400 facilities with more than 156,000 beds. Visions of profit potential have led to a flurry of mergers and acquisitions. During 1993, for example, Horizon Healthcare Corporation merged with the Greenery Rehabilitation Group and Sun Healthcare Groups Systems acquired Mediplex Group (Gilpin, 1994, p. F5). These two deals alone involved over 22,000 beds.

Banks, insurance companies, and law firms add to the cost of doing business. Banks finance capital construction and renovations and underwrite mergers and acquisitions. Insurance companies write health insurance policies and invest in the health care business while lawyers do considerable amounts of work for health care corporations, hospitals, physicians, and patients, ranging from malpractice work to corporate restructuring (Albrecht, 1992). These present arrangements are so profitable that the Health Insurance Association of America spent some $6.5 million on an ad campaign designed to fight any brand of health care reform that would dramatically alter their position in the marketplace (*Consumer Reports*, 1994, p. 117). All of these businesses make money on the volume and size of the transactions and typically pass on the costs to the consumer or the government. In 1990, for example, nursing home payments accounted for 38.2 percent of national Medicaid expenditures (Gilpin, 1994, p. F5). These profit margins and transaction costs drive up the costs of rehabilitation care in the hyperinflated marketplace and fuel the current health care crisis.

As a consequence of the corporate nature of these goods and services, people with disabilities must make purchasing decisions in a complex market about which they have little information. Individuals with disabilities are at a competitive disadvantage as consumers. As one veteran who lost a leg in the Vietnam War observed, "I have an entire closet full of artificial limbs and braces and a medicine cabinet jammed with drugs that I was prescribed or encouraged to buy. I don't even know what half of them are for." The disability and rehabilitation business is also discriminatory and inequitable. At present, slightly more than 80 million Americans are covered by some form of disability insurance under a tattered umbrella of forty different public and private programs, while the remainder have little or no coverage (Cheadle et al., 1994). As an unemployed recent college graduate told me, "I'm on my own and out of work. What will I do if I get sick or become disabled?" (Albrecht, 1993).

This picture characterizes the disability business in the United States. While much good has been accomplished in prolonging and improving the life of persons with disabilities, there is another side to the story. Few Americans appreciate what it is like to deal with disability until they personally experience dependency and discrimination as a result of their limitations and find themselves with little or no insurance to cover full rehabilitation (Susman, 1993). Those who are insured are usually overwhelmed by the prospect of managing their own disability when confronted with the disjointed health care system, labyrinths of bureaucracy, and incredible amounts of information needed to navigate the system.

THE AMERICANS WITH DISABILITIES ACT (PL 101-336)

While the powerful forces of the disability business can be daunting to a person with disabilities, consumers have recently shown that they can effectively unite to form an impressive stakeholder group. On a national level, disability activists were able to pull together their disparate interest groups under the aegis of the National Council on Disability to lobby skillfully for the passage of the Americans with Disabilities Act of 1990. This action demonstrated that persons with disabilities were becoming an increasingly sophisticated political force in Washington, knowledgeable in the ways of Capitol Hill and the White House.

The passage of the ADA marked the arrival of persons with disabilities as a political force and an empowered stakeholder group. The act and subsequent case law decisions based on it provided persons with disabilities legal remedies to enforce their rights and ensure their place in society. Persons with disabilities asked to be treated like other citizens, to be given educational and work opportunities, and not to be cut off from mainstream society by physical and social barriers. In short, persons with disabilities want to be included in the larger society; they want to be recognized as participating citizens in a multicultural society; they desire opportunities to be independent. In terms of politics, law, and public relations, they were successful. However, as

history demonstrates, having legal rights and a voice does not necessarily mean equality or access to needed services, or that mandates will ever be funded and enacted. These are the political issues before us today.

Persons with disabilities have become a formidable stakeholder group, but the effects of new laws and programs have yet to be fully felt at the grassroots level. Although the lives of persons with disabilities have improved, they still experience widespread discrimination, isolation, and poverty. And, like other Americans, they have incredible difficulties in acquiring and retaining health insurance adequate for their needs. They have little help and direction in seeking health care appropriate for their needs. They continually confront intractable government bureaucracies and health care businesses that seem to be more intent on perpetuating their own agendas and making profits than on helping persons with disabilities. Even with the law on their side, persons with disabilities find the American disability and rehabilitation system incredibly diffident, inefficient, and uncaring. While there are numerous personal exceptions to this rule, the expensive but disjointed system does not provide integrated, high-quality care to persons with disabilities at a reasonable cost. Given the level of expenditures and resources in the American health care system, this does not need to be the case. The ADA attempts to redress many of these problems but cannot do so effectively until disability and welfare constitute integral pieces of the American health care reform package. The ADA is but the first step in that direction.

The ADA was an anomaly, for it was a large piece of civil rights legislation supported and passed by the Bush administration at a time when Republicans were championing "trickle-down" Reaganomic economic policies and diminished government regulation of businesses. This law for people with disabilities had considerable political appeal not shared by earlier civil rights legislation. People with disabilities and families touched by disability belonged to both political parties (Berkowitz, 1994). Justine W. Dart Jr., for example, a close friend of Ronald Reagan, was a successful businessman, member of the National Council on Disability, and a wheelchair user who became a key Republican supporter of the ADA. Presidents Reagan and Bush were also touched by former Press Secretary James Brady's experiences with disability and rehabilitation resulting from the assassination attempt on President Reagan at the Washington Hilton. Then Senator Lowell Weicker (R-CT) and conservative columnist George Will were two other prominent Republicans who had family members with disabilities. Senators Robert Dole (R-KS) and John Kerrey (D-NE) live with disabilities dating from their military combat experience. All became strong supporters of the ADA. Senator Edward Kennedy (D-MA), who had a sister and a son with disabilities, led the way on the Democratic side of Congress, calling the act the "most critical legislation affecting individuals with disabilities ever considered by the Congress" (Berkowitz, 1994, p. 111).

The ADA passed for four important reasons. First, persons with disabilities, disability activists, and disability special interest groups like United Cerebral Palsy, the National Head Injury Foundation, the National Easter Seal Society and the Chicago Lung Association coalesced behind the leadership of the National Council on Disability to present a united lobbying effort for the bill. Second, many prominent politicians and business people of both parties had experienced disability personally or in their families so they were sympathetic to the cause. Third, in the course of discussing the act legislators became convinced that people with disabilities came from all social classes and racial ethnic groups and that they suffered discrimination in the workplace and in their daily lives. Finally, Republican politicians and business persons could portray the ADA as a cost-cutting measure. By providing appropriate health care and services, people with severe disabilities could be helped to live as independently as possible (and, therefore, be less of a burden on society). Many other persons with disabilities could be given technological and personal care assistance, education, job training, and employment opportunities that would enable these people to be self-supporting. As President Bush argued, "Excluding the millions of disabled who want to work from the employment ranks costs society literally billions of dollars annually in support payments and lost income revenues" (Berkowitz,

1994, p. 112). Given this consensus and support, he signed the ADA into law on July 26, 1990.

The Americans with Disabilities Act (ADA, PL 101-336) extended civil rights protections to people with disabilities. There are four major Titles to the legislation (U.S. Equal Employment Opportunity Commission and U.S. Department of Justice, 1991; Walk et al., 1993). Title I provides for equal employment opportunities for individuals with disabilities. It notes that a qualified person who can perform the essential functions of a job, with or without accommodation, shall not be discriminated against in regard to the job application procedure, hiring, advancement, compensation, or other conditions of employment. Under these provisions, employers have to make reasonable accommodations in the workplace unless such adjustments would place an undue hardship on the operation of the business. Such adjustments include barrier-free environments, accessible toilets, and technological aids like speaker phones and desks that accommodate wheelchairs.

Title II of the act addresses nondiscrimination on the basis of disability in the provision of state and local government services. It specifies specific requirements that insure accessibility of public buildings, rail and air transportation, and other means of public transportation. Good faith efforts must be demonstrated by government agencies to purchase or lease accessible vehicles.

Title III seeks to insure that persons will not be discriminated against on the basis of disability in public accommodations or in commercial facilities. This section of the law requires hotels, restaurants, theaters, Laundromats, museums, parks, zoos, day care centers, and professional offices of health care providers to be accessible. Architectural barriers are to be removed if this is "easily accomplishable and able to be carried out without much difficulty or expense." Where these standards are not met individuals can seek injunctive relief but not damages. The attorney general may bring suits with a maximum civil penalty of $50,000 for the first violation and $100,000 for a subsequent violation.

Title IV builds on the Communications Act of 1934 by requiring the Federal Communications Commission (FCC) to ensure that the intra- and interstate communications be designed and operated so that they can be efficiently used by people with hearing and speech impairments. These provisions, taken together, revolutionized the rights of persons with disabilities and gave them legal recourse to make their worlds and environments more hospitable. While laws do not change behavior, this act gives persons with disabilities powerful tools to facilitate their inclusion in society.

THE CONSEQUENCES OF THE AMERICANS WITH DISABILITIES ACT

The ADA has had a major impact on the treatment of people with disabilities in the United States as well as in many other countries. The United States, Canada, and Australia are unique among Western nations in having disability legislation based on the civil rights of its citizens. Among these nations, Canada led the way. Canada banned discrimination toward persons with disabilities under the Canadian Human Rights Act of 1977 and its 1985 amendments. In Australia, the Disability Discrimination Act of 1992 expanded the antidiscrimination legislation that already existed in most states and territories.

The European picture is different. In Britain, for example, repeated attempts to pass disability legislation based on the ADA have met with failure (Gooding, 1994). This is due in part to national differences in conceptions of welfare. In the European Community (EC), policies toward people with disabilities have been focused on providing economic support for disadvantaged groups and regions rather than on providing opportunities, inclusion strategies, and job training and employment. European nations have historically viewed disability as a welfare issue, not one to be approached from an equal rights perspective. However, passage of the ADA in this country has mobilized disability activist groups in Europe to put increased pressure on their respective governments to pass similar legislation.

In the United States, the civil rights legislation of 1964 and the *Griggs v. Duke Power Co.* 1971 Supreme Court decision provided the basis for the ADA rationale and law. Judicial interpretation of the Civil Rights Act developed two different doctrinal models. One, the

disparate treatment model based on civil rights legislation, focused attention on the intention of the employer and grounded decisions in formal equity analysis. The second model, resulting from the *Griggs v. Duke Power Co.* decision, recognized the inability of a law that focuses on the motives of individuals to challenge established discriminatory practices. In this decision, the Supreme Court devised a new doctrinal model that investigates consequences rather than intentions. The court interpreted the Civil Rights Act as prohibiting employment practices that have a discriminatory effect on protected classes unless the employer can justify them as being necessary for survival of the business. It was this second doctrinal model that was used to develop and argue for the ADA.

Within the United States, the ADA became the legal foundation for integration of persons with disabilities into the larger society. Unlike Europe, where no such encompassing legislation exists, the act gave Americans with disabilities rights, opportunities, and legal recourse to combat antidiscrimination measures. Yet, while the victory was sweet for disability activists, the reality of living with the act was often bitter. Persons with disabilities have had their lives improved and they have more opportunities than in the past, but they often have to fight for their rights every step of the way. The history of the previous disability legislation is that laws are frequently not enforced and mandates are unfunded (Cook, 1991). Despite legislation forcing integration of persons with disabilities into schools, residential housing facilities, and community services, for example, courts have often ruled in opposite directions. A federal appellate court recently ruled in Virginia that a school board could congregate services for students outside their neighborhood schools, compelling students with disabilities to ride in segregated buses every day to other schools (*Barnett v. Fairfax County School Board*, 1991). Similarly, the Supreme Court ruled in *Pennhurst State School and Hospital v. Halderman* (1981) that federal courts cannot enforce each section of the Rehabilitation Act of 1973 or the Education for All Handicapped Children Act of 1975 against a state agency.

In addition to these restrictions on the original intent of disability laws, federal agencies have been slow to publish administrative rules and enforce them (Cook, 1991, pp. 395–396). These actions of the federal and state governments serve to impede the application of laws and statutes that would improve the quality of life of persons with disabilities. During the Reagan administration, for example, the role of the Justice Department as a protector of the rights of institutionalized persons was substantially eroded (Dinerstein, 1984). Furthermore, congressional testimony repeatedly confirms that there is a lack of civil rights for persons with mental retardation and other disabilities in segregated state facilities (Enforcement of Section 504 of the Rehabilitation Act, 1984). While behavioral scientists suggest improved diagnostic and treatment systems to benefit persons with psychiatric and physical disabilities (Rogers, 1994), dramatic changes will not occur until government agencies and the courts conform with the spirit of disability laws and do not seek ways to circumvent their application and enforcement. To date, history shows that government and the courts have favored the interests of local governments and business over those of persons with disabilities when enforcement of the law came with some hardship or even reasonable economic costs.

The picture is not bleak, however. Many discriminatory practices have been altered. Architectural barriers have come down, job training and employment opportunities have expanded, transportation is more accessible, and more services are available to those with vision and hearing impairments (*Nelson v. Thornburgh*, 1983; *Rothschild v. Grottenhaler*, 1989). But the message is clear: persons with disabilities and others in their stakeholder group must be pro-active and ever vigilant that their hard-fought legislative gains are translated into effective programs and practices.

Aside from increased legal activity and reassessment, the ADA and related disability legislation have highlighted important social policy issues. The entire welfare system is being called into question. Under current welfare benefits, there is often a financial disincentive for persons with disabilities to work (Burns et al., 1994). The interrelationship among Social Security benefits for persons with disabilities, Medicare, and Medicaid are not carefully thought out or coordinated (Richardson, 1994). As a consequence, people with dis-

abilities and their potential employers are often caught in a bureaucratic maze of rules and regulations and conflicting incentives and disincentives. These impediments to rational action argue for an overhaul of the welfare system as well as the related health care system. The two must be coordinated or rational action is impossible for the person with disabilities and those employers and government officials who are trying to comply with laws and federal guidelines.

The ADA and discussion of its implications have also struck the raw nerves of what it means to be "politically correct" today. Is AIDS, for example, to be considered a disability and should persons with AIDS be covered under the ADA (Mitchell, 1986)? While persons with AIDS, with the exception of insured workers, are covered under the act, controversy continues over their inclusion. In the past, disability legislation and programs were typically aimed at more "traditional" disabilities like cerebral palsy, multiple sclerosis, spinal cord injuries, head injuries, and arthritis. Controversy arose when benefits for more stigmatized groups like persons with mental illness, Hansen's disease, and more recently AIDS were proposed. Also, disability today is more apt to be defined by functional limitations than disease category so those with AIDS, congestive heart failure, and asthma would qualify for benefits and services. These discussions involve diverse special interest groups and prejudices. The ADA has brought these discussions to the foreground. Politics, however, will likely decide the outcome of many of these issues.

The ADA also poses myriad problems for the health care community. Hospitals, physician offices, and therapy centers will have to be accessible. Health care providers will have to become more knowledgeable about the special problems of persons with disabilities (Best, 1992). Persons with disabilities, including the frail elderly, will have to have effective transportation to get to and from health care visits. Medical, nursing, and therapy schools will have to accommodate persons with disabilities as students (Helms and Helms, 1994). Similarly, colleges and universities will have to make it possible for persons with disabilities to matriculate, perform in classes, and graduate.

Finally, the ADA raises special problems for employers. There is a heated debate today over the ability of small businesses to pay health insurance for their employees, let alone include employees with disabilities into their insurance pool and accommodate them in the workplace. Larger businesses are concerned about what constitutes reasonable accommodation and compliance with the law. Employers are obviously concerned about trying to remain competitive in a world economy while fulfilling their civic and legal obligations. These questions will not be solved in a short time and the solution seems to require considerable cooperation among government, business, and persons with disabilities.

DISABILITY REFORM

Given the structure and dynamics of the disability business, what can be done to improve access, control costs, and guarantee reasonable standards of quality? The following discussion is based on four assumptions. First, the American political economy is so entrenched and powerful that it is unlikely to be altered in any significant way. In fact, recent reports indicate that the United States now leads Japan and Germany in labor productivity, is holding down labor costs, is controlling inflation, is reducing unemployment, has won back export markets, and leads the world in the production of computer chips. Analysts project that these trends will continue over the next several years (Nasar 1994, pp. F1, F6). With such a robust economy, a radical revolution in the political economy is unlikely (Lipset, 1994). Indeed, the contrary is true: if America is number one, why change anything?

Second, most stakeholders, those individuals and groups who will be affected by the outcomes of health care reform (Shadish et al., 1991), are vigorously resisting any fundamental changes because they are embedded and control one of the largest and most profitable businesses in the nation. There is no compelling reason for them to change (Molm et al., 1994). For many, their market encompasses the world. In fact, the larger health care corporations already compete effectively in and dominate selected niches in the multinational marketplace. These business are strong and profit-driven. Why should they compromise their survival and growth goals for humanitarian values or the well-being of per-

sons with disabilities? Federal and state governments similarly have little incentive to change because campaign contributions, lobbying forces, and support for reelection come from wealthy individuals and corporate stakeholder groups who defend the status quo. From January to October 1993, for example, the top five drug company political action committees contributed over $3.5 million to key members of Congress who could act to maintain their market position. The disenfranchised consumer group is the only stakeholder that suffers from "business as usual," and it has little knowledge or power to effect change.

Third, reform in the American disability system will need to come from a combination of bottom-up and top-down strategies. While there have been an increasing number of disability laws passed in the past twenty years, they do not have the intended effect if they are not enforced and if legislated programs are not properly funded. The history of disability legislation reveals that governments pass laws and institute programs but do not support them financially; and, they carefully restrict access to available public programs so that costs can be contained (Albrecht, 1992). At the same time, government agencies maintain their caseloads, regardless of intervention effectiveness, so that their organizations survive and individual jobs are protected. As a consequence, persons with disabilities often cannot get the help they need when they require it, resulting in deferred, more serious problems and increased dependency. Since those in power usually only perceive the world "top down" and do not have adequate feedback from those they touch, persons with disabilities need to be seen and heard. Consumers need to be part of the solution as well as part of the problem, but they cannot speak unless they have a voice.

Fourth, adjudicating disputes concerning the allocation of scarce goods and services in society presupposes a social context, and for some, a values framework within which decisions are made (Hechter, 1992; Priester, 1992). In elaborating national disability policy, it is important to understand the frames of reference used by the various stakeholders in arguing for specific policies and programs. Otherwise, disputes are not likely to be settled or compromises reached. These issues are foremost in the work of many contemporary thinkers who approach the allocation problem from different but related perspectives. Within the context of his rational choice theory, Coleman considers social rights and accountability and discusses the problems of holding institutions responsible for their actions and the incompatibility of their interests with individuals and their families (Coleman, 1990; Favell & Coleman, 1993). In *Local Justice* (1992) Elster provides a systematic analysis of the principles and procedures that institutions use in allocating scarce goods and imposing necessary burdens. In addressing the equity problem, Amartya Sen (1992) refers to the basic values of individual capabilities and freedom to achieve objectives in determining who should get what. James Q. Wilson (1993) contends that moral sense is what governs the social order and provides direction for the distribution of resources. Rawls does not agree. In *Political Liberalism* (1993), he argues that individuals in our multicultural society no longer share the same system of moral beliefs but can reach consensus based on a shared political conception of justice. He posits the concept of justice as fairness to direct the allocation of resources.

Conclusion

Regardless of their theoretical persuasion, these thinkers imply that social context, capabilities, values, and justice are likely to influence disability policy. I contend that an examination of the stakeholders and the dominant political economy will identify these different value systems and social forces. If we understand the forces at work in the disability business, we are more apt to devise strategies that will serve the needs of persons with disabilities.

REFERENCES

Albrecht, Gary L. (1992). *The disability business: Rehabilitation in America.* Newbury Park, CA: Sage.

Albrecht, Gary L. (1993). The social experience of disability. In Craig Calhoun & George Ritzer (Eds.), *Social problems.* New York: McGraw-Hill.

Albrecht, Gary L., & Ray Fitzpatrick. (1994). A sociological perspective on health-related quality of life research. *Advances in Medical Sociology, 5,* 1–22.

Albrecht, Gary L., & Paul C. Higgins. (1977). Rehabilitation success: The interrelationships of multiple criteria. *Journal of Health and Social Behavior, 18,* 36–45.

Albrecht, Gary L., & Judith A. Levy. (1991). Chronic illness and disability as life course events. *Advances in Medical Sociology, 2,* 3–16.

American Hospital Association. (1989). *Survey of medical rehabilitation hospitals and units—1988.* Chicago: American Hospital Association.

Bales, Virginia S. (1995). Commentary: Achieving comprehensive chronic disease programs. *Chronic Disease Notes and Reports, 8,* 1–4.

Barnett v. Fairfax County School Bd., 927 F.2d 146, 151 (4th Cir. 1991).

Batavia, Andrew I. (1993). Health care reform and people with disabilities. *Health Affairs, 12* (Spring), 40–57.

Berkowitz, Edward D. (1979). The American disability system in historical perspective. In Edward D. Berkowitz (Ed.), *Disability policies and government programs.* New York: Praeger.

Berkowitz, Edward D. (1987). *Disabled policy: America's programs for the handicapped.* Cambridge: Cambridge University Press.

Berkowitz, Edward D. (1989). Allocating resources for rehabilitation: An historical and ethical framework. *Social Science Quarterly, 70* (March), 40–52.

Berkowitz, Edward D. (1994). A historical preface to the Americans with Disabilities Act. *Journal of Policy History, 6* (1), 96–119.

Berkowitz, Edward D., & David H. Dean. (1990). Barrier free environments, congressional testimony. *Congressional Digest,* 157–162.

Best, Karen. (1992). The Americans with Disabilities Act: Its impact on your practice. *Colorado Medicine, 89* (May, Special Suppl.), 1–6.

Burns, Thomas J., Andrew I. Batavia, & Gerben DeJong. (1994). The health insurance work disincentive for persons with disabilities. *Research in Sociology of Health Care, 11,* 57–68.

Charmaz, Kathy. (1991). *Good days, bad days: The self in chronic illness and time.* New Brunswick, NJ: Rutgers University Press.

Cheadle, Allen, Gary Franklin, Carl Wolfhagen, James Savarino, P.Y. Liu, Charles Salley, & Marcia Waever. (1994). Factors influencing the duration of work-related disability: A population-based study of Washington State workers' compensation. *American Journal of Public Health, 84* (February), 190–196.

Chelimsky, Eleanor. (1993). The political debate about health care: Are we losing sight of quality? *Science, 262* (October 22), 525–528.

Coleman, James S. (1990). *Foundations of social theory.* Cambridge, MA: The Belknap Press of Harvard University Press.

Coll, Blanche D. (1969). *Perspectives in social welfare*. Washington, D.C.: U.S. Department of Health, Education, and Welfare.

Consumer Reports. (1994). Health care hucksters: What their ads say—and don't say. *Consumer Reports, 59*, 115–117.

Cook, Timothy M. (1991). The Americans with Disabilities Act: The move to integration. *Temple Law Review, 64* (Summer), 393–469.

Dinerstein, M. (1984). The absence of justice. *Nebraska Law Review, 63* (3), 680–722.

Elster, Jon. (1992). *Local justice*. New York: Russell Sage Foundation.

Enforcement of Section 504 of the rehabilitation act: Institutional care and services for retarded citizens. Hearing before the Subcommittee on Handicapped of the Senate Committee on Labor and Human Resources, Ninety-eighth Congress, 1st session.

Enthoven, Alain C. (1993). Why managed care has failed to contain health costs. *Health Affairs, 12* (Fall), 27–43.

Favell, Adrian. (1993). James Coleman: Social theorist and moral philosopher? *American Journal of Sociology, 99* (November), 590–613.

Feinstein, Jonathan S. (1993). The relationship between socioeconomic status and health: A review of the literature. *Milbank Quarterly, 71* (2), 279–322.

Gilpin, Kenneth N. (1994). Vital signs improve for the nursing home industry. *New York Times* (February 27).

Gooding, Caroline. (1994). *Disabling laws, enabling acts: Disability rights in Britain and America*. London: Pluto Press.

Griggs v. Duke Power Co., 401 US 424 (1971).

Grimby, Gunnar, Jane Finnstam, & Alan Jette. (1988). On the application of the WHO handicap classification in rehabilitation. *Scandinavian Journal of Rehabilitation Medicine, 20* (3), 93–98.

Hechter, Michael. (1992). Should values be written out of the social scientist's lexicon? *Sociological Theory, 10* (Fall), 214–230.

Helms, Lelia B., & Charles M. Helms. (1994). Medical education and disability discrimination: The law and future implications. *Academic Medicine, 69* (July), 535–543.

Hipplitus, P. (1985). Employment opportunities and services for youths with chronic illnesses. In N. Hobbes & J. M. Perrin (Eds.), *Issues in the care of children with chronic illness: A sourcebook on problems, services and policies*. San Francisco: Jossey-Bass.

Inglehart, John K. (1993). Health care reform: The labyrinth of Congress. *New England Journal of Medicine, 329* (November 18), 1593–1596.

Johnson, Robert J., & Frederic D. Wolinsky. (1993). The structure of health status among older adults: Disease, disability, functional limitation, and perceived health. *Journal of Health and Social Behavior, 34* (June), 105–121.

Kerr, Peter. (1993). A father's dream, a son's nightmare. *New York Times* (October 24), 3:1.

Kraus, L. E., & S. Stoddard. (1991). *Chartbook on work disability in the United States* (An InfoUse Report). Washington, D.C.: National Institute on Disability and Rehabilitation Research.

LaPlante, Mitchell P. (1991). The demographics of disability. *Milbank Quarterly, 69* (Suppl. 1/2), 57–77.

LaPlante, Mitchell P. (1993). *Disability, health insurance coverage, and utilization of acute health services in the United States*. Washington, D.C.: U.S. Department of Health and Human Services.

Levinsky, Norman G. (1993). The organization of medical care: Lessons from the Medicare end-stage renal disease program. *New England Journal of Medicine, 329* (November 4), 1395–1399.

Lipset, Seymour Martin. (1994). The social requisites of democracy revisited. *American Sociological Review, 59* (February), 1–22.

Louis Harris & Associates, Inc. (1986). *The ICD survey of disabled Americans: Bringing disabled Americans into the mainstream*. New York: Louis Harris & Associates.

Louis Harris & Associates, Inc. (1994). *National organization on disability/Harris survey of Americans with disabilities*. New York: Louis Harris & Associates.

Mathematica Policy Research. (1989). *Population profile of disability*. Washington, D.C.: U.S. Department of Health and Human Services.

Melville, Keith. (1994). *The health care explosion*. New York: McGraw-Hill.

Miller, David. (1991) *The Blackwell encyclopedia of political thought*. Oxford: Blackwell Publishers.

Mitchell, Patricia. (1986). Employment discrimination and AIDS: Is AIDS a handicap under Section 504 of the Rehabilitation Act? *University of Florida Law Review, 38* (Fall), 649–671.

Molm, Linda D., Theron M. Quist, and Phillip A. Wisely. (1994). Power and justice in social exchange. *American Sociological Review, 59* (February), 98–121.

Monahan, Colleen. (1988). Equipment/product standardization, safety and traceability. In *Final report of the consensus meeting on home respiratory care equipment*. Dallas: American Association of Respiratory Care.

Monahan, Colleen. (1991). *Notes on disability*. Chicago: State of Illinois, Division of Services for Crippled Children.

Nagi, Saad Z. (1965). Some conceptual issues in disability and rehabilitation. In Marvin B. Sussman (Ed.), *Sociology and rehabilitation* (pp. 100–113). Washington, D.C.: American Sociological Association.

Nasar, Sylvia. (1994). The American economy. *New York Times* (November 7), 13.

National Council on Disability. (1993). *Serving the nation's students with disabilities: Progress and prospects*. Washington, D.C.: National Council on Disability.

Nelson v. Thornburgh, 567 F. Supp. 369, 382 (E.D. Pa. 1985).

Oberman, C. Esco. (1965). *History of vocational rehabilitation in America*. Minneapolis: T. S. Denison.

Pennshurst State School and Hospital v. Halderman, 451 U.S. 1 (1981).

Pope, Andrew M., & Alvin R. Tarlov. (1991). *Disability in America: Toward a national agenda for prevention*. Washington, D.C.: National Academy Press.

Pope, Clyde. (1984). Disability and health status: The importance of longitudinal studies. *Social Science and Medicine, 19* (6), 589–593.

Priester, Reinhard. (1992). A values framework for health system reform. *Health Affairs, 11* (Spring), 84–107.

Rawls, John. (1993). *Political liberalism*. New York: Columbia University Press.

Richardson, Mary. (1994). The impact of the Americans with Disabilities Act on employment opportunity for people with disabilities. *Annual Review of Public Health, 15*, 91–105.

Rogers, E. Sally. (1994). The impact of the Americans with Disabilities Act upon rehabilitation research. *Journal of Disability Policies Studies, 5* (1), 25–43.

Rothschild v. Grottenhaler, 716 F. Supp. 796, 806 (S.D.N.Y. 1989).

Rusch, F. R., & L. A. Phelps. (1987). Secondary special education and transition from school to work: A national priority. *Exceptional Children, 53* (6), 487–492.

Sen, Amartya. (1992). *Inequality reexamined*. Cambridge, MA: Harvard University Press.

Shadish, William R., Jr., Thomas D. Cook, & Laura C. Leviton. (1991). *Foundations of program evaluation*. Newbury Park, CA: Sage.

Sharfstein, Joshua M., & Steven S. Sharfstein. (1994). Campaign contributions from the American medical political action committee to members of Congress: For or against public health? *New England Journal of Medicine, 330* (January 6), 32–37.

Sirrocco, Al. (1994). Nursing homes and board and care homes. *Advance Data, 244* (February 23).

Skocpol, Theda. (1992). *Protecting soldiers and mothers*. Cambridge, MA: The Belknap Press of Harvard University Press.

Social Security Administration. (1994). *Developing a world-class employment strategy for people with disabilities: A briefing for Commissioner Chater and Principal Deputy Commissioner Thompson*. Baltimore, MD: Social Security Administration.

Susman, Joan. (1993). Disability, stigma and deviance. *Social Science and Medicine, 38* (1), 15–22.

Teitlebaum, Robert. (1989). The supermeds. *Financial World* (June 10), 19–21.

U.S. Equal Employment Opportunity Commission and the U.S. Department of Justice. (1991). *Americans with disabilities handbook*. Washington, D.C.: U.S. Department of Justice.

U.S. House of Representatives. (1990). *Americans with Disabilities Act of 1990: Report together with minority views* (Report No. 101–485, Part 2). Washington, D.C.: U.S. Government Printing Office.

Verbrugge, Lois M., & Alan M. Jette. (1993). The disablement process. *Social Science and Medicine, 38* (1), 1–14.

Verbrugge, Lois, M., Joseto M. Reoma, & Ann L. Gruber-Baldini. (1994). Short-term dynamics of disability and well-being. *Journal of Health and Social Behavior, 35* (March), 97–117.

Walk, Eric E., Helen C. Ahn, Patricia M. Lumpkin, Shahriar A. Nabizadeh, & Richard F. Edlich. (1993). Americans with Disabilities Act. *Journal of Burn Care and Rehabilitation, 14* (January/February), 92–98.

Walsh, Matt. (1995). Health. *Forbes, 155*, 180–182.

Wilson, James Q. (1993). *The moral sense*. New York: The Free Press.

Wright, Tennyson J., & Paul Leung. (1993). *Meeting the unique needs of minorities with disabilities*. Washington, D.C.: National Council on Disability.

CHAPTER

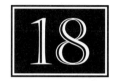

The Politics of Environmental Health

Barry G. Rabe

As adapted from Picket G. E., and Hanlon J. J. Public health: Administration and practice, 9th ed., 1990, St. Louis, Mosby-Year Book, Inc.

Few areas of public health policy are as riddled with ironies as environmental health. Environmental contamination constitutes a public health problem of long standing, yet one that constantly produces new wrinkles and challenges. It is a public health problem about which there is near unanimity among citizens that government must intervene, yet there is no consensus on the most appropriate methods of intervention. It is a public health problem that cannot be confined by local and state government boundaries, yet one about which the national government remains quite deferential to subnational and private-sector strategies. It is an area ripe for preventive strategies, yet one where reactive, crisis management approaches have prevailed. Finally, it is an area in which Health Departments and public health officials played a central, effective role in earlier decades but have seen their responsibilities diminish in more recent times in favor of officials from agencies with broad responsibilities for environmental and natural resource protection.

At the same time, few areas of public health policy pose a comparable set of opportunities for public health officials—and other individuals with a commitment to environmental health—to demonstrate a capacity to take action that will contribute to the public good. Whether examining the unfinished agenda of the 1960s and 1970s, which addressed water and air pollution with rigorous new legislation, or the diverse agenda of the 1980s and 1990s, which has included toxic substances, hazardous, nuclear, and biomedical wastes, indoor air pollution, ozone layer depletion, and global climate change, one finds questions in environmental health that defy simple remedies. Few nations approach the level of American resource commitment to environmental protection, which was nearly 2.5 percent of gross domestic product in the mid-1990s. But few observers contend that these substantial resources are efficiently or effectively applied to our most pressing environmental problems. Moreover, environmental policy commitments periodically receive intense political challenge, most evident in proposals in the 104th Congress that would dramatically scale back federal regulatory resources and authority. Thus while environmental policy is likely to remain high on the agendas of national and subnational governments for decades to come, there is considerable uncertainty over the focus and direction of future policy efforts.

This chapter examines the track record of recent government interventions, reviews the institutional and legislative infrastructures created to address environmental health, and outlines the tasks that lie ahead. It begins with an exploration of the nature of environmental health problems, reviewing progress and failure in past decades. In addition, it describes new and growing problems for which new policy remedies will be required. Second, the chapter considers the institutional and political response to environmental health problems over the past few decades. It devotes considerable attention to the ways in which authority for environmental health policy has been divided intergovernmentally (national, state, regional, local) and interorganizationally (public health, environmental superagency, natural resources, and agriculture, among others). It also considers the common practice of dividing policies and regulatory institutions by medium—air, land, and water—despite the fact that transfer, transport, and transformation of pollutants across these formal boundaries is commonplace. This discussion underscores the many lines of fragmentation in environmental health policy and management and explores both the strengths and weaknesses of such a pluralistic strategy. The chapter concludes with an analysis of alternative policy approaches in this area.

THE PROBLEMS OF ENVIRONMENTAL HEALTH

Human-made and natural environmental health threats come in many forms and pose many potential health problems. Foremost among these threats in re-

cent decades has been cancer, although exposure to various environmental contaminants may also result in genetic damage, birth defects, neurological effects, liver damage, infections, and injuries. In response, governments at all levels have developed a variety of methods, including animal bioassays and human epidemiologic studies, to measure and predict human risk. They have also devised a myriad of regulatory programs to attempt to control and minimize these risks.

Assessments of the effectiveness of these strategies must be couched in terms of extreme caution. There is neither a foolproof method for measuring the risk posed by a particular contaminant in a particular setting nor a certain regulatory method for minimizing risk and assuring protection of public health. Nonetheless, the experiences of recent decades do make possible some general assessments of environmental quality and the scope and severity of relatively new environmental health problems. In turn, they facilitate tentative assessments of the types of government regulatory interventions that may or may not be effective.

Areas of Progress

Perhaps the most encouraging twentieth-century developments in environmental health involve the tremendous advancements in sanitation achieved in the early 1900s and the substantial strides in reducing conventional air and water pollutants during the 1970s and 1980s. Public health officials and agencies were in the forefront of efforts to combat the enormous environmental health problems posed by unsafe sanitation systems. These problems proved particularly severe in industrialized urban areas that underwent rapid population growth in the late 1800s and early 1900s. Safe systems of sanitation and waste disposal lagged several decades behind this growth, and the public health community played a central role in securing its implementation.

Many of the public health or epidemiological accomplishments in the United States and certain other countries can be attributed to the sanitary measures that they have instituted. Included among these have been the spectacular reductions in typhoid fever, cholera, dysenteries, and summer diarrheas; the control of many milk- and food-borne infections; the control of malaria; and the elimination of yellow fever. It was not until the beginning of the present century that the chains of events involved in the transmission and perpetuation of these diseases became unraveled. Prompt steps were taken to break the links in these chains.

The nation's decision in the 1970s to combat a wide range of air and water pollution problems with unprecedented rigor and resource commitment led to serious assaults on several of the most obvious problems, many of which possessed a compelling environmental health component. These efforts went far beyond anything ever undertaken in these areas by the federal government or individual states. The Clean Air Act of 1970 and its subsequent amendments have established national ambient air quality standards (NAAQS), set an array of emissions standards for motor vehicles and industrial facilities, and required states to design and implement plans for air quality (Bryner, 1995). The Water Pollution Control Act of 1972 (now known as the Clean Water Act) and its later revisions imposed strict controls on industrial, municipal, and other sources of water pollution, established a program for wastewater discharge, and provided grants and loans for wastewater facility construction (Adler et al., 1993). Later pieces of legislation added new rigor and specificity to existing environmental regulation or addressed entirely new areas such as hazardous waste and toxic substances.

If not as sweeping a series of successes as had been attained in prior generations through new sanitation efforts, these legislative efforts have had a significant impact. If not measurable in lives saved, they have made at least some contribution to human health through improved environmental quality. Success has been particularly dramatic in reduction of the release of lead, particulates, sulfur dioxide, and automobile-related and other conventional pollutants to the air and reduction of suspended solids, bacteria, and oxygen-consuming materials discharged to surface waters. Overall emissions from automobiles have dropped markedly in recent decades due to implementation of clean air legislation, despite steady increases in the numbers of cars in use and a doubling of total mileage driven between 1970 and 1995. Cars produced in 1995, for example, release 98 percent less hydrocarbon emissions than their counterparts of the early 1970s.

In the area of surface water quality, which involves lakes and rivers as opposed to subsurface groundwater, conventional pollutants from industrial and municipal sources have received considerable regulatory attention, and some noteworthy successes have been registered. Water quality trends have been particularly encouraging for lead, dissolved oxygen, and fecal coliforms and streptococci (two common bacterial contaminants that are indicators of sewage pollution). Water bodies widely characterized as recently as twenty-five years ago as "dead," such as Lake Erie and the Cuyahoga River, have made notable comebacks, with significant improvements in many water quality indicators. Large regions with vital freshwater resources, such as the Great Lakes Basin and Chesapeake Bay, have registered encouraging improvements as well (Colborn et al., 1990; Horton & Eichbaum, 1991).

Future Challenges

Despite some heartening developments in improving environmental quality, potential threats to environmental health loom even greater today than they did on Earth Day in 1970. Incremental progress in water quality has been offset by growing concentrations of arsenic and cadmium, and minimal progress has been registered for metals such as chromium, iron, manganese, selenium, mercury, and zinc despite massive investments in water pollution control. Of even greater import is the growing recognition that early environmental regulatory efforts largely ignored a series of problems that may require massive new interventions by the public and private sectors in future decades. Many of these relate to the safe management of wastes, chemicals, and pesticides that are by-products of manufacturing, agriculture, household activity, and even environmental treatment processes. The United States generates approximately fifty thousand pounds of solid waste per person per year and by restricting traditional disposal methods (incineration or direct dumping into lakes, rivers, and oceans) has created a substantial waste management problem.

Approximately 200 million tons of hazardous waste are generated each year, and every plausible method of safe disposal has serious drawbacks. Land-based fills and surface impoundments allow wastes to seep into groundwater or vaporize into the air; deep-well injection poses serious groundwater contamination threats; incineration creates air pollution that could further harm water and land (Rabe, 1994). The federal Environmental Protection Agency, working through the Superfund program for cleanup of abandoned toxic waste sites, has already uncovered more than 25,000 abandoned dump sites that cause or have the potential to cause contamination. The agency also estimates the existence of more than 75,000 industrial landfills, nearly 75,000 mining waste sites, and more than 175,000 leaking underground storage tanks. Approximately one of every four Americans lives near a significant concentration of hazardous waste. Many of these wastes may pose serious environmental health threats, although assessments of the severity of the hazards remain subject to great scientific controversy. Site remediation has proven extremely difficult technologically and contentious politically, resulting in massive public and private expenditures to date but minimal progress (Hird, 1994; Church & Nakamura, 1993). These estimates do not touch on the problem of safe disposal of radioactive waste from plants that provide nuclear power or materials for nuclear weapons (Shrader-Frechette, 1993).

The 1970s assault on environmental degradation also tended to overlook hazardous substances such as chemicals and pesticides. By focusing so heavily on conventional pollutants, which were in many instances the most visible threats, national, state, and local governments devoted far less attention to toxic substances control. It is increasingly realized, however, that these substances are ubiquitous in air, water, land, and biosphere and that they may pose more serious public health problems than conventional pollutants. According to the inventories conducted under the 1976 Toxic Substances Control Act, more than sixty-three thousand chemical substances have been used commercially since 1975. In addition, new substances are introduced into commercial use far more rapidly than any national, state, or local program can evaluate their safety. The

National Institute of Occupational Safety and Health (NIOSH) has registered nearly sixty thousand chemical substances "that are known to have toxic effects at some level of exposure." These effects include irritation, mutation, reproductive effects, carcinogenesis, and death. However, it should be noted that many substances may not be particularly hazardous, and little is known about the health effects of a great many of them. Scientific understanding is particularly uncertain of the effects of the myriad possible combinations and permutations of these substances.

These sobering numbers are not intended to imply that a public health crisis owing to hazardous wastes and toxic substances is upon us. In fact, environmental scientists, industry leaders, and public health officials have little idea of how many Americans are at risk from exposure to these materials and how serious the health consequences might be. Rather, these figures are introduced to underscore the scope of potential human health effects and the nature of the challenge facing public- and private-sector leaders, including public health officials, who will have to make basic policy decisions concerning them in the face of considerable uncertainty. Unlike the triumphs over substandard sanitation early in this century, there will be no comparable scientific and political quick fix for the latest difficulties in environmental health.

THE EVOLUTION OF ENVIRONMENTAL POLITICS AND GOVERNANCE

Political systems respond to the public demands of the moment. In environmental health, this has resulted in a pattern of policy shifts dictated by problems or crises that have been seen as particularly serious at different points in time (Baumgartner & Jones, 1992). In the decade following World War II, concerns over natural resource abuse grew, and expanded government commitment to conservation soon followed, particularly through increased responsibilities for the U.S. Interior Department. In the late 1960s and early 1970s, concerns over visible environmental degradation in air and water led to formation of a national environmental agency and enactment of major new legislation related to air and water quality. In the late 1970s and throughout the 1980s, concerns mounted over hazardous wastes, toxic substances, and a series of even more far-reaching concerns, including stratospheric ozone layer depletion and global climate change. Mounting evidence indicates that a combination of natural and human-made gases, including chlorofluorocarbons, methane, carbon dioxide, and nitrous oxide, are depleting the earth's protective layer of stratospheric ozone. Not only does this increase the amount of dangerous ultraviolet radiation reaching life on earth, but these chemicals also act to trap radiative heat close to the Earth's surface. It is feared that this could substantially elevate atmospheric temperatures and have potentially severe consequences.

This series of perceived environmental problems has triggered political support for expanding government regulatory powers and increasing resources available for environmental protection purposes. In particular, growing authority has been amassed at national and state levels, as the once dominant role of local governments has been increasingly overshadowed by national and state legislation and agencies. Indeed, many environmental problems have begun to be addressed through international policy venues, such as pathbreaking agreements in the 1980s for industrialized nations to find substitutes for those chemicals likely to erode the stratospheric ozone layer. To be sure, the traditional local role has remained substantial, particularly in the implementation of various environmental health programs, but it has become increasingly dependent on national and state sources of funding and policy direction. Coordinating the efforts of these respective levels of government—and the multiple institutions active at each level—has proven to be a major stumbling block to effective environmental regulation.

Creation of New Programs and Agencies

The outcry over environmental contamination in the late 1960s fueled a social movement that placed enormous political pressure on Congress, President Richard Nixon, and state legislatures. As a result, there was substantial expansion of water and air pollution control programs, and Congress passed the National Environmental Policy Act (NEPA) in 1969. NEPA ushered in an era of "environmental impact statements" that were to take into account all anticipated environmental ramifications from proposed development projects supported by national government funding. Twenty-eight states subsequently responded with state environmental policy acts (or little NEPAs) of their own, several of which were far more detailed and rigorous than NEPA.

This new and expanded legislative commitment coincided with an executive branch decision to consolidate a wide range of environmental regulatory functions into a single agency. The Environmental Protection Agency emerged in 1970, with responsibility for all environmental media (air, water, and land) and most of the major pollution control programs. However, the agency was not the all-encompassing environmental superagency or vehicle of integration across media boundaries that many supporters of reorganization had recommended. Political resistance from individual program constituencies was too formidable to challenge, and the Nixon administration (especially then EPA administrator William Ruckelshaus) was eager to demonstrate its environmental commitment in some manner more dramatic than agency reorganization. As a result, the Departments of Interior, Health and Human Services, Agriculture, and Defense (and later Energy) retained considerable control over environmental regulatory functions that touched their immediate jurisdictions, and many previous dividing lines were perpetuated within the EPA (Marcus, 1980; Landy et al., 1994). Other agencies, such as the Nuclear Regulatory Commission, Consumer Products Safety Commission, Food and Drug Administration, and Occupational Safety and Health Administration, have also continued to play some direct role in environmental regulation.

As was the case with NEPA, many states quickly followed this national action by consolidating environmental regulatory responsibilities into new agencies. The Health Department soon ceased to be the dominant environmental regulatory agency in the majority of states, replaced after 1970 by a series of little EPAs modeled on the national agency or similarly structured environmental superagencies with broad jurisdiction. Much like the national EPA, the new state agencies achieved some degree of environmental program consolidation within a single agency but continued to share authority with a variety of other organizations. In Minnesota and Michigan, among other examples, nearly fifty separate agencies, boards, and commissions addressed some aspect of environmental regulation (Jessup, 1995). As a result, state agencies with responsibility for commerce, agriculture, natural resources, mining, economic development, and energy have continued to play a role in environmental regulation, often at cross-purposes with environmental regulatory agencies.

The federal EPA, much like its state-level counterparts, failed to resolve varying agency rivalries or coordinate different regulatory approaches. It has become an amalgamation of programs and divisions rather than a carefully integrated agency. The agency was built partly along program lines that adhered to divisions in environmental media (air versus water versus land) and partly along functional lines, such as standards, enforcement, and research, which transcended individual programs or media. This resulted in a divided agency in which programmatic concerns increasingly came to dominate cross-cutting functional ones (Rosenbaum, 1995; Landy et al., 1994). Moreover, the agency was restrained in any effort to integrate regulatory efforts by highly specific legislation and extensive congressional oversight, both of which reflected a fragmented congressional committee and subcommittee system, which tended to further subdivide national environmental policy. It received even more intense scrutiny in 1995, as Congress weighed a series of proposals that would dramatically reduce its staff and curtail its regulatory powers.

Air versus Water

Policy fragmentation was particularly evident in the two areas where tremendous expansion of national regulatory authority occurred in the 1970s: air and water pollution. Not only have they been studied separately and approached through differing legislation, but water pollution has consistently been addressed before air pollution at the national level. Regulations under federal legislation have continued to be issued much more

rapidly for water than for air. It is not surprising, therefore, that dramatically different national programs have evolved to address these two media. They are similar only in their extreme individual complexity. As political scientist Alfred Marcus has noted:

> In spite of the fact that air and water were in the same agency and for a time were in the same office, the two programs remained distinct and separate entities with different operating procedures and differing laws governing them. Their focus was not on the pollutant and its movement through the ecological chain. No efforts were made to determine where best to interdict the unhealthy, foul substances that needed elimination (Marcus, 1980).

The air and water pollution programs of the federal government continue to differ in many important respects. For example, the Clean Air Act established health-based national ambient air quality goals, while the Clean Water Act set technology-based effluent guidelines. Moreover, the water program emphasized the regulatory "carrot" of public works funding, whereas the air program emphasizes the regulatory "stick" of stringent requirements and few funding rewards. Even the political strategies adopted by the officials who operate the programs have differed considerably. Whereas the air program has attracted extensive public attention and controversy and its officials have tended to confront opposition directly, the water program has maintained a more modest political profile, responding to opposition in a less confrontational manner. This distinction is further evident in the early, and highly contentious, efforts to implement the far-reaching 1990 amendments to the Clean Air Act (Bryner, 1995). Provisions to impose new emissions-reduction technology on industry and to require states to develop extensive new auto emissions testing programs, for example, have generated considerable conflict.

Toxic Substances and Hazardous Waste

Various changes in the air and water programs and the enactment of a new wave of federal environmental programs in the 1970s and early 1980s did not bridge this fundamental, program-based gap. On the contrary, the emergence of legislation that did not address a single medium exclusively has served in some respects to fragment the system even further. For example, twenty-five separate federal laws address some aspect of toxic substances control and hazardous waste management; eight separate laws give EPA authority in toxic substances control. These programs are housed in several different national agencies, including EPA, the Food and Drug Administration, the Department of Transportation, the Department of Defense, the Department of Energy, and the Consumer Products Safety Commission. If not necessarily divided along medium lines, the management system that has resulted from this melange of programs has proven similarly complicated and cumbersome. Each incident or issue related to toxic substances control and hazardous waste management has required a different combination of program agencies. For example, national control of all exposures from the manufacture, use, and disposal of vinyl chloride would require the participation of five national agencies through fifteen national laws. Periodic efforts to foster better integration of these efforts, as in the Clinton administration's National Performance Review, have had minimal impact to date.

This continued proliferation of national legislation represents an exacerbation of the fragmented process of environmental policy formation that began with the earlier air and water programs. This is evident in such legislation as the 1976 Toxic Substances Control Act (TSCA); the 1976 Resource Conservation and Recovery Act (RCRA) and key 1984 amendments; the 1980 Comprehensive Environmental Response, Compensation, and Liability Act (CERCLA, or Superfund) and its succeeding 1986 Superfund Amendments and Reauthorization Act (SARA); the 1947 Federal Insecticide, Fungicide, and Rodenticide Act (FIFRA) and numerous subsequent amendments; and the 1973 Endangered Species Act (ESA). Each of these programs takes a separate cut at environmental problems: TSCA addresses premanufacture registration of toxic substances and authorizes EPA to ban certain substances; RCRA sets hazardous and solid waste disposal standards in close conjunction with states; CERCLA/SARA sets standards, determines responsibility, and implements cleanup of abandoned hazardous waste disposal sites; FIFRA oversees registration and monitoring of pesticides; and ESA creates a mechanism to determine animal and plant species that may be threatened with extinction and intervene to protect remaining survivors. As Joel Hirschhorn (1985) of the Congressional Office of Technology Assessment has noted, "These programs are not integrated in any sense. They are very fragmented and are not implemented in any sort of integrated fashion."

Congress versus Itself

Fragmentation in national environmental policy is not confined to the executive branch. The political institution responsible for creation of legislation, Congress, is itself fragmented, and it has directly impeded more integrative approaches. As early as 1970, committees dealing with environmental matters in both houses of Congress were divided along highly specialized, single-medium lines. No sooner did William Ruckelshaus become the first EPA administrator than he realized that he would have to deal with at least sixteen congressional subcommittees that had some jurisdiction over the agency's pollution control activities. Not only did these various bodies hold dramatically differing environmental responsibilities, but many were headed by members of the House and Senate who had already become wedded to a particular regulatory program or approach. Congressional leaders tend to build their environmental reputations through creation or expansion of specialized programs, with no responsibility for the ultimate fit between multiple programs. Proposals to enact or amend environmental legislation have been parceled out among specialized committees, with little coordination or interaction between them. By the early 1990s, at least twelve committees and fifty-four subcommittees in the House of Representatives alone played some role in environmental policy.

The fragmentation regularly results in delays and confusion in reaching consensus on environmental legislation, exemplified by the two-year process required to reauthorize and amend the Superfund program in the mid-1980s. Five full House committees and even more subcommittees assumed a role in some aspect of the reauthorization and encountered enormous difficulty in reaching common ground. As a result, the program was temporarily brought to a halt during 1986 after its funding ran out and was reinstituted only after a badly cobbled piece of legislation was approved, which proved full of internal contradictions and has fit poorly with other programs. Subsequent efforts to sort out this legislative mess have collapsed, most recently in late 1994. After two years of unusually constructive collaboration among industry, environmental groups, and other shareholders, a compromise proposal was scuttled as congressional Republicans blocked all environmental legislature pending before the November 1994 elections. The Clean Air Act underwent an even longer review, as far-reaching amendments were delayed nearly a decade before finally being approved in 1990, engulfing program implementation in considerable uncertainty throughout the 1980s (Bryner, 1995).

State Agency versus State Agency

Agency and legislative fragmentation in environmental regulation may be most evident at the national level, but it is not confined there. Although states have assumed increasingly prominent roles in environmental regulation in recent years, they have not, on the whole, been any more successful in integrating regulation along functional and across media lines than the national government. The emergence of dozens of new state environmental agencies has been only minimally effective in bringing various constituencies together in coordinated fashion. Indeed, many state efforts have been modeled after fragmented national forerunners. Fragmentation has been particularly evident in the implementation process, where states are often responsible for overseeing the approval of permits for various projects that will have some environmental impact. Each permitting, monitoring, and enforcement program, often medium-based and influenced by national policy, has its own internal logic and independent system of operation. As a result, very real trade-offs between media and regulatory strategies are not systematically taken into account.

Some states have responded to this problem with efforts to mesh the environmental programs under their jurisdiction. Permit coordination efforts have proven particularly popular, and more than thirty states have implemented such programs. Permits are a basic tool of environmental management in all states, as proposed development projects cannot begin until authorized agencies deem them in compliance with relevant regulatory requirements and provide a formal permit. Certain projects may require acquisition of dozens of such permits, ranging from those governing air and water pollution control to those for wetland and wildlife protection. State permit reforms have included developing master permit information forms, one-stop permitting processes, joint application procedures, mediation services, permit directories, permit information centers, and preapplication conferences. All of these have the common aim of streamlining the permit process, and they have attained some success in bringing together diverse regulatory constituencies into a unified focus. However, their overall impact has been far greater in smoothing the process for permit applicants than in integrating a management system that considers all environmental ramifications in an integrated fashion.

No two states have devised identical regulatory systems. Despite national government pressures and incentives for a certain degree of uniformity, approximately 70 percent of key state environmental legislation is not at all related to federal programs (Council of State Governments, 1994, p. 539). States thus retain considerable latitude in many areas of environmental policy. For example, the emergence of toxic substances control and hazardous waste management as a major public concern and challenge for state government has led to very different responses. In states such as Michigan, jurisdiction is divided among multiple agencies, with minimal policy integration or innovation occurring. By contrast, Minnesota has devised a multifaceted effort to integrate various regulatory functions with common goals of minimizing cross-media pollutant shifting and maximizing opportunities to prevent the generation of pollution. This activity involves systematic integration of permitting, enforcement, data reporting, and other functions, and has illustrated the potential for shifting toward a more integrated environmental regulatory order (Rabe, forthcoming).

State Innovators versus State Laggards

No two states are equally committed to environmental health, equally capable of effectively formulating and implementing regulatory programs, or equally adept at devising Minnesota-type policy innovations. Certain states have consistently emerged as leaders in devising innovative strategies for environmental health: California has been a pioneer in air pollution control and hazardous waste disposal; Minnesota has played a similar role in water pollution control and now regulatory integration; Illinois and New York have repeatedly proven leaders in cross-media integration of pollution control programs; North Carolina has championed preventive strategies of industrial waste reduction; New Jersey has taken dramatic steps in toxic substances control and biomedical waste management. These leadership roles can be attributed to the potential severity of environmental health problems in these states (such as air pollution in southern California and toxic substances in New Jersey) and to the political cultures of the states. States have often devised environmental policies that have served as models for other states or the nation.

Many evaluations of state environmental regulatory innovativeness and effectiveness have been attempted. In general, these tend to find significant differences across states and regions. For example, industrialized states of the Northeast, Upper Midwest, and Pacific Northwest consistently rank near the top in terms of regulatory rigor and commitment whereas the states of the Southeast and Southwest consistently fall toward the bottom. States such as California, Minnesota, New Jersey, New York, Massachusetts, Oregon, and Wisconsin are usually seen as the most dynamic and innovative, the most likely models for new approaches that may then diffuse regionally and nationally. By contrast, some states have continually been laggards in environmental health, taking new steps only when prodded by Washington. In fact, some states never appear near the top of any ranking scheme in any area of environmental policy (Lowry, 1992).

State-by-state variation is also evident in comparing the capacity and willingness of individual states to fund environmental regulatory programs. The states fund these efforts through a variety of mechanisms, including general tax revenues, bonds, user fees, and federal grants-in-aid. Many of them continue to face serious limitations on the amounts of funding they can be expected to generate for environment-related activities. In 1991, nine states spent less than $25 per capita on all environmental programs combined, whereas eleven spent more than $65 per capita on these programs. Those states that spent the least on average tend to be the ones most dependent on federal funding to carry out basic programs, making them especially vulnerable to proposed federal grant reductions. Such differences further illustrate the varied pattern in state performance that often emerges when regulatory authority is decentralized to that level (Ringquist, 1993; Lowry, 1992).

In turn, the ability of multiple states to work cooperatively toward a common environmental good is highly suspect. The problem of siting waste disposal facilities illustrates this problem, as states are increasingly reluctant to "host" facilities for solid, hazardous, biomedical, and radioactive wastes. Instead, they prefer to see wastes shipped elsewhere, preferably well beyond state boundaries. This has led to severe inequities in the distribution of burden for waste management by state and region, consistent with a long-standing pattern of state preference for waste—or pollutant—migration beyond their boundaries. States and communities that bear a disproportionate share of this burden contend increasingly that they serve as "magnets" for economic and racial reasons rather than out of any clear environmental strategy (Rabe, 1994). Such inequities in the "environmental balance of trade" between states is a growing source of intergovernmental tension and could be exacerbated by efforts to further decentralize environmental policy.

REGULATORY ALTERNATIVES FOR ENVIRONMENTAL HEALTH

Many areas of environmental health policy, unlike those in other spheres of health policy, remain in fairly early stages of development. As a result, many of the most influential agencies and programs remain fairly experimental in character and uncertain entities in terms of any demonstrated capacity to protect public health or the environment. In fact, the past quarter century is perhaps better thought of as an exploration of alternative regulatory methods, or tools, than as a definitive determination of what does and does not work in environmental regulatory policy. Not surprisingly, many of the prevailing approaches have been received with growing concern over their cost-effectiveness and with considerable skepticism about their capacity to achieve much in terms of public health or environmental protection. This has triggered a search for institutional arrangements and regulatory alternatives that may prove more successful. The following section will introduce some of the prevailing approaches and the most promising alternatives.

The arsenal of regulatory and managerial tools available for the protection of environmental health is formidable. It includes stringent regulatory controls with highly specific and demanding standards, many of which are backed by penalties for noncompliance, as well as more analytical and participatory measures intended to help public officials and the general citizenry make prudent policy decisions. No single regulatory approach is foolproof, and, in fact, more than a quarter century after the first Earth Day, the search for the proper mixture of regulatory approaches continues amid high uncertainty. How do we reduce environmental risk to scientifically, politically, economically, and socially "safe" levels? How do we reconcile the need for uniform compliance with national and international environmental objectives and the need for communities to devise locally tailored procedures to protect human health? We attempt to address such questions by examining a number of diverse approaches that have been undertaken in the name of protecting environmental health. This review will suggest that no single strategy has proven perfect, in terms either of overall capacity to safeguard human health or of likely cost-effectiveness. Instead, a confluence of such approaches is likely to prove necessary, given the diverse set of environmental health threats that exist and the array of existing legal and organizational mechanisms currently available to address them.

Imposing Strict Standards and Mandating Technological Advance: The Case of Clean Air

The national government's role in air pollution regulation is a classic example of the transformation from a regulatory system of high deference to local government and industry in the 1950s and 1960s to one of stringent national air quality goals and requirements in more recent decades. What was once a modest national presence, largely confined to research, limited funding assistance to states, and mediation of multistate conflicts, has become a model of "command-and-control" regulatory style, which concentrates considerable authority in federal government hands. What was once indifference to the types of pollution control technologies adopted and the rapidity with which they were put into use has become an ambitious scheme for prodding technological innovation and accelerating its widespread utilization.

Each version of federal air policy enacted between 1970 and 1990 has reflected a congressional commitment to transform the very nature of national regulatory policy in this area. All have demonstrated a sizable distrust of state and local governments, as well as the private sector. Rather than provide regulatory carrots of funding and other positive incentives, these pieces of legislation have established national primary and secondary air quality standards, set national emissions standards for stationary sources that required use of the "best available control technology," and created statutory deadlines for emission reductions. States have retained a direct role in the regulatory process but have been required to submit "state implementation plans" to the national government, which were intended to assure attainment of national air quality standards. Each legislative iteration has added further layers of specificity and, in many instances, regulatory rigor. The 1990 clean air legislation, for example, consists of more than one thousand pages of text with labyrinthine detail and complexity.

This constituted a federal regulatory undertaking of unprecedented ambition and scope. If fully implemented, it was expected to make radical improvements in air quality and to provide a permanent basis for promoting new pollution control technologies and responding to the emergence of new air quality threats. It was also thought likely to serve as a model for regulation in other environmental media, such as land and water, whereby the national government would attempt to bring all states and regions into uniform adherence to its standards.

The track record of such a regulatory approach is decidedly mixed. As noted earlier, emissions of a number of dangerous air pollutants have dropped since 1970, and much of this can be attributed to the national clean air legislation. Many new pollution control technologies have in fact been developed, such as the catalytic converter devices now standard in American automobiles. In addition, many industries with long-standing records of environmental abuse have been forced to introduce new pollution control devices, leading to significant air quality gains in some of the most polluted urban areas of the nation. Finally, these gains have been achieved at relatively modest direct cost to the public sector, including the national government. Direct government expenditures on air quality have been quite modest in comparison to those in other major regulatory areas, placing most of the burden on the private sector and, ultimately, on consumers of various goods.

Despite its bold preamble and lofty environmental goals, however, national clear air legislation has demonstrated a number of shortcomings. Many standards have neither been met nor, in some instances, approached, and implementation has proven extremely difficult. State and local governments have often resisted strict interpretation of the federal legislation and lacked the resources necessary to monitor and enforce it fully; they repeatedly have been caught in the middle between divergent demands from the national government and locally based industry. The clean air program has also tended to operate with minimal consideration for the overall environmental health ramifications of its

regulatory provisions and has, at times, only pushed pollutant problems into another medium (land or water) with less stringent regulation. For example, many air pollution control technologies generate highly toxic residues or sludges, which must then be disposed of through some other means.

Strict Standards and Substantial Funding Incentives: The Case of Clean Water

The national government's regulatory approach to water pollution featured somewhat similar rigor and specificity to that used for air, but has differed in at least one important respect from clean air legislation: it called for substantial direct expenditures by the national government (and other levels of government) to address some of the most severe water pollution problems facing the nation. Rather than a pure command-and-control strategy, which would deposit the vast majority of compliance costs on the private sector, the clean water approach emulated a public works strategy whereby government would open its coffers generously to advance clean water goals. In turn, subnational recipients of national grant moneys have looked more favorably upon this form of distributive policy than air programs, at least until fiscal cutbacks have begun in more recent years.

Much of the expanded governmental investment on behalf of clean water was concentrated in wastewater treatment plants, as the federal government offered grants for up to 75 percent of total construction costs to participating communities. This federal share jumped to 85 percent for innovative projects in 1977 before beginning to be scaled back during the 1980s. It was further reduced in 1987, when direct grants to states and localities were replaced with an intergovernmental loan fund. Such grants were never extended to private industries, which had to cover compliance costs for water regulations as well as those for air.

The availability of such major amounts of public funding has eased intergovernment and public–private tensions, although as in the case of strict clean air legislation, progress has been far slower than envisioned in the legislation of the early 1970s. Moreover, there has been growing concern over the appropriateness of concentrating scarce government dollars for environmental matters so overwhelmingly in the area of water pollution and relying so heavily on massive construction projects to reduce pollution. The focus of these government efforts on large industrial and sewage plants has tended to obscure other sources of water pollution, including uncontrolled pesticide runoffs from farmland, channel dredging, and—less visible but perhaps more health-threatening—toxic wastes from small businesses, industries, and individual residences. Indeed, a growing body of literature confirms that many of our most pervasive water pollution problems stem from these sources that have continued to go largely unexamined, much less regulated (Adler et al., 1993).

Environmental Assessment: The Case of Environmental Impact Statements

Not all of the national environmental initiatives of recent vintage have involved stringent command-and-control regulatory approaches. The National Environmental Policy Act of 1969 (NEPA) represented a markedly different approach, one that emphasized interdisciplinary planning in trying to minimize future environmental degradation. It relied on analytical skills and interagency cooperation rather than on strict standards and technology-forcing and was ultimately replicated by twenty-eight states that enacted their own counterpart legislation.

NEPA calls on all agencies of the national government to consider the environmental ramifications of their actions and to incorporate this consideration formally into their policymaking processes. Environmental impact statements were to provide a detailed environmental assessment for "proposals for legislation and other major Federal actions significantly affecting the quality of the human environment." These statements were to assess (1) the environmental impact of the proposed action; (2) any adverse environmental effects that could not be avoided should the proposal be implemented; (3) alternatives to the proposed action; (4) the relationship between local short-term environmental uses and the maintenance and enhancement of long-

term productivity; and (5) any irreversible commitments of resources that would be involved in the proposed action should it be implemented.

This was a tall order for government agencies, ranging from the Army Corps of Engineers to the Department of Health and Human Services, that had never before been asked to make such assessments. While philosophically appealing, given its vast scope, NEPA has suffered from many of the shortcomings that have made command-and-control regulatory approaches so attractive. It calls for thorough planning but lacks any precise measures of what is and is not environmentally appropriate activity, and it gives enormous leeway to individual agencies to weigh other pressing considerations against environmental ones. Moreover, NEPA is confined to activities sponsored by the federal government, excluding environmentally threatening activity that occurs through state and local government actions and in the private sector. It is widely viewed as having made some modest contributions to general environmental awareness but few tangible contributions to promoting environmental health.

Counterpart state programs vary greatly. Those in New York, Oregon, and Washington have proven particularly innovative in linking the environmental impact statements process to additional incentives and standards that appear to have proven more effective. For example, New York's State Environmental Quality Review Act represents an effort to integrate broad environmental assessment into virtually every aspect of the state's environmental policymaking and has been used aggressively by the state's Department of Environmental Quality. Many others largely replicate the experience of NEPA.

National Government as Direct Cleanup Agent: The Case of Superfund

The sheer volume of abandoned hazardous waste sites and the perceived potential threat they posed to human health necessitated a federal regulatory response that transcended both the command-and-control and environmental assessment styles that had prevailed earlier. As noted earlier, the seemingly ubiquitous nature of these sites caught the nation by surprise, and exact measures of their prevalence and potential health consequences remain elusive. Nonetheless, they constitute a new type of challenge for policymakers and represent the failure of the regulatory system in the decades before the late 1970s to address these waste disposal problems in a serious fashion. As a result, enormous public and private resources will have to be invested to clean up toxic messes that in many instances have been simmering for decades.

The national response to this problem has included enactment of Superfund, a multibillion-dollar program that enables the federal government to assess the severity of the abandoned site problem, rank the most serious environmental health hazards, and conduct far-reaching cleanups. It also sets detailed standards that guide the assessment and cleanup processes and has already been supplemented by a number of state government efforts that provide additional funding. This legislation not only involves government in the environmental cleanup process in a more direct, expansive way than ever before, but it also gives federal officials sweeping powers to attempt to determine liability for creating such environmental hazards. Government officials may either attempt to force responsible parties to clean up their own messes or initiate cleanup efforts and then sue responsible parties to recover the costs.

Since its inception, Superfund has suffered serious implementation problems. During the early years of the Reagan administration, leading environmental officials were accused of defining their authority under Superfund in minimalist terms and giving generous settlements (called "sweetheart deals") to industries responsible for abandoned sites. Enormous political controversy ensued, and Superfund became a political volleyball bounced between an executive branch committed to limited enforcement and a Congress committed to rigorous enforcement. This political conflict compounded a complicated process of assessment and intervention and allowed the program to accomplish very little in terms of successful site cleanups. This clouded record leaves Superfund's capacity as an effective regulatory tool largely uncertain.

Congress has continued to pump billions of dollars into this cleanup program, which in combination with state, local, and private-sector expenditures, has made it one of the largest environmental policy areas in terms of committed resources. However, no reliable technology exists for safely cleaning up many types of hazardous waste sites, and government officials have found it extremely difficult to assess liability and press cases that will hold up in court. Superfund has also received harsh criticism for consuming such a large share of scarce federal environmental funds given the wealth of other forms of expenditures that might afford greater environmental health benefit (Hird, 1994; Church & Nakamura, 1993).

ECONOMIC INCENTIVES: MAKING POLLUTERS PAY

Economists have long been among the harshest critics of the prevailing set of environmental regulatory approaches. Many tend to view command-and-control schemes and direct cleanup intervention as highly inefficient and as deterrents to innovation. They also tend to perceive other mechanisms, such as environmental assessment, as lacking the incentives necessary to secure broad commitment to improving environmental quality. Instead, they have devised proposals that would apply market-like incentives to the regulatory process. These incentive-based proposals would set specific pollution reduction timetables and monetary penalties for noncompliance but would give individual industries and other regulated sources great latitude in deciding how to meet them (Tietenberg, 1988; Schelling, 1983; Bryner, 1995; National Academy of Public Administration, 1994).

Congress, the federal EPA, and some states have become increasingly interested in these alternatives in recent years, as doubts over the efficacy of command-and-control provisions have mounted. The EPA completed a number of modest experiments designed to test some of these market-based strategies, particularly in the area of air quality regulation. These experiments go by an array of intriguing names, including "bubbles," "netting," "offsets," "banking," and "emissions trading," all of which significantly reshape incentives and opportunities for compliance with the Clean Air Act standards. Under the "bubble" approach, for example, an imaginary bubble covers multiple emissions points in an individual plant. The owners of the plant may choose which points are cheapest to clean up (and what methods are cheapest to achieve the cleanup) as long as overall reductions meet federal and state standards. This differs from the more rigid command-and-control approach, which offers no latitude for concentrating on the most cost-effective strategies. These early experiments established a precedent for expanded use of this approach in the 1990s. Under Title IV of the 1990 Clean Air Act amendments, an extensive market-based incentive system has been created to curb air emissions from coal-fired power plants that lead to acid rain. States and regions have also expanded their use of such tools, including California programs to reduce air emissions and Minnesota programs to reduce hazardous waste. Economic incentive programs are increasingly common in promoting recycling, such as through refundable deposits for beverage containers, auto tires, and batteries.

What begins as elegant theory is often difficult to translate into policy, and economic incentives have been no exception. This has been particularly evident in the more complex economic-based programs, such as emissions trading, rather than those involving more straightforward deposits and refunds. Implementation has been fraught with difficulties in the former instances, in part because of the enormous monitoring efforts that are required to determine compliance and (if necessary) set penalties. As a result, government oversight must be far more expansive than under command-and-control, where often the litmus test of compliance is simply use of a federally imposed technology rather than careful measurement of emissions. These approaches have also received scathing criticism from some environmental lobby groups that view them as a way to undermine regulatory rigor and appease industry. Nonetheless, careful analyses of these early experiments suggest that they hold considerable promise and could develop into a useful mechanism to promote

greater regulatory efficiency and flexibility (National Academy of Public Administration, 1994).

Prevention: Waste Reduction and Reuse

Regulatory strategies designed to reduce the amount of waste generated each year and promote its reuse or recycling would seem a natural component of a prevention-oriented environmental policy. However, preventive approaches have consistently been overshadowed at all levels of government by regulatory efforts designed to respond to existing problems and manage disposal of existing wastes rather than promote their reuse or reduce their generation.

The American track record in this area is particularly disappointing when compared with that of other Western democracies (Haigh & Irwin, 1990). The United States generates approximately three times as much hazardous waste per person as Germany, for example, in large part because of its comparatively modest—and recent—commitment to waste reduction and reuse. The Germans, like many of their Western European neighbors, have eschewed the land-based disposal techniques long preferred by the United States in favor of a variety of innovative strategies that are only beginning to be seriously considered in this country. These include programs requiring manufacturers to "take back" all packaging and related waste materials from their products for recycling or some form of reuse.

In the United States, local governments have perhaps been most active in this area, and many individual communities play an active role in recycling consumer wastes such as paper, glass, and metals. Recycling levels of such commodities now approaches 25 percent nationally, a dramatic jump in little more than a decade. State governments have supported a good deal of this activity, through grants, technical support, and, in some cases, the sorts of deposit systems discussed above. These sorts of efforts are beginning to be extended into chemicals, pesticides, and hazardous wastes. In recent years, the federal and many state governments have begun a variety of initiatives to promote waste reduction and reuse. All fifty states now provide small grants and technical assistance to private firms that have innovative waste reduction ideas and also operate waste exchange networks, whereby state officials provide information throughout the state on waste materials that may be reusable. In a number of other states, legislation has been enacted that either provides incentives for or mandates waste reduction or reuse, including some particularly far-reaching efforts being implemented in Minnesota, New Jersey, and New York (Rabe, in press). For example, New York has directly integrated waste reduction with its waste management process, requiring all generators of hazardous waste to complete a Waste Reduction Impact Statement (WRIS) before they are allowed to dispose of wastes. These statements call for comprehensive assessment of waste reduction alternatives and a schedule for implementing waste reduction plans. At the federal level, mandated "right-to-know" programs have begun to make information that is essential for preventive strategies more reliable and accessible than ever before. These programs require firms that use certain types and quantities of toxic materials to release information on their activities to the public each year. In turn, "pollution prevention" is being considered seriously in a number of federal program areas, propelled in part by the 1990 Pollution Prevention Act.

Risk Assessment

A growing issue in American environmental policy has been determining the best manner for introducing new methodological tools into the environmental regulatory process. Foremost among these tools is risk assessment, which at least in theory can quantitatively assess environmental health risk. If successful, such tools could facilitate a systematic consideration of the severity of various threats and the viability of alternative regulatory remedies.

One of the greatest political tests facing any expanded use of risk assessment is that it may threaten existing environmental agencies and officials who prefer to adhere to current practices. Some state and federal efforts to rank environmental risks by perceived severity have suggested that current policy priorities and resource allocation patterns are inverse to actual conditions, thereby posing a fundamental challenge to the prevailing order. Control over risk assessment development and application has already become a major battleground among federal agencies and in numerous states, with all relevant environmental agencies eager to exercise some influence over the way the process is devised and implemented. Not surprisingly, no two federal agencies or states have defined risk assessment in the same way or established identical institutional mechanisms for putting it into use.

Much as in the case of economic incentives, risk assessment comprises a promising but inexact set of methods for guiding regulatory priority setting and decision making. Its proponents credit it with great potential to analyze risk systematically and ultimately facilitate effective management of those risks and communication of their relative dangers to the public. Skeptics caution that it remains in a highly preliminary state of development and must also surmount a series of political and institutional hurdles before being adopted as a central environmental regulatory tool. As one leading analyst of risk assessment has cautioned, "In the face of scientific uncertainty and inadequate data, some interested parties magically invoke the term risk assessment in an effort to bring authority and confidence to an uncertain process" (Davies, 1984). Risk assessment received new consideration in the Republican-controlled 104th Congress, as opponents of the existing regulatory order sought to expand its use substantially and thereby deter new regulatory steps in the absence of overwhelming evidence that particular contaminants pose high risk.

Multinational Coordination

Environmental problems do not respect local, state, or national boundaries and may increasingly call for multinational approaches if substantial environmental health improvements are to occur. Just as uncontrolled air pollution emissions from Mexico threaten the health of American citizens, minimally controlled emissions from coal-burning power plants in the American Midwest exacerbate Canada's acid rain problems. Even more broadly, widespread destruction of Third World rainforests and rapid industrialization in Asia are likely to be leading contributors to global climate change, which may leave no continent, developed or otherwise, unscathed.

Nonetheless, multinational and international coordination on behalf of environmental health has proven elusive. Nations may be even less successful in this area than in negotiating common approaches to monetary policy, trade policy, and defense commitments. To date, few nations have proven willing to yield their sovereignty over internal environmental policy in favor of some broader cooperative approach. The role of the United Nations in this regard has been almost exclusively symbolic, like that of other broad institutions such as the World Health Organization and the Organization of American States. Even international institutions with considerable capacity to link economic development assistance to environmental health, such as the World Bank and the International Monetary Fund, have only recently begun to examine any potential involvement of this type.

Gradual progress on international environmental governance may be occurring, however, most notable to date in the historic, multinational agreement to attempt to reduce destruction of the stratospheric ozone layer (Benedick, 1991). This agreement binds signatories to development of substitutes for those chemicals most disruptive to ozone and transfer of new technology to developing nations. Comparable steps toward cooperation are also evident between neighboring nations of Western Europe and North America. The growing cohesion of individual European nations under the auspices of the European Economic Community (EEC) has led to major efforts to coordinate environmental regulatory programs and work cooperatively to protect environmental health. In North America, the Great Lakes Basin has served as a source for growing environmental cooperation between the Canadian and U.S. governments. The International Joint Commission has been increasingly active in attempting to reduce water pollution in the lakes and has been bolstered by a series of multinational regulatory and research initiatives, including a number of promising efforts launched by American states and Canadian provinces that border the Great Lakes. Most of these North American initiatives have moved gradually, in the face of enduring political disincentives to extensive collaboration, indicating that some progress may be possible in expanding the scope of regulatory efforts beyond national boundaries (Rabe & Zimmerman, 1995). Even trade policy has begun to be linked with environmental concerns, evident in the environmental "side agreement" to the North American Free Trade Agreement (NAFTA), which creates a series of measures for continental environmental protection.

NEW QUESTIONS AND CHALLENGES

The odyssey of American efforts to protect environmental health has featured numerous changes of course in recent decades. Once a fairly modest presence on the national political agenda, environmental policy has become a major domestic concern. Once the province of public health officials and agencies, it is now influenced by a myriad of laws, agencies, and interest groups. Once an area in which direct government expenditures were quite modest, it is likely to consume ever-increasing portions of scarce public-sector resources in future decades.

Following the expansion of national and state environmental regulatory efforts in the late 1960s and early 1970s, growing doubts emerged concerning their effectiveness. The Reagan administration posed a direct challenge to many areas of federal involvement, attempting to cut program funding and move toward a more voluntary compliance system. During the 1980s, however, most of its proposals for far-reaching deregulation were rejected, in large part because of overwhelming public support (as evident in public opinion surveys and growing participation in environmental groups) for rigorous environmental regulatory efforts. Some funding was cut at the federal level, but the basic infrastructure of federal programs was maintained. At the same time, many states began to expand dramatically their own involvement in environmental policy.

In the mid-1990s, however, a new set of challenges to the existing regulatory order has emerged. The 1994 national elections and the Republican-dominated 104th Congress in particular gave unprecedented visibility to strong opponents of the prevailing regulatory system. In response, Congress began to advance a series of bills intended to dramatically transform the way in which national and state governments address environmental protection. A common theme linking these initiatives was the view that existing regulations—and regulators—had become overzealous in pursuit of often-suspect environmental goals. Those holding such a view lamented the proliferation and growing stringency of regulations at national and state levels. One particularly strident and influential critic, Congressman Tom DeLay (R-TX), equated the EPA with the "the Gestapo" in July 1995. In seeking an alternative course, DeLay and his colleagues endorsed three types of options.

First, agencies could employ a dramatically expanded use of cost–benefit and risk assessment analysis. These tools would be expressly designed to create extremely high thresholds (of economic benefit from regulation and demonstrable health risk from human exposure to pollutants) that would have to be crossed before any regulatory action could be taken. Supporters of such provisions contend that these steps would require agencies to weigh economic and risk issues more systematically and allow them to set more reasonable regulatory priorities. Critics respond that thresholds for interventions are being set so high that virtually no regulatory activity could be justified. Moreover, they argue that the implementation of these analytic processes would become the dominant activity of regulatory officials, forcing them to neglect other essential duties, such as monitoring and enforcement.

Second, extensive provisions could be established requiring regulatory agencies to compensate citizens financially for any property value loss attributable to environmental regulations. Such legislation invokes the "takings" clause of the U.S. Constitution, which calls on government to compensate private holders of property seized for public purposes. If implemented, it could pose especially dramatic consequences on efforts to protect endangered species and ecologically sensitive areas such as wetlands. No systematic estimate of likely costs was produced for these legislative proposals, but many observers suggest that they would create a major disincentive for government to take certain types of regulatory actions because of extremely high costs. Although Arizona voters rejected such a proposal in a 1993 ballot initiative, twenty-four states were considering their own takings proposals in 1995.

Third, both the 104th Congress and the Clinton administration explored ways to streamline the environmental regulatory system. Both Republicans and Democrats heaped praise upon attorney Philip Howard's best-selling book, *The Death of Common Sense*, and used it to endorse their own simplification strategies (Howard, 1995). Howard contends that regulatory policy, particularly environmental protection, has become ossified due to overly detailed congressional interference in the drafting and oversight of regulation. The Clinton administration attempted to respond with its ongoing initiative to "reinvent government" and give agency officials greater latitude to pursue creative solutions to implementation problems. Congress responded with proposals to either simplify or eliminate significant sections of existing environmental legislation. One such tactic called for maintaining existing programs but eliminating all funding for implementation. This might prove less politically visible than outright termination but accomplish similar purposes, rendering federal legislation useless.

Conclusion

The long-term ramifications of these initiatives remain highly unclear. Earlier assaults on the prevailing environmental regulatory system, most notably in the early 1980s, triggered a huge public backlash. Membership in environmental advocacy groups soared, many efforts to pursue deregulation were thwarted, and many new programs were developed in response, especially at the state level. Public opinion surveys consistently indicate that the public overwhelmingly supports broad environmental protection goals and feels that both public and private sectors are not doing enough to realize them. In turn, there is broad support for propositions to streamline the current system and reduce regulatory excesses. Such sentiments, of course, are not always easy to reconcile in policy, as has been evident for the past quarter century.

REFERENCES

Adler, Robert W., Jessica C. Landman, & Diane M. Cameron. (1993). *The Clean Water Act 20 years later*. Washington, D.C.: Island Press.

Baumgartner, Frank, & Bryan Jones. (1992). *Agendas and instability in American politics*. Chicago: University of Chicago Press.

Benedick, Richard. (1991). *Ozone diplomacy*. Cambridge, MA: Harvard University Press.

Bryner, Gary C. (1995). *Blue skies, green politics: The Clean Air Act of 1990* (rev. ed.). Washington, D.C.: Congressional Quarterly.

Church, Thomas W., & Robert T. Nakamura. (1993). *Cleaning up the mess: Implementation strategies for Superfund*. Washington, D.C.: The Brookings Institution.

Colborn, Theodora E., et al. (1990). *Great Lakes, great legacy?* Washington, D.C.: Conservation Foundation.

Council of State Governments. (1994). *Book of the states, 1994–95*. Lexington, KY: Council of State Governments.

Davies, J. Clarence. (1984). *Risk assessment and risk control*. Washington, D.C.: Conservation Foundation.

DeWitt, John. (1994). *Civic environmentalism*. Washington, D.C.: Congressional Quarterly.

Haigh, Nigel, & Frances Irwin. (Eds.). (1990). *Integrated pollution control in Europe and North America*. Washington, D.C.: Conservation Foundation.

Hird, John A. (1994). *Superfund: The political economy of environmental risk*. Baltimore, MD: Johns Hopkins University Press.

Hirschorn, Joel. (1985). Presentation made to the Integrated National Hazardous Materials Workshop, Argonne National Laboratory, Argonne, IL.

Horton, Tom, & William M. Eichbaum. (1991). *Turning the tide: Saving the Chesapeake Bay*. Washington, D.C.: Island Press.

Howard, Philip K. (1995). *The death of common sense*. New York: Random House.

Jessup, Deborah Hitchcock. (1995). *Guide to state environmental programs* (rev. ed.). Washington, D.C.: Bureau of National Affairs.

Landy, Marc K., Marc J. Roberts, & Stephen R. Thomas. (1990). *The Environmental Protection Agency: Asking the wrong question*. New York: Oxford University Press.

Lowry, William R. (1992). *The dimensions of federalism: State governments and pollution control policies*. Durham, NC: Duke University Press.

Marcus, Alfred A. (1980). *Promise and performance: Choosing and implementing an environmental policy*. Westport, CT: Greenwood.

National Academy of Public Administration. (1994). *The environment goes to market*. Washington, D.C.: National Academy of Public Administration.

Rabe, Barry G. (1994). *Beyond NIMBY: Hazardous waste siting in Canada and the United States*. Washington, D.C.: The Brookings Institution.

Rabe, Barry G. (Forthcoming). An empirical examination of integrated environmental management. *Public Administration Review*.

Rabe, Barry G., & Janet B. Zimmerman. (1995). Beyond environmental regulatory fragmentation: Signs of integration in the case of the Great Lakes Basin. *Governance: An International Journal of Policy and Administration, 8* (January), 58–77.

Ringquist, Evan J. (1993). *Environmental protection at the state level: Politics and progress in controlling pollution*. Armonk, NY: M. E. Sharpe.

Rosenbaum, Walter. (1995). *Environmental politics and policy* (rev. ed.). Washington, D.C.: Congressional Quarterly.

Schelling, Thomas C. (Ed.). (1983). *Incentives for environmental protection*. Cambridge, MA: MIT Press.

Shrader-Frechette, K. S. (1993). *Burying uncertainty*. Berkeley: University of California Press.

Tietenberg, Thomas H. (1988). *Emissions trading: An exercise in reforming pollution policy*. Washington, D.C.: Resources for the Future.

Walker, David B. (1995). *The rebirth of federalism: Slouching toward Washington*. Chatham, NJ: Chatham House.

CHAPTER

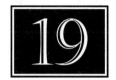

Rural Health Care Delivery
and Finance:
Policy and Politics

Keith J. Mueller

Approximately 25 percent of all U.S. citizens live in rural areas. While their needs for health care services do not differ appreciably from those of their urban counterparts, the health care delivery system differs considerably. Rural citizens, rural providers, and (most recently) general rural advocates have become political forces in U.S. health policy, both nationally and in many states. The issues that concern them, and the politics of how those issues are integrated into more general policies, are the subjects of this chapter.

The interplay of access, quality, and cost issues in developing health policies has a different meaning for rural health systems. The politics of interest group activities, described as either issue networks (Heclo, 1978) or policy communities (Peterson, 1993), is the arena in which rural interests have fared well since 1983. The shifting tides of how federalism is operationalized in U.S. health policy creates the need for rural interests to be sure of effective policy advocacy in state capitols as well as in Washington, D.C.

This chapter is organized into two major parts: the policy issues confronting rural health care delivery systems, and the politics of representing rural interests in policy debates.

POLICY ISSUES IN RURAL HEALTH CARE DELIVERY

The major policy issues in rural health care delivery are the needs of the population and sustaining the systems that deliver care.

The Needs of Rural Residents

The primary purpose of any health policy should be to promote the health and well-being of populations. To that end, current health status becomes a baseline by which progress can be judged. From a variety of indicators of health status, both general and specific to certain health conditions, any potential rural differential can be specified. There are reasons to believe that health conditions will differ, primarily related to different environments and lifestyles. The interaction between individual health care needs and the capabilities of the delivery system may also lead to rural–urban differences.

Using the 1990 census as the source of data, the economic conditions of rural residents are somewhat worse than those of their urban counterparts. Approximately 17 percent of rural residents live in households with incomes below the federal poverty level, compared with 12 percent of urban residents. Fortunately for rural residents, these disparities do not translate into an overall lower percentage of persons without health insurance. In 1992, the percent of uninsured was 17 percent for both urban and rural residents under age sixty-five (Employee Benefits Research Institute, 1994). Rural school-age children (ages 6–17), however, are more likely to be uninsured than the same aged children in urban areas (Porterfield & Scott, 1993). Moreover, because rural residents are more likely to have purchased health insurance either as individuals or through small employers, they are likely to pay higher premiums, co-insurance, and deductibles, and spend more of their own funds to purchase health care (Farley, 1985).

The comparative disadvantages of rural residents in the insurance marketplace can lead to lower utilization of health care services. Children in rural households with low incomes and not receiving public assistance are less likely to utilize physician care than urban children in the same circumstances (Levey et al., 1988). According to findings from a national interview survey, rural uninsured residents experience fewer physician visits than their urban counterparts (National Center for Health Statistics, 1991). There are, however, regional variations in these findings, as Comer and Mueller (1995) point out in their study of the insurance status of Nebraskans.

The relationship among insurance, underinsurance, and utilization of health care services has been documented in several studies. Uninsured persons are less likely to see a physician (Newacheck, 1989; Freeman et al., 1990; Hafner-Eaton, 1993), have a usual source of care, and be hospitalized when ill (Hafner-Eaton, 1993). In rural areas economic disadvantages are compounded by distance. When illness strikes, therefore, it can be even more debilitating. Rural residents also experience more days per year of restricted activity due to adverse health conditions and are more likely to report only fair or poor general health status (U.S. Office of Technology Assessment, 1990). Data from the 1989 National Health Interview Survey (NHIS) show higher rates of occurrence among rural residence for arthritis (9.7 per 100 vs. 7.4), absence of fingers or hands (0.49 per 100 vs. 0.25), liver disease (1.5 per 100 vs. 1.1), hernia (1.9 per 100 vs. 1.2), diabetes (2.5 per 100 vs. 1.7), high blood pressure (8.8 per 100 vs. 7.5), chronic sinusitis (16.4 per 100 vs. 13), and emphysema (0.86 per 100 vs. 0.32). Problems of access to health care services in rural areas can result in particular problems, such as inadequate screening of rural women for *C. trachomatous* (Ferris & Litaker, 1993). Similarly, cancers that can be detected through screening may go for longer periods before recognition in rural populations (Liff et al., 1991).

Rural residents reflect the nation's changing demographic composition, with the elderly representing an ever-increasing percentage of the population. The percent of the population age sixty-five and over is higher in rural areas than in urban areas, and higher still among farm populations. The percent of elderly who are poor is also higher in nonmetropolitan areas (Coward et al., 1992). Moreover, the incidence and prevalence of chronic health problems will only increase as this phenomenon continues.

Other "special" populations create demands for rural health care delivery systems. For example, migratory workers are low-income, mostly uninsured, and exposed to specific health risks related to their occupation. Migrant workers are more likely to experience gastroenteritis, parasitic infections, dermatitis, and musculoskeletal ailments (Slesinger, 1992). Rural minority populations in certain states may be left out of the mainstream patterns of health care delivery because they represent a very small percentage of the region's population and because their interactions with the delivery system may be very different (based on cultural definitions of illness).

While there is a natural tendency when considering health care policy to focus on the needy and ill, the majority of rural residents are insured, are under age sixty-five, are White, and lead "normal" lives. As a result, they may resist changes in the system, which they may perceive as threats to their current situations.

Implications

From the standpoint of public policy, this review of the characteristics of the rural population should provide the basis for considering specific interventions. Any health care delivery system should be capable of serving the basic needs related to emergency services and primary care. Even this fundamental level of services is not always accessible in rural areas, if accessibility is defined as within forty-five minutes of a person's residence. A health care system should also be able to facilitate the use of other more specialized services as needed.

In rural America, the principle of responding to population-based needs will mean paying special attention to the needs of the elderly, migratory workers, and children, among others. The reasons for disproportionate occurrences of adverse conditions should be specified, and then changes in the delivery and finance system targeted to meet identified needs. Examples of special efforts related to each population group are described below.

Policies for the rural elderly. Chief among the special needs of the elderly are assistance in completing activities of daily living, such as eating, bathing, and dressing. With community-based services the elderly can remain in their own homes, which could improve their quality of life. Unfortunately, formal community-based services such as adult day care services and congregate meal facilities are less available to rural residents than to their urban counterparts (Coward et al., 1992). Certain diseases plague the elderly as an age cohort. One of the best known of these is dementia, including Alzheimer's disease. Since this is a specialized condition, managing care for patients with dementia is a significant challenge to rural health systems, with the possible exception of those persons who are institutionalized. Rural areas do not have a sufficient number of trained professionals to deal with dementia as a special condition (Buckwalter, 1992). Therefore, this problem, as is true for mental health generally, will fall to the primary care provider.

Policies for migrant workers. Migrant workers in the United States present a special problem to rural health systems by the very nature of their transitory residence. They are not served by a single primary care provider throughout the year. In part as a response to this special problem, the Migrant Health Act was signed into law in 1962 to create a Migrant Health Program under Section 329 of the Public Health Service Act. Migrant health clinics have been created and funded under that act, but they serve only 13 percent of the target population (Slesinger, 1992). Problems include having enough clinics conveniently located near the populations, and reaching persons who are reluctant to utilize traditional medical services.

Policies related to children. Rural women are less likely than their urban counterparts to initiate prenatal care early in pregnancy (McManus & Newacheck, 1989), although subsequent rates of infant mortality do not differ. However, inadequate prenatal care, measured as onset and frequency, can have consequences for the health of children other than early death. Therefore, transportation and availability of physicians offering prenatal care, two of the leading rural barriers, are issues for policy resolution. To the extent that obstetrical care in rural areas is threatened by such factors as malpractice insurance premiums and loss of primary care physicians, perinatal outcomes for rural women are threatened (Nesbitt et al., 1989).

General population and policy. A focus on the groups needing improvements in the health care delivery system related to their special needs cannot overlook the majority of the population. For the majority of rural residents, public policy should focus on strengthening the delivery system where it may be weak now, such as medically underserved areas. These are areas where there are too few medical care professionals to serve the population. For most rural areas, though, policies should be related to sustaining what rural residents already have. That means helping local delivery systems make the necessary changes in financing and organization to remain viable in a time of increasingly intense economic competition among health insurance plans.

Sustaining the Rural Health Care Delivery System

In metropolitan areas one can find the complete spectrum of medical specialties, from primary care to the most sophisticated subspeciality. In rural areas, the system relies much more on the role of primary care providers, since many subspecialties simply are not there. Similarly, local rural hospitals do not pretend to offer the same array of services, particularly in tertiary care (such as sophisticated, technology-intensive surgeries), available in large metropolitan hospitals. Health care delivery involves more than doctors and hospitals, and the array of community-based services available in rural areas varies considerably. Rural and urban systems are of course integrated (especially for specialty care), but the needs of the rural system should be addressed separately.

According to many, rural health care delivery systems are anchored by local hospitals. While this paradigm is changing, sustaining emergency and acute care services associated with hospitals remains a paramount rural concern. The implementation of Medicare's prospective payment system (PPS) in the mid-1980s heightened concerns about the financial survival of small rural hospitals. These providers often rely quite heavily on Medicare for their finances, since for some, over 60 percent of their inpatient business is with Medicare beneficiaries (Mick & Morlock, 1990). The rate of rural hospital closure rose considerably in the years immediately following the advent of PPS, from fewer than ten closures in 1983 to forty in 1987 (Mullner & Whiteis, 1988). When the only hospital in a community closes, access to services is curtailed, and in some instances declines in health status have been documented (Bindman et al., 1990).

The financial problems of rural hospitals can be attributed to changes in the delivery of care. As more care shifted to outpatient settings, the percentage of unfilled beds increased. This in turn led to difficulties in financing a full array of acute care services, which required commitment to infrequently used equipment and personnel. A critical policy issue became facilitating changes in rural hospitals, from full-service acute care institutions to places offering emergency and short-term acute services only. Two resulting trends of the late 1980s and early 1990s were downsizing facilities and making maximum use of a smaller number of employees by cross-training persons to complete several tasks. These trends both require changes in public policies—changes in Medicare's "conditions of participation," which detail requirements for hospitals to be eligible for reimbursement, and changes in state government licensing requirements to allow different configurations of hospital services.

Another change in rural hospitals that is gaining increasing momentum as the next century approaches is the combining of several hospitals into a single network. These networks result in hospitals sharing responsibilities for services purchased jointly, such as mobile computer tomography scanners. Horizontal networks among hospitals may serve as building blocks for more comprehensive rural networks that may yield regional health managed care health plans.

An early example of a rural hospital network is the Rural Wisconsin Hospital Cooperative (RWHC), formed in 1979. The RWHC is a vehicle for joint ventures among eighteen small rural hospitals and an urban university hospital. The RWHC has grown in both size and scope of activities, and currently administers a health insurance plan—the Health Maintenance Organization (HMO) of Wisconsin (U.S. Office of Technology Assessment, 1990). Various rural hospital consortia have been developed, several with financial support from the Robert Wood Johnson Foundation. Typical activities have included shared services, primary/specialty clinics, marketing/public relations, and professional recruitment/development (Christianson et al., 1990).

Fully integrated rural health networks are those that have shared governance. As the debates about health reform unfolded in 1993–94, such networks seemed to be a viable means of implementing reform in rural areas. However, none existed at the time (Christianson & Moscovice, 1993). Recognizing that deficiency, many of the reform proposals, including the Health Security Act proposed by President Clinton, included assistance to rural communities and providers for the purposes of forming networks (Coburn & Mueller, 1995). State reforms also favored network development, and specific networks have evolved in Florida and elsewhere (Duncan et al., 1995).

A more severe problem for rural areas remains the chronic shortages of physicians and other health care professionals. As of June 30, 1994, there were 2,577 health professional shortage areas in the United States, with 45.2 million residents. For rural areas to achieve the standard physician-to-population ratio of one for every 3,500 persons, at least 5,085 additional primary care physicians would be required. Shortages have also been documented in several other health professions as well (e.g., dentistry, 1,115 areas requiring 3,592 professionals; and mental health, 832 areas requiring 4,033 professionals). For each profession, at least 70 percent of the shortage areas are in nonmetropolitan counties. This problem of physician shortages is occurring in spite of the national reality that there are too many specialist physicians for the needs of the population (Weiner, 1993). Moreover, a national trend toward greater use of primary care physicians in managed health care plans could even exacerbate the rural shortage problem. Newly trained primary care physicians, and some currently practicing in rural areas, may be attracted by higher salaries and more favorable working conditions to practice in urban areas.

Rural shortages also exist among the other health professions as well—some perhaps even more acute than that for primary care physicians. The allied health professions (e.g., physical therapy, medical technology, radiology technology, and occupational therapy), are in great demand in rural communities. The need for these professionals parallels the increasing numbers of elderly with needs for long-term care and rehabilitation from certain acute care treatments (e.g., heart surgery, joint replacements).

THE POLITICS OF REPRESENTING RURAL HEALTH INTERESTS IN POLICY DEBATES

The needs of rural citizens and rural health care providers can be addressed through public policies. There is general agreement among policymakers that government should help meet the needs of populations otherwise excluded from the benefits of health care delivery. Surely rural residents qualify for that attention. The rural health care delivery system has received attention from public policymakers at least since the Hill–Burton legislation passed in the 1940s, providing the funding to construct many of the hospitals that serve rural communities. National policies influence the training policies of academic health centers through Medicare payments for teaching, investment in scientific and medical research, and special programs for health professions training. State governments are involved through policies that license health professionals, fund medical and other health profession schools, and provide assistance to local communities.

Rural residents constitute only approximately 25 percent of the total population of the country, and in many states comprise an even smaller percentage. Therefore, for their interests to surface and be addressed in the political system, rural advocates must be particularly adept. During the past fifteen years, rural advocates have become visible and at times influential members of health policy issue networks.

Rural Influence in the National Government

Rural interests in general have always been represented effectively in Congress, as evident in the quadrennial debates surrounding authorization of the Farm Bill. To secure many of the benefits of that bill, however, rural representatives have been able to offer a trade within the same legislation, such as the food stamps program that benefits urban residents. Rural health interests have at times similarly benefited from other alliances with urban interests, such as the Hill–Burton program for health facilities construction, the National Health Services Corps, which places physicians in both urban and rural shortage areas, and the community health centers program, which provides direct assistance and favorable public program reimbursement to clinics in medically underserved areas.

The most successful policy ventures for rural interests, however, have resulted from a combination of traditional lobbying tactics by rural interests and the policy entrepreneurship of certain members of Congress. Rural concerns are expressed through a variety of interest groups. The umbrella organization for rural interests is the National Rural Health Association. Originally created in September 1978 as the National Rural Primary Care Association, the NRHA now has approximately 1,500 members representing health professionals, health educators and researchers, and health administrators. The NRHA utilizes lobbying, testimony before congressional committees, work with administrative agencies, and litigation as strategies to advocate for rural health (Mueller, 1995).

Rural hospitals are also represented by the Small and Rural Hospital Section of the American Hospital Association. During the twelve-year history of the prospective payment system (PPS), that section has provided analyses of the effects of the system. Of particular note, they have analyzed the effects of using different wage area definitions to determine the base rates. Historically general wage rates have been lower in rural areas, but in the medical field rural hospitals feel compelled to pay salaries comparable to those of urban institutions. Other general professional groups representing rural interests in national policy debates are the National Academy of Family Physicians, the National Association of Community Health Centers, the National Governors Association, and the National Council on State Legislatures.

Rural interests are represented in Congress through the activities of the 135-member Rural Health Care Coalition in the House of Representatives and the 50-member Rural Health Care Caucus in the Senate. The former was formed in 1987 and the latter in 1988. Each group is co-chaired by one member from each political party and the staff to those members comprise the coalition and the caucus. The House coalition, in most sessions, develops a package of legislative proposals that members introduce as the coalition's legislative agenda. The Senate caucus, on the other hand, does not introduce its own legislative package, preferring instead to function through the auspices of individual members, many of whom chair important committees or subcommittees.

The test of any interest group, or set of interests, is legislative success. The success should be related to issues of obvious concern. For rural health care interests, a direct financial challenge to their self-interests came in the 1980s. The enactment of the prospective payment system (PPS) for Medicare in 1983 was a jolt to rural hospitals and an inspiration for rural activism in national policies. The urban–rural difference in payment for identical services was significant and potentially devastating for many rural hospitals (Mick & Morlock, 1990). The attention focused on this particular policy issue did more than galvanize a rural constituency—it pointed out the need to increase the capacity to debate health care issues from the basis of data-driven analysis. The PPS differences between urban and rural payments originated from a research finding that historical cost differences between the two sets of hospitals could not be explained by other factors when subjected to sophisticated econometric modeling. To argue against that finding required presenting persuasive evidence that other forces were at work to explain those differences.

As a result of detecting an obvious disadvantage in policy discussions related to technical expertise, rural advocates pushed for federal funding for rural health research. That battle was at least partially won with the creation of an Office of Rural Health Policy in the Department of Health and Human Services. The first budget of the new office included support for a grant program to create centers for rural health research. Five centers were established in 1988, and two more were added in 1990. In addition to the centers, the push for rural health research resulted in set-asides earmarked for rural research in the budgets of the National Center for Health Services Research (NCHSR, now the Agency for Health Care Policy and Research [AHCPR]), the National Institutes for Mental Health, and the Health Care Financing Administration. These programs have increased the volume and quality of rural health research. As a result policymakers have more information and analysis about the critical issues affecting rural health care delivery and finance.

The Federal Office of Rural Health Policy's role in the administration includes reviews of regulations and programs of other agencies for the purpose of analyzing their potential impacts on rural health. Still the continuing vulnerability of rural programs in the federal budget was once again evident when it was proposed that the office's budget be reduced to zero by Republican members of the 104th Congress. The combination of work by rural health researchers and analysis by the office and others in administrative agencies lessens the possibilities that rural interests will again be caught flat-footed as they were when the PPS was enacted in 1983. Federal policy has become increasingly complex, particularly when concerns such as cost containment and improved access to services have to be balanced. Policy entrepreneurs speaking for rural interests need the ammunition supplied by basic research and policy analysis.

The existing representation of rural interests in Congress and the administration means that policy debates do not occur in the absence of rural input. As will be clear in a later section of this chapter, rural interests have been represented and considered in the debates about how the health care delivery and finance system should be systematically reformed. When compared to the pressing health policy concerns of the day, however, rural interests remain less important. For example, in a May 24, 1995 Hearing on Medicare and Managed Care before the House Ways and Means Subcommittee on Health (Ways and Means, 1995), the concern about how managed care and competition could be implemented in rural areas did not surface during the pre-

pared testimony of either the Prospective Payment Assessment Commission or the Physician Payment Review Commission. Only after questioning by Representative Christensen (R-NE) did those two witnesses offer their analyses.

The relatively weak position of rural interests was also evident in the fiscal year 1996 budget resolution passed by the House of Representatives in May 1995, which proposed eliminating the Office of Rural Health Policy, federal support for the Agency for Health Care Policy and Research (which includes centers for rural health policy and research, and centers for demonstrating managed care in rural areas), federal funding for projects to convert hospitals to differently configured organizations, and funding for health professions training. The debates about these programs are a tribute to the previous success of rural advocates in petitioning the federal government. Their proposed elimination is a testimony to the continued disadvantageous position of a collective interest that represents only 25 percent of the nation's population.

Rural policy successes of the late 1980s are attributable to the direct actions of policy champions in Congress, supported by the efforts of rural policy advocates. As noted by several policy scholars (see Mueller, 1993), during those years the process was such that individual policy entrepreneurs could incorporate modest program changes into omnibus legislation in Congress. Such was the case for rural programs, including the Rural Hospital Transition Grant program, which was inserted into the Omnibus Reconciliation Act of 1987 by Senator David Durenberger (R-MN). Other policies favoring rural interests were established as provisions of general programs. The most important examples were changes made to the Medicare prospective payment system to allow for higher payments for certain types of rural hospitals, such as regional referral centers (large institutions that receive patients referred by small rural hospitals) and sole community hospitals (at least thirty-five miles distant from other hospitals). Other refinements to that payment system included allowances for swing beds (both long-term care and acute care), changes in how wage areas are determined, and finally leveling the base payment rates between urban and rural hospitals. These changes instituted by Congress demonstrate the growing sophistication of rural interests and, more generally, congressional involvement in the details of policy implementation.

The executive branch has been active in addressing rural health issues as well. The funding agencies identified above have supported rural health research projects. The Federal Office of Rural Health Policy has provided technical assistance to state Offices of Rural Health, administered the program supporting research centers, staffed a national commission on rural health, and administered grants for special rural projects ("outreach") and demonstrations of telemedicine. The office has also completed special projects to further rural experimentation with managed care, network development, and health professions training. Programs elsewhere in the U.S. Department of Health and Human Services have been especially responsive to the most fundamental rural health needs—primary care, basic acute care services in hospitals, and emergency medicine.

Rural Influence in the States

As discussed previously, state government policies are critical to rural interests, especially policies that license professionals and institutions. Compared to the financial implications of federal policies, though, state policies do not seem as critical. For that as well as logistical reasons, rural influence is much less obvious in state capitols as compared to the nation's capitol. Issues of professional licensure are also of a different type than those of reimbursement for care and the distribution of grants. Grants and reimbursement are distributive policies, in which generally everyone can gain (Lowi, 1990). Professional licensure polices are more akin to Lowi's category of regulatory policy, and are certainly seen as threats to incomes of entrenched interests (Feldstein, 1977). Therefore, attempts to gain independent practice authority for nonphysician practitioners, for example, can be much more difficult than securing additional federal grant dollars.

Rural interests are represented in state policymaking by state associations that parallel national groups, particularly among the health professions. In debates about

the practice authorities of health professionals, the various professional organizations, such as nurses associations and state chapters of physician associations, are active in state politics. However, there are not fifty state rural health associations, or fifty small and rural hospital associations.

The process of state policy formation has been studied extensively by political scientists, with competing political and economic explanations of policy decisions. Political explanations combine variance in institutions with variations in party composition and electorate preferences to explain substantive decisions. Economic explanations claim that the resources available to decision makers will influence policy decisions. There can also be variation in explanations that is specific to the policy arena being considered. That is the case for health policy generally and for policies affecting rural areas specifically. In a study of state policies that provide technical assistance and flexible regulations for rural hospitals, legislative professionalism was found to be a statistically significant determinant of adoption of such policies, supporting the general argument that state institutional capacity is important. State expenditure per capita was also found to be a significant independent variable, lending support to economic determinism theories. The picture was completed, though, with a variable unique to this policy concern—the percent of the state's hospitals that were rural (Mueller, 1992).

Rural Interests in Health Reform Policies

The presence of rural interests in health policy discussions is illustrated by the debates surrounding President Clinton's Health Security Act and other attempts to revamp the health care delivery system during the 103rd Congress (1993–94). During that debate the rural concerns of availability of services, affordability of insurance, and equity in public programs were addressed to greater or lesser degrees by various proposals.

Politically, interests of rural Americans paled in comparison to the global concerns of how much money would be spent for health care, how involved the government would become in shaping the delivery system, and how and if universal financial access would be achieved. Those major issues, and partisan bickering, eventually could not be resolved. The major committees that debated reform proposals were chaired by members of Congress for whom rural constituents were not high priorities: Senate Finance (Moynihan [D-NY]), Senate Labor and Human Resources (Kennedy [D-MA]), House Ways and Means (Gibbens [D-FL], subcommittee chair Stark [D-CA]) and House Energy and Commerce (Dingel [D-MI], subcommittee chair Waxman [D-CA]). Therefore, securing provisions of interest to rural health care advocates was an uphill battle, but a battle for the most part won.

The general debates concerning the Clinton Health Security Act have been well chronicled elsewhere (see *Journal of Health Politics, 19* [Spring, 1994]). What is not as well known is the place of rural concerns in those debates. The Clinton White House task force that developed the plan included a special group working on rural health issues (Denton, 1993). Input for that group included the results of a special conference held in 1993 in Little Rock, Arkansas, which was attended by members of the administration (Campion et al., 1993). The president had been the governor of a rural state, so including rural concerns as issues during the task force deliberations was a natural focus, although certainly not the principal one. The Federal Office of Rural Health Policy helped inform those within the administration and others of the rural issues inherent in changing the methods of financing health care and reorganizing the delivery system. The office's activities included working with the task force, supporting special conferences, sponsoring analyses of major reform proposals (a series published by the author of this chapter), working with the National Advisory Commission on Rural Health, and sharing relevant research findings of the centers for rural health research.

The following provisions of the Health Security Act could be said to address rural health concerns:

- federal funding for planning and developing care systems
- inclusion of essential community providers in regional health plans

- tax credits for practitioners setting up practice in underserved rural areas
- funds for graduate medical education used to require 55 percent of all graduate residents be in primary care
- expansion of the National Health Service Corps
- Medicare bonus payments for primary care services in shortage areas
- special Medicare stipends for physicians practicing in rural hospitals in critical shortage areas
- additional grant funds for community and migrant health centers (Mueller, 1994)

Conversely, the following have been identified as inimical to rural interests:

- no requirements for the new National Board or federal agencies to include rural perspectives
- exclusion of undocumented aliens from basic coverage could adversely affect rural providers in migrant areas
- premium caps based on historical data could compel comparatively lower payments to rural providers
- National Quality Management Council not required to consult with rural interests (Mueller, 1994)

Rural interests were reflected in competing proposals for health reform. Table 19-1, taken from a report prepared by the Rural Policy Research Institute (RUPRI), assesses the rural implications of several major competing proposals for health reform in 1994 (Coburn et al., 1994). The various bills represented the "single-payer" option (Wellstone, [D-MN]), the moderate Republican alternative (Chafee [R-RI]), the conservative Republican alternative for insurance reform (Michael [R-IL]), the "pure" managed competition approach (Cooper [D-TN]), and the Clinton Health Security Act (Gephart [D-MO]).

Much of the legislation debated in 1993–94 included specific provisions targeted exclusively to rural interests. The influence of the House coalition and the Senate caucus were obvious in those provisions. The reform debates became increasingly contentious, making it important for supporters to secure and retain as many votes as possible. When rural concerns were presented

TABLE 19-1   Rural Implications of Competing Health Reform Proposals, 1994

Competing Health Reform Proposals	Rural Implications					
	Availability of Rural Providers	Availablility of Rural Facilities	Rural Health System Integration/ Coordination	Rural Influence, Involvement, Representation	Fiscal Climate	Scope of Insurance Benefits
S 491 Wellstone (D-MN)	Current decline will reverse fairly soon.	Will be enhanced.	Will not change, at best.	Will increase at local and state levels. Unclear at federal level.	Reimbusement provisions will improve short-term climate. Impact of cost control provisions unclear.	Will increase substantially.
S 1770 Chafee (R-RI)	Current decline will continue.	Will be enhanced assuming universal coverage achieved.	Will increase.	Will increase at state and federal levels. No change at local level.	Impact unclear. (Will depend on degree of universal coverage achieved.)	Will increase.
HR 3080 Michel (R-IL)	Current decline will continue.	Will be marginally enhanced.	Will not change.	Will decrease at local, state, and federal levels.	Will not change.	Will not change.
HR 3222 Cooper (D-TN)	Current decline will continue, followed by gradual increases.	Will be marginally enhanced; will be enhanced further if insurance coverage substantially extended.	Will be limited increase.	No change, or possible decreases at local, state, and federal levels.	Will not change for rural hospitals. Will improve for physicians.	Will increase somewhat.
HR 3600 Gephardt (D-MO) Clinton	Current decline will continue, followed by gradual increases.	Will be enhanced.	Will significantly increase.	Will increase at local and state levels. Unclear at federal level.	Reimbursement provisions will improve climate for providers. Impact of cost control provisions unclear.	Will increase substanially.

SOURCE: Rural Policy Research Institute: The Rural Perspective on National Health Reform Legislation, March 1994.

by members of Congress as prerequisites for their votes, they were included in the legislation. Rural interest groups were in agreement on basic principles they sought in national health reform, best presented as these written and published by the National Rural Health Association:

1. Universal access to comprehensive health care without financial barriers.
2. Federal government leadership in developing and financing a national health plan.
3. State and local self-determination for needs and preferences in plan design.

4. Encourage development of comprehensive local health care systems.
5. Assure consumer choice of financing intermediaries and providers of care.
6. Establish flexible payment systems and systems development mechanisms.
7. Provide policy direction and funding to educate and train a sufficient number and mix of appropriate health professionals.
8. Include quality assurance systems and accountability mechanisms to ensure reexamination of and improvement in health care service delivery (National Rural Health Association, 1992).

The principles focused on issues of access and system development, omitting cost, which is not perceived to be a severe problem in rural areas.

Technical support was available to Congress as members struggled with how to translate principles into specific legislative provisions. Their own congressional staffs had become more sophisticated in general health issues (Mueller, 1993), and for rural interests in particular. Supporting staff agencies of Congress, particularly the Office of Technology Assessment and the General Accounting Office, had developed rural expertise as evident in some of their leading publications. The administration, particularly the Office of Rural Health Policy, was also a source of expertise. External groups provided additional analysis. In particular, the Rural Policy Research Institute emerged during 1994 as a source of analysis. This group of university-based policy scientists is not associated with any particular lobbying group, but is instead supported in part by Congress to be a source of objective analysis of differential rural impacts of various policies, including health.

Rural advocates learned several important lessons about the federal policy process during the reform debates: argue from principles, find strength in numbers, use information and analysis, find effective champions and strategic allies, articulate concerns in a manner consistent with the dominant policy direction being taken, and be persistent. As evident in the 1994 election results, parties in power can change, and even before the elections the ideological flavor of policy was changing.

Therefore rural interests are best expressed as enduring principles, not as specific policy positions linked with current political fortunes. When those principles are widely supported, as in the two internal congressional groups, they are likely to be considered at all times during the policy debates. Specific analyses of legislative ideas should be based in empirical realities and scientific interpretations as much as possible.

When issues are as central as having health care available to rural residents, there should be members of Congress and others who are willing to carry forward the banner of rural health. The coalition and caucus serve that purpose. However, rural advocates were somewhat weakened in the 103rd Congress by not having among their champions any of the key committee chairmen. Other members of those committees, though were rural advocates; in the House, Payne (R-NJ) on Ways and Means and Cooper (D-TN) on Energy and Commerce, and in the Senate, Kerrey (D-NE) and Rockefeller (D-WV) on Finance and Harkin (D-IA) on Labor and Human Resources. In addition, prominent members of Congress highlighted rural concerns with special hearings and press conferences during the debates. Those members included Senators Daschle (D-SD), Chafee (R-RI), and Mitchell (D-ME); and Representatives Stenholm (D-TX) and Roberts (R-KS). The Committees on Agriculture of the two chambers were used as forums to emphasize rural concerns.

Of course the entire reform debate ended without resolution in 1994. So did rural interests invest too much time in a lost cause? If so, they were certainly in a large group of similarly situated interests. However, their energies were not misspent. In addition to the important lessons learned about how to succeed by really trying in the federal legislative process, rural advocates were able to focus attention on critical needs in rural health. Two in particular would reemerge quickly in the 104th Congress. First, the need to bolster the primary care workforce in rural areas became evident and is even more important as market forces are shifting to managed care plans. Second, rural health care systems need assistance if they are to restructure into effective networks that can support integrated health care plans for rural residents. During the end stages of the 1994 debates, legislation emerged from the Rural Health Coalition in the House of Representatives to provide assistance for network development in rural areas, and special grant programs were established in the AHCPR and HCFA for that purpose. Legislative proposals were discussed in both chambers that would use federal resources to influence programs that train health professionals to train more primary care professionals.

THE PRESENT AND FUTURE POLICY ISSUES IN RURAL HEALTH

The current issues in health policy are the same that were fought for during the reform debates—strengthening and retaining an effective delivery system in rural areas. These general concerns can be addressed with a collection of specific policies targeted to particular elements of the delivery system and designed to serve specific rural populations.

Filling the Gaps in the Delivery System

Attention remains focused on the two types of providers seen as fundamental building blocks in rural health systems—hospitals and primary care providers. Policies affecting hospitals were focused on Medicare reimbursement issues during the 1980s, and have evolved into policies designed to assist hospitals wanting to reconfigure the services they offer. State governments have been examining hospital licensure and Medicaid reimbursement policies with an eye toward sustaining services in rural areas (Mueller, 1992).

The federal government, under the Medicare PPS, created special categories of hospitals eligible for higher reimbursement than they would otherwise have received (sole community hospitals and rural referral centers). In the past five years, federal policymakers have focused on Medicare's conditions of participation, creating more flexibility for hospitals in eight rural states to change their capacity for providing a full array of acute care services. Two special programs were initiated: the Medical Assistance Facility (MAF) project in Montana and the Essential Access Care Facility/Rural Primary Care Facility (EACH/RPCH) program in seven

states. The former created a new category of facility, eligible for reimbursement by Medicare, which provides short-term, acute services in frontier counties, but need not have a physician on site or be fully staffed on site at all times. The EACH/RPCH program provided federal grants to hospital networks in which a large rural institution (EACH) is the hub, accepting referrals from small rural hospitals (RPCHs) that are equipped and staffed to provide short (less than seventy-two hours) acute care stays and emergency services. Both programs were designed to help rural communities retain the appropriate level of care in facilities that are no longer full-service acute care hospitals. This approach is not one of lowering the quality of care being offered in those communities. Rather it is one of correctly aligning the facility with the care being offered, removing imposition of unnecessary expenses.

Further policy developments can be expected that affect rural health care facilities. Both of the above federal programs were special demonstration projects; the basic conditions of participation in Medicare were waived, not changed. Therefore, one policy question before Congress is whether to make those changes permanent. Another issue is developing rules for reimbursing ambulatory care facilities in rural areas where clinics might replace hospitals.

Efforts to recruit and retain primary care providers (both physicians and nonphysician providers) in rural areas can be described for both state and federal policies. Both levels of government place emphasis on training the appropriate (usually primary care) professionals rural areas can then recruit. At the state level, policies can direct state-supported medical schools to graduate students interested in primary care. Minimum requirements to do so have been placed on medical schools in Washington, North Carolina, and Minnesota. State governments encourage students to choose rural communities for their initial professional practice sites by offering loan repayment plans. States provide assistance to communities trying to recruit primary care providers. The gamut of state policies related to recruiting and retaining primary care providers is evident in the policies introduced as part of health reform legislation in the states. Legislation was introduced in eleven states offering assistance to students choosing education in primary care, ten to assist in recruiting graduates to practice in rural communities, and eight to provide technical assistance to communities (Mueller & Dodson, 1993).

The federal government also encourages growth in primary care training programs, through special grant programs funded by the Health Resources and Services Administration (HRSA). Under authority provided in Titles VII and VIII of the Public Health Services Act, HRSA funds programs that train family medicine physicians, physician assistants, nurse practitioners, and nurse midwives. Interdisciplinary training programs are also eligible for assistance. From a rural perspective, though, these programs are too small in magnitude to counterbalance powerful federal incentives to train specialists. Specifically, Medicare reimbursement policies include special payments for graduate medical education (GME) that yield much higher revenues for specialty residencies than for primary care. In addition, the research support available for programs that feature advances in knowledge related to subspecialties offer far greater reward than grants for undergraduate medical training in primary care (Rosenblatt et al., 1993).

Just as provisions in state reform proposals would increase the emphasis on primary care training, a similar change in federal programs was suggested in reform legislation debated during the 103rd Congress. The most typical change was the proposal to require that at least 50 percent of GME support be to residencies in primary care (defined to include family medicine, general internal medicine, general pediatrics, and obstetrics/gynecology), and restrict the number of residencies to 110 percent of U.S. graduates (the current number is approximately 130%). Even more specific to rural interests, some legislation included bonus payments for residencies in ambulatory settings, which would more closely approximate the rural experience. Some reform proposals also increased Title VII and Title VIII (of the Social Security Act) funding, especially for programs that trained nonphysician primary care providers such as physician assistants, nurse practitioners, and nurse midwives. The changes in GME support and increases in Titles VII and VIII would increase the number of graduates in primary care, from whom rural

areas could recruit. The issue of funding medical education, however, remains a policy concern in Congress with changes in Medicare reimbursement advocated by Senator Kassebaum (R-KS), chair of the Labor and Human Resources Committee in the 104th Congress.

On the other hand, there is some evidence that the problems of training a disproportionate number of specialists may be self-correcting. During the 1992–95 period, there appeared to be an increasing tendency on the part of medical school graduates to choose residencies in primary care (Kahn et al., 1993). Until those students have completed their residencies and begun their practices, however, the effects on alleviating rural shortages cannot be determined.

Programs to fill other gaps in the rural health care delivery system are not as mature as those for hospitals and physicians. During the debates surrounding health reform, and since then, the need for other services has become more apparent. As policy discussions moved toward development of integrated delivery systems and comparisons of needs to existing supply were made, shortages became more obvious. Therefore we can expect attention to needs in mental health, geriatric health, allied health (therapists and others), and community services.

The Rural Transition for the Year 2000

The most important area of activity in rural health is the development of health care delivery networks, some based in rural areas and others based in urban areas but spreading to rural communities. Delivery networks can be the basis for developing and marketing managed care plans to rural residents. As of 1992, there were eleven states in which less than 5 percent of the population was enrolled in health maintenance organizations, and twelve in which enrollment was between 5 percent and 10 percent of the population. All of these are rural states, with Virginia the only one with over 70 percent of the population in metropolitan areas (Fuchs, 1994).

Network development has begun in some states, especially Florida, Minnesota, and Iowa. However, even in those states issues remain unresolved. The policy issues are important arenas for both federal and state activities. The issues can be thought of as structural, administrative, and financial. A major structural issue involves both federal and state anti-trust concerns. Can rural hospitals and physicians enter into formal agreements when doing so might mean a large percentage of the business in their community is "captured" by network plans? This is an issue that will not be resolved until there is sufficient case law to interpret legislative and administrative directives. A second structural issue has to do with network certification. Especially as networks develop health insurance plans, they will need to be certified by appropriate state government agencies. Networks may make decisions to reconfigure existing institutions as part of moving to a more effective delivery mode. As that occurs, states with certificate-of-need laws will need to think through the process of approving applications for approval under those laws.

Administrative issues facing networks include exploration of various schemes of sharing resources and governing authority. New entities may be needed, and as such will require approval from relevant public authorities. Public policies will also be important in providing technical assistance to rural providers and communities who are struggling with the administrative decisions they must make.

Financial issues will involve both generating start-up capital and receiving sufficient reimbursement. Start-up capital could be provided to rural networks under state or federal grant and loan programs. Insurance laws could be modified to permit lower requirements for capital reserves for rural networks, especially when providers share risk (e.g., agree to continue seeing patients if the plan fails). Technical assistance to rural networks could help them determine means of contracting with third parties for capital requirements. Once networks are operational and involved in selling health plans, a consistent flow of operating funds will of course be important. Therefore, the ongoing discussions of changes in Medicare and Medicaid reimbursement, especially changes to managed care and capitated payment, are important to rural networks. One novel approach might be to reimburse networks directly rather than only the providers in those networks.

A more complete discussion of the policy issues concerning rural networks can be found in publications of the University of Minnesota Rural Health Research Center (Casey et al., 1995). As networks are developed and begin to have operational experience, they will need to be evaluated. They can be assessed for their effects on efficiency, distribution of costs and benefits, and interorganizational activities (Moscovice et al., 1995).

Conclusion

This chapter has described current needs and policies related to the delivery and finance of health care in rural areas. An argument is made that needs of rural residents are different from those of their urban counterparts, based on the following variables: density of population, occupation, availability of health care services, and population demographics. While rural interests have always been present in national and state politics, their entry into the issue networks of health policy is more recent. The advent of Medicare's prospective payment system was a watershed event, marking an obvious need to strengthen representation of rural interests. Consistent with the political and policy environments of the 1980s and 1990s, rural interests have strengthened their analytical capacities and have established working relationships with policy entrepreneurs in the federal government (less so in state governments).

Responding to Rural Needs

Policies have been enacted in recent years that enhance access to medical services among rural residents. The Medicare hospital payment system has within it special categories that allow for higher payment to certain types of rural hospitals—sole community hospitals and rural referral centers. Furthermore, the difference between urban and rural base payments has been eliminated. The federal government is experimenting with new classifications of hospitals, and many states have enacted legislation enabling reconfiguration of small rural hospitals. These policies may help stabilize health care delivery systems. However, progress could be threatened with a new round of Medicare budget savings that includes lower levels of hospital reimbursement.

The need for health professionals to serve in rural shortage areas continues. This may be resolved in part through changes in the medical care marketplace that are inspiring more medical school graduates to choose careers in primary care. But moving those graduates into rural underserved areas at best would take years until residency training is completed and at worst even longer as urban-based health plans hire more primary care physicians. For at least the next few years, then, public policies that create incentives to practice in underserved areas remain important to rural health interests. Even more could be done, such as reforming the Medicare system of paying for graduate medical education and creating more state-based programs of assistance to health professionals locating in underserved areas.

The primary goal of public policy should be creating a sustainable system of health care services that improves the health of rural residents. Systems development is an important general purpose of policies, best exemplified by efforts to build rural health networks. Multiple policy issues need to be resolved before locally based networks will reach their full potential. An important role for both the federal government and the states will be to provide technical assistance to rural providers and community leaders who want to build their own networks rather than waiting for urban-based networks to absorb them.

Ultimately, any policy change should be designed to improve the health of residents. Specific health conditions that are more prevalent in rural than urban areas should be addressed. Special populations of rural residents, including the elderly, poor, minorities, and children should be targeted by specific policy interventions. For example, the health care problems of migrant farm workers present special challenges to public policy that have not yet been met by the creation of migrant health centers. As techniques for measuring quality of care and health status improve, changes in finance and delivery should be assessed vis-à-vis their impacts on those measures.

Successful Rural Health Policy: Can It Be Sustained?

Rural advocates have succeeded in placing their interests on the policy agenda in recent years, and have achieved at least modest success in policy enactments. But can this work be sustained, even enhanced? The simple answer is yes. The mere presence of the Rural Health Coalition in the U.S. House of Representatives and the Rural Health Caucus in the Senate assures continued attention to rural health issues. The successes of those two groups in the past twelve years, achieved with bipartisan support, are proof positive. Unless it falls prey to budget reductions the Federal Office of Rural Health Policy continues to monitor administrative decisions related to rural health. The growth in state offices of rural health (from a handful in 1990 to fifty in 1994 and in state rural health associations from a few to nineteen in 1994) will mean at least some increased attention to rural health issues in state governments.

The most important reason for optimism about the future of rural health, though, is that past policy successes have resulted in better placement of rural interests in the policy process. The ever-increasing analytical capacity of rural health advocates is attributable to the policies of the mid-1980s, which supported (and continue to support) rural health research centers, rural health researchers, and demonstration programs related to rural health systems. The quantity and quality of analytical activities that can contribute to policy debates has expanded geometrically since 1983. The issue network in health policy has expanded to include participants in rural health policy research and analysis.

Of course analysis still needs advocates. Rural interests have found policy entrepreneurs in Congress, through the Coalition and Caucus, to propose and pursue legislative initiatives. They have done so using the same legislative vehicles as others in the 1980s and 1990s—omnibus legislation that can be amended to include modest advances for rural health. Those advances have been quite modest in the context of a trillion-dollar federal budget.

The successes of rural health policy, however, are in jeopardy despite the growing strength of advocates. If politics becomes completely defined by ideology based on reducing government presence in any and all markets, rural programs are threatened. With the exception of community and migrant health clinics, the federal government is not involved directly in providing services to rural residents. Programs that assist others in providing services are more difficult to defend when deep budget cuts are made. Rural advocates have to rely on arguments of self-determination for rural providers and communities, and equity in terms of availability of services. These are powerful ideological arguments, often appealing to the same ideology that wants to reduce government spending. Those who champion rural interests in Congress and state legislatures can use these arguments as the basis for withholding their votes from other initiatives until basic rural demands are met.

REFERENCES

Bindman, Andrew B., Dennis Keane, & Nicole Lurie. (1990). A public hospital closes: Impact on patients' access to care and health status. *Journal of the American Medical Association, 264* (December 12), 2899–2904.

Buckwalter, Kathyrne C. (1992). *Mental and social health of the rural elderly.* Paper delivered at "Health and Aging in Rural America: A National Symposium," San Diego, September 13–15.

Campion, Daniel M., W. David Helms, & Nancy L. Barrand. (1993). Perspective: Health reform in rural areas. *Health Affairs, 12* (Fall), 76–80.

Casey, Michelle, Anthony Wellever, & Ira Moscovice. (1995). *Public policy issues and rural health network development* (Working Paper No. 8). Rural Health Research Center, University of Minnesota: Institute for Health Services Research.

Christianson, Jon, & Ira Moscovice. (1993). Health care reform and rural health networks. *Health Affairs, 12* (Fall), 58–75.

Christianson, Jon B., Ira S. Moscovice, Judy Johnson, John Kralewski, & Colleen Grogan. (1990). Evaluating rural hospital consortia. *Health Affairs, 9* (Spring), 135–161.

Coburn, Andrew F., Sam Cordes, Robert Crittendon, J. Patrick Hart, Keith Mueller, Wayne Myers, & Tom Ricketts. (1994). *The rural perspective on national health reform legislation.* Briefing reference document prepared for the congressional Rural Caucus and the House Rural Health Care Coalition (March 31). University of Missouri: Rural Policy Research Institute.

Coburn, Andrew F., & Keith J. Mueller. (1995). Legislative and policy strategies for supporting rural health network development: Lessons from the 103rd Congress. *Journal of Rural Health, 11* (Winter), 22–31.

Comer, John, & Keith Mueller. (1995). Access to health care: Urban–rural comparisons from a Midwest agricultural state. *Journal of Rural Health, 11* (Spring), 28–136.

Cornelius, L., K. Beauregard, & J. Cohen. (1991). Usual sources of medical care and their characteristics (AHCPR Pub. No. 91-0042). *National Medical Expenditure Survey Research Findings, 11.* Rockville, MD: Agency for Health Care Policy and Research.

Coward, Raymond T., D. K. McLaughlin, R. Paul Duncan, & C. Niel Bull. (1992). *An overview of health and aging in rural America.* Paper presented at "Health and Aging in Rural America: A National Symposium," San Diego, September 13–15.

Denton, Denise. (1993). Predicting the future of health care reform. *Rural Health Care, 15* (4), 3.

Duncan, R. Paul, Brian R. Klepper, Caren J. Krumerman, & Sandra L. Kuhn. (1995). Rural health networks in Florida. *Journal of Rural Health, 11* (Winter), 40–52.

Employee Benefits Research Institute. (1994). *Sources of health insurance and characteristics of the uninsured: Analysis of the March 1993 Current Population Survey* (EBRI Issue Brief No. 145). Washington, D.C.: Employee Benefits Research Institute.

Farley, Pamela J. (1985). Who are the underinsured? *Milbank Memorial Quarterly: Health and Society, 63* (Summer), 476–503.

Feldstein, Paul J. (1977) *Health associations and the demand for legislation: The political economy of health.* Cambridge, MA: Ballinger Publishing Co.

Ferris, Daron G., & Mark Litaker. (1993). Chlamydial cervical infections in rural and urban pregnant women. *Southern Medical Journal, 86* (June), 611–614.

Freeman, Howard E., Linda H. Aiken, Robert J. Blendon, & Christopher R. Corey. (1990). Uninsured working age adults: Characteristics and consequences. *Health Services Research, 24* (February), 811–823.

Fuchs, Beth C. (1994). Health care reform: Managed competition in rural areas. *CRS Report for Congress* (April 4). Washington, D.C.: Congressional Research Service, The Library of Congress.

Hafner-Eaton, Chris. (1993). Physician utilization disparities between the uninsured and insured: Comparisons of the chronically ill, acutely ill, and well nonelderly populations. *Journal of the American Medical Association, 269* (February 10), 787–792.

Heclo, Hugh. (1978). Issue networks and the executive establishment. In A. King (Ed.), *The new American political system* (pp. 87–124). Washington, D.C.: American Enterprise Institute.

Kahn, Norman B., Robert Graham, & Gordon Schmittling. (1993). Entry of U.S. medical school graduates into family practice residencies: 1992–1993 and three-year summary. *Family Medicine, 25,* 502–510.

Levey, Linda M., James P. Curry, & Samuel Levey. (1988). Rural–urban differences in access to Iowa City health services. *Journal of Rural Health, 4* (July), 59–72.

Liff, Jonathan M., Wong-Ho Chow, & Raymond S. Greenberg. (1991). Rural–urban differences in stage at diagnosis: Possible relationship to cancer screening. *Cancer, 67* (March 1), 1454–1459.

Lowi, Theodore. (1990). Distribution, regulation, redistribution: The functions of government. In Pietros Nivola & David Rosenbloom (Eds.), *Classic readings in American politics.* New York: St. Martin's.

McManus, Margaret A., & Paul W. Newacheck. (1989). Rural maternal, child, and adolescent health. *Health Services Research, 23* (February), 807–848.

Mick, Steven S., & Laura L. Morlock. (1990). America's rural hospitals: A selective review of the 1980s research. *Journal of Rural Health, 6* (Winter), 437–466.

Moscovice, Ira, Jon B. Christianson, & Anthony Wellever. (1995). Measuring and evaluating the performance of vertically integrated rural health networks. *Journal of Rural Health, 11* (Winter), 9–21.

Mueller, Keith J. (1992). State government policies and rural hospitals: Facilitating change. *Policy Studies Journal, 20* (1), 168–182.

Mueller, Keith J. (1993). *Health care policy in the United States.* Lincoln: University of Nebraska Press.

Mueller, Keith J. (1994). The Health Security Act. *National health reform legislation: Implications for rural health* (Brief No. 15), January. Omaha: Nebraska Center for Rural Health Research, University of Nebraska Medical Center.

Mueller, Keith J. (1995). National rural health association. In C. Ramsey (Ed.), *U.S. health policy groups: Institutional profiles* (pp. 359–362). Westport, CT: Greenwood Press.

Mueller, Keith J., & A. Dodson. (1993). *Health care reform: Effects on health professions.* Paper delivered at "Implementing Health Care Reform in Rural America: State and Community Roles," Des Moines, IA, December 2–5.

Mullner, R., & D. G. Whiteis. (1988). Closing rural hospitals: Issues and policy options. *Policy Forum.* 1(2).

National Center for Health Statistics. (1991). *Vital and health statistics: Current estimates from the National Health Interview Survey, 1990* (Series 10, No. 181). Hyattsville, MD: U.S. Department of Health and Human Services.

National Rural Health Association. (1992). *National health policy reform: The rural perspective.* Kansas City: National Rural Health Association.

Nesbitt, Thomas S., Roger A. Rosenblatt, F. A. Connell, & L. Gary Hart. (1989). Access to obstetric care in rural areas: Effect on birth outcomes. *Rural Health Working Paper Series* (Vol. 1, No. 4). WAMI Rural Health Research Center, University of Washington, Seattle, WA.

Newacheck, Paul W. (1989). Improving access to health services for adolescents from economically disadvantaged families. *Pediatrics, 84* (December), 1056–1063.

Peterson, Mark A. (1993). Political influence in the 1990s: From iron triangles to policy networks. *Journal of Health Politics, Policy and Law, 18* (Summer), 395–438.

Porterfield, S., & J. Scott. (1993). Health insurance in rural America. *Policy Research Summary.* Columbia, MO: Rural Policy Research Institute, University of Missouri.

Rosenblatt, Roger A., Michael E. Witcomb, Thomas J. Cullen, Denise M. Lishner, & L. Gary Hart. (1993). The effect of federal grants on medical schools' production of primary care physicians. *American Journal of Public Health, 83* (March), 322–328.

Slesinger, Doris. (1992). Health status and needs of migrant farm workers in the United States: A literature review. *Journal of Rural Health, 8* (March), 227–234.

Summer, L. (1991). *Limited access: Health care for rural poor.* Washington, D.C.: Center on Budget and Policy Priorities.

U.S. Office of Technology Assessment. (1990). *Health care in rural America.* Washington, D.C.: U.S. Government Printing Office.

Ways and Means, Committee on, Subcommittee on Health. (1995). Medicare managed care. Hearings. Washington, D.C.: U.S. Government Printing Office.

Weiner, J. P. (1993). The demand for physician services in a changing health care system: A synthesis. *Medical Care Review, 50* (Winter), 411–450.

CHAPTER

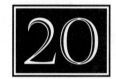

The Politics of AIDS

Leonard Robins and Charles Backstrom

The discovery of an unusual pattern of diseases among gays was reported in June 1981 (*CDC MMWR*, 1981). Initially called Gay-Related Immune Deficiency (GRID), it soon became clear that the problem was not limited to gays and the name was changed to Acquired Immunodeficiency Syndrome (AIDS).[1] Today, as nearly every reader of this chapter knows, AIDS is caused by the Human Immunodeficiency Virus (HIV), which is primarily transmitted by (1) intercourse (with anal intercourse being much more dangerous than vaginal intercourse, and transfer from men to women being easier than women to men); (2) shar-

ing contaminated needles between IV-drug users; (3) introducing contaminated blood by blood transfusions or spattering; and (4) transfer of the virus from pregnant mothers to their babies via the placenta, during labor, or through breastfeeding. HIV is not spread by casual contact, and condoms offer good, though not total, protection, as does bleaching needles. Testing the blood supply starting in 1985 in the United States has essentially eliminated the threat from blood transfusions.

In the United States, over 75 percent of new AIDS cases occur in two population groups: gays and IV-drug users. However, AIDS is growing fastest among women. In the underdeveloped world, AIDS is an overwhelmingly heterosexual disease almost equally prevalent among women and men.

AIDS is now one of the most widely known and feared diseases in the United States. Nearly half a million people have been diagnosed with AIDS through 1994, 60 percent of whom are now dead (*CDC*

We wish to thank Richard Danilla for helpful comments.

[1]In this chapter we refer to the virus as HIV, and reserve the term AIDS for the complex of diseases that appear because of the breakdown of the immune system. We also follow the Centers for Disease Control and Prevention (CDC) in no longer making a distinction between AIDS and the onset of symptoms not reaching the threshold of AIDS, which was once termed AIDS-Related Complex (ARC).

MMWR, 1995a). An additional six hundred thousand to eight hundred thousand people carry the HIV virus (*CDC MMWR*, 1992), with many not even knowing they are HIV-positive. Because of these numbers, even discovery of a vaccine, more effective drugs, or great reduction in all the various types of behaviors that spread the disease would eliminate AIDS as a major health problem until at best the end of the first decade of the twenty-first century.

An intense debate has developed over what is the appropriate public policy response to this epidemic. Because AIDS is nearly always terminal,[2] is a gruesome disease, its carriers can transmit the disease without themselves showing symptoms, and it primarily affects socially disdained groups of people, the disease is a special blend of sex, drugs, and death suffused with value dimensions that make health policy formation regarding it intensely political.

In an earlier article (Backstrom & Robins, 1989), we developed a conceptual framework for analyzing the political aspects of policy issues. The framework initially examines the goals of public policy. In the context of communicable diseases, there are five goals: research on how to prevent and treat the disease, comprehending the extent of the disease, finding those who have been exposed to the disease, preventing the disease's spread, and caring for persons with the disease.

The next step is to determine the public policy decisions required to meet the policy goals. We then ascertain the political problems involved in making effective policy decisions. Finally, recommended political strategies to overcome the political problems are considered.

This conceptual framework is here applied to AIDS (see Table 20-1).[3] Each policy goal is taken up in turn, beginning with the thrust of early writings on the subject. Next, current realities are contrasted with the early "conventional wisdom." Then present policy issues are examined, with special attention given to the political

---

[2]We are not here concerned whether the AIDS virus inevitably leads to AIDS and whether AIDS inevitably leads to death, because the very high percentages of both of those occurrences dictate the same public policy responses.

[3]An earlier version of this chart appeared in Backstrom & Robins, 1989.

dimensions of policy controversies. After completing this analysis, we present original research findings derived from our study of how the states make AIDS policy (Backstrom & Robins, 1992; Robins & Backstrom, 1993, 1994; Backstrom & Robins, 1995–96). As several of the chapters in this book indicate, the role of the states in health care is growing. In regard to AIDS policy, the states are more important policy players than is generally recognized.

Finally, the chapter concludes by indicating how the overall American polity, society, and health care system have affected AIDS policy, and, conversely, how experience with AIDS has affected the American polity, society, and health care system.

One final preliminary point. Public policy choices concerning AIDS should not be based primarily on abstract values. Rather, effective decision making will have to recognize that medical science and technologies concerning AIDS are rapidly evolving, and the resulting changes require adjustments in policy response.

RESEARCH TOWARD BIOMEDICAL PREVENTION AND TREATMENT

After an initially slow start that drew much deserved criticism from AIDS activists, funding for AIDS research grew dramatically, boosting the National Institute of Allergies and Infectious Diseases from a small division into one of the largest within the National Institutes of Health (NIH). Perhaps even more important, AIDS receives more research funding relative to the numbers of people it affects than other diseases.

This increase should not, in retrospect, have been surprising. Research funding is politically the easiest element of AIDS policy to achieve, for two reasons. First, the American public overestimates the ability to solve social and medical problems quickly by research leading to a technological "fix." Second, funding biomedical research to relieve human suffering is the form of action on which political consensus can be most easily reached. But even consensus behind support for funding was questioned in mid-1995, when Senator Jesse Helms (R-NC) argued that AIDS should receive less

TABLE 20-1 Current Political Issues of AIDS Policy

Goals of AIDS Policy	Policy Decisions Required	Political Problems of Decisions	Recommended Political Strategies
1. Research on prevention and treatment	a. Setting priorities for various types of research in overall program to counter AIDS	a. Pressure to focus on applied rather than basic research	a. Emphasize need for basic research to successfully develop vaccine and drugs
	b. Balance need for scientific proof with early release for clinical trials	b. Cannot deny persons facing death the chance to try drugs	b. Demonstrate that drugs must have real potential to be worth clinical trials
2. Comprehending the extent of AIDS	Determining probable trends in spread of AIDS	A needed focus on high-risk groups may lower general concern	Depict a general problem for all, but emphasize a great threat to some
3. Finding those who have been exposed	a. Deciding whom to test	a. Pressure to test widely can lead to overtesting	a. Rigorous targeting based on efficiency
	b. Voluntary or compulsory testing	b. Problems of classifying the problem as public health versus individual rights	b. Argue counterproductivity of compulsion in most circumstances
	c. Getting high-risk people located and tested	c. Fear of social and economic discrimination	c. Classify AIDS as a disability that cannot be discriminated against
	d. Home testing	d. Home testing means less counseling for HIV-positives	d. Accept trade-off of less counseling for more testing
4. Prevention of spread	a. Establishing the degree of personal restriction	a. Superficial attractiveness of quarantine	a. Stress individual responsibility as the norm, but use sanctions where necessary
	b. Getting high-risk people to define their behavior as risky and change it	b. Opposition to explicit messages targeting high-risk groups	b. Use nongovernment groups to design and communicate risks to identified target groups
	c. Providing the appropriate type of education	c. Objection to thorough sex education by certain ideologies	c. Emphasize AIDS as a health rather than moralistic question
	d. Assuring use of clean needles	d. Seeming to abet illegal behavior by providing clean needles	d. Argue clean needles help in AIDS reduction and in getting addicts into rehabilitation
5. Care of persons with AIDS	a. Limiting denial of insurance	a. Resistance by private insurers to absorbing costs of AIDS	a. Reform of private insurance
	b. Obtaining accessible, cost-effective, and quality care	b. Bias toward high-tech health care	b. Advocate San Francisco model

funds because those affected engage in "disgusting behavior" (*Congressional Record*, 1995).

Two current challenges threaten further increases in funding for research on AIDS. The first comes from those who feel that the explosion in funding for research on AIDS has resulted in an unfair deemphasis of research on diseases they find more serious. This "war of the diseases" may truly be a case of fighting the wrong enemy, because much biomedical research is basic in nature and has general applicability to many diseases. The knowledge gained from the study of the immune system—a key element in AIDS research—is, for example, likely to have real benefits for the treatment and possible cure of many other diseases.

The second challenge to funding for AIDS research comes from those who in principle strongly want to cut overall federal government spending. But rather than significantly retrenching AIDS research spending, this effort is likely to put a cap on it. In any event curbing spending growth would have been inevitable in the next few years; massive budget expansions for even the most worthwhile endeavor cannot continue indefinitely.

Research priorities—whether to emphasize basic or applied research—are another issue. Advocates of assigning highest priority to basic research argue that only through more long-term study of the immune system will we be able to develop an effective vaccine and drugs that will have a corrective impact. In contrast, those who advocate a high priority for applied research stress the immediate requirement of people living with AIDS for relief and the urgent need to rapidly try many types of vaccines to protect a new generation from getting AIDS.

The Food and Drug Administration Drug Approval Process

A related pressing biomedical research policy issue is the time it takes the Food and Drug Administration (FDA) to approve drugs for treating the symptomatic diseases of AIDS. One of the main early complaints of AIDS activists was that the FDA had been a "bottleneck" in getting effective drugs from the laboratory to the patient.

In recent years, however, the political pressures brought by persons living with AIDS (PLWAs) and their supporters have caused the FDA to drastically shorten and simplify the process required to gain approval for new AIDS drugs. A major change in FDA procedures was to allow putting drugs that have not yet been proven in the traditional way out for clinical trials in community-based projects. This allows people who are affected by the disease to volunteer for testing drugs without participating in the time-consuming, large-scale blind tests carried out in research settings—the so-called parallel track (Melnick et al., 1994).

It must be further pointed out that opposition to FDA overcaution is not unique to AIDS. Indeed it really is not the product of bureaucratic inertia, but rather results from prior congressional action—the Kefauver–Harris 1962 amendments to the Pure Food and Drug Act, which were triggered by the thalidomide scare and the resulting feeling that extraordinary care should be taken before new drugs are approved (Harris, 1964). Experts have long contended that negative health consequences due to excessive delays in introducing new drugs exceed the health benefits of delaying their introduction to safeguard against unanticipated negative side effects, or from using drugs that turn out to be ineffective (Fuchs, 1974).

Some AIDS activists who have developed expertise in the drug approval process have begun to believe that FDA standards have in certain circumstances become so lax that they result in useless and thus counterproductive science. As a result, proposed AIDS vaccines have been rejected for trial due to a widespread feeling that they would almost certainly be failures (Green, 1995). What this experience with FDA drug approval policy shows is the difficulty of reconciling the understandable simultaneous desires for both speedy success and sound science. Keeping an appropriate balance, however, is not and will not be easy.

Our view is that in the long run, science will likely be generally successful in preventing and treating AIDS. But HIV has become sufficiently seeded in the population that it is highly unlikely that vaccines and drugs will ever completely eliminate AIDS. Moreover, experience with other communicable diseases has shown that declining cases reduce fear, resulting in less than 100 percent usage of vaccines. In addition, drug-resistant strains appear. A truly "magic bullet" for AIDS is unlikely (Brandt, 1988).

COMPREHENDING THE EXTENT OF AIDS

Nearly every study of the initial indifference to AIDS emphasized the long delay in getting the Reagan administration to recognize its seriousness and significance. This indifference is usually attributed to hostility to those initially seen at risk—gays (Shilts, 1987).

While there is still considerable dispute about the scope and magnitude of the epidemic, all public policymakers now consider AIDS a very serious health issue demanding massive government endeavors.

The major concerns today regarding the incidence of AIDS are whether the explosive rise of infections among IV-drug users and their sexual partners can be reduced, whether a new generation of gay men will make the behavioral changes necessary to reduce the risk of exposure, and the chances that AIDS will become widely distributed among the rest of the population.

From 1986, when 65 percent of all new AIDS cases were among gay men (not including those who are also IV-drug users), the proportion so classified fell to 53 percent in 1994. During this same time period, the percentage of IV-drug users rose from 24 percent to 32 percent (counting gay IV-drug users). Thus the epidemic certainly has not peaked among drug users. Although there was a decline in the rate of increase of AIDS cases among gay men, only among white gay men did the number of new cases actually decrease. The rate of increase was dramatically higher among younger gay men (*CDC MMWR*, 1995c).

The segment of the population among which AIDS is rising fastest is women, who constituted 7 percent of new cases in 1985 but were 18 percent of new AIDS diagnoses in 1994. While about half of these were themselves IV-drug users, heterosexual infections of nonusing women accounted for 38 percent (*CDC MMWR*, 1995b).

The issue of paramount political importance in the spread of AIDS in the United States is whether there will be a major incursion of AIDS among the non-gay, non-IV-drug-user-related general population. Public health officials need to be very careful about the impressions they give as they try to lead the discussion on this issue. They must steer a careful course between downplaying the threat of AIDS and overdramatizing it. Relying on present statistics only could fail to warn the very sexually active population of the small but real chances of acquiring the disease through promiscuous sex. Yet overplaying this risk could incite unjustified panic or produce assertions of crying wolf from an increasingly cynical public.

To arouse sympathy and support for AIDS programs, many AIDS activists sloganeer that AIDS is equally everyone's concern. Yet, as Fumento (1990) has argued, this is not true because of the vastly lower risk outside the primary AIDS-carrying groups. Fumento pushes his argument too far, however, when he asserts that campaigns aimed at the general public might well have produced a belief among gays and IV-drug users that their risk of getting AIDS is no more than that of the general population.

The current consensus is that Fumento is technically right in that AIDS in the next few years is likely to be still largely confined to gays, bisexuals, IV-drug users, and the sexual partners of bisexuals and IV-drug users—that is, that AIDS will not become widely distributed among the rest of the population. It should, however, be equally emphasized that middle-class heterosexuals who ignore the possibility of AIDS could be making a fatal error.

Another marked trend in the spread of AIDS is its relative increase among people of color. Minorities constituted 58 percent of all new cases of the disease in 1994. African Americans, who comprise 12 percent of the total population, made up 39 percent of the AIDS cases. Hispanics, who constitute 10 percent of the population, account for 19 percent of new AIDS cases (*CDC MMWR*, 1995a).

The special growth of AIDS among African Americans is contributing to, but, it must be emphasized, is only one cause of the worsening status of African

American health in the United States (Rice & Winn, 1991). Clearly, the problem of AIDS in minority communities will not be solved in isolation from solutions to their overall health and socioeconomic problems.

FINDING THOSE WHO HAVE BEEN EXPOSED

It might seem obvious that the attempt to control AIDS should be based on public health methods traditionally used for other infectious diseases: surveillance of the disease's spread, testing those who are at high risk of contracting the disease, requiring reporting to public health officials the names of people with the disease, and tracing and treating their contacts. But AIDS differs from other infectious diseases in several notable respects. First, symptoms are long delayed, requiring getting people to test who don't feel or look sick. Second, those primarily at risk of acquiring the disease are engaging in behavior that is either illegal or morally frowned upon by large majorities of the public. Third, those having AIDS or even the HIV virus often report being subject to discrimination resulting in loss of jobs and housing. Finally, whereas diseases such as gonorrhea can be cured with penicillin, there is no cure for AIDS, though certain medications can slow the spread of the virus and opportunistic diseases. The one important exception to this is that if an infected mother during pregnancy takes AZT, the chances of her baby being born with HIV decreases from approximately 25 percent to 8 percent (*CDC MMWR*, 1994).

Testing

Gay activists, given their understandable fears of harassment by government agents and discrimination in civil society, were initially suspicious of all HIV testing programs. They have since become supportive of voluntary and anonymous testing, but typically oppose mandatory testing, mandatory reporting to public health authorities of those who test positive for the HIV virus, and programs of government contact tracing—partner notification (Bayer, 1989). While initially the impetus for this change was the growing realization of the serious threat that AIDS posed to gays, now the primary reason for support is the aforementioned development of drugs to delay the breakdown of the immune system and onset of some of the typically fatal opportunistic diseases associated with AIDS. Before these drugs there was no positive medical benefit to offer to induce individuals to determine their HIV status given the possible negative social consequences for doing so.

Nevertheless, gay leaders continue to insist strongly that unless testing is voluntary and anonymous, testing programs are doomed to failure, because at-risk populations will not cooperate but instead will go underground.

Analytically the debate over testing is usually framed in terms of *widespread, mandatory* testing. These two points, while related, are not interchangeable. One has to do with compulsion, the other with scope.

The political dimension of this question is that as long as the issue of massive mandatory testing is conceptualized as one of public health versus the right to privacy, the movement for massive mandatory testing will remain potent. If the issue is posed this way, AIDS is the classic kind of public health issue for which many politicians and the public are willing to override civil liberties. On the other hand, emphasizing the impracticality of mass testing can successfully derail it.

One can oppose mandatory testing of many very large groups solely on the basis of cost-effectiveness. Ultimately this was successfully done in Illinois and Louisiana, where laws requiring HIV tests before issuance of marriage licenses were repealed. In Illinois the incentive to overturn the law came from the demonstration that it cost over $200,000 for each case of the virus found. Additionally, requiring testing before marriage deprived counties bordering on Indiana and Wisconsin of approximately 20 percent of their expected marriage license fees as Illinois people saved money and hassle by marrying outside the state (Pierson and Egler, 1989).

Mandatory testing is also unwise for the two main groups at highest risk for AIDS—gays and IV-drug users. While it would certainly be desirable if members of these groups were tested, making testing compulsory could prove highly unproductive. Since members of these groups already have strong incentives to be "invisible," attempting to force them to test (no one has offered a practical proposal on how this could be done anyway) would only hurt the battle against AIDS by driving them away from the health care system.

The most controversial current issue involving widespread testing concerns pregnant women. Pregnant women in hospitals for delivery are often tested anonymously for HIV. Since this testing is done to estimate the incidence of AIDS in this group, the information gathered is not given to anyone, including the mothers. Growing numbers of medical and public officials now are calling for mandatory testing of birth mothers and informing them if they test positive. AIDS activists, however, remain skeptical, stressing that hospitals are less fastidious than public Health Departments about keeping such information confidential.

But testing at birth is too late. Instead, because (as was mentioned) taking AZT during pregnancy drastically lowers the transmission of HIV to the child, the CDC has issued guidelines that physicians and health institutions should strongly urge pregnant women to "voluntarily" test (*CDC MMWR*, 1995d).

Mandatory testing, however, need not necessarily involve large groups. One might well consider mandatory testing for certain high-risk and relatively easy-to-regulate populations, such as prisoners, although even testing prisoners is highly controversial because it might lead to discriminatory segregation.

The vital current challenge is how to increase the rate of voluntary testing among those likely to be carrying or acquiring the HIV virus. While nobody knows the exact number of persons with the HIV virus, it is generally agreed that a high percentage of asymptomatic people with the virus and those at high risk of getting it have not been tested.

Some groups welcome testing. One of these is emergency medical personnel who have been exposed to the blood of a patient. Typically they want to know as quickly as possible whether they might have been exposed to the HIV virus (Rhame, 1989). This results in calls for forced testing of accident victims who spill blood, although testing of the medical workers themselves is the only way to tell if they may have the virus.

Why do gays and IV-drug users and their advocates seem to have a different attitude toward testing? One argument has been the perception that such groups will suffer dire social and economic discrimination if they are known to carry the virus. Such possibilities include job loss, social discrimination, ostracism from family, loss of health insurance, and criminal charges; indeed, the threat is felt to be present just for having been tested, even if the test turns out to be negative.

The obvious response has been to seek to enact laws that forbid discrimination against those having the HIV virus. The Americans with Disabilities Act of 1989 includes AIDS as an unacceptable excuse for loss of employment. Trying to include gays under present general antidiscrimination statutes is never easy, and the hope that sympathy for those with AIDS might provide a great deal of additional support for passage has not often transpired.

It should be emphasized that other reasons for gays not to test are more powerful than fear of discrimination. Surveys have demonstrated that fear of finding out that they are HIV-positive is a far greater impediment to testing (Hoxworth et al., 1994).

A new policy question has been posed by development of at-home test kits. At present, the user has to send in the blood sample and obtain the results from a laboratory, so it is not completely anonymous. Testing at home presents the psychological issue of whether people should find out their status without the presence of a counselor. But there is no standing in the way of development of this technology, and the demand will be there, so it will not be possible to prevent people from using it regardless of the consequences. More positively, the price of less counseling may be overshadowed by the benefits of substantially increased testing.

Reporting

Absolute privacy of information about being tested and test results must be assured. Yet if high-risk persons do volunteer for testing, and test positive, failure to report results is a disservice to the larger society and indeed ultimately to the infected persons themselves. Yet this often occurs. The problem can be resolved only by gaining greater understanding and trust of public health officials when they assure that reported names, though not *anonymous* will remain *confidential*. Anonymity for those testing positive means that only they know they have the disease. Confidentiality means that those they don't want to know they have it don't in fact find out. While reporting a positive test to a Health Department sacrifices anonymity, true anonymity is really not desirable, for a person with the HIV virus obviously needs to be referred to a physician, and should be advised to seek the support of friends and other available services that will eventually be needed.

But quite in contrast is confidentiality. One's employers, workmates, and personal service vendors are not in danger and have no need to know one's HIV-virus status. Thus complete professionalism and legal protections to assure confidentiality are required. The highly successful record of public health agencies in maintaining confidentiality must be made known to diminish the exaggerated fears of breaches of professional responsibility in this regard.

Partner Notification

Overcoming resistance to testing and reporting is only the first task of public health authorities. Their traditional techniques also require tracing the sexual or needle-sharing contacts of those testing positive for HIV. Opposition to partner notification—telling others and trying to get them to test—is often greater than to getting oneself tested.

Some alternative test sites have stressed anonymity to the point of sacrificing all reporting and partner notification. Yet the case for the traditional public health approach is now clearly stronger than it was even as late as 1995. The already-mentioned new drug therapies, even given their severe limitations, mean that partner notification has moved beyond being an important component of health education to become a significant possible medical benefit to those being notified.

One possible way out of serious conflict over partner notification is for public Health Departments to persuade, and if necessary pressure, health providers and counselors to go beyond technical delivery of services and advocate to their patients the benefits of cooperating with the Health Department in partner notification. Increased reporting and partner notification obviously benefit the public's health, but will also ultimately benefit patients psychologically by enabling them to take a major step in helping fight AIDS. Conversely, if clinicians downplay the benefits of partner notification, patients are unlikely to cooperate, and if forced to name partners are likely to frustrate the whole effort by giving false names.

Our more positive view of the growing movement for increased testing/reporting/notification is largely a result of the fact that fifteen years of experience show that public Health Departments are responsible in handling sensitive information. But again this does not mean that widespread mandatory testing should or will occur, and more unfortunately, that all those with HIV will soon be testing, reporting, and notifying partners. More likely will be incremental improvements in carrying out these traditional public health initiatives.

PREVENTION OF SPREAD

Despite the difficulties faced by public health officials in implementing testing/reporting/tracing, this is not the core of the AIDS problem. Testing, reporting, and tracing by themselves do not prevent the spread of the HIV virus. And, as already noted, there is as yet no drug that can be given to those who test positive for HIV that will make them noncommunicable, as well as no vaccine that can be given to HIV-negative partners that will prevent them from getting the HIV virus. Only modification of risky behavior can prevent people from spreading or acquiring the HIV virus.

Restriction

AIDS activists were greatly apprehensive that fear of AIDS coupled with hatred for gays would lead to repressive physical restrictions like quarantine in the name of preventing the spread of the disease. They obviously oppose such proposals on principle, but they also warn that such extreme measures, or even milder restrictions, are counterproductive in that they will decrease cooperation by high-risk groups. Public health authorities also oppose most proposals for restriction, for such measures typically are both unfairly harsh and punitive and unlikely to be effective in this, the most individualistic society in the world. Successful opposition to restrictive proposals, however, lies in understanding the reasons for their appeal and responding to them in a manner that reduces that appeal.

The operative political reality is, as was true in the debate over mandatory testing, that as long as the issue is conceptualized as one of public health versus the right to privacy, the movement for repressive restrictions will remain strong. Proposals for restriction are politically attractive to many elected officials, because enacting them gives the appearance that public officials are being decisive in time of crisis. The battle could be lost unless the impracticality of most of the proposed restrictions is made the central issue.

Support for quarantine, for example, arises because of a false analogy of AIDS to other diseases, such as tuberculosis. Quarantine could rationally be urged for that disease, because an uninfected person can receive it merely by being in the same room with the carrier. AIDS is not, however, spread through casual contacts.

Some would attempt to restrict the spread of AIDS by defining the intentional spreading of AIDS as a crime. Another tack is to criminalize wanton promiscuity by a known HIV carrier. Unfortunately, these proposals by themselves could discourage testing, because not knowing one's status would appear to be a legal defense. So a third level of punishment is then suggested for transmission of the disease even without prior knowledge of one's virus status.

The task for health professionals is to emphasize that these are differing problems requiring different solutions. In fact, there is probably no need for new laws on the intentional spreading of AIDS, since assault is likely to be covered by present statutes. In the case of noncompliance by an HIV carrier who has been warned to stop his or her behavior, commitment procedures are now required by state statute. Public health authorities typically resist criminalizing transmission of HIV because they believe a punitive stance would seriously weaken the fight against AIDS by lessening cooperation

both in testing, reporting, and notification, and in programs of health education and behavior modification that are most essential to combat the disease.

But opposing on this principle all restrictions on dangerous behavior could boomerang. Unless action is taken against the few that might deliberately spread the disease, the public may well believe that public health officials are not doing enough to stop the spread of AIDS. Carefully delineating the behavior that is sought to be curbed, and tailoring reasonable and productive restrictions, should make thoughtful policy choices more probable. Moreover, taking action against the few serious offenders is an important symbolic effort to show that the public health guardians are alert (Backstrom & Robins, 1992).

Prevention

Effective voluntary programs of health education and behavior modification to prevent the spread of AIDS are currently the most important steps that can be taken in the fight against the disease. Unfortunately, actually stopping the spread of AIDS requires behavior changes of the most personal nature. Adjusting sexual activities and methods of drug use are extremely difficult.

Yet change is not impossible. As a result of AIDS, gays in recent years have greatly, though far from totally, reduced their risky behavior, demonstrating that change is possible in even such an elemental function as sexual behavior. This has been especially so for those who test positive for the HIV virus, but those who test negative also reduce their risk, though many fewer do so (Coates et al., 1987).

Significant permanent behavior change is facilitated by extensive professional counseling. But this type of counseling is very expensive because it involves face-to-face contact with a professional, usually one to one, or at most in small groups. The cost and the supply of trained personnel are practical limits. The alternative is training paraprofessionals and volunteers, which, in spite of a reduction in quality, would increase the possibility of more widespread behavior change.

Needle-sharing drug users present special problems in the control of AIDS. Already engaged in self-destructive behavior, they are the high-risk group least amenable to educational and counseling programs. Yet evidence indicates that even they are changing somewhat the manner in which they use needles as a result of their fear of AIDS (Green & Miller, 1987).

Rather than relying solely on promoting the use of bleach to (using the vernacular) "clean your works," most public health officials now favor reducing the risk of HIV transmission among IV-drug users by programs to provide free needles (for example, through needle exchange—requiring that a used needle be turned in before a clean one is handed out). All available empirical evidence shows that needle provision not only reduces AIDS, but also leads drug addicts to be more likely to apply for treatment programs (Lambert, 1988). The reason seems to be that such programs give addicts confidence that they can alter or modify their way of life and also a feeling of increased trust (or lessening of distrust) in the promise of public authorities that they want to help addicts overcome their addiction and not just punish them for their addiction.

These programs are controversial because to some they appear to legitimize and facilitate drug use. Still, support for them is growing, and while needle exchange is nowhere an overall state policy, it is formally a policy in several large cities and informal policy in several more.

Perhaps the most productive action that could currently be taken in preventing AIDS would be to expand drug treatment programs to handle the large numbers of abusers awaiting assistance (Presidential Commission on the Human Immunodeficiency Virus Epidemic, 1988). In 1995, however, Congress continued to pour more resources into prisons and punishing drug addicts rather than providing treatment facilities and personnel, which constitute the long-term solution to the problem.

Education

The most fundamental method of stopping the spread of AIDS is to educate people who are not infected about realistic actions they can take to avoid getting it. American public policy on AIDS education is in our judgment worse than in any other aspect of AIDS policymaking.

For example, efforts to require schools to conduct AIDS education often run into longstanding and increasingly well-organized opposition to any kind of public sex education. Unfortunately, pointing out that U.S. teenage girls have both the highest abortion and out-of-wedlock birth rates in the Western world, while not having any higher rate of sexual intercourse (Kantrowitz et al., 1987a) does not convince the opponents of effective sex education of its necessity. The most common fear of the opponents is that discussion of sexual behaviors appears to condone or even advocate them. The result is often teaching sex education in a bland, "scientific" way that offends no one but also accomplishes little. This style is especially problematic for AIDS education because public health practitioners believe anti-AIDS messages must be explicit enough to force people to identify their own behaviors as risky and to visualize themselves enjoying new practices (Brandt, 1988). The bulk of AIDS education is what is cynically described as AIDS 101—only a description of what AIDS is and a warning not to engage in sex. Indeed, it was only after the election of President Clinton that federal government educational advertising included open advocacy of the use of condoms. But Congress has prevented the federal government from including funding for private groups to conduct explicit demonstrations of gay sexual practices that are much safer than anal intercourse, and blocked the Department of Health and Human Services from putting out television public service announcements demonstrating how IV-drug users should clean their works. The result is that in the area of education the level of AIDS expenditures greatly overstates what the U.S. government is really doing to prevent AIDS.

Fairness also requires noting that in certain respects even AIDS educators fail to be realistic. For example, oral sex has a real, but much lower risk of AIDS transmission than anal sex. Yet AIDS organizations' educational materials usually advise avoiding both types of contacts equally. Critics of this approach to AIDS education insist that more honest, explicit directions would more realistically reduce truly risky behavior (Odets, 1994).

Two final points. First, education by public authorities is less persuasive than if done by private groups, especially by peers (Green & Miller, 1987). Therefore, subsidizing voluntary groups to carry out AIDS education makes sense, even though it certainly will not totally divert the opposition of groups who object to having public officials involved with sex education. Second, standardized educational materials are probably not sufficient to reach minorities. Messages will be more effective when tailored and delivered by people who understand specific cultural constraints and opportunities (DesJarlais et al., 1994).

CARE OF PATIENTS

AIDS activists were very critical of the initial response of the health care delivery system to the problem of caring for people with AIDS. They bitterly noted that those few physicians and institutions who were willing to treat AIDS patients were viewed as second-class citizens by the medical community. Again, they attributed this reaction to general homophobia among both providers and funders (Shilts, 1987).

AIDS activists also indicted the loss of health insurance or increases in premiums for those who test positive for the HIV virus as being both unjust and a barrier to testing and seeking medical care. They also complained about the acute-care emphasis of much of the treatment for AIDS, but in fairness this criticism can be made of our overall health care system. Finally, while AIDS patients are eligible, like others considered disabled, for Medicare after they have been diagnosed as having the disease for two years, many die before they can receive the funds.

Things have somewhat improved in recent years. First, an increasing percentage of care for people with AIDS is now community-based. The San Francisco model (the use of volunteers [often gays themselves]) to work with AIDS patients on a one-on-one basis to provide assistance in daily routine activities, emotional support, and help patient compliance) is increasingly recognized as the ideal—both in terms of high quality and low costs—to be striven for, and not only in caring for people with AIDS.

Second, increases in premiums or loss of insurance for people with AIDS are not indications of prejudice, but rather the result of the logic of unregulated competition, which inevitably leads to experience rating. Insurance companies can legally be forced to issue policies to persons with preexisting conditions (such as testing positive for the HIV virus), but given that in the United States medical care is not a right, the question can be asked why an exception should be made for AIDS. More validly, at least a few states forbid insurance companies from excluding persons from coverage who are thought to be at high risk of getting AIDS based on occupations stereotyped as attracting gays or ZIP code areas where many gays are known to reside (Hatch, 1989).

Third, associations of medical personnel and health institutions have reiterated the ethical and professional duty of providers to care for everyone—including AIDS patients (Goldsmith, 1987). This makes the role of state regulators in enforcing nondiscrimination—for example, against nursing homes that do not want to take AIDS patients—less politically controversial, because the government is acting against individuals and institutions who are not meeting their own industry's ethical and professional norms.

Projecting future costs of caring for people with AIDS is not simple. Clearly, costs will increase in coming years because, as previously noted, the number of those already carrying the HIV virus who develop the opportunistic diseases that signal AIDS will continue to climb. The real issue is whether the costs *per case* of treating individual AIDS cases—adjusted for medical price increases, which have gone up much faster than other prices—are likely to increase or decrease in coming years.

There are several ways to analyze this question, and the differing results they produce have differing implications for public policy. For example, the development of drugs that increase the period in which an HIV-positive person is asymptomatic will, unless they simultaneously shorten the period between the onset of full-blown AIDS and death, inevitably result in an increase in costs per AIDS case. Nonetheless, since asymptomatics (and early symptomatics under control with drug therapy) can continue to work and otherwise contribute to the economy, the development of such drugs is, even from a strictly economic viewpoint, clearly beneficial.

Conversely, medications that lengthen the period between the onset of full-blown AIDS and death by combatting the opportunistic diseases resulting from the breakdown in the immune system will inevitably increase the AIDS costs per patient without necessarily restoring their productivity and are thus much more problematic. Yet even in this instance, besides the humanitarian benefits, more familiarity with treating AIDS patients and increased use of the San Francisco model may result in cost savings that will outweigh the cost-increasing effects of medications that prolong the sickness phase of AIDS.

STATE POLICYMAKING ON AIDS

In the earlier chapter on the role of the states in health policymaking by Lipson (Chapter 8), the important growing role of the states was examined. Although federal expenditures on AIDS are as of now much greater than those of the states, and even the majority of state Health Department spending on AIDS comes from the Centers for Disease Control and Prevention, important aspects of AIDS policy, like health policy generally, are primarily set by the states.

The section that follows is based on results from research conducted by the authors on the role of the states in AIDS policymaking. The data are from surveys of state Health Department heads (forty-two of fifty responded), state legislative health committee chairs (sixty-eight of ninety-nine responded), and directors of state hospital associations (fifty-one of seventy-five responded).[4]

Three areas are examined: (1) the most influential state leaders in AIDS policymaking; (2) the policy preferences of state health officers and legislative health chairs; and (3) the most effective strategies for influencing AIDS policymaking. We conclude this section

[4]In addition, field interviews were conducted with AIDS policymakers in six states—Arizona, California, Georgia, Illinois, New York, and Minnesota. Fuller reports of the findings discussed here appear in Robins and Backstrom (1993, 1994) and Backstrom and Robins (1992, 1995).

with an overall assessment of the politics of AIDS policymaking in the states.

INFLUENCE

The relative influence of various leaders, organizations, and groups on AIDS policymaking, as assessed by state Health Department heads, legislative health committee chairs, and hospital association directors, is shown in Table 20-2.

Participants in AIDS policymaking fall into five general ranges of influence. Far and away the leading policymakers are state Health Departments—more than two-thirds of the respondents thought them very influential, and nearly all the rest said they were somewhat influential. The next most influential AIDS policymakers were seen to be elected leaders. Tops among these were legislative leaders, whom half of the respondents rated as very influential. The governor was seen as somewhat less influential on AIDS policy. At a distinctly lower level of influence stand health provider associations such as state medical associations—about a quarter of respondents thought they were very influential. Even lower in influence were affected groups; around one in ten respondents thought people living with AIDS were important policymakers. At the very bottom were ideological groups such as conservatives, with only one in fourteen respondents rating them as very influential.

Policy Preferences

Virtually all AIDS policymakers wanted to require AIDS education, but legislators were far more reluctant to authorize the state to publish explicit sex education materials. All favored encouraging noninstitutional care. Most favored forbidding discrimination against persons with HIV, and most favored prohibiting discrimination against gays, but the latter was not likely to be implemented. Only about half favored needle exchange at the time of this survey. About two-thirds resisted criminalizing risky sexual activities by HIV carriers. Most did not favor mandatory testing of large groups, but respondents were split on requiring reporting names of

TABLE 20-2 Relative Assessment of Influence of Various Participants in State AIDS Policymaking

Policy Participant	Very Influential			Some Influence		
	Health Dept.	Leg. Chair	Hosp. Assn.	Health Dept.	Leg. Chair	Hosp. Assn.
State administrators						
State Department of Health	59.5	67.6	72.3	38.1	30.9	25.5
Elected officials						
Legislative leaders	57.1	48.5	46.8	35.7	45.6	44.7
Governor	42.9	20.6	42.6	40.5	52.9	29.8
Health providers						
State medical association	23.8	29.9	19.1	61.9	62.7	40.4
State hospital association	14.3	25.0	23.4	64.3	61.8	46.8
Insurance industry	7.1	11.8	17.0	52.4	57.4	55.3
Affected groups						
Persons living with AIDS	9.5	15.2	6.4	40.5	43.9	34.0
Organized gay groups	9.5	10.3	6.4	54.8	29.4	34.0
Ideological organizations						
Conservative ideological groups	14.3	2.9	4.3	28.6	26.5	38.3
Liberal ideological groups	2.4	4.4	2.1	38.1	27.9	31.9
Mainline church leaders	4.8	1.5	4.3	47.6	35.3	34.8
Fundamentalist church leaders	2.4	0.0	6.5	35.7	20.6	23.9

Note: Number of respondents: state Health Departments (*n* = 42); legislative health chairs (*n* = 68); hospital association directors (*n* = 47). Responses are in percentages.

those testing positive, with half as many health chairs favoring it as Health Departments.

The overwhelming pattern that emerges from this review is that most state Health Departments and health committee chairs support an approach that generally stresses "cooperation and inclusion" with those at risk rather than a more punitive "contain and control" approach (Bayer & Kirp, 1992).

Strategies

To assess how state policymakers evaluated the policymaking process, they were asked to assess several proposed "conservative" and "liberal" strategies. Although their positions were not identical, views were fairly similar. Respondents thought arguments such as human interest in suffering people were useful; they thought the liberal ideology of emphasizing protection of civil liberties was likely to be counterproductive. Effective conservative strategies were seen to be protecting inno-

cent victims and the threat of AIDS to the general public. Conversely, only two in five thought emphasizing the differences between typical AIDS sufferers and the rest of the public would be productive, and fewer than a third thought stressing AIDS as an election issue would be an effective strategy.

Rather than take ideological stances, policymakers preferred to stress the impracticality of extreme programs in effective AIDS control.

Overall Assessment

Public officials in our surveys demonstrated that they were not mere pawns of public opinion and pressure. This finding was confirmed by our site visits. Health legislators were willing to take positions on AIDS policy that they thought might put their political careers at risk. They were willing to accept leadership from public health officials, who defined the AIDS problem as a scientific health issue to be addressed with careful steps, not broad reactions to panic. The result was that the details of AIDS policy were left to health professionals rather than being dealt with through partisan politics (Fox et al., 1989).

But enlightened Health Departments and committee chairs could not accomplish all they desired in AIDS policymaking. Many proactive AIDS policies could not overcome widespread attitudes about sexual and drug-using activities. Understandably, impatient AIDS activists often view the refusal of public officials to follow their policy desires as evidence that those officials were "the enemy." To the contrary, our research shows that the key to improved advocacy is the demonstration that change (or resistance to unwanted change) will have practical effects in fighting AIDS.

AIDS IN GENERAL PERSPECTIVE

We wish to conclude by examining AIDS (even if by necessity somewhat speculatively) in the overall context of the American political and social system generally and its health care system in particular. Our aim will be to answer two questions, which have three parts each: (1) how the American political and social systems and its health care system have shaped how we have dealt with AIDS, and (2) how AIDS has affected our overall political and social systems and health care system.

How Has the American Political System Affected AIDS?

In what ways, if any, has the American political system affected the formation of AIDS policy so that it developed differently from what might otherwise have been?

Perhaps the easiest way to present our views on this question is by contrasting them in part with those of Sandra Panem (1988) on how the U.S. government should have been organized to fight AIDS at the outset and how it should be organized to fight future health emergencies (Robins and Backstrom, 1989).

In brief, Panem argued that the United States' efforts against AIDS have not been coordinated; there has been no overall strategy regarding research, testing, tracking, or education, nor any overall plan for organizing and financing health care delivery to those suffering from AIDS.

Panem recommended reorganization under a "czar" of many federal agencies to bring about the necessary coordination to handle AIDS and any future emergencies. This would be intended to end the bureaucratic infighting among several National Institutes of Health (NIH), the Centers for Disease Control and Prevention (CDC), the Health Care Financing Administration (HCFA), the Health Services and Resources Administration (HSRA), the Alcohol, Drug Abuse and Mental Health Administration (ADAMHA), the Food and Drug Administration (FDA), the National Science Foundation (NSF), the Department of Veterans Affairs (VA), and the Department of Defense (DOD). An undersecretary in the Department of Health and Human Services for health emergencies was proposed as coordinator of all AIDS programs.

We would challenge this prescription on the grounds that single-agency (or czar) control might possibly sacrifice healthy multiple experimentation and competition in attacking AIDS. In more directly political terms, all of these agencies would be bitterly opposed to any czar. Even more important, the real czar of the executive branch—the president—is unlikely to favor a de facto delegation of authority.

Panem also advocated a large preappropriated emergency fund, with great executive flexibility as to how it could be used. This would bypass the slow bargaining of the federal budget process and soften the impact of health emergencies on local governments where they hit first. Yet even if Congress could be persuaded to tolerate a large fund lying around in a period of perpetual budget deficits, disputes would still arise as to whether a disease should be called an emergency, with attendant lobbying and political intervention. An enduring recrimination about AIDS is, after all, that it was not seen by appropriate federal agencies to be an emergency for some years. Moreover, at what point would a disease cease to qualify as an emergency?

Panem also wanted to sort out clearly the responsibilities of federal, state, and local governments, essentially bringing the latter under federal direction during health emergencies. But calling for federal government dominance in dealing with AIDS is, as noted earlier, contrary to the current trend toward delegating more functions to the states.

Two events in recent years confirm this analysis. First, in response to fears of unpreparedness for another health emergency like AIDS, Congress granted the Department of Health and Human Services a standing emergency fund. But the amount appropriated was only $15 million, less than 0.01 percent of the HHS health budget. Second, in response to a campaign promise, President Clinton appointed an official AIDS czar, Kristine Gebbie, former director of the Oregon and Washington State Health Departments. In fact, however, she was given little power or visibility, without even an executive order defining her responsibilities, and resigned before long in frustration over her inability to accomplish anything. Her successor, Patricia Fleming, has had more success, but is no czar.

Thus AIDS policymaking has been in broad consonance with the American political system. The result is that the localistic, incremental nature of AIDS policymaking is very much shaped by the general contours of the American political system. This is not to say that bold, aggressive action is impossible, but that typically it should not be expected. Advocates for effective AIDS policy who ignore the American political system's way of doing business put their entire effort in jeopardy.

How Has American Society Affected AIDS?

American values have also greatly shaped the American response to AIDS. As shown in the chapter on public opinion by Blendon and Brodie (Chapter 9), while a majority of Americans as measured by polls seem in the abstract to believe Americans have a right to guaranteed health care and economic security, those same polls show strong resistance to the increased taxes necessary to effectuate these rights.

Americans in their role as private individuals have been relatively warm and generous in their willingness to help those with AIDS, more than perhaps could have been expected given their biases against those most often afflicted. In their role as taxpayers, however, Americans have maintained their conservatism. Here also things have been pretty much as might have been predicted.

More positively, until now at least, there has not been the government repression against those with AIDS and gays in general that many greatly feared. Given the American emphasis on individual freedom and willingness to tolerate diversity, this also should not have been surprising.

Let us conclude this section with a conjecture. How would U.S. policy toward AIDS have differed if it had been a disease primarily of white heterosexuals? First, we believe it certainly would have been taken seriously earlier and more intensely by government at all levels and society as a whole. Second, while funding for biomedical research, would, we believe, have accelerated even faster than it did, it is unlikely that spending would *now* be at a considerably higher level than it is. Third, the pressures on the FDA would, we believe, have been even greater and therefore would probably have resulted in an even faster changing of its standards for drug approval, though again things would probably not be much different *now*.

While some of the policy problems in dealing with AIDS would have been greatly reduced if it had been a white, middle-class disease, some of the problems that did occur might in fact have been exacerbated. In particular, an argument can be made that if AIDS were a disease that struck randomly, pressures for restriction might have even been greater, for as long as AIDS was perceived as largely a disease of gays and drug users, there was less panic among the general public.

On balance, of course, public policy decisions would have been better if AIDS were a disease the majority of the public could perceive getting. But explaining AIDS policy—especially *now*—as almost solely a function of attitudes toward those most likely to get it would be a serious distortion.

How Has the Health System Affected AIDS?

AIDS policy has been greatly affected by the general characteristics of the nation's overall health care system. First, the problem of obtaining insurance and paying for health care for people with AIDS is only all too real, but this problem is not uniquely AIDS-specific. Individual employers and health insurers are increasingly seeking to screen applicants for drug use, alcoholism, and other diseases—not just AIDS. Moreover, as shown in the chapter on health access by Fraser (Chapter 13), there is a growing trend of employers either offering no insurance at all or requiring increasing cost sharing from their employees.

Second, although the French were at least equally responsible for the discovery of the HIV virus (Shilts, 1987), most of the major biomedical research on AIDS has been done in the United States, and it is likely that if a vaccine and cure are found for AIDS, they will be found here. There is nothing unusual in this, for the United States is far and away the world's leader in biomedical research, probably doing more than the rest of the world combined.

Finally, given the perceived weakness of public health in the United States (Institute of Medicine, 1988), the relative success so far experienced by public Health Departments in influencing the debate over AIDS is pleasantly surprising. Whether in the "hard" public health of testing, reporting, and tracing, or the "soft" public health of opposition to restrictions like quarantine and emphasis on voluntary action for behavioral change, public health department professionals have emerged as the group with the most influence in public policymaking on AIDS (Robins and Backstrom, 1994).

How Has AIDS Affected the Political System?

The reverse side of the question of how AIDS policy has been shaped by the general sociopolitical and health policy environments is how AIDS has affected American politics, society, and its health system. Without implying that AIDS has produced revolutionary effects, its overall impact can be fairly characterized as substantial.

Politically, the main impact of AIDS has probably been on the politics of the gay community. Prior to AIDS, its goals were first to "get government off the back of gays" and then to seek nondiscrimination laws. After AIDS, the goals of gay groups inevitably became more complex. They continued, of course, to seek nondiscrimination laws. They now, however, are deeply involved in government contacts, pressing for massive new funding for biomedical research, more rapid FDA approval of anti-AIDS drugs, and generous government funding for health care and social services for those with AIDS.

Some of this new political activity has taken the form of direct action—noisy demonstrations and sit-ins. In terms of general political affiliation, the gay perception of a highly inadequate (to say the least) response to AIDS by the Reagan and Bush administrations, along with the growing influence of the religious right in the Republican Party, led to gays giving even more support to the Democratic Party. But to be blunt, this has not been a total net gain for the Democrats. While the party gained increased support from an organized and generous constituency, they lost votes among those who dislike homosexuals.

Gays and lesbians as political interest groups have had a mixed record of success in obtaining legitimate objectives such as antidiscrimination laws. More important, their increased activities have resulted in an enhanced sense of efficacy, which is very helpful in decreasing the alienation and self-hatred among gays and lesbians.

How Has AIDS Affected Society?

Perhaps the most widely heralded contention about the effect of AIDS on American culture is that it has brought the sexual revolution to an end. Among gays, promiscuous sexual behavior had to change dramatically, and to a large but far from complete extent it has (Coates et al., 1987). Moreover, attempts at philosophically justifying anonymous sex in bathhouses as exemplifying a new and better "gay lifestyle" have largely ceased (Beauchamp, 1989). Whether these changes will be permanent is, of course, uncertain.

The effects on the heterosexual population of the fear of AIDS are, however, much more uncertain. The swinging lifestyle and the singles bar are less glorified than in the past, but there are several reasons for believing that the degree of overall change in heterosexual behavior is likely to be less than many have hoped.

For instance, men and women are delaying marriage, hoping first to complete their education or training and then successfully embark on their careers. The inevitable result is more sex outside marriage. Additionally, while the divorce rate has been slowly declining, the United States has by far the highest incidence in the world (Kantrowitz et al., 1987b). Thus urging sexual abstinence is not likely to be very effective. And polls indicate few of these adults engaging in unprotected multiple-partner sex characterized their behavior as risky (Laumann et al., 1994).

The argument here is not that changing values about sex are unimportant. Rather it is that widespread sex outside marriage is inevitably here to stay. Even the fear of AIDS cannot overcome this existential fact. The issue, then, is not whether AIDS will cause the end of the sexual revolution; it will not if this means greatly reduced sex. The hope and cautious prediction is that it ultimately will cause an increase in more responsible sexual behavior.

An additional important effect of AIDS on society is that Americans can no longer believe they are secure from plagues or epidemics. Comprehending and coping with AIDS itself presses the general public to the limits of its understanding and tolerance. Whether we will have learned enough from battling AIDS to handle further threats with some equanimity, or whether the difficulty of this struggle will cause people to react with heavy-handed, even cruel self-protective measures to the inevitable next crisis (McNeill, 1976) remains an open question that hopefully will not have to be answered soon.

Another and more controversial effect of AIDS on society is its effect on societal attitudes and actions toward gays. To imply a single, unidirectional effect would be inaccurate, for AIDS has more likely simultaneously increased hostility to gays and yet increased respect for them as human beings.

The negative effects are more direct and visible. First, there has been an increased number of reported acts of violence against gays (Barron, 1989). The reason, we suspect, is not an increase in homophobia, but that gays are more willing to report such acts and that gays are more open about their sexual orientation and thus present more potential targets. Less easily empirically quantifiable, but no less real, has been a growing understanding and acceptance of gays as a visible and more integral part of the larger community. This has risen as

more and more people are personally touched by relatives and friends who suffer and die from AIDS.

Whether this positive sentiment can soon overcome anti-gay hostility sufficiently to engender requisite support for passage in many jurisdictions of antidiscrimination laws to protect gays is problematic. Indeed, in 1994, Colorado voters overturned by referendum antidiscrimination ordinances protecting gays and lesbians in Boulder and Aspen. While the U.S. Supreme Court in one of its final decisions in the 1995–96 term gave homosexuals a major victory by declaring this unconstitutional, it did so on narrow grounds. It did not, moreover, extend to homosexuals the status of a protected class like blacks or women that was entitled to equal protection under law as a matter of right.

Finally, a noteworthy social effect of AIDS has been a shift in the values of gays toward greater emphasis on becoming a caring community (Altman, 1986). This raises their own feelings of worth and capacity and thereby is likely ultimately to increase their ability to effect personal and social change.

How Has AIDS Affected the Health System?

Finally, what effects has AIDS had on the health care system? First, as has been previously noted, public health professionals have been more influential in dealing with AIDS than many observers of that profession might have anticipated. AIDS has also affected public health professionals by forcing them to generally reconsider their legal powers. It turns out that alarmists' calls for new laws controlling the behavior of those testing positive for HIV are largely unnecessary because laws already on the books, typically dating back to the nineteenth century, give public health nearly dictatorial power (Gostin, 1986). In fact, public health professionals are telling appropriate legislators that such laws should either be repealed, modified to conform to modern concepts of fair procedure, or allowed to remain on the books as dead letters.

A second major change triggered by AIDS has occurred in the fields of biomedical and drug research. Women's groups rebelled when it became obvious that treatment trials and even the classification of symptoms that constituted the definition of AIDS excluded many women, in whom the course of the disease is somewhat different. In addition, the imbalance of federal effort on behalf of AIDS compared to breast cancer motivated women to demand increased funding to counter that disease. Women's groups modeled their lobbying efforts on the approach of AIDS activists and experienced similar success.

The acceleration of FDA procedures for approval and distribution of drugs for AIDS has also changed the general manner in which the FDA approves drugs. This seems to have happened for two main reasons. First, generally faster FDA approval was being increasingly advocated and already occurring to some extent. Second, the leadership of FDA found it easier to bureaucratically justify changes for AIDS drugs in the context of generally overhauling FDA procedures.

A third major issue was whether AIDS would foster fundamental revisions in the system for paying for health care in the United States. The gigantic forces that prevented health care reform in 1994 showed that the realities of a care crisis involving a single disease like AIDS had no impact. And, since any reasonable projection of AIDS costs would not have them becoming more than 5 percent of overall health care costs, AIDS will not likely ever be a factor in fundamental revisions in the system for paying for health care in this country.

Finally, AIDS care is likely to change as the disease continues to shift from predominantly white gays to African American and Hispanic IV-drug users. On the average the latter have fewer resources for obtaining private care than gays, and collectively they have no major community support networks. Hence, the models of effective and economical noninstitutional care provided for AIDS patients—done especially brilliantly in San Francisco—may not be as relevant for the new populations having AIDS. More positively, the San Francisco model has been extensively studied and likely will be emulated by other communities and for other diseases.

In summary, AIDS has affected as well as been affected by its broader environments, though not always as people had expected or thought. What is clear is that the effects of AIDS are subtle and deep. Health policy analysts must inevitably focus on the direct health effects of the disease, the number of cases, priorities in biomedical research, the modalities of testing, the effectiveness of education, and the costs of care. The observer of general policymaking and social trends will, however, both find much to learn from AIDS and have much to contribute to understanding how AIDS has affected our polity and society.

REFERENCES

Altman, Dennis. (1986.) *AIDS in the mind of America*. Garden City, NY: Anchor Press.

Backstrom, Charles, & Leonard Robins. (1989). The political elements in policymaking on AIDS. *New England Journal of Human Services, 9* (Summer), 13–19.

Backstrom, Charles, & Leonard Robins. (1992). *The Minnesota response to AIDS*. Minneapolis: Center for Urban and Regional Affairs, University of Minnesota.

Backstrom, Charles, & Leonard Robins. (1995–96). Public health policymaking: Perceptions of state legislators. *AIDS and Public Policy Journal, 10* (Winter), 238–248.

Barron, James. (1989). Homosexuals see 2 decades of gains, but fear setbacks. *New York Times* (June 25), 1:1.

Bayer, Ronald. (1989). *Private acts, social consequences: AIDS and the politics of public health*. New York: The Free Press.

Bayer, Ronald, & David L. Kirp. (1992). An epidemic in political and policy perspective. In David Kirp & Ronald Bayer (Eds.), *AIDS in the industrialized democracies: Passions, politics, and policies*. New Brunswick, NJ: Rutgers University Press.

Beauchamp, Dan E. (1989). *The health of the Republic: Epidemics, medicine, and moralism as challenges to democracy*. Philadelphia: Temple University Press.

Brandt, Allan. (1988). AIDS in historical perspective: Four lessons from the history of sexually transmitted diseases. *American Journal of Public Health, 78* (April), 367–371.

CDC MMWR [*Morbidity and Mortality Weekly Report*]. (1981) Pneumocystis pneumonia—Los Angeles. *30* (June 5), 250–252.

CDC MMWR. (1992). Projections of the number of persons diagnosed with AIDS and the number of immunosuppressed HIV-infected persons—United States, 1992–1994. *41* (December 15), 1–18.

CDC MMWR. (1994). Recommendations of the U.S. public health service task force on the use of Zidovudine to reduce perinatal transmission of Human Immunodeficiency Virus. *43* (August 5), 1–20.

CDC MMWR. (1995a). Update: Acquired Immunodeficiency Syndrome—United States, 1994. *44* (February 3), 64–67.

CDC MMWR. (1995b). Update: AIDS among women—United States, 1994. *44* (February 10), 81–84.

CDC MMWR. (1995c). Update: Trends in AIDS among men who have sex with men—United States, 1994. *44* (June 2), 401–404.

CDC MMWR. (1995d). U.S. public health service recommendations for Human Immunodeficiency Virus counseling and voluntary testing for pregnant women. *44* (July 7), 1–15.

Coates, Thomas, Stephen Morin, & Leon McKusick. (1987). Behavioral consequences of AIDS antibody testing among gay men. *Journal of the American Medical Association, 258* (October 9), 1889.

Congressional Record. (1995). Ryan White Act reauthorization. (July 26), S10716.

DesJarlais, Don C., Nancy S. Padian, & Warren Winkelstein Jr. (1994). Targeted HIV-prevention programs. *New England Journal of Medicine, 331* (November 24), 1451–1453.

Fox, Daniel M., Patricia Day, & Rudolph Klein. (1989). The power of professionalism: Policies for AIDS in Britain, Sweden, and the United States. *Daedalus, 118* (Spring), 93–112.

Fuchs, Victor. (1974). *Who shall live?* New York: Basic Books.

Fumento, Michael. (1990). *The myth of heterosexual AIDS.* New York: Basic Books.

Goldsmith, Marsha. (1987) AMA house of delegates adopts comprehensive measures on AIDS. *Journal of the American Medical Association, 258* (July 24), 425–426.

Gostin, Larry. (1986). The future of communicable disease control: Toward a new concept in public health law. *Milbank Quarterly, 64* (Suppl. 1), 79–96.

Green, Jesse. (1995). Who put the lid on gp100? *New York Times Magazine* (March 26), 50–82.

Green, John, & David Miller. (1987). The psychosocial impact of AIDS and Human Immunodeficiency Virus. In M. S. Gottlieb, D. J. Jeffries, D. Mildvan, A. J. Pinching, T. C. Quinn, & R. A. Weiss (Eds.), *Current topics in AIDS.* Chichester, UK: Wiley.

Harris, Richard. (1964). *The real voice.* New York: Macmillan.

Hatch, Michael. (1989). Personal interview with commissioner of commerce, State of Minnesota (July 12).

Hoxworth, Tamara, Richard Hoffman, David Cohn, & Arthur David. (1994). Anonymous HIV testing: Does it attract clients who would not seek confidential testing? *AIDS and Public Policy Journal, 10* (Winter), 182–189.

Institute of Medicine, National Academy of Sciences. (1988). *Confronting AIDS: Update 1988.* Washington, D.C.: National Academy Press.

Kantrowitz, Barbara, Mary Hager, Pat Wingert, Ginny Carroll, George Raine, Monroe Anderson, Deborah Witherspoon, Janet Huck, & Shawn Doherty. (1987a). Kids and contraceptives. *Newsweek, 109* (February 16), 54–58.

Kantrowitz, Barbara, Pat Wingert, Leanne Gordon, Renee Michael, Deborah Witherspoon, Eric Calonius, David Gonzalez, & Bill Turque. (1987b). How to stay married. *Newsweek, 110* (August 24), 52–57.

Lambert, Bruce. (1988). The free-needle program is under way and under fire. *New York Times* (November 13), 4:6.

Laumann, Edward O., John H. Gagnon, Robert T. Michael, & Stuart Michaels. (1994). *The social organization of sexuality: Sexual practices in the United States.* Chicago: University of Chicago Press.

McNeill, William. (1976) *Plagues and people.* Garden City, NY: Anchor Press.

Meinick, Sandra L., Renslow Sherer, Thomas A. Louis, David Hillman, Evelyn M. Rodriguez, Cheryl Lackman, Linnea Capps, Lawrence S. Brown Jr., Marcia Carlyn, Joyce A. Korvick, & Lawrence Deyton. (1994). Survival and disease progression according to gender of patients with HIV infection. *Journal of the American Medical Association, 272* (December 28), 1915–1921.

Odets, Walt. (1994). AIDS education and harm reduction for gay men: Psychological approaches for the 21st century. *AIDS and Public Policy Journal, 9* (Spring), 3–15.

Panem, Sandra. (1988). *The AIDS bureaucracy: Why society failed to meet the AIDS crisis and how we might improve our response.* Cambridge, MA: Harvard University Press.

Pierson, Rick, & Daniel Egler. (1989). Repeal of AIDS testing passes. *Chicago Tribune* (June 12), 1:1.

Presidential Commission on the Human Immunodeficiency Virus Epidemic. (1988). *Report.* Washington, D.C.: U.S. Government Printing Office.

Rhame, Frank, M.D. (1989). Personal interview with director of infection control, University of Minnesota Hospital and Clinic (June 21).

Rice, Mitchell, & Mylon Winn. (1991). Black health and the American health system: A political perspective. In Theodor J. Litman & Leonard Robins (Eds.), *Health politics and policy* (2nd ed.). Albany, NY: Delmar Publishers.

Robins, Leonard, & Charles Backstrom. (1989). Book review of Sandra Panem, *The AIDS bureaucracy: Why society failed to meet the AIDS crisis and how we might improve our response. Journal of Health Politics, Policy and Law, 14* (Summer), 428–431.

Robins, Leonard, & Charles Backstrom. (1993). Public policy and political perspectives of hospital associations on AIDS. *New England Journal of Human Services, 12* (4), 2–9.

Robins, Leonard, & Charles Backstrom. (1994). The role of state Health Departments in formulating policy: A survey on the case of AIDS. *American Journal of Public Health, 84* (June), 905–909.

Shilts, Randy. (1987). *And the band played on: Politics, people, and the AIDS epidemic.* New York: St. Martin's.

EPILOGUE

Health Politics and Policy: Additional Issues and Continuing Challenges for the Twenty-first Century

Leonard S. Robins

Health politics and policy in the 1970s, 1980s, and 1990s were dominated by two major issues. There is every reason to assume that both will continue to be of central importance for the foreseeable future. Health policy has primarily been about trying to control constantly increasing health care costs and reverse the trend in the rapidly growing number of persons without health insurance. Each of these has been extensively addressed by many of the authors in this volume.

Abortion and the right to die are also high on the nation's political agenda and need comment as well. The politics of abortion has in many ways been the most contentious social issue except for race since the *Roe v. Wade* decision in 1973. Although the likelihood of Roe's reversal has greatly diminished, the bitter divisions among the public, between the parties, and within the Republican Party clearly remain.

The issue of "death and dying" is clearly moving onto the political agenda and is likely to become a major political and policy issue in the twenty-first century. While seemingly identical to the abortion issue except that it occurs at the end of life rather than at the beginning of life, the politics of death and dying is in fact somewhat different.

THE POLITICS OF ABORTION

Having an abortion requires that, at a minimum, a woman consider the following issues:

- whether or not she wants to have a baby
- the relative safety of having a baby as opposed to the risks of having an abortion
- the relative cost of having a baby as opposed to that of having an abortion
- possible legal penalties associated with having an abortion as opposed to those associated with having a baby

In China, the government encourages women in a variety of official and unofficial ways to have abortions if they have had one child and that child is still alive. The government of the United States has never encouraged abortion, and throughout most of the twentieth century prior to 1973, most of the states—the level of government that had primary policy responsibility for this issue—made abortions illegal except under certain limited (usually very limited) circumstances.

In 1973, in *Roe v. Wade* the Supreme Court radically changed this. It made all abortions legal in the first trimester of pregnancy, severely limited the right of the states to restrict abortions in the second trimester, and granted considerable discretion to states only in the last trimester. Since the vast majority of abortions occur in the first trimester, the Supreme Court essentially created a full right to an abortion.

As a consequence of the *Roe* decision, those opposed to abortion rights had to limit themselves to actions designed to induce women to want to have their babies and the modification or reversal of *Roe*. If, for example, public hospitals are legally forbidden to perform abortions and physicians and hospitals are successfully pressured to not perform abortions, then a woman desiring to have one might reconsider because she feared the health consequences of a poorly performed abortion. Similarly, while abortions are much cheaper than pregnancies, if Medicaid refuses to pay for them for eligible women, they are more expensive to the woman and she may therefore decide to have the baby.

Between 1973 and 1989, the pro-life movement was politically stronger than the pro-choice movement. An increasing number of limitations on abortion were enacted, though they never were strong enough to limit the vast majority of abortions.

The reason for the strength of the pro-life movement was not its greater overall appeal to the public. While opinion polls gave a somewhat different picture of public opinion, depending on how the questions were asked, the majority of the public clearly wanted to keep abortions legal in most of the circumstances under which they occur. Instead, the key to the strength of the pro-life movement was the greater *intensity* of feeling on the part of the pro-life supporters in contrast to those who were pro-choice.

In its final decision of the 1988–89 term, the Supreme Court in *Webster v. Reproductive Health Services* limited the scope of *Roe* and gave the states greater discretion in limiting abortions. However, while the Court seemed to suggest that the reversal of *Roe* would be shortly forthcoming, in its final decision of the 1991–92 term, the Court in *Planned Parenthood v. Casey* shocked most observers by both reaffirming *Roe* and changing and improving the legal reasoning in support of it.

While the ultimate substantive result was a reaffirmation of the legal status quo, the politics of abortion had fundamentally changed after 1989. First, the dilution of *Roe* by the *Webster* case energized the pro-choice movement. Ordinarily, political disappointment leads to political apathy. In this case, however, it appears that *Roe* itself produced pro-choice apathy because the right of abortion appeared to be fully protected by the Court. The realization that this was no longer true brought an intensity to the pro-choice movement that almost matched that of the pro-lifers.

Second, even though most of the pro-choice leadership is politically liberal and most of the pro-life leadership is politically conservative, the recent success of the pro-choice movement has revolved around its ability to tap anti-big government sentiment. Public opinion polls typically show general support for abortion rights, but many circumstances under which people would be willing to limit the right to an abortion. Yet when people are asked whether they believe government should make the decision instead of a woman and her physician, they overwhelmingly say no.

Finally, while the Democratic Party has largely united behind *Roe*, the Republican Party remains bitterly divided on abortion. Most leading Republican politicians and the rank and file are pro-life, but many in the party elite are pro-choice. Perhaps most important, many of the most attractive moderate Republicans like Colin Powell are pro-choice and their nomination for president would likely result in a conservative, pro-life, third-party movement that would badly hurt the Republicans.

Thus while antipathy to *Roe*—a liberal, pro-choice decision—helped build the political strength of pro-lifers and indirectly helped the conservative movement and President Ronald Reagan dominate politics in the 1980s, a pro-choice position on the issue is more likely to be helpful to liberals in the political struggles of the first decade of the twenty-first century.

THE POLITICS OF DEATH AND DYING

There are at least three different and, despite superficial similarities, quite distinct subjects that fall within the death and dying rubric: medical care at the end of life, physician-assisted suicide, and euthanasia.

Euthanasia is not likely to be adopted anywhere in the United States in the near future. While many opponents of physician-assisted suicide argue that it will inevitably lead to euthanasia, and they may be right, the fact that euthanasia can be successfully used politically as the ultimate pejorative demonstrates that it is politically untenable for the foreseeable future. As a society, we are not even at the stage of developing specific public policy regarding euthanasia.

The reverse is true regarding medical care at the end of life. There is now overwhelming support for giving patients the right to refuse medical treatment. The most dramatic manifestation of our changed attitudes regarding end-of-life medical care is the evolution of public policy regarding living wills. Up until the mid-1980s, living wills were explicitly and consciously ignored by health providers in the vast majority of states where they were not legally recognized. Today, by contrast, they are, for all practical purposes, legal and universally encouraged everywhere in the United States.

What accounts for these changes in public policy? First, the growing longevity of the population coupled with the increased ability of medicine to delay death means that end-of-life medical care is now a regular, albeit not routine, issue that everyone can foresee facing on a personal basis. Second, end-of-life health care costs are now substantial. In the author's view, it is the desire of patients and their families to control end-of-life medical care decisions that is the driving force behind the public policy movement giving patients and their surrogates the right to deny care that in fact often delays death more than prolongs life. It should also be emphasized that religious doctrine often supports the view that there are times when it is appropriate for patients and their surrogates to terminate care. Catholic hospitals, for example, do not perform abortions, but dying hospitalized patients need not fear that Catholic theology will result in their being forced to endure painful end-of-life treatment.

While many physicians support a health care approach that emphasizes pain alleviation and patient autonomy rather than delaying death, many others view their primary imperative as saving life and consider a patient's death as a "defeat." A few also adopt this approach out of fear of being sued. Trends in medical education coupled with the growth in the hospice movement are likely to result, however, in growing acceptance of patient choice in end-of-life decision making and, when the choice is necessary, to favor pain alleviation rather than death delay.

Many of the groups supporting patient autonomy in end-of-life decisions do not support physician-assisted suicide. To the author's knowledge, all or nearly all major religions in the United States oppose physician-assisted suicide. The hospice movement opposes physician-assisted suicide in the belief that effective hospice care, stressing effective pain control and bonding with patients, eliminates all the reasons for suicide, except for depression, which itself is a clinically treatable condition. Finally, the American Medical Association and the vast majority of physicians in the United States officially and publicly oppose physician-assisted suicide.

At the time of this writing, physician-assisted suicide is only legal in one state (Oregon), but even there it has not gone into effect because its constitutionality has been challenged.

Despite all this, Dr. Jack Kevorkian has continued to advocate and participate in physician-assisted suicides and has repeatedly been acquitted in trials by jury in the State of Michigan. This has happened because the state's statute prohibiting physicians from assisting in a patient's suicide contains a clause excusing physicians if their actions were primarily trying to end the patient's "pain and suffering." Kevorkian's successful defense has rested on the contention that the result of suicide is only the by-product of actions taken to reduce pain and suffering.

In short, as individuals and as a society we are conflicted in our attitudes toward physician-assisted suicide. To the extent that physician-assisted suicide appears to be equivalent to euthanasia, we oppose it. Conversely, when it appears similar to patient choice in end-of-life treatment, we support it.

What will happen in the future? In the short run, the most probable outcome is a continuation of current trends. Specifically, physician-assisted suicide is likely to remain illegal, but will also be performed more frequently, though still rarely, on a de facto basis without punishment.

A long-range prediction is, of course, highly speculative. Nonetheless, on balance it seems likely that physician-assisted suicide will become much more acceptable. The main reason is, as with abortion, our ever greater hostility to "big government." In this context, the argument that government should not be allowed to interfere with the doctor–patient relationship is likely to prove persuasive in the most libertarian country in the world.

THE POLITICS OF INCREASING ACCESS AND CONTAINING COSTS

In 1994, the Clinton plan for national health insurance went down to ignominious defeat. Many political observers felt this was one of the main reasons for the major Republican triumph in the 1994 elections, which resulted in Republicans taking control of the United States House of Representatives for the first time in forty years.

In 1995, as part of their efforts to balance the budget congressional Republicans proposed major cuts and programmatic changes in Medicare and Medicaid. Both were vetoed by President Clinton. In the aftermath, it was clear that the proposed Republican changes were very unpopular with the public, resulting in a major increase in popularity for President Clinton and a sharp rise in negative attitudes toward the Republicans in Congress.

One of the most damning charges made by the Republicans against the Clinton plan was that by promoting managed competition it would decrease patients' choice of physicians. Similarly, one of the strongest attacks made by the Democrats against the Republican plan was that by promoting managed care, it would decrease patients' choice of physicians. While the plans differed in many important ways, both did in fact provide strong incentives for managed care.

Instead of merely thinking, "oh well, that's politics," a better assumption is that there were understandable reasons for these actions and reactions and to see what we can learn from them.

First, resistance to dramatically overhauling the American medical care system is great. Evans in this volume eloquently demonstrates that one person's cost containment is another's income reduction. Thus, while medical care cost increases elicit growing concern among policy experts and fear and anger among the public, they also paradoxically increase the extent of vested interests having a stake in the status quo and willing to go to great lengths to defend it. For example, while Lammers in this volume shows that President Clinton directed more of his time and energy to health issues than any previous president, his efforts at promoting change, as Hinkley shows, were dwarfed by the resources devoted by the Health Insurance Association of America and the National Federation of Independent Businesses in opposing his plan.

Another main element of support for those resisting change is public opinion. Blendon and Brodie in this volume demonstrate that when public opinion is carefully analyzed, it is much less supportive of major change than many politicians and policy experts realize. There is no need to repeat their analysis, but it is important to expand it by noting that one price of evidence they present that indicates relative dissatisfaction with the American health system in fact demonstrates the opposite. Specifically, they compare relative satisfaction and dissatisfaction with their medical care system by the publics in the United States, Canada, and Germany. In this comparison (and in several previous surveys Blendon has conducted on this subject), the most dissatisfaction is shown in the United States.

On the surface, this would seem to be an argument for change. In fact, however, for purposes of political change, comparative dissatisfaction is irrelevant. The big issue is whether the public in any given country is *relatively* satisfied or dissatisfied. By this criterion, Blendon's surveys show that more people in the United States are satisfied than dissatisfied with their medical care systems. Moreover, those who are relatively satisfied tend to have higher social status and income and thus greater political influence than those who are relatively dissatisfied.

Despite the strong resistance to change, it is highly unlikely that attempts at comprehensive reform will go into hibernation for twenty years as they did after failed efforts in the 1970s, 1950s, and 1930s. This is true for several reasons.

First, the number of uninsured is likely to grow. This is true even if action is taken that makes insurance coverage more portable. The continued drift in employment from unionized large manufacturing firms to nonunionized small firms providing services means a continuing shift of employment to those sectors of the workforce least likely to be covered by health insurance. Additionally, a conscious climate of conservatism discouraging employers from providing fringe benefits is another reason for believing that the number of workers and their families covered by relatively comprehensive health insurance is likely to continue to decline.

Second, the ability of hospitals and other health providers to provide uncompensated care is likely to shrink. Fraser in this volume shows the growth in the

amount of uncompensated care in recent years. Since one of the main ways managed care contains costs is by not paying extra premiums to help hospitals and other providers pay for their uncompensated care, the continued growth of managed care means less and less ability for providers to pay for such services.

These two trends mean there will be inevitable medical care cost pressures on government even if managed care succeeds in controlling overall medical care costs to the extent that they do not constitute a growing percentage of the gross national product. Government activism in health care finance and efforts to control *its* health care costs are thus likely to increase, even if national health insurance itself remains off the agenda.

While short-term political calculations are likely to keep national health insurance off the political agenda during the remainder of the 1990s, long-term political strategy suggests that it will ultimately return to center stage. The findings of Blendon and Brodie do not provide support for the view that advocating major change is good politics, but they also suggest that *after enactment* national health insurance is likely to be quite popular. More broadly, it would be an important example of government working in providing a service that is of concern to and benefiting the entire population rather than a program perceived to only be of benefit to the poor or minorities.

But at the end of the day the question of how to get over the hump of initial opposition to fundamental health reform still remains. On a tactical level, while the Clinton strategy of going beyond the labor–liberal base by working to achieve business support was not well managed, it was also probably fundamentally flawed. The understandable antigovernment ideology of business and its fear of setting a precedent by supporting government control and regulation is likely to mean that the neutrality of business is the best national health insurance advocates can hope for.

A more likely ally would be the provider community. For decades, as Morone notes in this volume, health professionals fought the idea of losing power to government only to see it transferred to the market. It is not at all clear that either health professionals' interests or their ideological preferences make market power preferable to government power.

It must be admitted that the provider community (nurses being an exception, as Hinckley notes in this volume) has shown little interest in supporting any national health insurance program that has effective cost-containment provisions. Whether they would be willing to accept compromise national health insurance proposals from a labor–liberal coalition seeking a true alliance is unknown. Unfortunately, however, it has not been tried since each has viewed the other as its primary enemy in medical care politics and policy. This may have been true in the past, but is surely no longer true today.

One final point. While Medicare was politically popular, the key to its enactment was the election of an overwhelmingly Democratic and liberal Congress and president. The issue of Medicare helped get them elected, but it was not the main reason for their election. It was after the passage of Medicare, as Brandon notes in this volume, that the elderly became a more conscious and cohesive interest group. Perhaps national health insurance will also have to wait for a political climate conducive to major health reform, but as Morone argues in this volume, it will importantly redound to the political benefit of those who are responsible for its enactment.

APPENDIX

A Chronology and Capsule Highlights of the Major Historical and Political Milestones in the Evolution of the Relationship of Government Involvement in Health and Health Care in the United States

Theodor J. Litman

1730 American seamen (then British subjects) are taxed to pay for hospital care.

1760 New York City adopts licensure requirement for physicians to practice medicine.

1772 New Jersey legislature adopts an act to regulate medical practice requiring that all persons wishing to practice medicine be examined and approved by any two judges of the Supreme Court. This act serves as a colonial prototype of later state boards of medical examiners.

1776 The first national disability-related law, the Pension Act of 1776, providing compensation to soldiers and sailors who lost a limb or became so disabled by a war injury that they could not work, is enacted, granting half pay for life or as long as the disability lasts.

1780 Virginia taxes seamen for hospital care.

1798 The Fifth Congress passes act to tax seamen for health care and establishes the U.S. Marine Hospital Service to provide medical care for sick and disabled seamen—in essence, the first prepaid medical care program in the United States.

1809 The Commonwealth of Massachusetts adopts the nation's first compulsory vaccination (smallpox) law.

1846 In response to a call from the New York State Medical Society, a preliminary meeting of delegates from medical societies and colleges from throughout the United States is held at New York University to explore the establishment of a national physicians' organization (a forerunner of the American Medical Association—AMA).

1847 The American Medical Association is established. Under its charter, representation is to be comprised of delegates from state, county, and local medical societies, institutions, and medical colleges in a fixed numerical ratio.

1854 Congress passes a bill providing for federal financing of the indigent insane, signifying the first federal action dealing with public welfare. The measure, however, is vetoed by President Pierce on the grounds that the federal government should not be involved in any welfare program.

1855 The first state board of health is established in Louisiana (Freedman, 1951).

1872 The American Public Health Association (APHA) is founded.

1878 The National Quarantine Act is passed.

1891 The National Confederation of State Medical Examining and Licensing Boards is founded.

1899 The classic legal recognition for the practice of state aid to church-related welfare institutions such as hospitals is given by the U.S. Supreme Court in the case of *Bradfield v. Roberts* 175 US 299 (1899).

1902 The Public Health Service is reorganized and renamed the Public Health and Marine Hospital Service.

1904 A uniform curriculum, recommended to all faculties, is adopted by the National Confederation of State Medical Examining and Licensing Boards.

1905 The U.S. Supreme Court upholds the constitutionality of Massachusetts Compulsory Vaccination Law [*Jacobson v. Commonwealth of Massachusetts* 197 US 11 (1905)].

1906 The first bill to establish a national children's bureau is introduced.

1906 PL 59-384, the Pure Food and Drug or "Wiley" Act, is passed prohibiting the transport of adulterated and misbranded foods and drugs in interstate commerce.

1908 Although limited in that it only applies to women working in heavy industry and to the length of the shift, the Supreme Court in *Muller v. Oregon* upholds a ten-hour workday for female industrial workers, justifying its ruling on the basis of the state's interest in protecting the "mothers of the race" and the principle that gender is a valid basis for legislative classification. The Court's justification serves as the precedence under which fetal protection policies are instituted, defended, and upheld by the courts over the next eighty years.

1909 President Theodore Roosevelt calls together a conference (later to be known as the first White House Conference on Children) of some two hundred professional and lay leaders interested in the care of dependent children.

1910 The Flexner Report, commissioned by the Carnegie Foundation, condemns the current state of medical education in the United States and proposes major reforms that are to transform medical education from a guild apprenticeship model to a university-hospital-based enterprise modeled after that of the Johns Hopkins University.

1912 On a vote of 54 to 20 with 17 not voting in the Senate and 177 to 17 with 190 not voting in the House, a bill calling for the establishment of a children's bureau is passed and approved by President Taft.

1912 Social insurance, including health insurance, is endorsed in the platform of the Progressive Party and espoused by its candidate, Theodore Roosevelt.

1912 The Public Health and Marine Hospital Service is renamed the U.S. Public Health Service.

1913 The American College of Surgeons (ACS) is formed to further a more structured examination of surgical practice in the United States.

1916 Samuel Gompers, one of organized labor's early patriarchs, reaffirms his opposition to any form of government-sponsored compulsory health insurance as infringing on labor's right to bargain.

1917 Congress passes an amendment to the War Risk Insurance Act to provide medical benefits to veterans with service-connected disabilities.

1917 The AMA's house of delegates passes a resolution stating principles to be followed in government health insurance plans.

1918 First federal grants are given to states for public health services.

1920 The AMA's house of delegates reverses its position, declaring its unequivocal opposition to compulsory health insurance.

1920 Congress passes the first Vocational Rehabilitation Act. Passage rests less on humanitarian than utilitarian terms; that is, it would put people on the productive tax rolls.

1920 The Snyder Act (PL 66-141) is the first federal legislation pertaining to health care for Native Americans. The act directs the Bureau of Indian Affairs under the supervision of the secretary of the interior to direct, supervise, and expend funds appropriated by Congress for the "benefit, care and assistance of the Indians throughout the United States."

1920 Several state commissions study a standard bill for health insurance and conclude that it is neither needed nor wanted. State interest then wanes.

1921 Congress enacts (PL 67-97) the first Maternity and Infancy Act (Sheppard–Towner), which provided grants to states to develop health services for mothers and children. The act is a prototype for federal grants-in-aid to the states.

1924 Congress passes the World War Veteran's Act, providing more liberal hospital benefits to all war veterans.

1924 A bill to remove a prohibition against contraceptives and information on contraception fails to win congressional approval.

1929 The first Blue Cross plan in the United States is established at Baylor University, Dallas, Texas.

1929 Assailed and opposed in Congress as "drawn chiefly from the radical, socialistic, behavioristic philosophy of Germany and Russia" and denounced by the AMA as an "imported socialistic scheme," the Sheppard–Towner Act is allowed to lapse.

1930 The National Institute of Health (NIH) is created as the administrative home for the medical research of the Public Health Service (PHS).

1932 The report of the Committee on the Cost of Medical Care (CCMC) is published calling for the organization of the U.S. medical services on a group practice, prepayment basis. Despite the preeminence of its compilers and extensive documentation, the report is rejected out of hand by the AMA as socialistic and inimical to the best interests of the people of the United States.

1933 Enactment of the Federal Emergency Relief Act affords the first federal financing of medical care for the aged as funds are made available to states through the Federal Emergency Relief Administration (FERA) to pay medical expenses for people receiving relief. However, in most states, only emergency medical and dental care is provided for.

1935 On January 17, President Franklin D. Roosevelt sends to Congress the report of the President's Committee on Economic Security, which is to form the basis of the Social Security Act (PL 74-271) (SSA) passed later that year. The report endorses the principle of compulsory national health insurance (NHI) but makes no specific program recommendations. In his accompanying message, the president states that he is not planning to recommend adoption of "so-called health insurance at this time." His decision not to recommend national health insurance reportedly is based, in part, on the fear that opposition to it would endanger passage of the entire Social Security Act, and, in part, on the belief that the nation's medical facilities were inadequate to sustain such a program and needed to be beefed up first through public health facility grants and other similar efforts.

1935 On July 15, the first government health insurance bill is introduced in Congress—the Epstein Bill sponsored by Senator Capper.

1935 Congress passes and the president signs (August 14) the Social Security Act (PL 74-271), which includes provisions for grants-in-aid to states for maternal and child care, aid to crippled children, aid to the blind, the aged, and other health-impaired people.

1935 The first National Health Survey is conducted.

1936 Congress authorizes federal regulation of industrial safety in companies doing business with the government through passage of the Walsh–Healy Act (PL 74-846).

1937 The first categorical institute, the National Cancer Institute, is established under the National Cancer Institute Act (PL 75-244).

1938 The National Health Conference calls for expansion of public health services, provision of medical services to people at the lowest income levels at public expense, and medical insurance at the state level for the rest of the population.

1938 The LaFollette–Bulwinkle Act (venereal disease—VD control) (PL 75-540) provides grants-in-aid to states and other authorities to investigate and control VD.

1938 The federal Food, Drug, and Cosmetic Act (PL 75-717) extends federal authority to act against adulterated and misbranded food, drugs, and cosmetic products, banning new drugs until approved by the federal Food and Drug Administration (FDA).

1939 Senator Robert Wagner (D-NY) introduces a bill based on recommendations of the 1938 National Health Conference calling for federally subsidized state medical care compensation. No action is taken, however.

1939 The Public Health Service is transferred from the Treasury Department to the new Federal Security Agency by the Reorganization Act of 1939 (PL 76-19).

1939 The AMA, the District of Columbia Medical Society, and the Harris, Texas Medical Society are indicted for violation of the Sherman Antitrust Case over their efforts to restrict physicians in prepaid group practice from practicing medicine.

1940 After a lengthy trial, the AMA and the District of Columbia Medical Society are found guilty of restraint of trade in their battle against prepaid medicine. Despite their legal reversal, organized medicine is successful in getting legislation passed at the state level prohibiting the corporate practice of medicine. Many such restrictions remain in existence today and limit the growth and development of health maintenance organizations (HMOs).

1941 The Nurse Training Act (PL 77-146) gives schools of nursing support to increase their enrollments and help strengthen their facilities.

1941 The Physicians Forum, a liberal-based physicians' organization, is formed by dissident members of the New York County Medical Society to work for the adoption of compulsory health insurance.

1942 Rhode Island becomes the first state to pass a health insurance law.

1942 A *Fortune* magazine poll reports that 75 percent of the public favors national health insurance.

1943 The first Wagner (Sen. Robert, D-NY), Murray (Sen. James E., D-MT), Dingell (Rep. John D., Sr., D-MI) Bill (S 1161, HR 2861) calling for sweeping revisions and broadening of the Social Security Act, including a compulsory national health system for people of all ages financed through a payroll tax, is introduced in the Senate and the House. No action is taken on the measure, however, by the Seventy-eighth Congress. Opponents call the bill "the most virulent scheme ever to be conjured out of the mind of man" and depict a revised version to mean "the end of freedom for all classes of Americans."

1944 President Roosevelt, in his January 11 State of the Union Address, outlines an Economic Bill of Rights, which includes "the right to adequate care and the opportunity to achieve and enjoy good health." Although interpreted by many to imply that the president favored a national health insurance system, no subsequent recommendations of any such enabling legislation to Congress is forthcoming.

1944 The APHA adopts a set of principles on comprehensive health care for all people in the United States financed through social insurance supported by general taxation or by general taxation alone.

1944 All public health service authorities are consolidated into a single statute (42 U.S. Code) under the Public Health Service Act (PL 78-410).

1945 Wagner, Murray, and Dingell reintroduce the same broad bill that they had sponsored in 1943.

1945 On November 19, President Harry S. Truman sends a message on health legislation to Congress calling for comprehensive, prepaid medical insurance for all people of all ages, to be financed through a 4 percent rise in the Social Security Old Age and Survivors Insurance Tax. His proposal is quickly introduced in the Senate and House by Senators Wagner and Murray and Representative Dingell. The bill, however, languishes in Congress and no action is taken.

1946 The National Mental Health Act (PL 79-487) authorizes major federal support for mental health research, diagnosis, prevention, and treatment, establishes state grants-in-aid for mental health, and changes the PHS Division of Mental Health to the National Institute of Mental Health.

1946 Recognizing a shortage in health care services and the antiquated status of the nation's hospital facilities, Congress enacts the Hospital Survey and Construction Act (PL 79-725) (Hill–Burton) providing for national direct support for the development of community hospitals, ostensibly rural facilities, and for the first time attempts to mandate, at least, rudimentary standards for construction and the insistence on regional planning. At the same time, however, the act carries a hidden time bomb that only comes to light thirty some years later, that is, a requirement that recipients provide a "reasonable volume of services to those unable to pay"—a free care obligation—and make their facilities "available to all persons residing in their service areas"—a community service obligation.

1946 The Communicable Disease Center is established in Atlanta, Georgia, and the Census Bureau's Division of Vital Statistics is transferred to the Public Health Service as the National Office of Vital Statistics.

1946 California passes a compulsory health insurance act.

1948 The National Health Act (PL 80-655) establishes the National Heart Institute, pluralizing NIH.

1949 Flushed with success after upset victories in the 1948 presidential and congressional elections that found the Democratic Party in control of both houses of Congress plus the White House, President Truman again calls for compulsory national health insurance in his January 5 State of the Union Address.

1949 Hearings on bills embodying the proposals sponsored by Senators Murray and Wagner (S 1679) and Representative Dingell and others (HR 43121) produces bitter controversy and heavy lobbying on both sides of the issue.

1949 The AMA sets up a $3.5 million war chest and mobilizes a massive campaign to defeat what they consider to be socialized medicine and a threat to the free practice of medicine in the United States, using the talents of the California public relations firm of Whitaker and Baxter for a fee of $100,000 and assessing each physician $25 to support their efforts. No congressional action in either house is taken.

1950 The president repeats his earlier request for compulsory national health insurance, but again no congressional action is forthcoming. Instead, Congress moves to help the states provide medical care for welfare recipients supported by the four federal–state public assistance programs for the indigent, that is, Old Age Assistance (OAA), Aid to Dependent Children (ADC), Aid to the Blind (AB), and Aid to the Permanently and Totally Disabled (APTD). Amendments to the Social Security Act provide for federal sharing with the states in vendor payments, that is, payments to providers as well as the direct payments of living expenses to recipients.

1950 PL 81-507 establishes the National Science Foundation as an autonomous entity and strengthens the concept of federal support for university-based research in physical, medical, and social sciences.

1951 Durham–Humphrey amendments (PL 8-2-215) establish a category of prescription drugs requiring labeling and medical supervision.

1952 The Joint Commission on Accreditation of Hospitals (JCAH) is established.

1952 A bill (S 3001, HR 7484-85) is introduced in Congress by Senator Murray and Representatives Dingell and Celler (Emanuel D., D-NY) calling for the payment of hospitalization costs for retired people and their dependents or survivors under the Social Security Old Age and Survivors Insurance (OASI) system. No action is taken, however.

1953 The Federal Security Agency (FSA) is transformed into the Department of Health, Education, and Welfare (DHEW) and elevated to cabinet status.

1954 The Hill–Burton Act is amended (PL 83-482, Medical Facilities Survey and Construction Act) to expand the scope of the program to include nursing homes, rehabilitation facilities, chronic disease hospitals, and diagnostic or treatment centers.

1954 Responsibility for maintenance and operation of Indian health facilities is placed in PHS rather than the Bureau of Indian Affairs (PL 83-568).

1955 The U.S. Major trade unions—the American Federation of Labor (AFL) and Congress of Industrial Organization (CIO)—merge (AFL-CIO) and set health insurance for the aged as a top priority.

1955 The American Hospital Association's board of trustees passes a resolution recommending federal subsidies to the states to begin voluntary health insurance programs for older people, and the concept is approved by the association's house of delegates.

1955 PL 84-377 (Polio Vaccination Assistance Act) provides assistance to state vaccination programs.

1956 The Social Security Act is further amended to permit separate federal matching funds for medical care payments on an individual basis in addition to cash assistance.

1956 The Dependents Medical Care Act (PL 84-569) sets up CHAMPUS program of primarily inpatient medical care for military dependents.

1956 PL 84-911, the Health Amendments Act of 1956, constitutes the first federal legislation addressed specifically to the question of health manpower, authorizing traineeships for public health personnel and advanced training for professional nurses.

1956 The National Health Survey Act (PL 84-652) provides for a continuing survey and special sickness and disability-studies of the U.S. population.

1956 PL 84-941 transfers responsibility for the Library of Medicine to the Public Health Service.

1957 The Forand (Rep. Aime J., D-RI) Bill (HR 9467) calling for an increase in the Social Security OASI payroll tax to provide for up to 120 days of combined hospital and nursing home care as well as necessary surgery for aged OASI beneficiaries is introduced. Although no action is taken by Congress, the Forand bill begins to draw increasing public interest and debate. Both the American Hospital Association (AHA) and American Nurses Association (ANA) endorse the bill.

1958 The AMA sets up the joint council to improve the health care of the aged comprised of the AMA, AHA, the American Dental Association (ADA), and the American Nursing Home Association, which concludes that the health care of the aged does not need improvement. Not represented in the council is the ANA, which in 1957 had supported in principle the Forand bill.

1958 PL 85-929, the Food Additive Amendment to the Food, Drug, and Cosmetics Act, requires premarketing clearance for new food additives, establishes a generally recognized as safe (GRAS) category, and prohibits under the so-called Delaney clause the approval of any additive "found to induce cancer in man or animal."

1958 The Small Business Administration is authorized to provide loans to nursing homes through the Small Business Act and the Small Business Investment Act.

1958 A program of formula grants to schools of public health is established (PL 85-544).

1959 The House Ways and Means Committee holds hearings on Forand's reintroduced bill, but no action is taken.

1959 Blue Cross negotiates a contract with the Civil Service Commission to provide health insurance coverage for federal employees under PL 86-352, Federal Employees Health Benefits Act. The contract serves as a foot-in-the-door and a prototype for Blue Cross's later involvement in Medicare–Medicaid.

1960 The Forand bill becomes a major political issue, supported by organized labor and liberal Democrats and opposed by the AMA, most Republicans including President Eisenhower, most business and insurance groups, and political conservatives.

1960 On March 31, the House Ways and Means Committee on a 17 (Dem. 7, Rep. 10) to 8 (Dem. 8, Rep. 0) vote to table the Forand bill. Voting in favor of killing the bill are Committee Chairman Wilber D. Mills (D-AK) and six other southern representatives.

1960 On May 4, in testimony before the Ways and Means Committee, the Eisenhower administration unveils its own "Medicare" program, which it proposes will help the needy aged meet the costs of catastrophic illness without using the compulsory national health insurance feature proposed under the Forand bill. Under the administration's plan, federal matching grants would be offered to the states to help them pay for a varied list of specified medical, hospital, and nursing costs for elderly persons with incomes of $2,500 a year or less ($3,800 for a couple). Individuals would have the option of receiving cash payments to help them purchase private commercial health insurance.

1960 In August, Congress passes the Kerr (Sen. Robert S., D-OK)–Mills (Rep. Wilbur D.) Bill (PL 86-778—Title XVI of the Social Security Act) providing additional federal matching funds to the states for vendor payments under the Old Age Assistance Act as well as federal matching funds for the medically needy aged, creating a new public assistance category—Medical Assistance for the Aged (MAA). The significance of the MAA program (Bernard and Feingold, 1970) lay in (1) its recognition of medical indigence, (2) its introduction of open funding by the federal government, and (3) the introduction of some minimal standard to the substance and administration of public assistance medical care.

1961 The White House Conference on Aging is held and the issue of medical care to the elderly is debated.

1961 The King–Anderson bill, embodying President Kennedy's proposal to provide health insurance for the elderly through the Social Security system is introduced in both houses of Congress by Senator Anderson (Clinton, D-NM) and Representative King (Cecil, D-CA) [*Note:* As a senator, the president had earlier sponsored a Senate version of the Forand bill (S 2915).] Although normally an administration's legislative initiatives are sponsored by the highest-ranking member of the president's party on the committee with jurisdiction over it, since both Senate Finance Committee chairman Harry F. Byrd (D-VA) and Ways and Means chairman Mills were opposed to the president's proposal, the bill carried the sponsorship of Congressman King and Senator

Anderson. The latter had earlier proposed a revised version of the Forand–Kennedy bill in the Senate Finance Committee in 1960 but it was rejected. Hearings on the proposed legislation are held by the Ways and Means Committee but no action is taken.

1962 The AMA sets up AMPAC, a political action committee analogous to the AFL-CIO's COPE to fight the Kennedy proposal for medical care for the aged.

1962 PL 87-692, Health Services for Agricultural Migratory Workers Act, authorizes federal aid to clinics serving migratory agricultural workers and their families.

1962 PL 87-781, Kefauver–Harris drug amendments, requires improved manufacturing practices, better reporting, assurances of efficacy, as well as safety and strengthened regulation of the drug industry.

1962 On January 3, the AHA drops its opposition to federal funding, averring that the source of funding is of secondary importance and federal assistance a necessity.

1962 Continued inaction by the House Ways and Means Committee leads Senator Anderson to offer a revised version of the administration's medical care for the aged proposal as an amendment on the floor of the Senate, to the Public Welfare Amendment (HR 10606) that already had been passed by the House. The Anderson amendment, co-sponsored by five Republicans, headed by Senator Jacob K. Javits (R-NY), proposes a one-quarter of one percent increase on the OASDI payroll tax on each employer and employee and three-eighths of one percent on the self-employed, as well as a rise to $5,200 in the wage base for the tax, with additional revenues to be earmarked to pay for all or most of the costs of a long list of hospital (90 days inpatient care), nursing home (180 days, skilled care), and diagnostic services for people sixty-five years of age and older eligible for OASDI old age benefits, as well as certain other people not otherwise eligible for OASDI benefits.

1962 On July 17, in a dramatic roll call vote, Senate Republicans and southern Democrats unite to kill the Anderson amendment on a 52 (Dem. 21, Rep. 31) to 48 (Dem. 43, Rep. 5) vote.

1963 The Health Professions Educational Assistance Act (PL 88-129) provides construction money for health professions schools, funds tied to increase enrollment requirements to assist with the school's operating expenses, plus loans and scholarship programs. It authorizes support to medical schools for the first time and establishes the presence of the federal government in health-related educational institutions.

1963 The Blue Cross Association of America, under the leadership of its president, Walter McNerney, issues a report in support of government financing of medical care for the aged, noting the problem the high cost of health care poses for the elderly, hospitals, and third-party carriers.

1963 PL 88-156, Maternal and Child Health and Mental Retardation Planning Amendments, initiates a program of comprehensive maternity, infant care, and mental retardation prevention.

1963 PL 88-164, Community Mental Health Centers Construction Act, seeks to bring comprehensive mental health services to patients in their own communities and further deinstitutionalization.

1963 PL 88-206, Clean Air Act, authorizes direct grants to state and local governments for air pollution control and establishes federal enforcement in interstate air pollution.

1963 The AMA raises several million dollars to fight Medicare.

1964 PL 88-525 authorizes the food stamp program for low-income people to purchase nutritious foods for a balanced diet.

1964 PL 88-581, Nurse Training Act, provides a special federal effort for training professional nursing personnel.

1964 The Hill–Burton act is amended to set aside moneys for the modernization and replacement of health care facilities.

1965 Congress amends the Social Security Act (PL 89-97) providing for medical care for the elderly

(Medicare—Title 18) and grants to the states for medical assistance to the poor (Medicaid—Title 19), on a vote of 307 to 116 in the House and 70 to 24 in the Senate, and President Lyndon B. Johnson signs it into law on July 30. The act also extends Social Security coverage to physicians.

1965 The conservative Association of American Physicians and Surgeons urges its 16,500 members not to cooperate with the program. The AMA, on the other hand, cautions against a physicians' boycott. The legislative defeat leads to the forced retirement of Dr. Morris Fishbein, former editor of the *Journal of the American Medical Association* (1924–49) and the long-time, erstwhile spokesman of organized medicine as executive secretary of the AMA. He is replaced by Dr. Frank Blasingame, who later is summarily dismissed in 1968.

1965 PL 89-239 amends the Public Health Service Act and establishes a nationwide network of regional medical programs (RMPs) for heart disease, cancer, and stroke. The legislation is an outgrowth of the President's Commission on Heart Disease, Cancer, and Stroke headed by Dr. Michael DeBakey.

1965 PL 89-272, Clean Air Act Amendments, provides for federal regulation of Motor Vehicle Exhaust (Title I) and establishes a program of federal research and grants-in-aid in solid waste disposal (Title II).

1965 PL 89-290, Health Professions Educational Assistance Amendments, provides scholarships, loans, and construction aid to schools of medicine, osteopathy, and dentistry. Introduces provision of 50 percent forgiveness of loans for service in personnel shortage areas.

1965 Congress authorizes a program of special project grants for health of school and preschool children under Title V of the Social Security Act Amendments (PL 89-97), including the delivery of compulsory health services to low-income children. Out of this legislation come the Children and Youth (C and Y) projects and clinics administered through the Maternal and Child Health Service (Lewis et al., 1976).

1965 PL 89-73, The Older Americans Act, establishes an Administration on Aging within DHEW headed by a commissioner of aging appointed by the president. It declares ten objectives for older people, which are the joint responsibility of federal, state, and local governments.

1965 PL 89-92, The Federal Cigarette Labeling and Advertising Act, requires that all cigarette packages or containers offered for sale in the United States must bear the warning statement: "Caution: Cigarette Smoking May be Hazardous to Your Health." The new law preempts the field of cigarette labeling, precluding any federal, state, or local authority in the area.

1966 An amendment (PL 89-749) to the Office of Economic Opportunity (OED) legislation formalizes the Comprehensive Health Services program, including the provision for the establishment of neighborhood health centers.

1966 PL 89-749, The Comprehensive Health Planning Act, is passed to promote comprehensive planning for health services, personnel, and facilities in federal-state-local partnership.

1966 PL 89-614 broadens eligibility to CHAMPUS and extends benefits beyond inpatient care.

1966 PL 89-642, Child Nutrition Act, establishes a federal program of research and support for child nutrition, including authorization for school breakfast program.

1966 PL 89-751, Allied Health Professions Personnel Act, provides initial effort to support the training of allied health workers.

1967 Amendment to the Social Security Act (PL 90-248) seeks to raise the quality of care provided in nursing homes, establishing a number of conditions of nursing home participation under Medicare and Medicaid. Creates a new class of facility—the intermediate care facility. Establishes educational requirements for long-term care facility administrators (Kennedy amendment). The latter constitutes the first time that educational requirements for licensure are mandated by legislative fiat at the federal level.

1968 PL 90-407 amends the National Science Foundation to include major support of applied research in the sciences.

1968 PL 90-490, Health Manpower Act, authorizes formula institutional grants for training all health professionals and adds pharmacy and veterinary medicine to the professions covered.

1968 The Social Security Act is amended to strengthen the nursing home enforcement activities of the individual states. No federal matching funds may be paid to any nursing home that does not fully meet state requirements for licensure. States are also required, as part of their medical assistance program for skilled nursing home care, to evaluate each patient's needs prior to admission, followed by regular and periodic inspections of the care being given to medical assistance patients in nursing homes.

1969 PL 91-173, Federal Coal Mine Health and Safety Act, provides for protection of the health and safety of coal miners.

1969 PL 91-190, National Environmental Policy Act, creates the Council on Environmental Quality to advise the president on environmental matters; requires preparation of environmental impact statements before major federal actions.

1969 In an effort to slow the rise in Medicaid costs, the secretary of DHEW issues regulations setting an upper limit (75th percentile of customary charges) on fees to be paid to individual practitioners.

1969 Amidst a hail of legislative and newspaper criticism of the Medicaid program and the fees physicians receive under it, New Mexico becomes the first state in the nation to drop out of the program as the state legislature adjourns without appropriating funds for the program for the coming fiscal year. In doing so, the legislature directs state officials to seek reentry into the program on a reduced basis, providing the five basic services—a reduction in the scope of the program that would disqualify it from receiving federal matching funds.

1970 PL 91-222, Public Health Cigarette Smoking Act, bans cigarette advertising from radio and television.

1970 The Communicable Disease Center is renamed the Center for Disease Control (CDC), and its functions are broadened under PL 91-464 to address other preventable conditions in addition to infectious disease.

1970 PL 91-596, Occupational Safety and Health Act (OSHA), provides federal program of standard setting and enforcement to assure safe and healthful conditions in the workplace.

1970 PL 91-616 establishes National Institute of Alcohol Abuse and Alcoholism and provides comprehensive aid program to states and localities.

1970 PL 91-623, Emergency Health Personnel Act, provides for assistance to health manpower shortage areas through the establishment of the National Health Service Corps.

1971 In his February health message to Congress, President Nixon introduces the notion of health maintenance organizations (HMOs) as the cornerstone of his administration's national health insurance proposal.

1971 The health industry is singled out for special stringent controls under the Economic Stabilization Act (and is the last segment of the economy to be relieved of such controls three years later).

1971 PL 92-157, Comprehensive Health Manpower Training Act, covering programs for students in medicine, osteopathy, dentistry, veterinary medicine, optometry, pharmacy, and podiatry replaces institutional formula grants with capitation grants. Provides for schools to receive a fixed sum of money for each student in return for agreeing to increase its enrollment by a specified percentage. Adds interest subsidies and loan guarantees to outright grants for construction (the sole previous financing mechanism under earlier programs) as the federal government assumes an active role in the funding of primary care. The act is the most comprehensive piece of health manpower legislation to date. A shift from support to control is evident (Losteller and Chapman, 1979).

1972 PL 92-303 amends the Federal Coal Mine Health and Safety Act, providing benefits and other assistance for coal miners suffering from black lung disease.

1972 PL 92-426 establishes a Uniformed Services University of the Health Sciences and an Armed Forces Health Professions Scholarship program.

1972 PL 92-433, The National School Lunch and Child Nutrition Amendments, adds funds to support nutritious diets for pregnant and lactating women and for infants and children (the WIC program).

1972 PL 92-541 authorizes the Veterans Administration (VA) to help establish eight state medical schools and provides grant support to existing medical schools.

1972 PL 92-573, Consumer Product Safety Act, creates the Consumer Product Safety Commission and transfers enforcement of hazardous substances, flammable fabrics, poison prevention packaging acts to the commissions.

1972 PL 92-585, Emergency Health Personnel Act Amendments of 1972, establishes Public Health and National Health Services Corps scholarships.

1972 PL 92-603, amendments of the Social Security Act, establishes, over the bitter opposition of organized medicine, professional standards review organizations (PSROs) to monitor the need and quality of care rendered to recipients of federal health programs. Extends health insurance benefits to the disabled and end-stage renal disease patients.

1972 PL 93-154, Emergency Medical Services Systems Act, provides aid to state and localities to establish coordinated cost-effective emergency medical service (EMS) systems.

1972 Blue Cross, at McNerney's urging and in response to public pressure concerning conflict of interest, severs formal ties with AHA.

1973 PL 93-222, Health Maintenance Organization Act, provides assistance for the establishment and expansion of HMOs. Authorizes $375 million over a five-year period for grants, loans, and loan guarantees for feasibility studies, development studies, and initial operations for new and existing HMOs.

1973 Congress passes the Older Americans Act that shifts the Administration on Aging from HEW's Social and Rehabilitation section to the Office of the Secretary, establishes the National Clearinghouse for Information on Aging, creates the Federal Council on Aging, and authorizes funds for the establishment of gerontology centers and grants for training and research in the field of aging.

1973 The National Institute of Occupational Safety and Health (NIOSH) is incorporated into the Center for Disease Control.

1973 The Supreme Court (*Roe v. Wade*, 410 U.S. 113, 93 S. Ct. 705) declares laws outlawing abortion unconstitutional.

1974 PL 93-247, Child Abuse Prevention and Treatment Act, creates a National Center on Child Abuse and Neglect, and authorizes research and demonstration grants to states and other private and public agencies.

1974 PL 93-296, Research in Aging Act, establishes National Institute on Aging within the National Institutes of Health (NIH).

1974 PL 93-523, Safe Drinking Water Act, requires the Environmental Protection Agency to set national drinking water standards and aid states and localities in their enforcement.

1974 Moss (Sen. Frank, D-UT) Senate Subcommittee on Nursing Homes issues an extensive report detailing abuses in the nursing home industry.

1974 Hawaii becomes first state in the nation to enact comprehensive health care reform legislation (Hawaii Prepaid Health Care Act of 1974) mandating that all employers offer their employees and their dependents a basic health care package. Although nullified by the passage of ERISA later that year (see next page), Congress grants the state a special exemption, permitting the program to operate as long as it is not changed without congressional approval.

1974 PL 93-406, the Employee Retirement Income Security Act (ERISA), is signed into law. Although originally intended to protect workers' pension rights, health and medical benefits are placed under its exclusive domain almost as an afterthought. Because it contains no substantive standards for health benefits and precludes the states from imposing their own, it provides self-insured employers and their insurance plans protection from interference by either the state or the beneficiaries of the plans and proves to be a serious obstacle to later efforts by the states to enact health care reform.

1974 Louisiana becomes last state in the Union to license chiropractors. The U.S. Office of Education gives the Chiropractic Commission on Education the power to accredit chiropractic colleges. Congress sets aside $12 million of NIH's annual budget to ascertain the scientific merits and basis for chiropractic, and chiropractic fees are declared reimbursable under Medicare.

1975 PL 93-641, the National Health Planning and Resources Development Act, sets up national designation of local health systems areas and authorizes major federal reorganization of health planning programs. Establishes a national certificate-of-need (CON) program.

1975 Rhode Island enacts the first state catastrophic health insurance program.

1975 In the face of soaring medical malpractice insurance premiums and the flight of commercial insurers from the state, which threatens to leave its health care providers bereft of coverage, the California state legislature passes a landmark Medical Injury Claims Reduction Act (MICRA) calling for a variety of tort reforms and limitations on the malpractice awards a plaintiff can receive.

1976 PL 94-484, Health Professions Educational Assistance Act, requires medical schools to have 50 percent of their graduates nationally entering primary residencies by 1980. Continues capitation payments but no longer requires enrollment increases as a condition for funding. Mandates that recipient schools reserve positions in their classes for U.S. students studying at foreign medical schools as a condition for receiving federal financial support. The latter provision is heatedly opposed by the U.S. medical schools as an unwarranted infringement on their right to determine admissions. Northwestern, Indiana, and Yale Universities announce that they will not comply even if it should mean loss of federal funding.

1976 Medicare and Medicaid are transferred from the Social Security Administration and Social and Rehabilitation Service (SRS) and combined into a new agency, the Health Care Financing Administration (HCFA).

1976 In a unanimous decision, the Supreme Court rules (*Bellotti v. Baird*) that states may require minors seeking abortions to obtain parental consent under certain circumstances. In two other cases, it rules 6–3 that states cannot require a woman seeking an abortion to obtain her husband's consent (*Planned Parenthood of Central Missouri v. Danforth*) and by a 5–4 vote, it decides that an unmarried minor does not need written parental consent to receive an abortion. States, however, may still require a woman to sign a consent form.

1976 Over the strenuous opposition of the hospital industry, Congress tightens up the immigration rules amending the Immigration and Nationality Act (Sections 101 and 212) to restrict the entry of alien physicians into the United States and imposes stringent constraints on the licensure of foreign medical graduates, including the requirement of passage of the VISA and/or FLEX exam, declaring that "there is no longer an insufficient number of physicians and surgeons in the United States" and that "there is no further need for affording preference to alien physicians and surgeons in admission to the United States."

1977 PL 95-210, Rural Health Clinic Act, extends Medicare and Medicaid coverage to new health practitioners in rural clinics.

1977 In both *Maher v. Roe* and *Beal v. Doe*, the Supreme Court on a vote of 6–3 rules that states may prohibit the use of public funds for medically unnecessary abortions. In addition, in another case (*Poelker v. Doe*) the Court decides 6–3 that public hospitals may refuse to perform abortions.

1977 The Carter administration proposes placing a cap (9%) on increases in hospital revenues to be reimbursed by federal programs by limiting what they can spend. The industry counters by proposing its own voluntary program, deemed voluntary effort (VE).

1977 In PL 95-215, Health Professions Education Amendments, bowing to medical school pressure, Congress repeals the requirement that medical schools, as a condition of receiving capitation funds, must reserve an adequate number of positions in their classes for U.S. citizen foreign medical students (USFMS).

1978 The DHEW secretary, Joseph Califano, issues controversial bed supply guidelines to control excess hospital bed capacity in the United States. Rural and western sections of the country take strong exception, seeing the proposal as a further intrusion of the federal government on what they consider to be a local or state matter.

1979 The Supreme Court decides 8–1 in *Bellotti v. Baird* that states cannot require a minor to obtain parental consent.

1980 The Department of Education is split off as a separate department from DHEW and the remainder is renamed the Department of Health and Human Services (DHHS).

1980 Medicare and Medicaid amendments of the Omnibus Reconciliation Act of 1980 (PL 96-499) results in significant changes in both programs, including simplification of methods for state reimbursement of nursing homes, increased funding for state Medicaid fraud-control units, changes in utilization review requirements, coverage of nurse midwife services, reimbursement under both programs for hospital swing beds, and a measure for state enrollment in Medicare Part B.

1980 The Center for Disease Control is reorganized and renamed Centers for Disease Control.

1980 The Supreme Court rules 5–4 in both *Harris v. McRae* and *Williams v. Zbarz* that neither the federal nor state governments are constitutionally required to provide funds for abortions for poor women.

1981 President Reagan proposes the consolidation of twenty-six categorical health programs into two large block grants. Instead, Congress responds by creating four health block grants: preventive health (combining eight programs: home health, rodent control, water fluoridation, health education, risk reduction, health incentive grants, emergency medical services, rape crisis centers, and hypertension), health services, primary care, and maternal and child health care, authorizing all for three years or until the end of fiscal year 1984 (the Omnibus Budget Reconciliation Act of 1981, [PL 97-35]). Several other programs originally targeted for block grants, that is, family planning, childhood immunization, VD research and treatment, migrant health center, tuberculosis, primary care research and demonstrations, retain their categorical status, and a new adolescent family life program is authorized.

1981 Capitation grants to schools of medicine, osteopathy, dentistry, veterinary medicine, optometry, podiatry, pharmacy, and nursing are eliminated.

1981 The provision for free medical care for merchant seamen is eliminated as of October 1, 1981, with existing public health hospitals slated for closure by end of fiscal year 1982.

1981 In a 6–3 decision, the Supreme Court (*H. L. v. Matheson*) upholds a Utah statute requiring a physician to notify a minor's parents before performing an abortion.

1982 President Reagan proposes in a single bold stroke to create a "New Federalism," transferring responsibility of many human services to the states.

1982 The Office of Management and Budget considers proposals to trim the cost of Medicare by requiring the elderly to demonstrate need as a condition of receiving benefits. The introduction of a means test is acknowledged to constitute a significant change in the program, making Medicare less of an insurance program and more of an income assistance one.

1982 Congress passes the Tax Equity and Fiscal Responsibility Act (TEFRA) authorizing Medicare reimbursement for hospice services.

1982 The State of Arizona implements a new and experimental Medicaid program known as the Arizona Health Care Cost Containment System (AHCCS). Its predominant feature is its reliance on competitive bidding to establish a complete acute care delivery system for its indigent population and to set capitated reimbursement rates for participating providers.

1982 The Health Resources and Services Administration is established through the merger of the Health Resources Administration and the Health Services Administration.

1982 Congress seeks to encourage and facilitate the development and approval of drugs for rare diseases and conditions by passage of the PL 97-414, the Orphan Drug Act.

1982 The Supreme Court affirms its earlier 1977 decision (*Bates v. State Bar of Arizona*) striking down the prohibitions of professional associations against advertising by their members. The ruling lets stand a 1979 Federal Trade Commission (FTC) order (*American Medical Association v. Federal Trade Commission*) banning the AMA from prohibiting advertising by its members.

1982 Congress passes PL 97-248, the Tax Equity and Fiscal Responsibility Act (TEFRA), which seeks to control costs by placing limits on total hospital costs per discharge adjusted to reflect each hospital's case mix. Places a ceiling on the annual rate of increase in total costs per discharge while providing a token incentive payment for hospitals that operate below the established limits. Also authorizes Medicare payments for hospice services but includes a "sunset provision," which allows the benefit to expire in 1986.

1982 Congress declines to kill PSROs (professional standards review organizations), transforming them into PROs (peer review organizations) instead.

1983 Congress establishes a new Medicare hospital prospective payment (reimbursement) system based on the use of diagnosis-related groups (DRGs) as part of the 1983 Amendments to the Social Security Act (PL 98-21), signed into law June 1983.

1983 On September 1, the Health Care Finance Administration ushers in a new era of Medicare hospital reimbursement with the publication of regulations implementing the DRG-based prospective payment system.

1983 The Supreme Court strikes down (6–3) a city ordinance (*City of Akron v. Akron Center for Reproductive Health*) requiring a fourteen-hour waiting period and counseling for a woman. The decision also rules against requiring that all abortions be performed in a hospital and that minors must obtain parental consent without the option of a judicial waiver. In another case (*Planned Parenthood Association of Kansas City v. Ashcroft*) the Court decides that states cannot require all second-trimester abortions be performed in a hospital.

1984 Under the Deficit Reduction Act of 1984 (PL 98-369) Congress extends health insurance coverage to poor pregnant women, breaking down the financial barriers that had kept them from obtaining prenatal care. For the first time, Medicaid coverage is not limited to welfare eligibility. Instead, prenatal care services for women who do not have health insurance and whose incomes are too low to afford medical care will be paid for by Medicaid. It also imposes a temporary (fifteen months) freeze on physician fees under Medicare.

1984 Amendments to the Child Abuse Prevention and Treatment Act (PL 98-457) involving the states and infant care review committees in medical decisions about the treatment of handicapped newborns are passed.

1985 The Balanced Budget and Emergency Deficit Control Act (H.J. Res. 372, PL 99-177), otherwise known as Gramm–Rudman, Hollings, mandates that if projected deficits exceed predetermined targets, federal spending is to be reduced according to a prescribed formula.

1985 The Reagan administration seeks and Congress rejects placement of a cap on the exclusion of the amount contributed by an employer to a worker's health benefit plan from the employee's taxable income.

1985 As part of the Consolidated Omnibus Budget Reconciliation Act of 1985 (COBRA), PL 99-272, hospice care is made a permanent part of the Medicare program. Payment rates under the program are raised and the states are given the ability to provide hospice services under the Medicaid program. In addition, employers are required to continue health insurance for employees and their dependents who otherwise would lose their eligibility because of reduced work hours or termination of employment. Coverage is also extended to survivors and separated or divorced spouses of workers. Continuation of employer contributions, however, is not required.

1985 In addition to the above, COBRA-85 also establishes the Physician Payment Review Commission (PPRC) to advise Congress on physician payment policies for Medicare, and prohibits medically unjustified patient transfers (patient dumping). In the case of the latter, however, HCFA does not issue implementing regulations until eight years later, on June 22, 1994.

1985 Massachusetts, using its licensure powers, passes the nation's first full-fledged' ban on balanced billing of Medicare patients, banning such billing as a condition of licensure.

1986 Secretary of Health and Human Services Otis Bowen submits recommendations to the president calling for the expansion of federal health programs to provide coverage for catastrophic care.

1986 Congress enacts two omnibus budget bills: COBRA, the Consolidated Omnibus Budget Reconciliation Act, and SOBRA, the Sixth Omnibus Budget Reconciliation Act. Both seek to clean up Medicare's prospective payment system for hospitals and gradually close some of the more gaping holes in Medicaid.

1986 PL 99-272, PL 99-509. (Medicare), inner-city hospitals serving a "disproportionate" share of poor patients are given a Medicare payment boost of as much as 15 percent. Payments for graduate medical education (GME), however, are scaled back, with direct GME support of residents and interns limited to five years of postgraduate work. Attempts to end support for foreign medical graduates fails, but passage of a tough new qualification test is required.

1986 New penalties are imposed on hospitals that transfer (dump) poor patients to public and other facilities. Medicare hospice benefit is made permanent, and restrictions are imposed on the growth of the Part A deductible. Physician fees are frozen for nearly three years and placed under federal controls beginning in 1987.

1986 PL 99-278, PL 99-509 (Medicaid). Administration proposal to put the lid on federal Medicaid funding is rejected twice. Under COBRA, Medicaid coverage is mandated for pregnant women in two-parent families with an unemployed breadwinner. SOBRA, on the other hand, encourages coverage for pregnant women in families with incomes below the poverty line.

1986 Omnibus Health Act (PL 99-660). States are allowed to offer coverage to all pregnant women, infants up to one year of age, and, on a phased-in basis, children up to five years of age with incomes up to the federal poverty line.

1986 In a twelfth-hour package of health bills, Congress provides for a federal vaccine injury compensation system (National Childhood Vaccine Injury Act) that would bypass the courts, limiting out-of-court awards to income losses plus $250,000 for pain and suffering or death; affords members of peer review committees protection from most damage suits filed by physicians whom they discipline; mandates (Health Care Quality Improvement Act) creation of a national physician malpractice and discipline databank to which physicians and hospitals are required to report information on licensure actions and malpractice claims paid; repeals PL 93-641, the 1974 National Health Planning and Resource

Development Act, effective January 1, 1987, throwing responsibility for certificate-of-need programs to the states.

1987 Passage of the Omnibus Budget Reconciliation Act (PL 100-203) provides a number of significant changes in the Medicaid program, including additional options for children and pregnant women. Requires states to extend coverage to children up to age six with an option of allowing for coverage up to age eight. Encourages the provision of Medicaid clinic services to the homeless at shelters, soup kitchens, and other such locations.

Also substantially amends and adds to the Medicaid nursing home law by eliminating the old law's distinction between skilled nursing facilities (SNFs) and intermediate care facilities (ICFs) and repeals its requirement that states pay less for ICF than SNF services. Requires that facilities maintain or enhance the quality of life of each resident and operate a quality assurance program, conduct and periodically update a standardized assessment of each resident's functional capacity; mandates that by October 1, 1990, nursing homes serving Medicaid patients provide twenty-four hour nursing, including at least one registered nurse on duty eight hours a day, seven days a week plus one licensed nurse on duty twenty-four hours per day seven days per week, plus employment of at least one full-time social worker in facilities of more than 120 beds. Nurses' aids are required to have at least seventy-five hours of preservice training. While states may waive these requirements, each must have in effect by July 1 a preadmission screening program for all mentally ill or mentally retarded individuals to determine the appropriateness of placement in an SNF or ICF as well as review all mentally ill or mentally retarded nursing home residents to determine whether continued placement is appropriate.

In addition, OBRA-87 authorizes states to provide home and community-based care to persons age sixty-five and over who otherwise would likely require care in a skilled nursing or interme-

diate care facility without prior treatment in such facilities. Finally, the act calls for the secretary of health and human services to establish federal qualifications for nursing home administrators.

1987 The National Health Service corps (NHSC) program (PL 100-177) is reauthorized and amended. Under a new loan repayment program, students who have completed their training or are in their final year may have up to $20,000 ($25,000 if Native Americans) of their educational and related loans repaid by the federal government in return for providing services to designated needy areas. The law also authorizes payment to states for loan repayment programs in which the state is responsible for 25 percent of program costs. Repayment for students who default on their scholarships since obligation is set at three times the amount of the scholarship, plus interest.

1987 The era of federal involvement in local regulation of health care capital spending ends as HHS terminates Section 1122 Capital review agreements with sixteen states and the Virgin Islands. Begun in 1972, the program was the oldest federal effort at capital regulation and provided a separate capital review system operated by the states with some help from HHS. Coupled with the repeal of the 1974 National Health Planning and Resource Development Act in 1986, the Reagan administration appears to have succeeded in its goal of dismantling the federal health planning apparatus.

1987 Following passage of the House's own version in late July, the Senate on an 86–11 vote, October 27, virtually assures ultimate enactment of a catastrophic insurance measure. The two bills (HR 2470; S 1127), remarkably similar in scope, attempt to limit out-of-pocket expenditures by the elderly for Medicare-covered services. Both offer expanded coverage of short-term nursing home and home health care; both seek to finance the new benefits by taxing the upper-income elderly while charging the rest of the nation's 32 million beneficiaries relatively minor amounts. In addition, over the opposition of both the prescription drug industry and the Reagan administration, both provide, for the first time, coverage of prescription drugs.

1987 Following an eleven-year court battle, the AMA, American College of Surgeons, and American College of Radiologists are found guilty of antitrust and conspiracy in their efforts to restrain the practice of chiropractic medicine.

1987 Congress replaces the National Health Service Corps Scholarship program with a loan repayment plan to keep medical students from defaulting on their government loans.

1987 Senator Edward Kennedy (D-MA) introduces legislation that would require employers to provide a minimum package of health benefits to any worker employed 17.5 hours or more a week and extends such coverage to spouses and dependents. The proposal draws support from some members of the automobile industry, but most corporations and small businesses, as well as the Reagan administration, oppose it.

1987 Oregon becomes the first state in the Union to limit organ transplants to kidneys and corneas under its Medicaid program. The decision arises after the state legislature opts for expanding its prenatal care program at the expense of providing additional funds for organ transplants. In so doing, the legislature makes explicit their preference, within the constraints of limited public resources, for investing in preventive services that can benefit many, rather than spend large sums for high-tech procedures that would benefit only a few.

1987 The Reagan administration is accused of attempting to exert political control over government-funded health services research. In testimony before a congressional committee, the former director of the National Center for Health Services Research tells of efforts by the administration to stifle research that is not in agreement with its political aims, including recommending the creation of research agenda boards made up of political appointees to screen all research projects.

1987 The surgeon general's annual report on smoking asserts for the first time that inhalation of cigarette smoke by nonsmokers (passive smoking) is a cause of disease, including lung cancer. The report calls for the establishment of smoke-free worksites.

1988 Enactment of PL 100-360, the Catastrophic Coverage Act, marks the largest expansion of the Medicare program in twenty-three years. The act, which passes 328 (230 Dem., 98 Rep.) to 72 (9 Dem., 63 Rep.) in the House and 86 (52 Dem., 34 Rep.) to 11 (0 Dem., 11 Rep.) in the Senate, is aimed at shielding Medicare's 32 million beneficiaries from catastrophic hospital and physicians' bills related to acute illness and provides Medicare's first broad coverage of outpatient prescription drug costs. It does not, however, cover the costs associated with long-term care, the principal source of health care costs for the elderly. Even more controversial is its financing. For the first time in the program's history, enrollees themselves will pick up the tab for the entire cost of the program. This change represents a departure from the original idea of the program—that its costs would be funded by contributions made during the working years to one that seeks to balance the contributions of workers with those of retirees. Under terms of the legislation, the program is to be funded entirely by enrollee premiums, with 37 percent of the cost to be covered by a fixed monthly premium and the remainder by an income-related, supplemental premium—an income surtax to be paid by an estimated 40 percent of the enrollees.

1988 In the largest mailing on health ever done in the United States, some 45 million pieces, the Department of Health and Human Services sends out informational materials on the dangers of AIDS and methods of prevention to every residential address in the country.

1988 The Institute of Medicine issues its report on the status of public health in the United States. While finding much to commend in the nation's public health efforts, the twenty-six-member committee notes an even longer list of "problems," including citizen ignorance of what public health protection does for them, the difficulty public health officials have in communicating the urgency of prevention and other efforts to the public and its elected representatives, and the disorganization within and lack of coordination among agencies that carry out public health activities.

1988 The Department of Health and Human Services publishes rules that family planning clinics that receive federal funds may not do anything to assist women to obtain an abortion or increase the availability or accessibility of abortion for family planning purposes. The action is immediately challenged in the courts by Planned Parenthood, the American Public Health Association, the National Family Planning and Reproductive Health Association, as well as other advocacy groups.

1988 Massachusetts enacts the first law in the nation to mandate competitive, universal health insurance coverage of an entire state's population.

1988 In a unanimous decision, the Supreme Court (*West v. Atkins*) confirms the right of prisoners to adequate health care in prisons and makes it clear that the constitutional mandate to provide such care is the same whether given by a full-time state employee or is contracted out.

1988 After initial controversy and delay, the Presidential Commission on the Human Immune Deficiency Virus epidemic (AIDS) issues its final report to President Reagan. Emphasizing that in general the nation's response has been seriously deficient, the report proposes nearly five hundred recommendations including a call for a national law barring discrimination against persons with AIDS, AIDS-related complex, and those infected with the AIDS virus; a federal law penalizing improper disclosure of HIV-antibody test results; increased federal and state funds for drug abuse treatment; expedited consideration of AIDS budget requests from the Public Health Service; expanded access to voluntary HIV testing; and new efforts to provide less expensive noninstitutional care to AIDS patients.

1988 Minnesota becomes the first state in the nation to create a children's health insurance program (the Minnesota Children's Health Plan) that does not rely on Medicaid expansions to extend coverage to uninsured children.

1988 California passes Proposition 99, a voter initiative providing for a 25 cent a pack cigarette tax to fund anti-tobacco programs.

1988 The Federal Fair Housing Amendment extends protection from discrimination in housing to persons with disabilities as a group. This marks the first time that the antidiscrimination principle regarding persons with disabilities is extended to the private sector.

1989 For the first time the federal government (Health Care Financing Administration) releases information on the quality of the nation's more than 15,000 nursing homes.

1989 The Senate Finance Committee splits its health subcommittee in two in order to ease its workload. Responsibility for Medicaid and making health insurance coverage available to the nation's uninsured is to be handled by the subcommittee on Health and Families and the Uninsured, and oversight of Medicare budget issues and the search for ways to cover the cost of long-term nursing home care is to rest with the subcommittee on Medicare and long-term care.

1989 As part of the Omnibus Budget Reconciliation Act of 1989 (PL 101-239) Congress calls for the establishment of the Agency for Health Care Policy and Research (AHPR) to succeed the National Center for Health Services Research and Health Care Technology Assessment (NCHSR). The purpose of the new agency is to enhance the quality, application, and efficiency of Health Care Services and improve access to services.

1989 The Omnibus Budget Reconciliation Act of 1989 (PL 101-239) contains a provision requiring the states to extend Medicaid coverage to all pregnant women and children up to the age of six, in families with incomes up to 133 percent of the federal poverty line ($13,380 for a family of four) beginning April 1, 1990. In addition, states are given the option of extending such coverage to pregnant women with family incomes up to 185 percent of poverty.

1989 In a series of 5–4 votes in a Missouri case (*Webster v. Reproductive Health Services*) a divided Supreme Court gives states broad powers to limit a woman's right to an abortion but stops short of reversing its 1973 decision legalizing abortion. The decision upholds the state's right to prohibit the use of public facilities to perform abortions as well as require a physician to perform viability testing if there is a reason to believe a woman is twenty or more weeks pregnant.

1989 Oregon passes historic legislation increasing Medicaid eligibility to all individuals living below the federal poverty line, mandating insurance coverage for all the state's uninsured and creating a Health Services Commission to analyze and rank according to costs and benefits 709 medical services to be included in a basic health care package to be provided to persons covered under the state's Medicaid program. The impetus for the legislation is the Oregon Medicaid Priority-Setting Project. The Oregon proposal is the first attempt to rank treatments by effectiveness, cost, and quality of life and in so doing embodies an explicit form of rationing.

1989 In response to intense pressure (over 5 million cards, letters, petitions, and telegrams) from senior citizen groups and individuals (primarily upper- and middle-income elderly), upset over its funding provisions that would require many of them to pay an income tax surtax, the House votes 360 to 66 to repeal and the Senate, 73 to 26 to sharply cut back on the 1988 Catastrophic Coverage Act. Efforts by the Senate to save several features of the act (i.e., unlimited inpatient hospital coverage, thirty-eight days of home health care per spell of illness, eighty hours a year of respite care, unlimited hospice care, $50 in coverage toward mammography screening for elderly and disabled women, as well as some Medicaid protection for low-income elderly and poor pregnant women and infants) in the Conference Committee fail and the law, passed just sixteen months earlier, is repealed. As a result of the congressional action, Medicare's previous Part A deductible and co-payment requirements as well the requirement of a three-day hospital stay in order to be eligible for skilled nursing home care are revived. The final vote to repeal (360–66 in the House and 99–0 in the Senate) marks the first time in its history that Congress has rescinded major social benefits it had created.

1989 In its continuing effort to try to hold down costs, Congress adopts as part of its Medicare physician reforms, included under the fiscal year 1990 budget legislation, a new volume performance standard (VPS) and directs the Department of Health and Human Services to establish a Medicare relative value scale (RVS) fee schedule, with a five-year phase-in.

1990 PL 101-336, the Americans with Disabilities Act (ADA), is adopted, providing income support, rehabilitation opportunities, and civil rights to persons with disabilities, prohibiting discrimination on the basis of disability in employment, public services, and public accommodations. The law requires employers to make "reasonable accommodations" for disabled workers; stores, restaurants, doctors' offices, and other facilities to make "readily achievable" modifications to accommodate the disabled; and buses as well as trains be accessible to the disabled.

1990 The bipartisan authored Ryan White Comprehensive AIDS Resources Emergency (CARE) Act (PL 101-381) is passed and signed into law. Named for a young Indiana schoolboy afflicted with the disease, the act is intended to help urban areas (sixteen epicenters, including San Francisco and New York City) and states hardest hit by the disease to cope with the exploding and expensive cost of care and treatment. The legislation authorizing formula-based and competitive supplemental grants to cities and states represents the largest dollar investment specifically for HIV-related outpatient medical services to date.

1990 PL 101-508, OBRA-90, expands Medicaid coverage to all children in poverty, adding an estimated 5 million persons to the program by the end of the decade. It also provides a new earned income tax credit to assist low-income working families to purchase private health insurance.

1990 For the first time (HR 5835-H Rept 101-964), responsibility for overseeing the regulation of the medigap market is assigned to the federal government, dramatically changing the rules for selling supplementary health insurance to the nation's elderly. A key feature of the legislation is the standardization of insurance offerings, with carriers permitted to sell only ten specified benefit packages. The medigap reform puts teeth into an earlier 1980 law by replacing a voluntary certification program with one that requires all policies be approved by either the state or the federal government.

1990 President Bush signs into law PL 101-629, the Safe Medical Devices Act amendment to the 1976 Federal Food, Drug, and Cosmetic Act. The legislation gives the Food and Drug Administration new authority to regulate the safety and effectiveness of medical devices and diagnostic products.

1990 Over the vehement objections of the pharmaceutical industry, Congress requires drug manufacturers to provide discounts to state Medicaid programs as they have done for hospitals, HMOs, the Department of Veterans Affairs, and other bulk purchasers of prescription drugs. But while the new law requiring pharmaceutical companies to give Medicaid their "best price" is estimated to save the government some $700 million, representatives of hospitals, nursing homes, HMOs, and other providers, including the VA, military hospitals, community and migrant health centers, and family planning clinics, complain that their drug prices jumped as much as 100 percent since the Medicaid rebate began, as drug makers sought to offset the discounted Medicaid prices by shifting the cost to other buyers. Remedial legislation is introduced in Congress the following year.

1990 In a 6–3 decision, the Supreme Court rules (*Ohio v. Akron Center for Reproductive Health*) that states may require a minor to notify one parent or obtain a judicial waiver in order to obtain an abortion. It also upholds (*Hodgson v. Minnesota*) state laws requiring parental consent before a teenage girl can get an abortion.

1991 Harris Wofford (D-PA), a comparative political unknown, upsets Richard Thornburgh, former governor and attorney general under the Bush administration, in a special election to succeed the late John Heinz, a fellow Republican, by calling for enactment of legislation providing universal access to health care. The victory shakes up both parties and puts health care reform on the legislative agenda.

1991 The American Medical Association abandons its long-held opposition to federal intervention in health care, calling for the enactment of national health care reform in its May 15 (Vol. 265) issue of the *Journal of the American Medical Association*.

1991 In a move hailed by women's groups, Congress agrees to provide medical coverage for mammograms to detect breast cancer. The coverage, which is tacked onto the final version of the 1991 Budget Reconciliation bill, was not originally in either the House or Senate bill, although it had been included in the ill-fated 1988 Medicare Catastrophic Coverage Act. The legislative fiat is credited to the perseverance of Representative Mary Rose Oskar (D-OH), who hectored the congressional leadership into including the provision in the final bill.

1991 Senate Majority Leader George Mitchell (D-ME) introduces a comprehensive health care reform plan (S 1227), called "Health America," which advocates a play-or-pay approach to covering the uninsured, requiring employers to either insure their workers or pay the government to do it for them. Co-sponsors are Senators Kennedy (D-MA), Rockefeller (D-WV), and Riegle (D-MI). House Democrats foreshadowing things to come are divided over a number of proposals.

1992 Secretary of Health and Human Services (HHS) Louis Sullivan, M.D., rejects Oregon's request for a federal waiver to rank some 700 medical services and eliminate coverage of 122 of them under the Medicaid program in order to free up funding to nearly double the number of residents in the state eligible for coverage under the program. The decision, made at the highest levels of the Bush administration, involves HHS, the Justice Department, and the Office of the White House Counsel and turns on interpretation of the 1990 Americans with Disabilities Act, which is designed to protect the physically and mentally disabled from bias in workplaces, housing, and public accommodations including health care. The decision comes nearly a year after Oregon submitted its application for the waiver of fifteen separate Medicaid rules, including one barring states from discriminating among patients on the basis of their diagnosis.

1992 Medicare, breaking a thirty-six-year tradition, agrees to eliminate the disparity in how it pays rural and urban physicians and begins paying them under a single fee system.

1992 In a strong break from past practices, the health insurance industry calls for a new federal law that would require coverage for all Americans, define a basic set of benefits, and try to contain health care costs by limiting tax breaks for purchase of insurance.

1992 Congress passes the Veterans Health Care Act of 1992 (PL 102-585) requiring the Department of Veterans Affairs hospitals to establish "suitable" indoor and outdoor smoking areas that have appropriate heating and air conditioning. The law is a major setback to progress made by the department's nationwide hospital smoke-free policy, implemented in 1991, puts the VA hospitals out of step with public and private hospitals, and supersedes the Joint Commission on Accreditation of Health Care Organizations' smoke-free hospital accreditation standard.

1992 The Supreme Court, with only two dissenting votes (Justice Sandra Day O'Connor and Harry Blackmun), refuses to hear an appeal of a deceased AIDS patient whose medical benefits were slashed from $1 million to $5,000 shortly after he revealed his illness to his employer (*Greenberg v. H & H Music Company*). The original case, *McGann v. H & H Music Company*, reveals a large loophole in federal and state laws governing medical benefits underwritten by employers. Although the Employee Retirement Income Security Act of 1974 (ERISA), which regulates pensions and employee benefits, specifically states that employers may not discriminate against any employee for exercising any right to which they are entitled under the company's plan, both the federal district court and the federal court of appeals ruled that the company had an absolute right under ERISA to change the terms of the health plan. In refusing to even consider the appeal, the Court gives companies that fund their own health insurance plan the right to sharply cut the benefits paid for AIDS and other catastrophic conditions. Not only may such companies refuse to provide coverage for certain costly illnesses but they may drop all coverage after an employee reveals his or her illness.

1992 In *Planned Parenthood of Southeastern Pennsylvania v. Casey*, the Court reaffirms a woman's right to an abortion but allows states to impose some restrictions (i.e., parental consent, a twenty-four-hour waiting period for all women seeking abortions in the state) but not husband notification.

1992 New Jersey's twelve-year-old hospital reimbursement system that imposes a surcharge on all inpatient hospital bills to fund care for the state's nearly one million uninsured is struck down by a federal judge as in violation of the 1974 Employee Retirement Income Security Act because it requires self-funded group health plans to pay for individuals who are not beneficiaries of the plan.

1993 President Clinton orders the federal government to make it easier for states to obtain federal waivers of the Medicaid program to introduce new health care programs for the poor. His goal is to add greater flexibility to a health care system that is often constrained by federal regulations by loosening the red tape that has hindered states from seeking to experiment and innovate.

1993 In an unprecedented move, the president expands the role of the First Lady by naming his wife, Hillary Rodham Clinton, to head a new White House Task Force on Health Reform that is charged with developing a bill within one hundred days. Release of the Clinton proposal, however, is delayed until September, when before a televised joint session of Congress the president outlines his proposal, calling for the establishment of purchasing alliances, an employer mandate, price controls, universal coverage, and federal subsidies for early retiree coverage. In response, the health insurance industry, namely, the Health Insurance Association of America (HIAA), launches a series of "Harry and Louise" television commercials attacking the president's plan.

1993 After much delay and several false starts, the Health Security Act of 1993 (S 1757), all 1,342 pages of it, is formally introduced in Congress on November 20. Ninety-nine Democrats join Majority Leader Richard Gephardt (D-MO) in sponsoring the House bill and thirty senators, including Vermont Republican James Jeffords, sign on with Majority Leader George Mitchell (D-ME) in the Senate.

1993 The U.S. Chamber of Commerce drops its opposition to managed competition if some relief is given to small business. Earlier, the AMA's request to the First Lady to formally participate in the president's 536-member Task Force on Health Reform is rebuffed. Later the White House is sued to divulge the names of task force members.

1993 After initial rejection under the Bush administration, Oregon receives approval from the Department of Health and Human Services under the Clinton administration to test its plan (originally filed in 1991) for eliminating (rationing) some medical services in exchange for extending enrollment of its Medicaid population to cover 120,000 poor persons not currently eligible under the program. Approval is conditioned on the state revising its list of covered conditions and treatments to comply with HHS's interpretation of the Americans with Disabilities Act.

1993 How businesses account for health care costs changes dramatically as the impact of the Financial Accounting Standards Board's Rule 106 is fully realized. Under the rule companies are required to account for future obligations for retiree health benefits during the period in which they are incurred rather than at some time in the future. Business responses to the rule include increasing or completely shifting the cost of premiums to retirees, instituting defined employer contributions to retiree health care plans, increasing deductibles and co-payments for retirees, and tightening eligibility criteria for coverage.

1993 The federal Equal Employment Opportunity Commission declares that employers may not refuse to hire people with disabilities because of concern over health insurance costs and that disabled workers must be given equal access to any health insurance provided to other employees. The commission's statement offers the first indication of how it will apply the 1990 Americans with Disabilities Act.

1993 PL 103-66, the Omnibus Budget Reconciliation Act (OBRA-93), calls for a record five-year cut in Medicare funding, an end to return on equity (ROE) payments to proprietary skilled nursing facilities for capital expenditures, reductions in the previously established rate of increase in payment rates for hospice care, and dramatic cuts in laboratory fees by changing the formula for reimbursement. The law also includes the Comprehensive Childhood Immunization Act, which provides $585 million to support the provision of vaccines for the immunization of children eligible for Medicaid, those that are uninsured, or Native American.

1993 In a end-of-the-year (December 28) announcement, HCFA notifies the states that Medicaid must cover abortions for women who are victims of rape or incest as well as for women whose lives are endangered by their pregnancies. The last-minute notice implements congressional action aimed at easing restrictions imposed by the sixteen-year-old Hyde Amendment barring federal funding of abortions except in cases when the woman's life is at risk. The announcement causes considerable controversy, drawing angry reactions from operators of state Medicaid programs as well as some Hill staffers who question whether the administration's action reflects congressional intent. Earlier the president, reversing the position of his predecessor, signs an executive order removing the ban against abortion counseling in federally financed family planning clinics and the use of fetal tissue in research.

1994 As opposition mounts in Congress, the president says he will compromise on everything in his health reform proposal but universal coverage. Business opposition, however, intensifies as the Business Roundtable, U.S. Chamber of Commerce, and the National Association of Manufacturers formally reject the Clinton plan. In the meantime, the Congressional Budget Office reports that the proposed package is seriously underfinanced. In March, congressional leaders declare one of the key elements of the Clinton bill—purchasing alliances—dead. On September 26, the curtain falls on health care reform as the Senate majority leader, George Mitchell, formally lays to rest health reform for the year.

1994 Over the objections of both the AMA (the Oregon Medical Association was divided on the issue) and the Catholic Church, Oregon voters approve Measure 16, the Death with Dignity Act. The ballot initiative represents a legal acceptance of physician-assisted suicide that is without precedent in the United States. Central to the law is the stipulation that a physician may only write a prescription for the fatal drug. The patient must get the drug and take it. Lethal injection, mercy killing, or active euthanasia are specifically proscribed. The law applies to patients with terminal illnesses who are eighteen years of age and older, residents of the state, and not expected to live more than six months.

1994 Despite warnings by the California Medical Association, the California Association of Hospitals and Health Systems, and the California Teachers Association that passage would endanger public health, create a police-state mentality, leave uneducated children unsupervised, increase crime, and cause the state to lose $10 billion of federal funding for Medicaid and AFDC, California voters approve Proposition 187, which requires publicly funded health care facilities to deny care to illegal immigrants and report them to government officials.

1994 California establishes the first statewide voluntary health insurance purchasing alliance HIPC (Health Insurance Plan of California), providing insurance to small businesses with between five and fifty full-time employees.

1994 Specifically side-stepping First Amendment free speech issues, the Supreme Court unanimously rules that the twenty-four-year-old Racketeer Influenced and Corrupt Organizations Act (RICO) anti-racketeering law can be used against abortion protesters, even if they do not have a strictly economic motive. The ruling allows the National Organization for Women (NOW) to return to the lower courts and sue abortion clinic blockaders for millions of dollars in damages.

1994 Accusing insurers and managed care companies of trying to "take over the examining room" and denying some medical care to boost profits, the AMA unveils a proposal it contends will protect consumers and their physicians from insurance coverage decisions driven by cost. Introduced by Senator Paul Wellstone (D-MN), an advocate of a tax-financed Canadian-style health system and an unlikely ally, the Patient Protection Act would require insurers to detail which procedures are covered under their policies and to set up an appeals process for doctors dropped from a health network for prescribing costly treatment.

1994 Civil rights and health groups join in a law suit (*Madison-Hughes v. Shalala*) charging federal officials with failure to comply with the Civil Rights Act of 1964 by not requiring health providers to collect or report race/ethnicity data that could document their compliance with antidiscrimination regulations.

1994 State voters overwhelmingly reject Proposition 186, California's single-payer initiative under which providers would have been paid by the state rather than by insurance companies. The plan, which was vigorously opposed by the insurance industry and hospitals, would have been financed in part by a payroll tax of up to 8.9 percent, an income tax surcharge of 2.5 percent, and a $1 per pack cigarette tax.

1994 Following a campaign that featured their "Contract with America," Republicans score a stirring victory in the midterm elections, winning majorities in both houses of Congress as well as at the state level. The election is heralded as a new "Republican revolution."

1995 Upon taking control of both houses of Congress for the first time in forty years, Republicans propose major cuts and changes in the Medicare and Medicaid programs, including the provision for medical savings accounts in Medicare and conversion of Medicaid into a block grant program. They also seek roll-backs in environmental protection laws, nursing home regulations, and limits on the powers of the Federal Food and Drug Administration.

1995 The Pew Health Professions Commission calls for the closing of 20 percent of the nation's medical schools by the year 2005 and a cutback of 25 percent in training slots for physicians, registered nurses, and pharmacists in order to reduce a projected surplus of such personnel. The AMA, the American Nurses Association, and the Association of American Medical Colleges (AAMC) claim the projections are overblown.

1995 The Medicare Part A (Hospital) trust fund runs a deficit for the first time since 1972, one year earlier than expected.

1995 The U.S. Supreme Court (*New York et al. v. Travelers Insurance Company*) unanimously broadens the state's powers to regulate employee benefit plans, upholding a New York surcharge on hospital rates paid by commercial insurers and HMOs. The ruling gives state lawmakers new recourse against ERISA, the Employee Retirement Income Security Act. The landmark decision is the first case to significantly narrow the ERISA preemption, holding that insurers are still subject to state regulations such as surcharges whose effect on costs is indirect.

1995 Two years after adopting what had been hailed as the most complete health care delivery reform legislation in the nation, the Washington State legislature votes to nullify most of the mandates called for in the 1993 Health Services Act before they can take effect.

1995 House Republicans seek to scrap federal regulations adopted seven years earlier (1987) that set standards for nursing home care, including staffing levels, nutrition guidelines, and rules governing the use of physical restraints, but are rebuffed by party moderates in the Senate, who join the Democrats in defeating their efforts.

1995 In a long-awaited ruling (*Lee v. Oregon*) Oregon's landmark law legalizing physician-assisted suicide, which had been approved by a 51 percent to 49 percent margin in the November 1994 election (Ballot Measure 16), is struck down by a U.S. district court judge. The law is held to be unconstitutional on the grounds that it provides insufficient safeguards for vulnerable patients and unfairly discriminates against the terminally ill, and as such is in violation of the equal protection clause of the Fourteenth Amendment to the Constitution. The decision, which is appealed to the 9th Circuit Court of Appeals in San Francisco, is expected to eventually end up before the U.S. Supreme Court. *Note:* The Oregon law is the first in the world to actually legalize physician-assisted death.

1995 The Senate, after three days of continuous debate and a record thirty-eight roll-call votes, on a 52–47 largely party-line vote (only Maine Republican Senator William Cohen breaking ranks to vote against the measure) follows the House (227–203) in passing a far-reaching budget bill calling for unprecedented cutbacks and restraints on Medicare and Medicaid. The legislation, however, is vetoed by the president.

1995 The House votes to criminalize a late-term (after twenty weeks) abortion procedure, and to subject physicians who perform it to civil suits, fines, and up to two years in prison. The House action marks the first time since the *Roe v. Wade* decision that Congress has tried to curb an abortion procedure. On a 54–44 vote, the Senate agrees to the ban unless the mother's life is in danger. The legislation is vetoed by the president.

1996 Proposed major revisions in Medicare and Medicaid are at the heart of a budget stalemate between the Republican-controlled Congress and President Clinton, with both sides far apart on total Medicaid savings and the Republicans' desire to end current coverage guarantees for welfare beneficiaries. Continued squabbling between the two sides over cuts in Medicare, Medicaid, and other related social programs leads to a budget impasse and a temporary shutdown of the federal government.

1996 An Institute of Medicine report, "The Nation's Physician Workforce: Options for Balancing Supply and Requirements," calls for a freeze in the number of U.S. medical schools, their class size, and a reduction in the number of residency slots by limiting access to graduate medical education for international medical graduates and to more closely match the number of residency positions to the level of graduates of U.S. medical schools. The report comes on the heels of an earlier (1995) proposal by the Pew Health Professions Commission to cut the physician supply by closing 20 percent of the nation's medical schools and reducing Medicare Graduate Medical Education (GME) allowances to hospitals to 110 percent of U.S. graduates.

1996 The Clinton administration announces final rules requiring the states to enforce their laws barring the sale of tobacco to minors or lose their federal antidrug abuse funding. The long-delayed regulations were mandated by Congress in 1992 in legislation known as the Synar amendment, named after its chief House sponsor, the late Congressman Mike Synar (D-OK).

1996 A bill (S 1028), the Health Insurance Reform Act, is introduced in the Senate, co-sponsored by Senators Kassebaum (R-KS) and Kennedy (D-MA) and Congressman Pete Peters (D-FL). The bill calls for small-group market health insurance reform that would protect consumers from insurance abuses and improve access to coverage. The package, which is opposed by the health insurance industry, includes reforms outlined earlier in model legislation drafted by the National Association of Insurance Commissioners (NAIC) in 1990 and included in several health reform bills introduced in the 103rd Congress as well as adopted piecemeal in many of the states (i.e., guaranteed renewal and portability of coverage, limits on waiting periods for coverage of preexisting conditions, and conversion from group to individual coverage). The bill is written to apply to self-funded employer-sponsored health plans as well as independent insurers. Following months of delay in which the bill (passed earlier 267–151 in the House) is held captive by the deft use of the senatorial hold by conservative Republicans backed by the health insurance industry, it finally passes in the Senate on a 100–0 vote and is sent off to a joint House–Senate conference committee to resolve differences between the two bodies. The Senate's rare unanimity of support, however, is misleading as opponents sought to place themselves on record as favoring the legislation in advance of the upcoming fall election, in the hope that it will either be revised to their liking in the conference committee or be scuttled altogether. Key points of contention are the House's provision for medical savings accounts (MSAs) and the Senate's inclusion of mental health benefits.

After several months of continued heated partisan wrangling, Congress on a vote of 421–2 in the House (Representatives Pete Stark [D-CA] and Pat Williams [D-MT] dissenting) and 98–0 in the Senate, agrees to make health insurance coverage portable from job to job and curtail exclusions based on preexisting medical conditions. The final legislation, renamed the Health Insurance Portability and Accountability Act of 1996, affords workers employed by companies that offer health insurance to their employees guaranteed accessibility to "affordable" health insurance in the event that they change jobs or become unemployed. This guarantee of accessibility holds regardless of whether they have any preexisting medical problems, with the determination of affordability (i.e., regulation of premiums) left to the states. The measure also guarantees renewability as long as premiums are paid; prohibits insurers from charging higher insurance rates to new workers with potentially expensive medical problems; allows the self-employed to take a tax deduction for 80 percent of their health insurance premium costs versus the then current 30 percent; allows tax deductibility for medical expenses related to long-term care and tax breaks for employers providing long-term care coverage. In addition, in perhaps its most contentious provision it creates a Republican-sponsored four-year experimental trial permitting about 750,000 self-employed or persons working for companies of fifty or fewer workers, on a first come, first serve basis, to put money into medical savings accounts covered by a high-deductible catastrophic illness insurance policy, with earnings and contributions to be tax-free. Eliminated from the original Kassebaum–Kennedy bill, however, is a provision backed by members of both parties that would have required insurers to provide the same level of coverage for mental disorders as they do for other health problems, thus leaving them able to continue their practice of providing a much narrower range of mental health benefits.

1996 The number of Americans without health insurance reaches an unprecedented 42 million, up from 39 million just three years earlier.

REFERENCES

Becker, Dorothy D., & Ruth R. Johnson. (1980). *Chronology health professions legislation, 1956–1979* (DHHS Publication No. [HRA] 80-69). Bureau of Health Professions. Washington, D.C.: U.S. Government Printing Office.

Berliner, Howard S. (1973). The origins of health insurance for the aged. *International Journal of Health Services, 3* (3), 465–474.

Bernard, Sydney E., & Eugene Feingold. (1970). The impact of Medicaid. *Wisconsin Law Review, 2*, 726–755.

Blendon, Robert, et al. (Eds.). (1976). *Baselines for setting health goals and standards*. Papers on the National Health guidelines (DHEW Publication No. [HRA] 76-640). Washington, D.C.: U.S. Government Printing Office.

Brown, Lawrence D. (1986). Introduction to a decade of transitions. *Journal of Health Politics, Policy and Law, 11* (4), 569–583.

Chapman, Carleton B., & John M. Talmadge. (1970). Historical and political background of federal health care legislation. Health care: Part I. *Law and Contemporary Problems, 35* (Spring), 334–347.

Chapman, Carleton B., & John M. Talmadge. (1971). The evolution of the right to health concept in the United States. *Pharos, 34* (1), 30–51.

Congressional Quarterly. (1963). Medical care for the aged. *Congressional Quarterly special report*. Washington, D.C.: Congressional Quarterly Service, Inc.

Corning, Peter A. (1969). *The evolution of Medicare . . . from idea to law*. Office of Research and Statistics, Social Security Administration, Department of Health, Education and Welfare. Research Report No. 29. Washington, D.C.: U.S. Government Printing Office.

Feingold, Eugene. (1966). *Medicare: Policy and politics*. San Francisco, CA: Chandler Publishing Co.

Fishbein, Morris. (1947). *A history of the American Medical Association*. Philadelphia: W. B. Saunders Co.

Freedman, Ben. (1951). The Louisiana State Board of Health. *American Journal of Public Health, 41* (Fall), 1279–1285.

Freund, Deborah A., & Edward Neuschler. (1986). Overview of Medicaid capitation and case management initiatives. *Health Care Financing Review* (Annual Suppl.), 21.

Gardner, John W., Wilbur J. Cohen, & Ralph K. Huitt. (1965). *1965: Year of legislative achievements in health, education and welfare*. Office of the Secretary, DHEW. Washington, D.C.: U.S. Government Printing Office.

Langwell, Kathryn M., & James P. Hadley. (1986). Capitation and the Medicare program: History, issues and evidence. *Health Care Financing Review* (Annual Suppl.), 9–20.

Lewis, Charles E., Rashi Fein, & David Mechanic. (1976). *A right to health*. New York: John Wiley & Sons.

Longest, Buford B., Jr. (1994). *Health policymaking in the United States*. Ann Arbor, MI: AUPHA Press/Health Administration Press.

Losteller, John O., & John E. Chapman. (1976). The participation of the United States government in providing financial support for medical education. *Health Policy and Education*, 27–65.

Mariner, Wendy. (1992). Problems with employer-provided health insurance—the Employee Retirement Income Security Act and health care reform. *New England Journal of Medicine, 327* (December 30), 1682–1685.

Pegels, C. Carl. (1981). *Health care of the elderly*. Germantown, MD: Aspen Systems Corporation.

Sommerville, Janice. (1993). The more things change. *American Medical News* (October 11), 7.

Wilson, Florence A., & Duncan Newhauser. (Eds.). (1985). *Health services in the United States* (2nd ed.). Cambridge, MA: Ballinger.

BIBLIOGRAPHY

Theodor J. Litman

GENERAL REFERENCE GUIDES TO CONGRESS, LEGISLATION, HEALTH POLICY, AND GOVERNMENT AFFAIRS

Current Government Documents and Publications

Bills and Resolutions

One free copy of all legislation is printed daily after it is introduced and is available from one's member of Congress. One free copy of a bill, committee report, conference report, or public law may be obtained by sending a request along with a self-addressed mailing label to either the Senate Document Room B-04, Hart Senate Office Building, Washington, DC 20510, or House Document Room 1B-18, Annex #2, U.S. Capitol, Washington, DC 20515.

Committee Reports

When each piece of legislation goes to the floor, it is accompanied by a report that generally analyzes the bill, describes its purposes, and states the view of the committee's members as to the desirability of its enactment. Available from the publications clerk of the appropriate committee.

Congressional Directory

Issued annually. Contains brief biographical sketches of each member of Congress, complete rosters of standing and special committee assignments by members, as well as maps of all congressional districts. Also lists major executives of all government agencies and members of the diplomatic corps. Available from the Superintendent of Documents, Government Printing Office (GPO), Washington, DC 20402.

The Congressional Record

Published in its present form since 1973, it is the official record of the proceedings and debates of the U.S. Congress. Provides a verbatim transcript, subject to revision by members of Congress, of the proceedings and floor debates of the U.S. Senate and House of Representatives, including extension of remarks and materials inserted at the request of members of Congress. Bound sets consist of fifteen to twenty parts per year, including a separate index and, since 1947, *Daily Digest volumes*. A *Daily Digest* is included at the back of each issue. Single copies may be obtained for a modest fee from the Congressional Record Office, H-112, U.S. Capitol, Washington, DC 20515.

Digest of Public General Bills

Cumulative compilation providing a brief description of each public bill introduced during the session. Published approximately five times per year. Indexed by subject matter. Available from the Government Printing Office (GPO).

Federal Register

Published five days each week. Contains notices of proposed rule making as well as proposed regulations and changes and all legal documents of the executive branch. Available from the Government Printing Office (GPO).

Forum

Bimonthly publication. Official magazine of the Health Care Financing Administration (HCFA). Covers all aspects of health care financing as well as HCFA programs and activities. Available from the Government Printing Office (GPO).

General Accounting Office Reports

Issued on an irregular basis by the General Accounting Office (GAO), the investigative and program auditing arm of Congress, pursuant to a special request by a congressional committee. Single copies may be obtained free of charge by writing the U.S. General Accounting Office, Document Handling and Information Services Facility, PO Box 6015, Gaithersburg MD 20884-6015. A free monthly listing of reports with summaries may be obtained by writing the General Accounting Office, 441 G Street NW, Washington, DC 20548.

Health Care Financing Review

A quarterly publication of the Health Care Financing Administration's Office of Research and Demonstrations. Presents statistics on Medicare, Medicaid, national health expenditures, and related subjects, as well as reports on agency-supplied research, demonstration, and evaluation projects. Available from ORDS, HCFA, C-3-11-07, 7500 Security Boulevard, Baltimore, MD 21244-1850, or http://www.hcfa.gov

Index to U.S. Government Periodicals

Published quarterly. Index to articles appearing in periodicals produced by over one hundred federal departments and agencies.

Monthly Catalog of U.S. Government Publications

Monthly publication with annual cumulative index. Lists every document published by the federal government that is made available to the public, including House and Senate documents, hearings, and reports, as well as those of federal departments and agencies. Available from the Government Printing Office (GPO).

Rules of the House and Senate

Published separately for the House and Senate at least once each Congress. Provides a useful reference on jurisdiction of committees, procedures in handling of legislation, precedents, and the like.

Social Security Bulletin

Official monthly publication of the Social Security Administration. Offers feature articles, regular reports, notes, statistics, and analyses of public and private expenditures for hospital care and physician services. Provides review of private health insurance and Medicare and Medicaid experience. Available from the Government Printing Office (GPO).

U.S. Government Manual

Issued annually. Official handbook of the federal government. Describes purposes and programs of most government agencies, including listings of top personnel. Contains brief references to the statutory authority for federal programs by department or agency as well as organization charts and statements of purpose of various administrative units in the executive branch and the names and titles of principal administrative officers.

U.S. Government Printing Office's GPO Access Internet Service

Provides access to GAO reports from October 1994 to date, the *Congressional Record Index* from 1992 to date, and the full text of the *Congressional Record* from 1994 to date. Web address is http://www.access.gpo.gov/su_docs/aces/aaces001.html

U.S. Statutes at Large

Official edition of federal laws arranged numerically in order of enactment. Includes subject and name index, list of bills enacted into law, guide to legislative history of bills enacted, and tables of laws affected. Usually consists of one or more volumes for each legislative session.

Nongovernment Sources and Publications

Almanac of American Politics

Contains biographies, group ratings, committee assignments, voting records, and lobby interests of members of Congress as well as political, demographic, and economic makeup of each member's state or district. Published by *National Journal*, 1501 M Street NW, Washington, DC 20005.

Commerce Clearing House Congressional Index

Weekly looseleaf publication. Lists, indexes, summarizes, and reports progress of bills and resolutions in Congress. Pending measures are indexed by number, subject, author, and headline term. Voting records of members of Congress on each bill and status tables of action taken on each bill in the House and Senate are given. Published by Commerce Clearing House, 4025 W. Peterson Avenue, Chicago, IL 60646-6085.

Congress and the Nation

Volume 1 (1945–64), Volume 2 (1965–68), *Congressional Quarterly*. A 3,100-page, two-volume set. Documents all major legislative actions and national political campaigns from 1945 to 1968. Published by *Congressional Quarterly*, Inc.

Congressional Information Service (CIS)

Index to Publications of the U.S. Congress. Private commercial reference work that abstracts and indexes all congressional committee hearings and all House and Senate reports, documents, and special publications. Available from Congressional Information Service, 4520 East-West Highway, Bethesda, MD 20814.

Congressional Quarterly Almanac

Published each spring since 1945. Presents a thorough review of the legislative and political activity of each session of Congress, as well as a summary of the terms of the U.S. Supreme Court. Published by *Congressional Quarterly*, Inc., 1414 22nd Street NW, Washington, DC 20037.

Congressional Quarterly Weekly Report (CQ)

Weekly report, published since 1945, of major congressional actions in the House and Senate. Contains all roll call votes taken in each chamber plus weekly political roundups. Includes rosters, updated committee and subcommittee assignments, presidential texts, and so on. Published by *Congressional Quarterly*, Inc. 1414 22nd Street NW, Washington, DC 20037.

Congressional Quarterly's Guide to the Congress of the United States

A 1,000-page volume documenting the origins, development, and operations of the U.S. Congress. Explains how Congress works, including its powers, pressures on it, and prospects for change. Published by *Congressional Quarterly*, Inc., 1414 22nd Street NW, Washington, DC 20037.

Congressional Staff Directory

Published annually. Contains biographical sketches of many members of Congress and staffs, lists of employees of members and committees. Published by Staff Directories, Ltd., Mount Vernon, VA 22121-0062.

The Health Care 1000

An annual directory published by Faulkner and Gray, profiling the leading one thousand health care policymakers, advisers, opinion leaders, and organizations in the United States. Includes their addresses, telephone numbers, background data, and critical information on the budget and programs they control. Available from the Healthcare Information Center, 1133 Fifth Street NW, Washington, DC 20005.

Health Legislation and Regulation

A newsletter published fifty times a year by Faulkner and Gray, Inc., on the activities of the federal government in health. Formerly a McGraw-Hill publication, it is noted for its detailed briefings and ongoing analyses of congressional health care developments, providing detailed reports on the federal health budget, insurance coverage, and interviews with congressional health leaders. Includes comprehensive summaries of major health legislation and regulations as well as updates on new bills in Congress. Available from Faulkner and Gray, Healthcare Information Center, 133 Fifteenth Street NW, Suite 450, Washington, DC 20005.

Intergovernmental Health Policy Project (IHPP)

Devoted exclusively to research on health and health-related law and programs in the fifty states, and funded principally by contracts from the Health Care Financing Administration and the U.S. Public Health Service. IHPP is based at George Washington University, 2021 K Street NW, Suite 800, Washington, DC 20006. Publications include:

Focus/On. Published six times a year, each issue presents a thorough analysis of a single topic of major interest to state health policymakers and providers. Pre-

pared by leading health care policy researchers and writers, the reports present the latest thinking on the topic and describe current policy and practice.

Health Care Reform: 50 State Profiles. A 260-page, 1995 special report compiled by the Project staff, which describes the current status of universal access, cost containment, and delivery systems in the fifty states. Provides a comprehensive overview of state reform activities, followed by state-by-state summaries covering thirteen categories of reform: comprehensive reform and financing proposals, medical high-risk pools, tax incentives and medical savings accounts, regulation of physician fees and practice, hospital cooperative agreements and anti-trust issues, purchasing alliances and accountable health plans, insurance market reform, Medicaid, data collection and disclosure, and cost containment.

State Health Notes. A unique biweekly newsletter devoted to state health legislation and policy trends. Covers recent legislative and administrative developments in the states. Provides up-to-date information on significant health policy trends and innovations occurring in the states, including analysis of significant federal and state health legislation and regulations, descriptions and reviews of major public health programs, highlights of innovative state programs, summaries of congressional activity in the health arena, and important findings and recommendations from the latest health policy research carried out by the states.

Managed Medicare and Medicaid News

Formerly *Health Care Reform Week.* Its name was changed in 1995 reportedly to better reflect the editorial direction of the publication, namely, to provide more news and analyses of changes in the federal, state, and private sectors that are transforming the Medicare and Medicaid programs. Published forty-eight times a year by United Communications Group, PO Box 90608, Washington, DC 20090-0608.

Medicine and Health

A weekly (fifty issues a year) newsletter published by Faulkner and Gray, Inc. Formerly a McGraw-Hill publication, it provides brief coverage of health care developments in Congress, HHS, and the executive branch, as well as reports on health care providers, associations, and insurers, including the current status and probable fate of health bills on Capitol Hill. A special four-page section called "Perspectives" offers a provocative analysis of a different topic each week. Available from Faulkner and Gray's Healthcare Information Center, 133 Fifteenth Street NW, Suite 450, Washington, DC 20005.

National Health Council's Government Relations Handbooks

Congress and Health

An introduction to the legislative process and its key participants. Provides description of how a bill becomes a law. Gives practical information on how to determine the current status of a bill. Lists committees and subcommittees having significant impact on health legislation, including a brief description of their jurisdictions as well as names, photographs, and phone numbers of the six most important health subcommittees and the names of their staff members who handle health issues. Available from National Health Council, Inc., 350 Fifth Avenue, Suite 1118, New York, NY 10118.

Congressional Staff Aides for Health Legislation

Directory of the names, addresses, and phone numbers of senators and representatives and their staff aides assigned responsibility for health matters. Available from National Health Council (see above).

National Health Directory

Published annually. Directory of more than six thousand key health and medical officials within Congress, including health legislative aides, federal agencies, state governments, federal regional offices, and congressional districts. Complete list of members of the six major congressional committees on health; current titles, addresses, and phone numbers of health decision makers in offices of the governor, state agencies, and state legislators. Available from Aspen Publishers, Inc., 200 Orchard Ridge Drive, Gaithersburg, MD 20878.

National Journal Report

Weekly periodical reviews congressional activities, lobbying, campaign, and policy issues. Includes chart of roll call votes. Spotlights federal officials and election campaign reports and analyzes executive action. Especially informative is the discussion on health policy issues by John Iglehart.

Private Health Organizations' Government Relations Directory

Lists major private health organizations and groups with major interest in health policy as well as names and phone numbers of their staffs assigned to lobby in Washington, D.C. Available from National Health Council (see this page).

Reforming the Health Care System: State Profiles

Compiled and published annually since 1990 by the American Association of Retired Persons' (AARP) Division of Legislation and Public Policy's Public Policy Institute (PPI). Offers a snapshot of the health care landscape in each state by presenting nearly ninety key indicators, depicting major health care system characteristics of each of the fifty states and selected measures of each state's efforts to address health care problems within its system. Provides national statistics for purposes of comparison. For each state, information is presented in a standard four-page format on demographic data, health status, utilization of services, administration and quality, expenditures and financing, resources available, health care coverage including insurance status, managed care, and Medicaid and health care reform. Data are presented for each individual state and by state rankings. Available from Public Policy Institute, American Association of Retired Persons, 601 E Street NW, Washington, DC 20049.

State Health Watch

An independent monthly publication of SHW Inc. devoted to covering state legislative and administrative activities in the field of health. Available from SHW Inc., 668 Sunny Hill Road, Yardly, PA 19067.

State Initiatives in Health Care Reform

A newsletter on state health care reform activities by the Alpha Center, a nonprofit health policy center specializing in the dissemination of health research and demonstration findings to national, state, and local policymakers under a grant from the Robert Wood Johnson Foundation. Available from Alpha Center, 1350 Connecticut Avenue NW, Suite 1100, Washington, DC 20036.

States of Health

A newsletter providing coverage of state health care reform issues. Published six times a year by Families USA, 1334 G Street NW, Washington, DC 20005.

Washington Health Record

A weekly publication (fifty issues) originally published by McGraw-Hill but, like *Medicine and Health* and *Health Legislation and Regulation*, is now distributed by Faulkner and Gray, Inc. Each issue lists presidential proclamations, federal regulations and notices, and legislative activities, including committee and floor actions on House and Senate bills. Available from Faulkner and Gray's Healthcare Information Center, 1133 Fifteenth Street NW, Washington, DC 20005.

Additional Sources

American Medical News

Weekly tabloid-size newspaper published by the AMA. Distributed free to association members as part of their dues and offered on subscription basis to others. Covers policy positions and activities of organized medicine at both the national and state levels as well as government actions of interest to the medical profession.

Drug Research Reports (The Blue Sheet)

A weekly newsletter published by a commercial firm, providing special coverage of government activities in the drug, medical, and allied research fields. Reports on congressional committee hearings and health bills and reviews on congressional and executive branch actions in the area of health and health care.

The Nation's Health

Tabloid-size newspaper of the American Public Health Association. Contains reports of current status of state and federal actions in the field of health and health care and comments on government activities as they relate to the public's health.

THE POLITICS OF HEALTH AND HEALTH CARE

Begun, James W., & Ronald C. Lippincott. (1982). A case study in the politics of free-market health care. *Journal of Health Politics, Policy and Law, 7* (Fall), 667–687.

Belkin, Gary S. (1994). Numbers and politics of health care. *Journal of Health Politics, Policy and Law, 19* (Spring), 3–6.

Bellin, Lowell E. (1980). The intellectual decline of the health care left. *Medical Care, 18* (September), 960–968.

Bergman, Abraham B. (1988). *The discovery of sudden infant death syndrome: Lessons in the practice of political medicine.* Seattle: University of Washington Press.

Bergtheld, Linda A. (1990). *Purchasing power in health: Business, the state and health care politics.* New Brunswick, NJ: Rutgers University Press.

Blendon, Robert J., Tracey Stelzer Hyams, & John Benson. (1996). Health care and the 1996 election. *Inquiry, 33* (Spring), 10–14.

Blumenthal, David, & Robert A. Berenson. (1989). Health care issues in presidential campaigns. *New England Journal of Medicine, 321* (September 28), 908–912.

Borisoff, Mindy J., & J. Stuart Showalter. (1994). Health politics and policy: Survey of U.S. health administration courses. *Journal of Health Administration Education, 12* (Spring), 215–219.

Brown, J. H. U., & Southwest Research Consortium. (1978). *The politics of health care.* Cambridge: Ballinger.

Brown, Lawrence D. (1991). Knowledge and power: Health services research as a political resource. In Eli Ginzberg (Ed.), *Health services research: Key to health policy.* Cambridge, MA: Harvard University Press.

Brown, Lawrence D. (1993). Conference summary: The changing policies and politics of urban health. *Health Affairs, 12* (Winter), 233–236.

Brown, Lawrence D. (1994). Politics, money and health-care reform. *Health Affairs, 13* (Spring, 2), 175–184.

Cater, Douglass, & Philip R. Lee (Eds.). (1972). *Politics of health.* New York: Medcom Press.

Edelman, Murray. (1974). The political language of the helping professions. *Politics and Society, 4* (3), 295–310.

Facchinetti, Neil J., & W. Michael Dickson. (1982). Access to generic drugs in the 1950's: The politics of a social problem. *American Journal of Public Health, 72* (May), 468–475.

Falcone, David. (1976). The challenge of comparative health policy for political science. *Journal of Health Politics, Policy and Law, 1* (Summer), 196–213.

Fox, Daniel M. (1986). *Health policies, health politics: The British and American experience, 1911–1965.* Princeton, NJ: Princeton University Press.

Fox, Daniel M. (1990). Health policy and the politics of research in the United States. *Journal of Health Politics, Policy and Law, 15* (Fall), 481–499.

Fox, Daniel M., & Robert Crawford. (1979). Health politics in the United States. In Howard E. Freeman, Sol Levine, & Leo G. Reeder (Eds.), *Handbook of medical sociology* (3rd ed., pp. 392–411). New York: The Free Press.

Goldsmith, Seth B. (1973). Political party platform planks: A mechanism for participation and prediction. *American Journal of Public Health, 63* (July), 594–601.

Gray, Bradford. (1993). The legislative battle over health services research. *Health Affairs, 11* (4), 38–66.

Hadley, Jack. (1995). Politics versus policy analysis. *Inquiry, 32* (Summer), 127–129.

Helms, Robert B. (1993). *Health care policy and politics: Lessons from four countries.* Washington, D.C.: AEI Press.

Hodgson, Godfrey. (1976). The politics of health care: What is it costing you? In David Kotelchuck (Ed.), *Prognosis negative, crisis in the health system* (pp. 304–316). New York: Vintage Books.

Iglehart, John K. (1995). Republicans and the new politics of health care. *New England Journal of Medicine, 332* (April 6), 972–975.

Immergut, Ellen M. (1992). *Health politics: Interests and institutions in western Europe.* Cambridge: Cambridge University Press.

Jacobs, Lawrence R. (1995). The politics of America's supply state. *Health Affairs, 14* (Summer), 143–157.

Kaufman, Herbert. (1966). The political ingredient of public health services: A neglected area of research. *Milbank Memorial Fund Quarterly, 44* (October), 13–34.

Krause, Elliott. (1971). Health and the politics of technology. *Inquiry, 8* (September), 51–59.

Lee, Philip R., & A. E. Benjamin. (1988). Health policy and the politics of health care. In Stephen J. Williams & Paul R. Torrens (Eds.), *Introduction to health services* (3rd ed., pp. 457–479). New York: John Wiley & Sons.

Lepawsky, Albert. (1967). Medical science and political science. *Journal of Medical Education, 42* (October), 905–917.

Lewis, Irving J. (1969). Science and health care—the political problem. *New England Journal of Medicine, 281* (October 16), 888–896.

Luft, Harold S. (1991). Translating U.S. HMO experience to other systems. *Health Affairs, 10* (Fall), 172–186.

Makinson, Larry. (1992). Political contributions from the health and insurance industries. *Health Affairs, 11* (Winter), 119–134.

Margolis, Richard J. (1974). Where does it hurt?: America's medical crisis and the politics of health reform. *The New Leader, 57* (April 15), 3–35.

Marmor, Theodore R. (1989). *Rhetorical excess and American health politics: The debate about the tax exemption of nonprofit hospitals.* Chicago, IL: University of Chicago, The Center for Health Administration Studies.

Marmor, Theodore R., Amy Bridges, & Wayne L. Hoffman. (1978). Comparative politics and health policies: Notes on benefits, costs, limits. In Douglas E. Ashford (Ed.), *Comparing public policies: New concepts and methods* (Vol. 4, pp. 59–80). Beverly Hills, CA: Sage.

Marmor, Theodore, & Andrew B. Dunham. (1982). Political science and health. In Thomas Choi & Jay Greenberg (Eds.), *From social science approaches to health services research* (pp. 55–80). Ann Arbor, MI: Health Administration Press.

Marmor, Theodore R., & Andrew B. Dunham. (1983). Political science and health services administration. In Theodore R. Marmor (Ed.), *Political analysis and American medical care* (pp. 3–44). New York: Cambridge University Press.

Marmor, Theodore R., Donald A. Wittman, & Thomas C. Heagy. (1976). Politics, public policy and medical inflation. In Michael Zubkoff (Ed.), *Health: A victim or cause of inflation* (pp. 299–316). New York: Prodist.

McFarlane, Deborah R., & Larry J. Gordon. (1992). Teaching health policy and politics in U.S. schools of public health. *Journal of Public Health Policy, 13* (Winter), 428–434.

McKinlay, John B. (Ed.). (1973). *Politics and law in health care policy.* New York: Prodist.

McKinlay, John B. (Ed.). (1981). *Politics and health care: A Milbank Reader, No. 6.* Cambridge: MIT Press.

Mechanic, David. (1974). *Politics, medicine and social science.* New York: John Wiley & Sons.

Mendeloff, John. (1985). Bioethical commissions: "Muddling through" and the "slippery slope." *Journal of Health Politics, Policy and Law, 10* (Spring), 81–92.

Middleton, William J. (1974). Politics of liberating the health system. *The Black Scholar, 5* (May), 16–25.

Millman, Michael L. (1977). *Politics and the expanding physician supply.* Unpublished Ph.D. diss., Columbia University.

Navarro, Vicente. (1976). Social class, political power and the state: Their implications in medicine—Parts 1 and 2. *Journal of Health Politics, Policy and Law, 1* (Fall), 256–284.

Navarro, Vicente. (1994). *The politics of health policy.* Oxford, UK: Blackwell Publishers.

Patel, Kant, & Mark E. Rushefsky. (1995). *Health care politics and policy in America.* Armonk, NY: M. E. Sharpe.

Powell, John E. (1976). *Medicine and politics: 1975 and after.* Turnbridge Wells, UK: Pitman Medical.

Record, Jane Cassels. (1977). Medical politics and medical prices: The relation between who decides and how much it costs. In Kenneth M. Friedman & Stuart H. Rakoff (Eds.), *Toward a national health policy: Public policy and the control of health care costs.* Cambridge, MA: Lexington Books.

Riska, Elianne, & James A. Taylor. (1978). Consumer attitudes toward health policy and knowledge about health legislation. *Journal of Health Politics, Policy and Law, 3* (Spring), 112–123.

Silver, George A. (1976). Medical politics, health policy, party health platforms, promise and performance. *International Journal of Health Services, 6* (2), 331–343.

Swanson, Bert E. (1972). The politics of health. In Howard E. Freeman, Sol Levine, & Leo G. Reeder (Eds.), *Handbook of medical sociology* (2nd ed., pp. 435–455). Englewood Cliffs, NJ: Prentice-Hall.

Taylor, Peter. (1984). *The smoke ring: Tobacco, money, and multinational politics.* New York: Pantheon Books.

Vaillancourt Rosenau, Pauline. (1994). Health politics meets postmodernism: Its meaning and implications for community health organizing. *Journal of Health Politics, Policy and Law, 19* (Summer), 303–334.

Weaver, Jerry L. (1973). Health care costs as a political issue: Comparative responses of Chicanos and Anglos. *Social Science Quarterly, 53* (March), 846–854.

Weissert, Carol, & William G. Weissert. (1996). *Governing health: The politics of health policy.* Baltimore, MD: Johns Hopkins University Press.

Weller, G. R. (1977). From "pressure group politics" to "medical-industrial complex": The development of approaches to the politics of health. *Journal of Health Politics, Policy and Law, 1* (Winter), 444–470.

Wildavsky, Aaron. (1977). Doing better and feeling worse: The political pathology of health policy. *Daedalus, 106* (Winter), 105–123.

Zola, Irving K. (1975). In the name of health and illness: On some sociopolitical consequences of medical influence. *Social Science and Medicine, 9* (February), 83–87.

Abortion and Reproductive Health

Brodie, Janine, Shelley A. M. Gavigan, & Jane Jenson. (1992). *The politics of abortion: Representations of women in Canada.* New York: Oxford University Press.

Byrnes, Timothy A., & Mary C. Segars. (1991). *The Catholic Church and the politics of abortion: A view from the states.* Boulder, CO: Westview Press.

Cates, Willard, David A. Grimes, & L. Lynn Hogue. (1995). Topics for our times: Justice Blackmun and legal abortion—a besieged legacy to women's reproductive health. *American Journal of Public Health, 85* (September), 1204–1206.

Cook, Elizabeth Adell, Ted G. Jelen, & Clyde Wilcox. (1992). *Between two absolutes: Public opinion and the politics of abortion.* Boulder, CO: Westview Press.

Craig, Barbara H., & David M. O'Brien. (1993). *Abortion and American politics.* Chatham, NJ: Chatham House.

Epstein, Lee, & Joseph F. Kobylka. (1992). *The Supreme Court and legal change: Abortion and the death penalty.* Chapel Hill: University of North Carolina Press.

Gordon, Linda. (1975). The politics of birth control. *International Journal of Health Services, 5* (2), 253–278.

Hafner-Eaton, Chris, & Laurie K. Pearce. (1994). Birth choices, the law, and medicine: Balancing individual freedoms and protection of the public's health. *Journal of Health Politics, Policy and Law, 19* (Winter), 813–836.

Hoefler, James. (1994). *Deathright: Culture, medicine, politics and the right to die.* New Brunswick, NJ: Westview Press.

Hood, Howard, Igor I. Kavass, & Charles O. Galvin. (Eds.). (1991). *Abortion in the United States: A compilation of state legislation* (Vols. 1–2). Buffalo, NY: William S. Hein and Co.

Joffe, Carole. (1995). *Doctors of conscience: The struggle to provide abortion before and after* Roe v. Wade. Boston, MA: Beacon Press.

Judges, David P. (1993). *Hard choices, lost voices: How the abortion conflict has divided America, distorted constitutional rights, and damaged the courts.* Chicago, IL: Ivan R. Dee.

Karson, Stephen M. (1984). *Abortion: Politics, morality, and the Constitution: A critical study of* Roe v. Wade *and* Doe v. Bolton *and a basis for change.* Latham, MD: University Press of America.

Littlewood, T. B. (1979). *The politics of population control.* South Bend, IN: University of Notre Dame Press.

Mariner, Wendy K. (1992). The Supreme Court, abortion and the jurisprudence of class. *American Journal of Public Health, 82* (November), 1556–1562.

McKeegan, Michele. (1992). *Abortion politics: Mutiny in the ranks of the right.* New York: The Free Press, Macmillan.

Paige, Constance, & Elisa B. Karnofsky. (1986). The antiabortion movement and baby jane doe. *Journal of Health Politics, Policy and Law, 11* (Summer), 255–270.

Roemer, Ruth. (1971). Abortion law reform and repeal: Legislative and judicial developments. *American Journal of Public Health, 61* (March), 500–509.

Schneider, Carl E., & Maris A. Vinovskis. (1980). *The law and politics of abortion.* Lexington, MA: Lexington Books.

Staggenborg, Suzanne. (1991). *The pro-choice movement: Organization and activism in the abortion conflict.* New York: Oxford University Press.

Steinhoff, Patricia G., & Milton Diamond. (1977). *Abortion politics: The Hawaii experience*. Honolulu: University of Hawaii Press.

Wing, Kenneth R. (1993). The principles and principals of abortion compromise. *Journal of Health Politics, Policy and Law, 18* (Winter), 967–982.

AIDS

Anderson, Warwick. (1991). The New York needle trial: The politics of public health in the age of AIDS. *American Journal of Public Health, 81* (November), 1506–1517.

Andrulis, Dennis P. (1989). *Crisis at the front line: The effects of AIDS on public hospitals*. Washington, D.C.: The Brookings Institution.

Arno, Peter S., Karen Bonuck, & Michael Davis. (1995). Rare diseases, drug development, and AIDS: The impact of the Orphan Drug Act. *Milbank Quarterly, 73* (2), 231–252.

Arno, Peter S., & Karyn L. Feiden. (1992). *Against the odds: The story of AIDS drug development, politics and profits*. New York: HarperCollins.

Backstrom, Charles, & Leonard Robins. (1989). The political elements in policymaking on AIDS. *New England Journal of Human Services, 9* (Summer), 13–19.

Backstrom, Charles, & Leonard Robins. (1992). *The Minnesota response to AIDS*. Minneapolis: University of Minnesota Center for Regional Affairs.

Backstrom, Charles, & Leonard Robins. (1995). Public health policymaking: Perceptions of state legislators. *AIDS and Public Policy Journal, 10* (Winter), 238–248.

Bayer, Ronald. (1988). *Private acts, social consequences: AIDS and the politics of public health*. New York: The Free Press.

Bayer, Ronald. (1991). AIDS: The politics of prevention and neglect. *Health Affairs, 10* (Spring), 87–97.

Bosk, Charles L., & Joel E. Frader. (1990). AIDS and its impact on medical work: The culture and politics of the shop floor. *Milbank Quarterly, 68* (Suppl. 2), 257–279.

Buchanan, Robert J. (1988). State Medicaid coverage of AZT and AIDS-related policies. *American Journal of Public Health, 78* (April), 432–436.

Daniels, Norman. (1992). HIV infected health care professionals: Public threat or public sacrifice? *Milbank Quarterly, 70* (1), 3–42.

Daniels, Norman. (1995). *Seeking fair treatment: From the AIDS epidemic to national health care reform*. New York: Oxford University Press.

Falco, Mathea, & Warren I. Cikins. (Eds.). (1989). *Toward a national policy on drug and AIDS testing*. Washington, D.C.: The Brookings Institution.

Feldman Douglas A. (Ed.). (1994). *Global AIDS policy*. Westport, CT: Bergin and Garvey, Greenwood Publishing.

Fox, Daniel M. (1990). Chronic disease and disadvantage: The new politics of HIV infection. *Journal of Health Politics, Policy and Law, 15* (Summer), 341–356.

Fox, Daniel M., & E. H. Thomas. (1989). *Financing care for persons with AIDS: The first studies, 1985–1988*. Frederick, MD: University Publishing Group.

Fox, Renée C., Linda H. Aiken, & Carla M. Messikomer. (1990). The culture of caring: AIDS and the nursing profession. *Milbank Quarterly, 68* (Suppl. 2), 226–256.

Francis, Donald. (1994). Insulating public health from extremist politics—Do we need boards of health? *American Journal of Public Health, 84* (May), 720–721.

Fumento, Michael. (1990). *The myth of heterosexual AIDS: How a tragedy has been distorted by the media and partisan politics*. New York: Basic Books.

Glantz, Leonard H., Wendy K. Mariner, & George J. Annas. (1992). Risky business: Setting public health policy for HIV-infected health care professionals. *Milbank Quarterly, 70* (1), 43–80.

Gostin, Lawrence O. (Ed.). (1990). *AIDS and the health care system*. New Haven, CT: Yale University Press.

Green, Jesse, Gerald M. Oppenheimer, & Neil Wintfeld. (1994). The $117,000 misunderstanding: Repercussions of overestimating the cost of AIDS. *Journal of Health Politics, Policy and Law, 19* (Spring), 69–90.

Griggs, John. (Ed.). (1987). *AIDS: Public policy dimensions*. New York: United Hospital Fund of New York.

Hellinger, Fred J. (1988). National forecasts of the medical care costs of AIDS: 1988–1992. *Inquiry, 25* (Winter), 469–484.

Hummel, Robert F., William F. Leavy, Michael Rampolla, & Sherry Chorost. (Eds.). (1988). *AIDS: Impact on public policy. An international forum: Policy, politics, and AIDS*. New York: Plenum.

Hurley, Peter, & Glenn Pinder. (1992). Ethics, social forces, and politics in AIDS-related research: Experience in planning and implementing a household HIV seroprevalence survey. *Milbank Quarterly, 70* (4), 605–628.

Judson, Franklyn N., & Thomas M. Verhon Jr. (1988). The impact of AIDS on state and local Health Departments: Issues and a few answers. *American Journal of Public Health, 78* (April), 387–393.

Kaplan, Edward H., & Margaret L. Brandeau. (Eds.). (1994). *Modeling the AIDS epidemic: Planning, policy, and prediction*. New York: Raven Press.

Kayal, Philip M. (1993). *Bearing witness: Gay men's health crisis and the politics of AIDS*. Boulder, CO: Westview Press.

Kirp, David L., & Ronald Bayer. (Eds.). (1992). *AIDS in the industrialized democracies: Passions, politics, and policies*. New Brunswick, NJ: Rutgers University Press.

Krieger, Nancy. (1988). AIDS funding: Competing needs and the politics of priorities. *International Journal of Health Services, 18* (4), 521–542.

Krieger, Nancy, & Joyce C. Lashoff. (1988). AIDS policy analysis and the electorate: The role of schools of public health. *American Journal of Public Health, 78* (April), 411–417.

Krieger, Nancy, & Glen Margo. (Eds.). (1994). *AIDS: The politics of survival*. Amityville, NY: Baywood Publishing.

Lee, Philip R., & Peter S. Arno. (1986). The federal response to the AIDS epidemic. *Health Policy, 6* (3), 259–267.

Mariner, Wendy K. (1995). AIDS phobia, public health warnings, and lawsuits: Deterring harm or rewarding ignorance. *American Journal of Public Health, 85* (November), 1562–1568.

Mechanic, David., & Linda H. Aiken. (1989). Lessons from the past: Responding to the AIDS crisis. *Health Affairs, 8* (Fall), 16–32.

Merson, Michael H. (1992). AIDS: The world situation. *Journal of Public Health Policy, 13* (Spring), 18–26.

Misztal, Barbara A., & David Moss. (1990). *Action on AIDS: National policies in comparative perspective*. Westport, CT: Greenwood Publishing.

Murray, Thomas H. (1990). The poisoned gift: AIDS and blood. *Milbank Quarterly, 68* (Suppl. 2), 205–225.

Nelkin, Dorothy. (1991). AIDS and the news media. *Milbank Quarterly, 69* (2), 293–308.

Panem, Sandra. (1988). *The AIDS bureaucracy: Why society failed to meet the AIDS crisis and how we might improve our response*. Cambridge, MA: Harvard University Press.

Perrow, Charles, & Mauro F. Guillen. (1990). *The AIDS disaster: The failure of organizations in New York and the nation*. New Haven: Yale University Press.

Philipson, Tomas J., & Richard A. Posner. (1993). *Private choices and public health: The AIDS epidemic in an economic perspective*. Cambridge, MA: Harvard University Press.

Pollack, Michael. (1994). *The second plague of Europe: AIDS prevention and sexual transmission among men in western Europe*. Binghampton, NY: Harrington Park Press.

Rabin, Judith A. (1986). The AIDS epidemic and gay bathhouses: A constitutional analysis. *Journal of Health Politics, Policy and Law, 10* (Winter), 729–748.

Richland, Jordan H. (1988). Role of state health agencies in responding to AIDS. *Public Health Reports, 103* (May/June), 267–272.

Robins, Leonard, & Charles Backstrom. (1993). Public policy and political perspectives of hospital associations on AIDS. *New England Journal of Human Services, 12* (4), 2–9.

Robins, Leonard, & Charles Backstrom. (1994). The role of state Health Departments in formulating policy: A survey on the case of AIDS. *American Journal of Public Health, 84* (June), 905–909.

Roemer, Ruth. (1971). Abortion law reform and repeal: Legislative and judicial developments. *American Journal of Public Health, 61* (March), 500–509.

Rogers, David E., & Eli Ginzberg. (Eds.). (1989). *Public and professional attitudes toward AIDS patients: A national dilemma.* Boulder, CO: Westview Press.

Rothman, David J., & Harold Edgar. (1990). Drug approval and AIDS: Benefits for the elderly. *Health Affairs, 9* (Fall), 123–130.

Rowe, Mona, & Caitlin C. Ryan. (1987). *AIDS: A public health challenge, state issues, policies and programs.* Washington, D.C.: Intergovernmental Health Policy Project, George Washington University.

Rowe, Mona, & Caitlin C. Ryan. (1988). Comparing state-only expenditures for AIDS. *American Journal of Public Health, 78* (April), 424–431.

Rudzinski, Karen A., Katherine M. Marconi, & Martha M. Mckinney. (1994). Federal funding for health services research. *Health Affairs, 13* (Summer), 261–266.

Rundall, Thomas G., & Katheryn A. Phillips. (1990). Informing and educating the electorate about AIDS. *Medical Law Review, 47* (Spring), 3–13.

Scitovsky, Anne A. (1988). The economic impact of AIDS in the United States. *Health Affairs, 7* (Fall), 32–45.

Shilts, Randy. (1987). *And the band played on: Politics, people and the AIDS epidemic.* New York: St. Martin's Press.

Singer, Eleanor, Theresa F. Rogers, & Mary Corcoran. (1987). The polls—A report: AIDS. *Public Opinion Quarterly, 51* (Winter), 580–595.

Thomas, Stephen B., & Sandra Crouse Quinn. (1991). The Tuskegee Syphilis study, 1932 to 1972: Implications for HIV education and AIDS risk education programs in the black community. *American Journal of Public Health, 81* (November), 1498–1504.

Zuercher, Andrea. (1990). A look at the latest U.S. AIDS projections. *Health Affairs, 9* (Summer), 163–170.

Cancer

Eisenberg, Lucy. (1971). The politics of cancer. *Harpers, 243* (November), 100–105.

Epstein, Samuel S. (1978). *Politics of cancer.* San Francisco: Sierra Club Books.

Hixson, Joseph. (1976). *The patchwork mouse, politics and intrigue in the campaign to conquer cancer.* Garden City, NY: Anchor Press/Doubleday and Co.

Lally, John J. (1977). Social determinants of differential allocation of resources to disease research: A comparative analysis of crib death and cancer research. *Journal of Health and Social Behavior, 18* (June), 125–138.

Levine, Adeline G. (1982). *Love canal, politics and people.* Lexington, MA: Lexington Books.

Markle, Gerald E., & James C. Peterson. (Eds.). (1980). *Politics, science and cancer: The Laetrile phenomenon.* Boulder, CO: Westview Press.

Proctor, Robert N. (1995). *Cancer wars: How politics shapes what we know and don't know about cancer.* New York: Basic Books.

Rettig, Richard A. (1977). *Cancer crusade: The story of the National Cancer Act of 1971.* Princeton, NJ: Princeton University Press.

Rushefsky, Mark E. (1986). *Making cancer policy.* Albany: State University of New York Press.

Strickland, Stephen P. (1972). *Politics, science and dread disease: A short history of United States medical research policy.* Cambridge, MA: Harvard University Press.

Whelan, Ellen Haas. (1980). Government: Hindrance or help in the cancer war? In Bernard H. Siegan (Ed.), *Government, regulation and the economy.* Lexington, MA: Lexington Books.

Competition and Regulation

Altman, Drew. (1978). The politics of health care regulation: The case of the National Health Planning and Resources Development Act. *Journal of Health Politics, Policy and Law, 2* (Winter), 560–580.

Anderson, Gerard F., Robert Heyssel, & Robert Dickler. (1993). Competition vs. regulation: Its effect on hospitals. *Health Affairs, 12* (Spring), 70–80.

Arnould, Richard J., Robert F. Rich, & William D. White. (Eds.). (1993). *Competitive approaches to health care reform.* Washington, D.C.: Urban Institute Press.

Ashby, John L., Jr. (1984). The impact of hospital regulatory programs on per capita costs, utilization and capital investment. *Inquiry, 21* (Spring), 45–59.

Avellone, Joseph C., & Francis D. Moore. (1978). The Federal Trade Commission enters a new arena: Health services. *New England Journal of Medicine, 299* (August), 478–483.

Barth, Peter S. (1987). *The tragedy of black lung: Federal compensation for occupational disease.* Kalamazoo, MI: Upjohn Institute for Employment Research.

Battistella, Roger M., & Thomas P. Weil. (1986). Pro-competitive health policy: Benefits and perils. *Frontiers of Health Services Management, 2* (May), 3–27.

Bauer, Morris L. (1988). Regulating physician supply: The evolution of British Columbia's Bill 41. *Journal of Health Politics, Policy and Law, 13* (Spring), 1–26.

Bazzoli, Gloria J., David Marx Jr., Richard J. Arnould, & Larry M. Manheim. (1995). Federal antitrust merger enforcement standards: A good fit for the hospital industry? *Journal of Health Politics, Policy and Law, 20* (Spring), 137–170.

Bice, Thomas W. (1984). The politics of health care regulation. In Theodor J. Litman & Leonard S. Robins (Eds.), *Health Politics and Policy* (1st ed., pp. 274–289). New York: John Wiley & Sons.

Brennan, Troyen A., & Donald M. Berwick. (1996). *New rules: Regulation, markets, and the quality of American health care.* San Francisco: Jossey-Bass.

Bromberg, Michael D. (1993). Flexibility in antitrust enforcement. *Health Affairs, 12* (Fall), 150–151.

Brown, Lawrence D. (1992). Political evolution of federal health care regulation. *Health Affairs, 11* (Winter), 17–37.

Campbell, Ellen S., & Gary M. Fournier. (1993). Certificate-of-need: Deregulation and indigent hospital care. *Journal of Health Politics, Policy and Law, 18* (Winter), 905–926.

Celnicker, Arnold C. (1990). An economic and antitrust analysis of the distribution of medical products. *American Journal of Law and Medicine, 16* (4), 499–524.

Chesney, James D. (1982). The politics of regulation: An assessment of winners and losers. *Inquiry, 19* (Fall), 235–245.

Christoffel, Tom, & Katherine K. Christoffel. (1989). The Consumer Product Safety Commission's opposition to consumer product safety: Lessons for public health advocates. *American Journal of Public Health, 79* (March), 336–339.

Clark, Robin E., & Robert A. Dorwart. (1992). Competition and community mental health agencies. *Journal of Health Politics, Policy and Law, 17* (Fall), 517–540.

Cohen, Harris S. (1975). Regulating politics and American medicine. *American Behavioral Scientist, 19* (1), 122–136.

Curran, William, Richard Steele, & Ellen Ober. (1975). Government intervention on increase. *Hospitals, 49* (May 16), 57–61.

Danzon, Patricia M. (1994). *Global budgets versus competitive cost-control strategies.* American Enterprise Institute: Special Studies in Health Reform. Waldorf, MD: AEI Press.

Day, Patricia, & Rudolf Klein. (1987). The regulation of nursing homes: A comparative perspective. *Milbank Memorial Fund Quarterly, 65* (3), 303–347.

Dranove, David, & Kenneth Kone. (1985). Do states rate setting regulations really lower hospital expenses? *Journal of Health Economics, 4* (June), 159–165.

Eby, C. A., & Donald R. Cohodes. (1985). What do we know about rate setting? *Journal of Health Politics, Policy and Law, 10* (Summer), 299–327.

Eisenberg, John M. (1994). If trickle-down physician workforce policy failed, is the choice now between the market and government regulation? *Inquiry, 31* (Fall), 241–249.

Enthoven, Alain C. (1989). Effective management of competition in the FEHBP. *Health Affairs, 8* (Fall), 33–50.

Feldstein, Paul J. (1986). The emergence of market competition in the U.S. health care system: Its courses, likely structure and implications. *Health Policy, 6* (1), 1–20.

Field, Marilyn J., & Bradford H. Gray. (1989). Should we regulate "utilization management"? *Health Affairs, 8* (Winter), 103–112.

Finkler, Merton D. (1987). State rate setting revisited. *Health Affairs, 6* (Winter), 82–89.

Fox, Daniel M. (1994). Two fringe discourses in search of influence on policy. *Journal of Health Politics, Policy and Law, 19* (Winter), 809–812.

Frankford, David M. (1994). Scientism and economism in the regulation of health care. *Journal of Health Politics, Policy and Law, 19* (Winter), 773–800.

Fuchs, Victor R. (1988). The "competition revolution" in health care. *Health Affairs, 7* (Summer), 5–24.

Gaumer, Gary L. (1984). Regulating health professionals: A review of the empirical literature. *Milbank Memorial Fund Quarterly, 62* (Summer), 380–416.

Glaser, William A. (1993). The competition vogue and its outcomes. *Lancet, 341* (March 27), 805–812.

Grabowski, Henry G. (1976). *Drug regulation and innovation* (Evaluative Studies No. 28). Washington, D.C.: American Enterprise Institute for Public Policy Research.

Graddy, Elizabeth. (1991). Interest groups or the public interest—why do we regulate health occupations? *Journal of Health Politics, Policy and Law, 16* (Spring), 25–50.

Greenberg, Warren. (1988). *Competition in the health care sector: Ten years later.* Durham, NC: Duke University Press.

Greenberg, Warren. (1991). *Competition, regulation and rationing in health care.* Ann Arbor, MI: Health Administration Press.

Hackey, Robert B. (1992). Trapped between state and market: Regulating hospital reimbursement in the northeast states. *Medical Care Review, 49* (Fall), 355–388.

Hackey, Robert B. (1993). Commentary: New wine in old bottles: Certificate of need enters the 1990s. *Journal of Health Politics, Policy and Law, 18* (Winter), 927–936.

Hackey, Robert B. (1993). Commentary: Regulatory regimes and state cost containment programs. *Journal of Health Politics, Policy and Law, 18* (Summer), 491–502.

Helms, Robert B. (Ed.). (1993). *Health policy reform: Competition and controls.* Waldorf, MD: AEI Press.

Joskow, Paul. (1984). *Controlling hospital costs: The role of government regulation.* Cambridge, MA: MIT Press.

Kavaler, Florence, Howard R. Kelman, & Alan P. Brownstein. (1980). Regulating health care: Prospects for the future. *Journal of Public Health Policy, 1* (September), 230–240.

Kennedy, Donald. (1983). Health, science, and regulation: The politics of prevention. *Health Affairs, 2* (Fall), 39 51.

Krause, Elliott A. (1975). The political context of health service regulation. *International Journal of Health Services, 5* (4), 593–608.

Kronick, Richard, David C. Goodman, John Wennberg, & Edward Wagner. (1993). The marketplace in health care reform: The demographic limitations of managed competition. *New England Journal of Medicine, 328* (January 14), 148–152.

Levin, Arthur. (1981). *Regulating health care: The struggle for control.* New York: Academy of Political Science.

Levine, Adeline G. (1982). *Love canal: Science, politics, and people.* Lexington, MA: Lexington Books.

Leyerle, Betty. (1994). *The private regulation of American health care.* Armonk, NY: M. E. Sharpe.

Luft, Harold S. (1985). Competition and regulation. *Medical Care, 23* (May), 383–400.

MacSheoin, Thomas. (1985). The dismantling of U.S. health and safety regulations under the first Reagan administration: A bibliography. *International Journal of Health Services, 15* (4), 585–608.

Marks, Harry M. (1995). Revisiting the origins of compulsory drug prescriptions. *American Journal of Public Health, 85* (January), 109–115.

McCaffrey, David P. (1982). *OSHA and the politics of health regulation*. New York: Plenum.

McCall, Nelda, Thomas Rice, & Arden Hall. (1987). The effect of state regulations on the quality and sale of insurance policies to Medicare beneficiaries. *Journal of Health Politics, Policy and Law, 12* (Spring), 53–76.

Melhaldo, Evan M. (1988). Competition versus regulation in American health policy. In Evan M. Melhaldo, Walter Feinberg, & Harold W. Swartz (Eds.), *Money, power and health care* (pp. 15–102). Ann Arbor, MI: Health Administration Press.

Melnick, Glenn A., Jack Zwanziger, & Tom Bradley. (1989). Competition and cost containment in California. *Health Affairs, 8* (Summer), 129–136.

Mendeloff, John M. (1979). *Regulation safety: An economic and political analysis of occupational safety and health policy*. Cambridge, MA: MIT Press.

Mendeloff, John M. (1988). *The dilemma of toxic substance regulation: How overregulation causes underregulation*. Cambridge, MA: MIT Press.

Mendeloff, John M. (1991). Commentary: On the feasibility of strict and extensive rulemaking. *Journal of Health Politics, Policy and Law, 16* (Spring), 19–24.

Merrill, Jeffrey, & Catherine McLaughlin. (1986). Competition versus regulation: Some empirical evidence. *Journal of Health Politics, Policy and Law, 10* (Winter), 613–623.

Merrill, Richard A. (1994). Regulation of drugs and devices: An evolution. *Health Affairs, 13* (Summer), 47–69.

Metzenbaum, Howard M. (1993). Antitrust enforcement: Putting the consumer first. *Health Affairs, 12* (Fall), 137–143.

Meyer, Jack A. (Ed.). (1987). *Incentives versus controls in health policy*. Washington, D.C.: American Enterprise Institute for Public Policy Research.

Miller, Robert G. (1996). Health system integration: A means to an end. *Health Affairs, 15* (Summer), 92–106.

Miller, Robert H. (1996). Competition in the health systems: Good news and bad news. *Health Affairs, 15* (Summer), 107–120.

Moore, Gordon T. (1994). Will the power of the marketplace produce the workforce we need? *Inquiry, 31* (Fall), 276–282.

Morford, Thomas G. (1988). Nursing home regulation: History and expectations. *Health Care Financing Review, Supplement* (December), 129–132.

Morrisey, Michael A., Frank A. Sloan, & Samuel A. Mitchell. (1983). State rate setting: An analysis of some unresolved issues. *Health Affairs, 2* (Summer), 36–47.

Mosher, James F., & Lawrence M. Wallack. (1981). Government regulation of alcohol advertising: Protecting industry profits versus promoting the public health. *Journal of Public Health Policy, 2* (December), 333–353.

Paringer, Lynne, & Nelda McCall. (1991). How competitive is competitive bidding? *Health Affairs, 10* (Winter), 220–230.

Pauly, Mark V. (1988). Is medical care different? Old questions, new answers. *Journal of Health Politics, Policy and Law, 13* (Summer), 227–238.

Reinhardt, Uwe E. (1994). Planning the nation's health workforce: Let the market in. *Inquiry, 31* (Fall), 250–263.

Rice, Donald. (1981). Government regulation of the hospital industry in Colorado. *Journal of Public Health Policy, 2* (March), 58–69.

Rice, Thomas, & Kathleen Thomas. (1992). Evaluating medigap standardization regulations. *Health Affairs, 11* (Spring), 181–193.

Robinson, James C., & Mita K. Gincomini. (1992). A reallocation of rights in industries with reproductive health hazards. *Milbank Quarterly, 70* (4), 587–604.

Robinson, James C., & Dalton G. Paxman. (1991). Technological, economic, and political feasibility in OSHA's air contaminants standard. *Journal of Health Politics, Policy and Law, 16* (Spring), 1–18.

Rolph, Elizabeth S., Paul B. Ginsburg, & Susan D. Hosek. (1987). The regulation of preferred provider arrangements. *Health Affairs, 6* (Fall), 32–45.

Safriet, Barbara J. (1994). Impediments to progress in health care workforce policy: License and practice laws. *Inquiry, 31* (Fall), 310–317.

Samuel, Frank E. Jr. (1991). Safe medical devices act of 1990. *Health Affairs, 10* (Spring), 192–195.

Schramm, Carl J. (1986). Revisiting the competition/ regulation debate in health care cost containment. *Inquiry, 23* (Fall), 236–242.

Schramm, Carl J., Steven C. Renn, & Brian Biles. (1986). Controlling hospital cost inflation: New perspectives on state rate setting. *Health Affairs, 5* (Fall), 22–33.

Schwartz, Theresa M. (1975). Protecting consumer health and safety: The need for coordinated regulation among federal agencies. *George Washington Law Review, 43* (May), 1031–1076.

Seplaki, Les. (1994). *Cost and competition in American medicine: Theory, policy and institutions.* Lanham, MD: University Press of America.

Sloan, Frank A. (1983). Rate regulation as a strategy for hospital cost control: Evidence from the last decade. *Milbank Memorial Fund Quarterly, 61* (Spring), 195–221.

Smith, Barbara E. (1987). *Digging our own graves: Coal miners and the struggle over black lung disease.* Philadelphia: Temple University Press.

Smith, David W., Stephanie L. McFall, & Michael B. Pine. (1993). State rate regulation and inpatient mortality rates. *Inquiry, 30* (Spring), 23–33.

Spitz, Bruce, & John Abramson. (1987). Competition, capitation and case management: Barriers to strategic reform. *Milbank Memorial Fund Quarterly, 65* (3), 348–370.

Vistnes, Gregory. (1995). Hospital mergers and antitrust enforcement. *Journal of Health Politics, Policy and Law, 20* (Spring), 175–190.

Wallack, Stanley S., Kathleen Carley Skwara, & John Cai. (1996). Redefining rate regulation in a competitive environment. *Journal of Health Politics, Policy and Law, 21* (Fall), 489–510.

Weissert, William G., Jennifer M. Elston, Melissa Constable Musliner, & Elizabeth Mutran. (1991). Adult day care regulation: Déjà vu all over again. *Journal of Health Politics, Policy and Law, 16* (Spring), 51–66.

Zwanziger, Jack. (1995). The need for an antitrust policy for a health care industry in transition. *Journal of Health Politics, Policy and Law, 20* (Spring), 171–174.

Cost Containment

Abel-Smith, Brian. (1984). *Cost containment in health care: A study of twelve European countries 1977–1983* (Occassional Papers on Social Administration No. 73). Bedford, UK: London Square Press, Brookfield Publishing Company.

Abel-Smith, Brian. (1992). Cost containment and new priorities in the European community. *Milbank Quarterly, 70* (3), 393–416.

Abel-Smith, Brian. (1992). *Cost containment and new priorities in health care.* Brookhead, VT: Ashgate.

Abel-Smith, Brian, & Elias Mossialos. (1994). Cost containment and health care reform: A study of the European union. *Health Policy, 28* (May), 89–132.

Birch, Stephen. (1988). DRGs U.K. style: A comparison of U.K. and U.S. policies for hospital cost containment and their implications for health status. *Health Policy, 10* (2), 143–154.

Birenbaum, Arnold. (1993). *Putting health care on the national agenda.* Westport, CT: Praeger.

Blendon, Robert J., & Jennifer N. Edwards. (Eds.). (1991). *System in crisis: The case for health care reform* (Vol. 1). Washington, D.C.: Faulkner & Gray, Inc.

Blendon, Robert J., & Tracey Hyams. (1992). *Reforming the system: Containing health care costs in an era of universal coverage* (Vol. 2). Washington, D.C.: Faulkner & Gray, Inc.

Christensen, Sandra. (1991). Did 1980's legislation slow Medicare spending? *Health Affairs, 10* (Summer), 135–142.

Christianson, Jon B., Bryan Dowd, John Kralewski, Susan Hayes, & Catherine Wisner. (1995). Managed care in the Twin Cities: What can we learn? *Health Affairs, 14* (Summer), 114–130.

Christianson, Jon B., & Diane G. Hillman. (1986). *Health care for the indigent and competitive contracts: The Arizona experiment.* Ann Arbor, MI: Health Administration Press.

Christianson, Jon B., Diane G. Hillman, & Kenneth R. Smith. (1983). The Arizona experiment: Competitive bidding for indigent medical care. *Health Affairs, 2* (3), 88–103.

Christianson, Jon B., & Kenneth R. Smith. (1985). *Current strategies for containing health care expenditures.* Bridgeport, CT: Robert B. Luce, Inc.

Davis, Karen, Gerard F. Anderson, Steven C. Renn, Diane Rowland, Carl J. Schramm, & Earl Steinberg. (1985). Is cost containment working? *Health Affairs, 4* (Fall), 81–94.

Davis, Karen, Gerard F. Anderson, Diane Rowland, & Earl P. Stenberg. (1990). *Health care cost containment.* Baltimore, MD: Johns Hopkins University Press.

Davis, Karen, Karen Scott Collings, & Cynthia Morris. (1994). Managed care: Promise and concerns. *Health Affairs, 13* (Fall), 178–185.

Enthoven, Alain C. (1993). Why managed care has failed to contain costs. *Health Affairs, 12* (Fall), 27–43.

Evans, Robert G. (1986). Finding the levers, finding the courage: Lessons for cost containment in North America. *Journal of Health Politics, Policy and Law, 11* (4), 585–615.

Fraser, Irene. (1985). Medicare reimbursement for hospice care: Ethical and policy implications of cost-containment strategies. *Journal of Health Politics, Policy and Law, 10* (Fall), 565–578.

Fuchs, Victor. (1986). Has cost containment gone too far? *Milbank Memorial Fund Quarterly, 64* (3), 479–488.

Ginsburg, Paul B. (1989). Physician payment policy in the 101st Congress. *Health Affairs, 8* (Spring), 5–20.

Ginsburg, Paul B. (1993). Expenditure limits and cost containment. *Inquiry, 30* (Winter), 389–399.

Ginsburg, Paul B., Philip R. Lee, William C. Hsiao, Victor G. Rodwin, James S. Todd, & William A. Glaser. (1989). Perspectives on physician payment reform. *Health Affairs, 8* (Winter), 67–96.

Ginsburg, Paul B., Lauren B. LeRoy, & Glenn T. Hammons. (1990). Medicare physician payment reform. *Health Affairs, 9* (Spring), 178–188.

Ginsburg, Paul B., & Kenneth E. Thorpe. (1992). Can all-payer rate setting and the competitive strategy coexist? *Health Affairs, 11* (Summer), 73–86.

Glaser, William A. (1989). The politics of paying American physicians. *Health Affairs, 8* (Fall), 129–146.

Glaser, William A. (1993). How expenditure caps and expenditure targets really work. *Milbank Quarterly, 71* (1), 97–128.

Gold, Marsha, Karyn Chu, Suzanne Felt, Mary Harrington, & Timothy Lake. (1993). Effects of selected cost-containment efforts: 1971–1993. *Health Care Financing Review, 14* (Spring), 183–226.

Grumbach, Kevin, & Thomas Bodenheimer. (1990). Reins or fences: Physicians' view of cost containment. *Health Affairs, 9* (Winter), 120–126.

Grumbach, Kevin, & Thomas Bodenheimer. (1994). Painful vs painless cost control. *Journal of American Medical Association, 272* (November 9), 1458–1464.

Gutterman, Stuart, Stuart H. Altman, & Donald A. Young. (1990). Hospital finances in the first five years of PPS. *Health Affairs, 9* (Spring), 125–134.

Hackey, Robert B. (1993). Commentary: Regulatory regimes and state cost containment programs. *Journal of Health Politics, Policy and Law, 18* (Summer), 491–502.

Hall, William J., & Paul F. Griner. (1993). Cost-effective health care: The Rochester experience. *Health Affairs, 12* (Spring), 58–69.

Health Care Financing Review. Selected annotated references by topic for each of the five cost-containment efforts. *Health Care Financing Review, 14* (Spring), 215–225.

Kildreth, Elizabeth, & Alan B. Cohen. (1993). Strategic choices for cost containment under a reformed U.S. health care system. *Inquiry, 30* (Winter), 372–388.

Langwell, Kathryn. (1993). Price controls: On the one hand . . . and on the other. *Health Care Financing Review, 14* (Spring), 5–10.

Lave, Judith R. (1985). Cost containment policies in long-term care. *Inquiry, 22* (Spring), 7–23.

Lomas, Jonathan, Catherine Fooks, Thomas Rice, & Roberta J. LaBelle. (1989). Paying physicians in Canada: Minding our Ps and Qs. *Health Affairs, 8* (Spring), 80–102.

Long, Stephen H., & W. Pete Welch. (1988). Are we containing costs or pushing on a balloon? *Health Affairs, 7* (Fall), 113–117.

Martin, Cathie Jo. (1993). Together again: Business, government, and the quest for cost control. *Journal of Health Politics, Policy and Law, 18* (Summer), 359–394.

McCall, Nelda, Douglas Henton, Susan Haber, et al. (1987). Evaluation of Arizona health care cost containment system, 1984–85. *Health Care Financing Review, 9* (Winter), 79–90.

McCarthy, Carol M. (1988). DRGs—five years later. *New England Journal of Medicine, 318* (June 23), 1683–1686.

McCombs, Jeffrey S. (1989). A competitive bidding approach to physician payment. *Health Affairs, 8* (Spring), 50–64.

McCue, Jack D. (Ed.). (1989). *The medical cost-containment crisis: Fears, opinions, and facts.* Melrose Park, IL: Health Administration Press.

Mechanic, David. (1985). Cost containment and the quality of medical care: Rationing strategies in an era of constrained resources. *Milbank Memorial Fund Quarterly, 63* (Summer), 453–475.

Melnick, Glenn A., Jack Zwanziger, & Tom Bradley. (1989). Competition and cost containment in California. *Health Affairs, 8* (Summer), 129–136.

Menges, Joel. (1986). From health services research to federal law: The case of DRGs. In Marion Ein Lewin (Ed.), *From research into policy. Improving the link for health services* (pp. 20–23). Washington, D.C.: American Enterprise Institute for Public Policy Research.

Neumann, Peter J., & Magnus Johannesson. (1994). From principle to public policy: Using cost-effectiveness analysis. *Health Affairs, 13* (Summer), 206–214.

Organization for Economic Cooperation and Development. (1995). *New orientation in health care policies: Improving cost control and effectiveness.* Washington, D.C.: OECD Publications and Information Center.

Pauly, Mark V. (1995). When does curbing health costs help the economy? *Health Affairs, 14* (Summer), 68–82.

Pauly, Mark V., John M. Eisenberg, Margaret Higgins Radany, M. Haim Erder, Roger Feldman, & J. Sanford Schwartz. (1992). *Paying physicians: Options for controlling cost, volume and intensity of services.* Ann Arbor, MI: Health Administration Press.

Raphaelson, Arnold H. (1978). Politics and economics of hospital cost containment. *Journal of Health Politics, Policy and Law, 3* (Spring), 87–111.

Rasell, M. Edith. (1995). Cost-sharing in health insurance: A reexamination. *New England Journal of Medicine, 332* (April 27), 1164–1168.

Rice, Thomas. (1992). Containing health care costs in the United States. *Medical Care Review, 49* (Spring), 19–65.

Rosko, Michael D., & Robert W. Broyles. (1986). The impact of the New Jersey all-payer DRG system. *Inquiry, 23* (Spring), 67–75.

Sammons, James H. (1989). Physician payment reform: Don't forget the patient. *Health Affairs, 8* (Spring), 132–137.

Sapolsky, Harvey M. (1986). Prospective payment in perspective. *Journal of Health Politics, Policy and Law, 11* (4), 633–645.

Schramm, Carl J. (1986). State hospital cost containment: An analysis of legislative initiatives. *Indiana Law Review, 19* (4), 919–954.

Schramm, Carl J., & Jon Gabel. (1988). Prospective payment—some retrospective observations. *New England Journal of Medicine, 318* (June 23), 1681–1682.

Schwartz, William B., & Daniel N. Mendelson. (1992). Why managed care cannot contain hospital costs—without rationing. *Health Affairs, 11* (Summer), 100–107.

Schwartz, William B., & Daniel N. Mendelson. (1994). Eliminating waste and inefficiency can do little to contain costs. *Health Affairs, 13* (Spring), 224–238.

Sheingold, Steven H. (1986). Unintended results of Medicare's national prospective payment rates. *Health Affairs, 5* (Winter), 5–21.

Shortell, Stephen M., Robbin R. Gillies, & David A. Anderson. (1994). The new world of managed care: Creating organized delivery systems. *Health Affairs, 13* (Winter), 46–64.

Thompson, Lawrence H. (1992). Observations on "cost containment and new priorities in the European community" by Brian Abel-Smith. *Milbank Quarterly, 70* (3), 417–422.

Welch, W. Pete. (1989). Prospective payment to medical staffs: A proposal. *Health Affairs, 8* (Spring), 34–49.

White, Joseph. (1993). Markets, budgets, and health care cost control. *Health Affairs, 12* (Fall), 44–57.

Wood, Juanita B., & Carroll L. Estes. (1990). The impact of DRGs on community-based service providers: Implications for the elderly. *American Journal of Public Health, 80* (July), 840–843.

Zedlewski, Sheila R., Gregory P. Acs, & Colin W. Winterbottom. (1992). Play-or-pay employer mandates. *Health Affairs, 11* (Spring), 62–83.

Disability and Rehabilitation

Albrecht, Gary L. (1992). *The disability business: Rehabilitation in America.* Newbury Park, CA: Sage.

Batavia, Andrew I. (1993). Health care reform and people with disabilities. *Health Affairs, 12* (Spring), 40–57.

Berkowitz, Edward D. (1976). *Rehabilitation: The federal government's response to disability, 1935–1954.* Unpublished Ph.D. diss., Northwestern University. Also, New York: Arno Press. (1980).

Brandt, Allan M. (1978). Polio, politics, publicity and duplicity: Ethical aspects in the development of the Salk vaccine. *International Journal of Health Services, 8* (2), 257–270.

Burgdorf, Robert L., Jr. (1991). Equal access to public accommodations. *Milbank Quarterly, 69* (Suppl. 1/2), 183–213.

Chiang, Yen-Pin, Laurie J. Bassi, & Jonathan C. Javitt. (1992). Federal budgetary costs of blindness. *Milbank Quarterly, 70* (2), 319–340.

Daunt, Patrick. (1991). *Meeting disability: A European response.* New York: Cassell.

Driedger, Diane. (1989). *The last civil rights movement: Disabled People's International.* New York: St. Martin's.

Gooding, Caroline. (1995). *Disabling laws, enabling acts: Disability rights in Britain and America.* Boulder, CO: Westview Press.

Gostin, Lawrence O. (1992). The Americans with Disabilities Act and the U.S. health system. *Health Affairs, 11* (Fall), 248–256.

Howards, Irving, Henry P. Brehm, & Saad Z. Nagi. (1980). *Disability: From social problem to federal program.* New York: Praeger.

Jones, Nance Lee. (1991). Essential requirements of the act: A short history and overview. *Milbank Quarterly, 69* (Suppl. 1/2), 25–54.

Katzmann, Robert A. (1991). Transportation policy. *Milbank Quarterly, 69* (Suppl. 1/2), 214–237.

Krause, Elliott A. (1976). The political sociology of rehabilitation. In Gary L. Albrecht (Ed.), *The sociology of physical disability and rehabilitation* (pp. 210–222). Pittsburgh: University of Pittsburgh Press.

Morris, Robert. (Ed.). (1981). *Allocating health resources for the aged and disabled: Technology versus politics.* Lexington, MA: Lexington Books.

Oliver, Mike. (1990). *The politics of disablement: A sociological approach.* New York: St. Martin's Press.

Percy, Stephen L. (1989). *Disability, civil rights, and public policy: The politics of implementation.* Tuscaloosa: University of Alabama Press.

Reisine, Susan, & Judith Fifield. (1992). Expanding the definition of disability: Implications for planning, policy, and research. *Milbank Quarterly, 70* (3), 491–508.

Rivlin, Alice M., & Joshua M. Wiener. (1988). *Caring for the disabled elderly: Who will pay?* Washington, D.C.: The Brookings Institution.

Roper, William L. (1992). Americans with Disabilities Act: Lessons for the future. *Health Affairs, 11* (Fall), 257–258.

Scotch, Richard K. (1984). *From good will to civil rights: Transforming federal disability policy.* Philadelphia: Temple University Press.

Springarn, Natalie Davis. (1976). *Heartbeat: The politics of health research.* Washington, D.C.: Robert B. Luce.

Stone, Deborah. (1984). *The disabled state.* Philadelphia: Temple University Press.

Tanenbaum, Sandra, & Robert E. Hurley. (1995). Disability and the managed care frenzy: A cautionary note. *Health Affairs, 14* (Winter), 213–219.

Weaver, Carolyn L. (1991). *Disability and work: Incentives, rights, and opportunities.* Waldorf, MD: AEI Press.

West, Jane. (1991). The social and policy context of the act. *Milbank Quarterly, 69* (Suppl. 1/2), 3–24.

West, Jane. (Ed). (1991). The Americans with Disabilities Act: From policy to practice. *Milbank Quarterly, 69* (Suppl. 1/2).

Yelin, Edward H., & Patricia P. Katz. (1994). Making work more central to work disability policy. *Milbank Quarterly, 72* (4), 593–620.

Drugs

Avden, Jerry. (1990). The elderly and drug policy: Coming of age. *Health Affairs, 9* (Fall), 6–19.

Blank, Charles H. (1974). Delaney clause: Technical naivete and scientific advocacy in the formulation of public health policies. *California Law Review, 62* (July–September), 1084–1120.

Bloom, Bernard S. (1992). Issues in mandatory economic assessment of pharmaceuticals. *Health Affairs, 11* (Winter), 197–201.

Blumberg, Linda J., & Gail R. Wilensky. (1988). Pharmaceuticals in developing countries. *Health Affairs, 7* (Fall), 175–179.

Burstall, M. L. (1991). Europe after 1992: Implications for pharmaceuticals. *Health Affairs, 10* (Fall), 157–171.

Campbell, Rita Ricardo. (1976). *Drug lag; Federal government decision making* (No. 55). Stanford, CA: Hoover Institution Press.

Fincham, Jack E., & Albert I. Wertheimer. (1991). *Pharmacy and the U.S. health care system.* Binghampton, NY: The Haworth Press, Inc.

Freiman, Paul E. (1990). New drug legislation: A response from the pharmaceutical industry. *Health Affairs, 9* (Fall), 110–113.

Gondek, Kathleen. (1994). Prescription drug payment policy: Past, present, and future. *Health Care Financing Review, 15* (Spring), 1–8.

Greenberg, Daniel S. (1976). Report of the president's biomedical panel and the old days at the FDA. *New England Journal of Medicine, 294* (May 27), 1245–1246.

Kleiman, Mark A. R. (1992). *Against excess: Drug policy for results.* New York: Basic Books.

Landau, Richard L. (Ed.). (1973). *Regulating new drugs.* Chicago, IL: University of Chicago, Center for Policy Study.

Levine, Harry G., & Craig Reinerman. (1991). From prohibition to regulation: Lessons from alcohol policy for drug policy. *Milbank Quarterly, 69* (3), 461–494.

Orzack, Louis, Kenneth I. Kaitin, & Louis Lasagna. (1992). Pharmaceutical regulation in the European community: Barriers to single market integration. *Journal of Health Politics, Policy and Law, 17* (Winter), 847–867.

Peltzman, Sam. (1974). *Regulation of pharmaceutical innovation: The 1962 amendments* (Research Evaluative Studies No. 15). Washington, D.C.: American Enterprise Institute for Public Policy Research.

Pryor, David. (1990). A prescription for high drug prices. *Health Affairs, 9* (Fall), 101–109.

Rock, Paul E. (Ed.). (1977). *Drugs and politics.* New Brunswick, NJ: Transaction Books.

Schondelmeyer, Stephen W., & Joseph Thomas III. (1990). Trends in retail prescription expenditures. *Health Affairs, 9* (Fall), 131–145.

Schroeder, Richard C. (1975). *The politics of drugs: Marijuana to mainlining.* Washington, D.C.: Congressional Quarterly.

Schur, Claudia L., Marc L. Berk, & Penny Mohr. (1990). Understanding the cost of a catastrophic drug benefit. *Health Affairs, 9* (Fall), 88–100.

Silverman, Milton, & Philip R. Lee. (1974). *Pills, profits and politics.* Berkeley: University of California Press.

Walsh, Diana Chapman, Philip J. Cook, Karen Davis, Marcus Grant, Pekka Sulkunen, George E. Vaillant, & Thomas L. Delbanco. (1989). The cultural dimensions of alcohol policy worldwide. *Health Affairs, 8* (Summer), 48–62.

Wardell, William M., & Louis Lasagna. (1975). *Regulation and drug development.* Washington, D.C.: American Enterprise Institute for Public Policy Research.

Wisotsky, Steven. (1990). *Beyond the war on drugs: Overcoming a failed public policy.* Buffalo, NY: Prometheus Books.

Environmental and Occupational Health (see also Competition and Regulation)

Adler, Robert W., Jessica C. Landman, & Diane M. Cameron. (1993). *The Clean Water Act 20 years later.* Washington, D.C.: Island Press.

Bryner, Gary C. (1995). *Blue skies, green politics: The Clean Air Act of 1990.* Washington, D.C.: Congressional Quarterly Press.

Church, Thomas W., & Robert T. Nakamura. (1993). *Cleaning up the mess: Implementation strategies for Superfund*. Washington, D.C.: The Brookings Institution.

Donnelly, Patrick G. (1982). The origins of the Occupational Safety and Health Act of 1970. *Social Problems, 30* (October), 13–25.

Gordon, Larry J. (1995). Environmental health and protection: Century 21 challenges. *Journal of Environmental Health, 57* (January/February), 28–34.

Hays, Samuel P., in collaboration with Barbara D. Hays. (1987). *Beauty, health and permanence: Environmental politics in the United States, 1955–1985*. New York: Cambridge University Press.

Hird, John A. (1994). *Superfund: The political economy of environmental risk*. Baltimore, MD: Johns Hopkins University Press.

Kakonen, Jyrki. (Ed.). (1993). *Perspectives on environmental conflict and international politics*. New York: Pinter.

Kemp, Ray. (1992). *Issues in environmental politics: The new politics of radioactive waste disposal*. New York: Manchester University Press.

Landy, Marc., Marc J. Roberts, & Stephen R. Thomas. (1990). *The Environmental Protection Agency's asking the wrong question*. New York: Oxford University Press.

Lowry, William R. (1992). *The dimensions of federalism: State governments and pollution control policies*. Durham, NC: Duke University Press.

Marcus, Alfred A. (1980). *Promise and performance: Choosing and implementing an environmental policy*. Westport, CT: Greenwood Press.

Rabe, Barry G. (1990). Legislative incapacity: The congressional role in environmental policy-making and the case of Superfund. *Journal of Health Politics, Policy and Law, 15* (Fall), 571–590.

Rabe, Barry G. (1994). *Beyond NIMBY: Hazardous waste siting in Canada and the United States*. Washington, D.C.: The Brookings Institution.

Reich, Michael R. (1991). *Toxic politics: Responding to chemical disasters*. Ithaca, NY: Cornell University Press.

Ringquist, Evan J. (1993). *Environmental protection at the state level: Politics and progress in controlling pollution*. Armonk, NY: M. E. Sharpe.

Rosenbaum, Walter. (1995). *Environmental politics and policy*. Washington, D.C.: Congressional Quarterly.

Rosner, David, & Gerald Markowitz. (1991). *Deadly dust: Silicosis and the politics of occupational disease in twentieth-century America*. Princeton, NJ: Princeton University Press.

Szasz, Andrew. (1984). Industrial resistance to occupational safety and health legislation. *Social Problems, 32* (December), 103–116.

Walker, Bailus, Jr. (1990). Environmental health policies in the 1990s. *Journal of Public Health Policy, 11* (Winter), 438–448.

Weale, Albert. (1992). *Issues in environmental politics: The new politics of pollution*. New York: Manchester University Press.

Wysong, Earl. (1992). *High risk and high stakes: Health professionals, politics and policy*. Westport, CT: Greenwood Press.

Health Care Finance (see also Medicare and Medicaid; National Health Insurance and Health Care Reform)

Aaron, Henry J. (1991). *Serious and unstable condition: Financing America's health care*. Washington, D.C.: The Brookings Institution.

Aaron, Henry J. (1993). Budget limits and managed competition: Allies, not antagonists. *Health Affairs, 12* (Fall), 132–136.

Aaron, Henry J. (1994). Health spending analysis: Thinking straight about medical costs. *Health Affairs, 13* (Winter), 7–13.

Anderson, Gerard F. (1985). National medical care spending. *Health Affairs, 5* (Fall), 123–130.

Anderson, Gerard F. (1986). Payment reform in the United States. *Health Policy, 6* (4), 321–328.

Bast, Joseph L., Richard C. Rue, & Stuart A. Wesbury Jr. (1993). *Why we spend too much on health care . . . and what we can do about it*. Latham, MD: University Press of America.

Bodenheimer, Thomas, & Kevin Grumbach. (1992). Financing universal health insurance: Taxes, premiums, and the lessons of social insurance. *Journal of Health Politics, Policy and Law, 17* (Fall), 439–462.

Bodenheimer, Thomas, & Kevin Grumbach. (1994). Paying for health care. *Journal of the American Medical Association, 272* (August 24, 31), 634–639.

Bodenheimer, Thomas, & Kevin Grumbach. (1994). Reimbursing physicians and hospitals. *Journal of the American Medical Association, 272* (September 28), 971–977.

Bovbjerg, Randall R. (1995). Review essay: The high cost of administration in health care: Part of the problem or part of the solution? *Journal of Law, Medicine, and Ethics, 23* (Summer), 186–194.

Delnoij, Diana M. (1994). *Physician payment systems and cost control.* Utrecht, Netherlands: Netherlands Institute of Primary Health Care.

Eastaugh, Steven R. (1987). *Financing health care. Economic efficiency and equity.* Dover, MA: Auburn House Publishing Co.

Enthoven, Alain. (1988). Managed competition in health care and the unfinished agenda. *Health Care Financing Review* (Suppl.), 105–119.

Epstein, Arnold M., & David Blumenthal. (1993). Physician payment reform: Past and future. *Milbank Quarterly, 71* (2), 193–216.

Feldman, Roger. (1988). Health care: The tyranny of the budget. In David Boaz (Ed.), *Assessing the Reagan years.* Washington, D.C.: CATO Institute.

Fuchs, Victor. (1986). Has cost containment gone too far? *Milbank Memorial Fund Quarterly, 64* (3), 479–488.

Getzen, Thomas E. (1992). Population aging and the growth of health expenditures. *Journal of Gerontology, 47* (3), 98–104.

Ginsburg, Paul B. (1989). Physician payment policy in the 101st Congress. *Health Affairs, 8* (Spring), 5–20.

Glaser, William A. (1984). Juggling multiple payers: American problems and foreign solutions. *Inquiry, 21* (Summer), 178–188.

Glaser, William A. (1987). *Paying the hospital: The organizational dynamics and effects of differing financial arrangements.* San Francisco, CA: Jossey-Bass.

Glaser, William A. (1989). The politics of paying American physicians. *Health Affairs, 8* (Fall), Commentary: 67–86; Response: 87–96; Text: 129–146.

Glaser, William A. (1993). How expenditure caps and expenditure targets really work. *Milbank Quarterly, 71* (1), 97–128.

Gold, Steven D. (1992). One approach to tracking state and local health spending. *Health Affairs, 11* (Winter), 135–144.

Hadley, Jack, & Stephen Zuckerman. (1991). *Determinants of hospital costs: Outputs and regulations in the 1980s.* Washington, D.C.: Urban Institute.

Henke, Klaus-Dirk, Margaret A. Murray, & Claudia Ade. (1994). Global budgeting in Germany: Lessons for the United States. *Health Affairs, 13* (Fall), 7–21.

Holahan, John, Linda J. Blumberg, & Stephen Zuckerman. (1994). Strategies for implementing global budgets. *Milbank Quarterly, 72* (3), 399–430.

Holahan, John, & Sheila Zedlewski. (1992). Who pays for health care in the United States? Implications for health system reform. *Inquiry, 29* (Summer), 231–248.

Hsiao, William C. (1995). Medical savings accounts: Lessons from Singapore. *Health Affairs, 14* (Summer), 260–266.

Huskamp, Haiden A., & Joseph P. Newhouse. (1994). Is health spending slowing down? *Health Affairs, 13* (Winter), 32–38.

Kanaan, Susan Baird. (1991). Financing policy for mental health services. *Health Affairs, 10* (Summer), 207–211.

Langwell, Kathryn, & Lyle M. Nelson. (1986). Physician payment systems: A review of history, alternatives and evidence. *Medical Care Review, 43* (Spring), 5–58.

Lazenby, Helen C., Katharine R. Levit, Daniel R. Waldo, Gerald S. Adler, Suzanne W. Letsch, & Cathy A. Cowan. (1992). National health accounts: Lessons from the U.S. experience. *Health Care Financing Review, 13* (Summer), 89–104.

Letsch, Suzanne W. (1993). Datawatch: National health care spending in 1991. *Health Affairs, 12* (Spring), 94–110.

Levit, Katharine R. (1994). Delving into health expenditure trends. *Health Affairs, 13* (Winter), 44–45.

Levit, Katharine R., Cathy A. Cowan, Helen C. Lazenby, Patricia A. McDonnel, Arthur L. Sensenig, Jeane M. Stiller, & Darleen K. Won. (1994). National health spending trends: 1960– 1993. *Health Affairs, 13* (Winter), 14–31.

Levit, Katharine R., & Mark S. Freeland. (1988). National medical care spending: Datawatch. *Health Affairs, 7* (Winter), 124–136.

Levit, Katharine R., Mark S. Freeland, & Daniel Waldo. (1990). National health care spending trends: 1988. *Health Affairs, 9* (Summer), 171–184.

Levit, Katharine R., Helen C. Lazenby, Cathy A. Cowan, & Suzanne W. Letsch. (1993). Health spending by state: New estimates for policy making. *Health Affairs, 12* (Fall), 7–26.

Levit, Katharine R., Helen C. Lazenby, Suzanne W. Letsch, & Cathy A. Cowan. (1991). National health care spending: 1989. *Health Affairs, 10* (Spring), 117–130.

Levit, Katharine R., Helen C. Lazenby, & Lekha Sivarajam. (1996). Health care spending in 1994: Slowest in decades. *Health Affairs, 15* (Summer), 130–144.

Massaro, Thomas A., & Yu-Ning Wong. (1995). Positive experience with MSAs in Singapore. *Health Affairs, 14* (Summer), 267–272.

McMenamin, Peter. (1987). Medicare Part B: Rising assignment rates, rising costs. *Inquiry, 24* (Winter), 344–356.

Monaco, Ralph M., & John H. Phelps. (1995). Health care prices, the federal budget, and economic growth. *Health Affairs, 14* (Summer), 248–259.

Moreno, Jonathan D. (Ed.). (1990). *Paying the doctor: Health policy and physician reimbursement.* Westport, CT: Auburn House.

Morrisey, Michael A. (1994). *Cost shifting in health care: Separating evidence from rhetoric.* Waldorf, MD: AEI Press.

Newhouse, Joseph P., Geoffrey Anderson, & Leslie L. Roos. (1988). Hospital spending in the U.S. and Canada. *Health Affairs, 7* (Winter), 6–16.

Pauly, Mark V. (1993). U.S. health care costs: The untold true story. *Health Affairs, 12* (Fall), 152–159.

Peden, Edgar A., & Mark S. Freeland. (1995). Historical analysis of medical spending growth, 1960–1993. *Health Affairs, 14* (Summer), 235–247.

Redelmeier, Donald A., & Victor R. Fuchs. (1993). Hospital expenditures in the United States and Canada. *New England Journal of Medicine, 328* (March 18), 772–728.

Reinhardt, Uwe E. (1989). Health care spending and American competitiveness. *Health Affairs, 8* (Winter), 5–21.

Ron, Aviva. (1886). Sharing in the financing of health care: Government, insurance and the patient. *Health Policy, 6* (1), 87–101.

Roper, William L. (1989). Financing health care: A view from the White House. *Health Affairs, 8* (Winter), 97–102.

Schieber, George J., & Jean-Pierre Poullier. (1986). International health care spending: Datawatch. *Health Affairs, 5* (Fall), 111–122.

Schieber, George J., & Jean-Pierre Poullier. (1991). International health spending: Issues and trends. *Health Affairs, 10* (Spring), 106–117.

Schieber, George J., Jean-Pierre Poullier, & Leslie M. Greenwald. (1992). U.S. health expenditure performance: An international comparison and data update. *Health Care Financing Review, 13* (Summer), 1–88.

Schieber, George J., Jean-Pierre Poullier, & Leslie Greenwood. (1993). Health spending, delivery, and outcomes in OECD countries. *Health Affairs, 12* (Summer), 120–129.

Schondelmeyer, Stephen W., & Joseph Thomas III. (1990). Trends in retail prescription expenditures. *Health Affairs, 9* (Fall), 131–145.

Schramm, Carl J., Steven C. Renn, & Brian Biles. (1986). Cost inflation: New perspectives on state rate setting. *Health Affairs, 5* (Fall), 22–33.

Somers, Anne R. (1985). Financing long-term care for the elderly: Institutions, incentives, issues. In Institute of Medicine, National Research Council (Ed.), *America's aging: Health in an older society* (pp. 182–233). Washington, D.C.: Institute of Medicine, National Academy Press.

Terris, Milton. (1991). Global budgeting and control of hospital costs. *Journal of Public Health Policy, 12* (Spring), 61–71.

Terris, Milton. (1992). Budget cuting and privatization: The threat to health. *Journal of Public Health Policy, 13* (Spring), 27–41.

Thorpe, Kenneth E. (1993). The American states and Canada: A comparative analysis of health care spending. *Journal of Health Politics, Policy and Law, 18* (Summer), 477–490.

U.S. Congress, Office of Technology Assessment. (1993). *International health statistics: What the numbers mean for the United States*. Washington, D.C.: U.S. Government Printing Office.

U.S. Congress, Office of Technology Assessment. (1994). *International comparisons of administrative costs in health care*. Washington, D.C.: U.S. Government Printing Office.

Waldo, Daniel R., & Sally T. Sonnefeld. (1991). U.S./Canadian health spending: Methods and assumptions. *Health Affairs, 10* (Summer), 159–165.

Waldo, Daniel R., Sally T. Sonnefeld, Jeffrey A. Lemieux, & David R. McKusick. (1991). Health spending through 2030: Three scenarios. *Health Affairs, 10* (Winter), 231–242.

Wiener, Joshua M., Steven B. Clauser, & David L. Kennell. (Eds.). (1995). *Persons with disabilities: Issues in health care financing and service delivery*. Washington, D.C.: The Brookings Institution.

Wiley, Miriam M. (1992). Hospital financing reform and case-mix measurement: An international review. *Health Care Financing Review, 13* (Summer), 119–131.

Winterbottom, Colin, David W. Liska, & Karen M. Obermaier. (1995). *State-level databook on health care access and financing* (2nd ed.). Washington, D.C.: Urban Institute Press.

Zwanziger, Jack, Geoffrey M. Anderson, Susan G. Haber, Kenneth E. Thorpe, & Joseph P. Newhouse. (1993). Comparison of hospital costs in California, New York and Canada. *Health Affairs, 12* (Summer), 130–139.

Health Insurance and the Un- and Underinsured

Health Insurance

Blendon, Robert J., Jennifer M. Edwards, & Ulrike S. Szalay. (1991). Perspectives: Future of private health insurance. Health insurance industry in the year 2001. *Health Affairs, 10* (Winter), 170–177.

Bowler, M. Kenneth. (1987). Changing politics of federal health insurance programs. *PS, 20* (Spring), 202–211.

Cantor, Joel C., Stephen H. Long, & M. Susan Marquis. (1995). Private employment-based insurance in ten states. *Health Affairs, 14* (Summer), 199–211.

Chollet, Deborah. (1994). Employer-based health insurance in a changing work force. *Health Affairs, 13* (Spring), 315–326.

Cohodes, Donald R. (1991). Insurance reform: Industry, heal thyself! *Health Affairs, 10* (Winter), 178–180.

Cunningham, Peter J., & Alan C. Monheit. (1990). Insuring the children: A decade of change. *Health Affairs, 9* (Winter), 76–90.

Davis, Karen, Karen Scott Collins, Cathy Schoen, & Cynthia Morris. (1995). Choice matters: Enrollees' views of their health plans. *Health Affairs, 14* (Summer), 99–112.

Enthoven, Alain. (1984). A new proposal to reform the tax threat of health insurance. *Health Affairs, 3* (Spring), 21–39.

Evans, Robert G. (1987). Public health insurance—the collective purchase of individual care. *Health Policy, 7* (115), 115–134.

Fein, Rashi. (1986). *Medical care, medical costs: The search for a health insurance policy*. Cambridge, MA: Harvard University Press.

Feldman, Roger, & Bryan Dowd. (1992). Employee-sponsored health insurance in 1991. *Health Affairs, 11* (Winter), 172–185.

Field, Marilyn J., & Harold T. Shapiro. (Eds.). (1993). *Employment and health benefits.* Washington, D.C.: National Academy Press.

Flynn, Patrice. (1994). COBRA qualifying events and elections, 1987–1991. *Inquiry, 31* (Summer), 215–220.

Fox, Daniel M., & Daniel C. Schaffer. (1987). Tax policy as social policy: Cafeteria plans, 1978–1985. *Journal of Health Politics, Policy and Law, 12* (Winter), 609–664.

Frank, Richard G., David S. Salkever, & Steven S. Sharfstein. (1991). A look at rising mental health insurance costs. *Health Affairs, 10* (Summer), 116–123.

Freedman, Benjamin, & Francoise Baylis. (1987). Purpose and function in government-funded health coverage. *Journal of Health Economics, 12* (Spring), 97–112.

Fronstin, Paul, Sara C. Snider, William S. Custer, & Dallas L. Salisbury. (1994). The cost of providing health care benefits to early retirees. *Health Affairs, 13* (Spring, 2), 246–254.

Gabel, Jon, Steven DiCarlo, Steven Fink, & Gregory deLissovoy. (1989). Employer-sponsored health insurance in America. *Health Affairs, 8* (Summer), 116–128.

Gabel, Jon, Steven DiCarlo, Cynthia Sullivan, & Thomas Rice. (1990). Employer-sponsored health insurance, 1989. *Health Affairs, 9* (Fall), 161–175.

Gabel, Jon, Roger Formisano, Barbara Lohr, & Steven DiCarlo. (1991). Tracing the cycle of health insurance. *Health Affairs, 10* (Winter), 48–61.

Gabel, Jon, Derek Liston, Gail Jensen, & Jill Marstellar. (1994). The health insurance picture in 1993: Some rare good news. *Health Affairs, 13* (Spring), 328–336.

Garnick, Deborah W., Ann M. Hendricks, Kenneth E. Thorpe, Joseph P. Newhouse, Karen Donelan, & Robert J. Blendon. (1993). How well do Americans understand their health coverage? *Health Affairs, 12* (Fall), 204–212.

Hall, Mark A. (1992). Political economics of insurance market reform. *Health Affairs, 11* (Summer), 108–124.

Helms, W. David, Anne K. Gautheir, & Daniel M. Campion. (1992). Mending the flaws in the small-group market. *Health Affairs, 11* (Summer), 7–27.

Holahan, John, Colin Winterbottom, & Shruti Rajan. (1995). A shifting picture of health insurance coverage. *Health Affairs, 14* (Winter), 253–264.

Holmes, Martin. (1984). Tax policy and the demand for health insurance. *Journal of Health Economics, 3* (December), 203–221.

Jecker, Nancy S. (1993). Can an employer-based health insurance system be just? *Journal of Health Politics, Policy and Law, 18* (Fall), 657–673.

Long, Stephen H. (1987). Public versus employment-related health insurance: Experience and implications for black and non-black Americans. *Milbank Memorial Fund Quarterly, 65* (Suppl. 1), 200–212.

Long, Stephen H., & M. Susan Marquis. (1996). Some pitfalls in making cost estimates of state health insurance coverage expansions. *Inquiry, 33* (Spring), 85–91.

Mariner, Wendy. (1992). Problems with employer-provided health insurance—the Employee Retirement Income Security Act and health care reform. *New England Journal of Medicine, 327* (December 3), 1682–1685.

McCall, Nelda, Thomas Rice, & Arden Hall. (1987). The effect of state regulations on the quality and sale of insurance policies to Medicare beneficiaries. *Journal of Health Politics, Policy and Law, 12* (Spring), 53–76.

Mechanic, David. (1989). Consumer choice among health insurance options. *Health Affairs, 8* (Spring), 138–148.

Meiners, Mark R., & Stephen C. Goss. (1994). Passing the "laugh test" for long-term care insurance partnerships. *Health Affairs, 13* (Winter), 225–228.

Miller, Irwin. (1996). *American health care blues: Blue Cross, HMOs, and pragmatic reform since 1960.* New Brunswick, NJ: Transaction Publishers.

Monheit, Alan C., & Pamela Farley Short. (1989). Mandating health coverage for working Americans. *Health Affairs, 8* (Winter), 22–38.

Morrisey, Michael A., Gail A. Jensen, & Stephen E. Henderlite. (1990). Employer-sponsored insurance for retired Americans. *Health Affairs, 9* (Spring), 57–73.

Morrisey, Michael A., Gail A. Jensen, & Robert J. Morlock. (1994). Datawatch: Small employers and the health insurance market. *Health Affairs, 13* (Winter), 149–161.

Newacheck, Paul W., Dana C. Hughes, & Miriam Cisternas. (1995). Children and health insurance: An overview of recent trends. *Health Affairs, 14* (Spring), 244–254.

Newhouse, Joseph P., & The Insurance Experiment Group. (1994). *Free for all? Lessons from the RAND health insurance experiment.* Cambridge, MA: Harvard University Press.

Nyman, John A. (1994). Feasibility of long-term care insurance partnerships. *Health Affairs, 13* (Winter), 220–224.

Rice, Thomas, & Kenneth E. Thorpe. (1993). Income-related cost sharing in health insurance. *Health Affairs, 12* (Spring), 21–39.

Rogowski, Jeannette A. (1992). Insurance coverage for drug abuse. *Health Affairs, 11* (Fall), 137–148.

Schur, Claudia L., & Amy K. Taylor. (1991). Health insurance and the two-worker household. *Health Affairs, 10* (Spring), 155–163.

Stone, Deborah A. (1993). The struggle for the soul of health insurance. *Journal of Health Politics, Policy and Law, 18* (Summer), 287–318.

Sullivan, Cynthia B., & Thomas Rice. (1991). The health insurance picture in 1990. *Health Affairs, 10* (Summer), 104–115.

Wiener, Joshua M., Laurel Hixon Illstom, & Raymond J. Hanley. (1994). *Sharing the burden: Strategies for public and private long-term care insurance.* Washington, D.C.: The Brookings Institution.

Wilensky, Gail R., Pamela J. Farley, & Amy K. Taylor. (1984). Variations in health insurance coverage: Benefits versus premiums. *Milbank Memorial Fund Quarterly, 62* (Winter), 53–81.

Zarkin, Gary A., Steven A. Garfinkel, Francis J. Potter, & Jennifer J. McNeill. (1995). Employment-based health insurance: Implications of the sampling unit for policy analysis. *Inquiry, 32* (Fall), 310–319.

Zellers, Wendy K., Catherine G. McLaughlin, & Kevin D. Frick. (1992). Small-business health insurance: Only the healthy need apply. *Health Affairs, 11* (Spring), 174–180.

Medical Savings Accounts

Chollet, Deborah. (1995). Why the Pauly/Goodman proposal won't work. *Health Affairs, 14* (Summer), 273–274.

Hall, Mark A. (1995). Managed competition meets tax-neutrality. *Health Affairs, 14* (Summer), 274.

Hsiao, William C. (1995). Medical savings accounts: Lessons from Singapore. *Health Affairs, 14* (Summer), 260–266.

Keeler, Emmett, Jesse K. Malkin, Dana P. Goldman, & Joan L. Buchanan. (1996). Can medical savings accounts for the nonelderly reduce health care costs? *Journal of the American Medical Association, 275* (June 5), 1666–1671.

Massaro, Thomas A., & Yu-Ning Wong. (1995). Positive experience with MSAs in Singapore. *Health Affairs, 14* (Summer), 267–272.

Michels, Len M. (1995). MSAs and risk segmentation. *Health Affairs, 14* (Summer), 275.

Pauly, Mark V., & John C. Goodman. (1995). Medical savings accounts: The authors respond. *Health Affairs, 14* (Summer), 277–279.

Schweitzer, Maurice, John C. Hershey, & David A. Asch. (1996). Individual choice in spending accounts: Can we rely on employees to choose well? *Medical Care, 34* (June), 583–593.

Steuerle, C. Eugene. (1995). Designing a nondiscriminatory tax credit. *Health Affairs, 14* (Summer), 276.

Un- and Underinsured

Berk, Marc L., Leigh Ann Albers, & Claudia L. Schur. (1996). The growth in the U.S. uninsured population: Trends in Hispanic subgroups, 1977–1992. *American Journal of Public Health, 86* (April), 572–576.

Billings, John, & Nina Teicholz. (1990). Uninsured patients in District of Columbia hospitals. *Health Affairs, 9* (Winter), 158–165.

Black, Jeanne T. (1986). The employed uninsured and the role of public policy. *Inquiry, 23* (Summer), 209–212.

Blumberg, Mark S. (1994). Impact of extending health care coverage in the United States. *Health Affairs, 13* (Winter), 181–192.

Bovbjerg, Randall P., & William G. Kopit. (1986). Coverage and care for the medically indigent: Public and private options. *Indiana Law Review, 19* (4), 857–917.

Bowler, M. Kenneth. (1987). Changing politics of federal health insurance programs. *PS, 20* (Spring), 202–211.

Brown, Lawrence D. (1990). Medically uninsured: Problems, policies, and politics. *Journal of Health Politics, Policy and Law, 15* (Summer), 413–426.

Butler, Patricia A. (1989). *Too poor to be sick: Access to medical care for the uninsured.* Washington, D.C.: American Public Health Association.

Cartland, Jenifer D. C., & Beth K. Yudkowsky. (1993). State estimates of uninsured children. *Health Affairs, 12* (Spring), 144–151.

Cohodes, Donald R. (1986). America: The home of the free, the land of the uninsured. *Inquiry, 23* (Fall), 227–235.

Davis, Karen, & Diane Rowland. (1983). Uninsured and underserved: Inequities in health care in the United States. *Milbank Memorial Fund Quarterly, 61* (Spring), 149–176.

de la Torre, Adela, Robert Friis, Harold R. Hunter, & Lorena Garcia. (1996). The health insurance status of U.S. Latino women: A profile from the 1982–1984 HHANES. *American Journal of Public Health, 86* (April), 533–537.

Diehr, Paula, Carolyn W. Madden, Allen Cheadle, Diane P. Martin, Donald L. Patrick, & Susan Skillman. (1996). Will uninsured people volunteer for voluntary health insurance? Experience from Washington State. *American Journal of Public Health, 86* (April), 529–532.

Feder, Judith, Jack Hadley, & Ross Mullner. (1984). Falling through the cracks: Poverty, insurance coverage, and hospital care for the poor, 1980 and 1982. *Milbank Memorial Fund Quarterly, 62* (Fall), 544–566.

Friedman, Emily. (1991). The uninsured from dilemma to crisis. *Journal of the American Medical Association, 265* (May 15), 2491–2495.

Fronstin, Paul. (1995). Children without health insurance: An analysis of the increase of uninsured children between 1992 and 1993. *Inquiry, 32* (Fall), 353–359.

Holahan, John, & Sheila Zedlewski. (1991). Expanding Medicaid to cover uninsured Americans. *Health Affairs, 10* (Spring), 45–61.

Long, Stephen H. (1987). Public versus employment-related health insurance: Experience and implications for black and non-black Americans. *Milbank Memorial Fund Quarterly, 65* (Suppl. 1), 200–212.

Long, Stephen G., & M. Susan Marquis. (1994). The uninsured "access gap" and the cost of universal coverage. *Health Affairs, 13* (Spring, 2), 211–220.

Monheit, Alan C., Michael M. Hagan, Marc L. Berk, & Gail R. Wilensky. (1984). Health insurance for the unemployed: Is federal legislation needed? *Health Affairs, 3* (Spring), 101–111.

Monheit, Alan C., Michael M. Hagan, Marc L. Berk, & Pamela J. Farley. (1985). The employed uninsured and the role of public policy. *Inquiry, 22* (Winter), 348–364.

Moyer, M. Eugene. (1989). A revised look at the number of uninsured Americans. *Health Affairs, 8* (Summer), 102–110.

Mulstein, Suzanne. (1984). The uninsured and the financing of uncompensated care: Scope, costs, and policy options. *Inquiry, 21* (Fall), 214–229.

Regula, Ralph. (1987). National policy and the medically uninsured. *Inquiry, 24* (Spring), 48–56.

Reinhardt, Uwe E. (1987). Health insurance for the nation's poor. *Health Affairs, 6* (Spring), 101–112.

Reinhardt, Uwe E. (1993). Reforming the health care system: The uninsured dilemma. *American Journal of Law and Medicine, 19* (1/2), 21–36.

Rice, Thomas, & Jon Gabel. (1986). Protecting the elderly against high health care costs. *Health Affairs, 5* (Fall), 5–21.

Rowland, Diane, Barbara Lyons, Alina Salganicoff, & Peter Long. (1994). A profile of the uninsured in America. *Health Affairs, 13* (Spring, 2), 283–287.

Thorpe, Kenneth E. (1988). Uncompensated care pools and care to the uninsured: Lessons from the New York prospective hospital reimbursement methodology. *Inquiry, 25* (Fall), 354–363.

Weissman, Joel S., & Arnold M. Epstein. (1994). *Falling through the safety net: Insurance status and access to health care.* Baltimore, MD: Johns Hopkins University Press.

Wilensky, Gail R. (1987). Viable strategies for dealing with the uninsured. *Health Affairs, 6* (Spring), 33–46.

Health Maintenance Organizations

Bauman, Patricia. (1976). The formulation and evolution of the health maintenance organization policy, 1970–1973. *Social Science and Medicine, 10* (March/April), 129–142.

Brown, Lawrence D. (1983). *Politics and health care organization: HMO's as federal policy.* Washington, D.C.: The Brookings Institution.

Falkson, Joseph L. (1980). *HMO's and the politics of health system reform.* Chicago: American Hospital Association and Robert J. Brady Co.

Hellinger, Fred J. (1995). Any-willing-provider and freedom-of-choice laws. *Health Affairs, 14* (Winter), 297–302.

Moran, Donald W. (1981). HMO's, competition and the politics of minimum benefits. *Milbank Memorial Fund Quarterly/Health and Society, 59* (2), 190–208.

Schlesinger, Mark. (1986). On the limits of expanding health care reform: Chronic care in prepaid settings. *Milbank Memorial Fund Quarterly, 64* (2), 189–215.

Health Policy (see also Rationing)

Aday, Lu Ann, Charles E. Bagley, David R. Lairson, & Carl H. Slater. (1993). *Evaluating the medical care system: Effectiveness, efficiency and equity.* Ann Arbor, MI: AUPHA/Health Administration Press.

Anderson, Gerard F. (1992). Courts and health policy: Strengths and limitations. *Health Affairs, 11* (Winter), 95–110.

Anderson, Odin W. (1989). *The health services continuum in democratic states: An inquiry into solvable problems.* Ann Arbor, MI: Health Administration Press.

Axinn, June, & Mack J. Stern. (1985). Age and dependency: Children and the aged in American social policy. *Milbank Memorial Fund Quarterly, 63* (Fall), 648–670.

Bailey, Mary Ann. (1984). "Rationing" and "American health policy." *Journal of Health Politics, Policy and Law, 9* (Fall), 489–501.

Battistella, Roger M., & Robert J. Buchanan. (1987). National health policy: Efficiency–equity syncretism. *Social Justice Review, 1* (3), 329–360.

Bauman, Patricia. (1976). The formulation and evolution of the health maintenance organization policy, 1970–1973. *Social Science and Medicine, 10* (March/April), 129–142.

Bayer, Ronald, & Jonathan D. Moreno. (1986). Health promotion: Ethical and social dilemmas of government policy. *Health Affairs, 5* (Summer), 72–85.

Beauchamp, Dan E. (1988). *Health of the republic: Epidemics, medicine, and moralism as challenges to democracy.* Philadelphia: Temple University Press.

Beauchamp, Tom, & Ruth Faden. (1979). The right to health and the right to health care. *Journal of Medicine and Philosophy, 4* (2), 118–131.

Bell, Nora. (1979). The scarcity of medical resources: Are there rights to health care? *Journal of Medicine and Philosophy, 4* (1/2), 158–169.

Birenbaum, Arnold. (1993). *Putting health care on the national agenda.* New York: Praeger.

Blendon, Robert J., Carl J. Schramm, Thomas W. Maloney, & David E. Rogers. (1981). An era of stress for health institutions: The 1980s. *Journal of the American Medical Association, 245* (May 8), 1843–1845.

Blumstein, James F., & Michael Zubkoff. (1979). Public choice and health: Problems, politics and perspectives on formulating national health policy. *Journal of Health Politics, Policy and Law, 4* (Fall), 382–413.

Bodenheimer, Thomas S., & Kevin Grumbach. (1994). *Understanding health policy: A clinical approach.* Stamford, CT: Appleton & Lange.

Bossert, Thomas. (1985). Health policy and international agencies in Central America. *Political Science Quarterly, 9,* 441–453.

Bowler, M. Kenneth. (1987). Changing politics of federal health insurance programs. *PS, 20* (Spring), 202–211.

Brown, Jonathan B., & Richard B. Saltman. (1985). Health capital policy in the United States: A strategic perspective. *Inquiry, 22* (Summer), 122–131.

Brown, Lawrence D. (1978). The formulation of federal health care policy. *Bulletin of the New York Academy of Medicine, 54* (January), 45–58.

Brown, Lawrence D. (1979). *The scope and limits of equality as a normative guide to federal health care policy* (Reprint No. 350). Washington, D.C.: The Brookings Institution.

Brown, Lawrence D. (1986). Introduction to a decade of transition. *Journal of Health Politics, Policy and Law, 11* (4), 569–583.

Brown, Lawrence D. (1987). *Health policy in transition: A decade of health politics, policy and law.* Durham, NC: Duke University Press.

Brown, Lawrence D. (1988). *Health policy in the United States: Issues and options* (Occasional Paper No. 4). New York: Ford Foundation.

Brown, Lawrence D. (1990). The deconstructed center: Of policy plagues on political houses (Commentary). *Journal of Health Politics, Policy and Law, 15* (Summer), 427–434.

Brown, Lawrence D. (1993). Conference summary: The changing policies and politics of urban health. *Health Affairs, 12* (Winter), 233–236.

Cassel, Christine K., Mark A. Rudberg, & S. Jay Olshansky. (1992). Price of success: Health care in an aging society. *Health Affairs, 11* (Summer), 87–99.

Chapman-Walsh, Diana. (1990). The shifting boundaries of alcohol policy. *Health Affairs, 9* (Summer), 47–62.

Coddington, David, J. Keen, Keith D. Moore, & Richard L. Clarke. (1990). *The crisis in health care: Costs, choices and strategies.* San Francisco, CA: Jossey-Bass.

Dallek, Geraldine. (1988). Frozen in ice: Federal health policy curing the Reagan years. *PAC Bulletin* (Summer), 4–14.

Davis, Karen. (1981). Reagan administration health policy. *Journal of Public Health Policy, 2* (December), 321–332.

deKervasdóue, Jean, John R. Kimberly, & Victor G. Rodwin. (Eds.). (1985). *The end of an illusion: The future of health policy in Western industrialized nations.* Berkeley: University of California Press.

Desario, Jack P. (1987). Health issues and policy options. *PS, 20* (Spring), 226–231.

Dobson, Allen, & Ronald Bialek. (1985). Shaping public policy from the perspective of a data builder. *Health Care Financing Review, 6* (Summer), 117–134.

Dobson, Allen, Donald Moran, & Gary Young. (1992). Role of federal waivers in the health policy process. *Health Affairs, 11* (Winter), 72–94.

Doty, Pamela. (1986). Family care of the elderly: The role of public policy. *Milbank Memorial Fund Quarterly, 64* (1), 34–75.

Dunham, Andrew B., & Theodore Marmor. (1978). Federal policy in health: Recent trends and different perspectives. In Theodore J. Lowi & Alan Stone (Eds.), *Nationalizing government: Public policies in America.* Beverly Hills, CA: Sage.

Etheredge, Lynn. (1984). An aging society and the federal deficit. *Milbank Memorial Fund Quarterly, 62* (Fall), 521–543.

Etheredge, Lynn, & Stanley Jones. (1991). Managing a pluralist health system. *Health Affairs, 10* (Winter), 93–105.

Falcone, David. (1976). The challenge of comparative health policy for political science. *Journal of Health Politics, Policy and Law, 1* (Summer), 196–213.

Falcone, David, Robert Broyles, & Steven R. Smith. (1994). American health policy in temporal and cross-national perspective. In Stuart Nagel (Ed.), *The encyclopedia of policy studies.* (2nd ed.). New York: Marcel Dekker.

Fein, Rashi. (1980). Social and economic attitudes shaping American health policy. *Milbank Memorial Fund Quarterly, 58* (Summer), 349–385.

Fein, Rashi. (1986). *Medical care: Medical costs: The search for a health insurance policy.* Cambridge, MA: Harvard University Press.

Fein, Rashi. (1990). Entitlement to health services reappraised. *Bulletin of New York Academy of Medicine, 66* (July/August), 319–328.

Foreman, Christopher H. Jr. (1994). *Plagues, products, and politics: Emergent public health hazards and national policy making.* Washington, D.C.: The Brookings Institution.

Fox, Daniel M. (1986). The consequences of consensus: American health policy in the twentieth century. *Milbank Memorial Fund Quarterly, 64* (1), 76–99.

Fox, Daniel M. (1986). *Health policies, health politics: The British and American experience, 1911–1965.* Princeton, NJ: Princeton University Press.

Fox, Daniel M. (1990). Health policy and the politics of research in the United States. *Journal of Health Politics, Policy and Law, 15* (Fall), 481–500.

Fox, Daniel M. (1991). The Milbank Quarterly and health services research, 1977–1990. *Milbank Quarterly, 69* (2), 185–198.

Fox, Daniel M. (1993). *Power and illness: The failure and future of American health policy.* Berkeley: University of California Press.

Fox, Daniel M., & Daniel C. Schaffer. (1989). Health policy and ERISA: Interest groups and semi-preemption. *Journal of Health Politics, Policy and Law, 14* (Summer), 239–268.

Freeman, Richard. (1995). Prevention and government: Health policy making in the United Kingdom & Germany. *Journal of Health Politics, Policy and Law, 20* (Fall), 745–766.

Friedland, Robert B., Lynn M. Etheredge, & Bruce C. Vladeck (Eds.). (1994). *Social welfare policy at the crossroads: Rethinking the roles of social insurance, tax expenditures, mandates and means-testing.* Washington, D.C.: National Academy of Social Insurance.

Fuchs, Beth C., & John F. Hoadley. (1987). Reflections from inside the Beltway: How Congress and the president grapple with health policy. *PS, 20* (Spring), 212–220.

Fuchs, Victor R. (1993). *The future of health policy.* Cambridge, MA: Harvard University Press.

Furino, Antonio. (Ed.). (1992). *Health policy and the Hispanic.* Boulder, CO: Westview Press.

Garber, Alan M., & Judith L. Wagner. (1991). Practice guidelines and cholesterol policy. *Health Affairs, 10* (Summer), 52–66.

Ginzberg, Eli. (1982). The future supply of physicians: From pluralism to policy. *Health Affairs, 1* (Fall), 6–19.

Ginzberg, Eli. (1984). The monetization of medical care. *New England Journal of Medicine, 310* (May 3), 1162–1165.

Ginsberg, Eli. (Ed.). (1991). *Health services research: Key to health policy.* Cambridge, MA: Harvard University Press.

Ginzberg, Eli, & Miriam Ostow. (1985). *The coming physician surplus: In search of a public policy.* Savage, MD: Rowman and Littlefield Publishers, Inc.

Goggin, Malcolm L. (1987). *Policy design and the politics of implementation: The case of child health care in the American states.* Knoxville: University of Tennessee Press.

Graig, Laurene A. (1993). *Health of nations: An international perspective on U.S. health care reform* (2nd ed.). Washington, D.C.: Congressional Quarterly, Inc.

Greenwald, Leslie M. (1992). Meaning in numbers. *Milbank Quarterly, 14* (3), 6–9.

Hadley, Jack. (1995). Politics versus policy analysis. *Inquiry, 32* (Summer), 127–129.

Havighurst, Clark C. (1988). *Health care law and policy: Readings, notes and questions.* Westbury, NY: Foundation Press.

Helms, Robert B. (Ed.). (1993). *Health care policy and politics: Lessons from foreign countries*. Washington, D.C.: AEI Press.

Hudson, Robert B. (1993). Social contingencies, the aged, and public policy. *Milbank Quarterly, 71* (2), 253–278.

Huefner, Robert P., & Margaret P. Battin. (Eds.). (1992). *Changing to national health care: Ethical and policy issues*. Salt Lake City: University of Utah Press.

Ibrahim, Michel A. (1985). *Epidemiology and health policy*. Rockville, MD: Aspen Systems Corp.

Iglehart, John K. (1992a). The American health care system. *New England Journal of Medicine, 326* (April 2), 962–967.

Iglehart, John K. (1992b). Desperately seeking solutions. *Milbank Quarterly, 14* (3), 2–5.

Iglehart, John K. (1994). Changing course in turbulent times: An interview with David Lawrence. *Health Affairs, 13* (Winter), 65–77.

Ingraham, Norman R. (1961). Formulation of public policy in medical care: Dynamics of community action at local level. *American Journal of Public Health, 51* (August), 1144–1151.

Jacobs, Lawrence R. (1993). *The health of nations: Public opinion and the making of American and British health policy*. Ithaca, NY: Cornell University Press.

Jajich-Toth, Cindy, & Burns W. Roper. (1991). Basing policy on survey data: Proceed with caution. *Health Affairs, 10* (Summer), 170–172.

Johnston, J. Bruce, & Uwe E. Reinhardt. (1989). Addressing the health of a nation: Two views. *Health Affairs, 8* (Summer), 5–23.

Kars-Marshall, Cri, Yvonne W. Spronk-Boon, & Marjan C. Pollemans. (1988). National health interview surveys for health care policy. *Social Science and Medicine, 26* (2), 223–233.

Katz, Aaron, & Jack Thompson. (1996). The role of public policy on health care market change. *Health Affairs, 15* (Summer), 77–91.

Kissick, William L. (1994). *Medicine's dilemmas: Infinite needs versus finite resources*. New Haven, CT: Yale University Press.

Klein, Rudolph. (1981). Economic versus political models in health care policy. In John B. McKinlay (Ed.), *Issues in health care policy* (pp. 66–79). Cambridge, MA: MIT Press.

Kleiman, Mark A. R. (1992). *Against excess: Drug policy for results*. New York: Basic Books.

Klein, Rudolph. (1990). Research, policy, and the National Health Service. *Journal of Health Politics, Policy and Law, 15* (Fall), 501–524.

Kohler, Peter O. (1994). Specialists/primary care professionals: Striking a balance. *Inquiry, 31* (Fall), 289–295.

Kronenfeld, Jennie Jacobs, & Marcia Lynn Whicker. (1984). *U.S. national health policy: An analysis of the federal role*. New York: Praeger.

Leader, Helah, & Marilyn Moon. (Eds.). (1988). *Changing America's health care system: Proposals for legislative action*. Washington, D.C.: American Association of Retired Persons, Public Policy Institute.

Lee, Philip R., & A. E. Benjamin. (1988). Health policy and the politics of health care. In Stephen J. Williams & Paul R. Torrens (Eds.), *Introduction to health services* (3rd ed., pp. 457–479). New York: John Wiley & Sons.

Lee, Philip R., & Carroll L. Estes. (Eds.). (1990). *The nation's health* (3rd ed.). Boston, MA: Jones and Bartlett.

Lee, Philip R., & Carroll L. Estes. (Eds.). (1994). *The nation's health* (4th ed.). Boston, MA: Jones and Bartlett.

Leigh, J. Paul, & Christine Hunter. (1992). Health policy and the distribution of lifetime income. *Milbank Quarterly, 70* (2), 341–360.

Lewin, Marion Ein. (Ed.). (1985). *The health policy agenda: Some critical questions*. Washington, D.C.: American Enterprise Institute.

Lewin, Marion Ein. (Ed.). (1986). *From research into policy: Improving the link for health services*. Washington, D.C.: American Enterprise Institute for Public Policy Research.

Light, Paul. (1985). *Artful work: The politics of Social Security reform*. New York: Random House.

Lipsky, Michael, & Marc A. Thibodeau. (1990). Domestic food policy in the United States. *Journal of Health Politics, Policy and Law, 15* (Summer), 319–340.

Longest, Beaufort B., Jr. (1994). *Health policy making in the United States*. Ann Arbor, MI: AUPHA Press/Health Administration Press.

Mann, Thomas, & Norman Ornstein. (Eds.). (1995). *In intensive care: How Congress shapes health policy*. Washington, D.C.: American Enterprise Institute and The Brookings Institution.

Marmor, Theodore R. (1986). American medical policy and the "crisis" of the welfare state: A comparative perspective. *Journal of Health Politics, Policy and Law, 11* (4), 617–631.

Marmor, Theodore R., Amy Bridges, & Wayne L. Hoffman. (1978). *Comparative politics and health policies: Notes on benefits, costs and limits*. In Douglas E. Ashford (Ed.), *Comparing public policies: New concepts and methods* (Vol. 4, pp. 59–80). Beverly Hills, CA: Sage.

Marmor, Theodore R., & Jon B. Christianson. (1982). *Health care policy: A political economy approach*. Beverly Hills, CA: Sage.

Marmor, Theodore R., & James A. Morone. (1983). The health programs of the Kennedy–Johnson years: An overview. In Theodore R. Marmor (Ed.), *Political analysis and American medical care* (pp. 131–154.). New York: Cambridge University Press.

Marmor, Theodore R., Donald A. Wittman, & Thomas Heagy. (1976). Politics, public policy and medical inflation. In Michael Zubkoff (Ed.), *Health: A victim or cause of inflation* (pp. 299–316). New York: Prodist.

Mason, James O. (1990). A prevention policy framework for the nation. *Health Affairs, 9* (Summer), 22–29.

McAllister, William. (1994). Concrete fictions and hegemonic methodologies: Doing policy research in government. *Journal of Health Politics, Policy and Law, 19* (Spring), 91–106.

McAuliffe, William E. (1990). Health care policy issues in the drug abuser treatment field. *Journal of Health Politics, Policy and Law, 15* (Summer), 357–386.

McKinlay, John B. (Ed.). (1981). *Issues in health care policy: A Milbank reader*. Cambridge, MA: MIT Press.

McLachlan, Gordon, & Alan Maynard. (Eds.). (1982). *The public/private mix for health*. London: Nuffield Provincial Hospitals Trust.

Mechanic, David. (1981). Some dilemmas in health care policy. *Milbank Memorial Fund Quarterly/Health and Society, 59* (Winter), 80–94.

Mechanic, David. (1986). *From advocacy to allocation: The evolving American health care system*. New York: The Free Press.

Melhaldo, Evan M., Walter Feinberg, & Harold W. Swartz. (Eds.). (1988). *Money, power and health care*. Ann Arbor, MI: Health Administration Press.

Meyer, Jack A. (1985). *Incentives versus controls in health policy: Broadening the debate*. Washington, D.C.: American Enterprise Institute.

Meyer, Jack A., & Marion Ein Lewin. (Eds.). (1987). *Chart up the future of health care: Policy, politics and public health*. Washington, D.C.: American Enterprise Institute for Public Policy Research.

Mick, Stephen S. (1987). Contradictory policies for foreign medical graduates. *Health Affairs, 6* (Fall), 5–18.

Mitchell, Faith, & Claire Brindis. (1987). Adolescent pregnancy: The responsibilities of policy makers. *Health Services Research, 22* (August), 399–437.

Moreno, Jonathan D. (Ed.). (1990). *Paying the doctor: Health policy and physician reimbursement*. Westport, CT: Auburn House.

Morone, James A. (1990). American political culture and the search for lessons from abroad. *Journal of Health Politics, Policy and Law, 15* (Spring), 129–143.

Morone, James A. (1990). Epilogue: Tales of trouble. *Journal of Health Politics, Policy and Law, 15* (Summer), 435–440.

Morone, James A. (1992). The bias of American politics: Rationing health care in a weak state. *University of Pennsylvania Law Review, 140* (5), 1923–1938.

Morone, James A., & Janice M. Goggin. (1995). Introduction—health policies in Europe: Welfare states in a market era. *Journal of Health Politics, Policy and Law, 20* (Fall), 557–570.

Morris, Jonas. (1986). *Searching for a cure: National health policy*. Berkeley: Morgan Publishing Co.

Mueller, Keith J. (1993). *Health care policy in the United States.* Lincoln: University of Nebraska Press.

National Leadership Commission on Health Care. (1989). *For the health of a nation: A shared responsibility. Report of the national leadership commission on health care.* Ann Arbor, MI: Health Administration Press.

Navarro, Vicente. (1987). Federal health policies in the United States: An alternative explanation. *Milbank Memorial Fund Quarterly, 65* (1), 81–110.

Omenn, Gilbert S. (1990). Prevention and the elderly: Appropriate policies. *Health Affairs, 9* (Summer), 80–93.

Otten, Allen L. (1992). The influence of the mass media on health policy. *Health Affairs, 11* (Winter), 111–118.

Patrick, Donald L., & Jennifer Erickson. (1993). *Health status and health policy: Allocating resources to health care.* New York: Oxford University Press.

Peterson, Mark A. (1993). Political influence in the 1990s: From iron triangles to policy networks. *Journal of Health Politics, Policy and Law, 18* (Summer), 395–438.

Potter, Margaret A., & Beaufort B. Longest Jr. (1994). The divergence of federal and state policies on the charitable tax exemption of nonprofit hospitals. *Journal of Health Politics, Policy and Law, 19* (Summer), 393–420.

Powell, Francis D. (1994). Government participation in physician negotiations in German economic policy as applied to universal health care coverage in the United States. *Social Science and Medicine, 38* (1), 35–43.

Raffel, Marshal W., & Norma K. Raffel. (1987). *Perspectives on health policy: Australia, New Zealand, United States.* New York: John Wiley & Sons.

Reinhardt, Uwe E. (1991). Breaking American health policy gridlock. *Health Affairs, 10* (Summer), 96–103.

Reinhardt, Uwe E. (1992). The United States: Breakthroughs and waste. *Journal of Health Politics, Policy and Law, 17* (Winter), 637–666.

Rhodes, Robert P. (1992). *Health care politics, policy, and distributive justice: The ironic triumph.* Albany: State University of New York Press.

Rhoads, Steven E. (Ed.). (1980). *Valuing life: Public policy dilemmas.* Boulder, CO: Westview Press.

Rice, Thomas. (1992). Trading off access to enhance welfare. *Health Affairs, 8* (Summer), 96–101.

Riska, Elianne, & James A. Taylor. (1976). Consumer attitudes toward health policy and knowledge about health legislation. *Journal of Health Politics, Policy and Law, 6* (2), 331–343.

Rochefort, David A. (1986). *American social welfare policy: Dynamics of formulation and change.* Boulder, CO: Westview Press.

Rodwin, Marc A. (1993). *Medicine, money and morals: Physicians' conflicts of interest.* New York: Oxford University Press.

Roemer, Ruth. (1988). The right to health care—gains and gaps. *American Journal of Public Health, 78* (March), 241–247.

Rosenberg, Paul M. (1994). Federal and state policies on the charitable tax exemption of nonprofit hospitals. *Journal of Health Politics, Policy and Law, 19* (Summer), 421–422.

Rosner, David. (1995). Power and illness: The failure and future of American health policy by Daniel M. Fox. *Journal of Health Politics, Policy and Law, 20* (Fall), 816–819.

Sass, Hans-Martin, & Robert U. Massey. (Eds.). (1988). *Health care systems, moral conflicts in European and American public policies.* Higham, VA: Kluwer Academic Publishing Co.

Schlesinger, Mark S., & Tae-Ku Lee. (1993). Is heath care different? Popular support of federal health and social policies. *Journal of Health Politics, Policy and Law, 18* (Fall), 551–628.

Schroeder, Steven A. (1994). Managing the U.S. health care workforce: Creating policy amidst uncertainty. *Inquiry, 31* (Fall), 266–275.

Sherrill, Robert. (1995). The madness of the market: Dangerous to your health. *The Nation* (January 9, 16), 45–72.

Shortell, Stephen M., & Uwe E. Reinhardt. (Eds.). (1992). *Improving health policy and management: Nine critical research issues in the 1990s.* Ann Arbor, MI: Health Administration Press.

Siegler, Mark. (1979). A right to health care: Ambiguity, professional responsibility and patient liberty. *Journal of Medicine and Philosophy, 4* (2), 148–157.

Silver, George A. (1978). Ordering social objectives: National Health Service and national health insurance as policy options in organizing the medical care system. *Yale Journal of Biology and Medicine, 5,* 177–184.

Sisk, Jane E. (1993). Improving the use of research-based evidence in policy making: Effective care in pregnancy and childbirth in the United States. *Milbank Quarterly, 71* (3), 477–496.

Sorian, Richard. (1988). *The bitter pill: Tough choices in America's health policy.* Washington, D.C.: McGraw-Hill.

Starr, Paul. (1983). Medical care and the pursuit of equality in America. In president's commission for the study of ethical problems in medical and biomedical behavior research. *Securing access to health care* (Vol. 2, pp. 3 49). Washington, D.C.: U.S. Government Printing Office.

Stone, Deborah A. (1988). *Policy paradox and political reason.* Glenview, IL: Scott, Foresman and Co.

Straetz, Ralph A., & Marvin Lieberman. (1974). Health policy studies by political scientists. *Policy Studies Journal, 3* (Winter), 195–200.

Straetz, Ralph A., Marvin Lieberman, & Alice Sardell. (1981). *Critical issues and health policy.* Lexington, MA: Lexington Books.

Torrens, Paul R. (1988). Historical evolution and overview of health services in the United States. In Stephen J. Williams & Paul R. Torrens (Eds.), *Introduction to health services* (3rd ed., pp. 3–32). New York: John Wiley & Sons.

VanEtten, Geert, & Frans Rutten. (1986). The social sciences in health policy and practice. *Social Science and Medicine, 22* (11), 1187–1194.

Waters, William J., & John T. Tierney. (1984). Hard lessons learned. *New England Journal of Medicine, 311* (November 8), 1251–1252.

Weeks, Lewis E., & Howard J. Berman. (1985). *Shapers of American health care policy: An oral history.* Ann Arbor, MI: Health Administration Press.

Weissert, Carol S., & Jack H. Knott. (1995). Foundations' impact on policy making: Results from a pilot study. *Health Affairs, 14* (Winter), 275–286.

Weissert, Carol S., Jack H. Knott, & Blair E. Stieber. (1994). Education and the health professions: Explaining policy choices among the states. *Journal of Health Politics, Policy and Law, 19* (Summer), 361–392.

Wikler, Daniel. (1991). What has bioethics to offer health policy? *Milbank Quarterly, 69* (2), 233–252.

Willis, David P. (1989). *Health policies and black Americans.* New Brunswick, NJ: Transaction Publishers.

Wilsford, David. (1995). States facing interests: Struggles over health care policy in advanced, industrial democracies. *Journal of Health Politics, Policy and Law, 20* (Fall), 571–614.

Wisotsky, Steven. (1990). *Beyond the war on drugs: Overcoming a failed public policy.* Buffalo, NY: Prometheus Books.

Woolhandler, Steffie, & David U. Himmelstein. (1991). The deteriorating administrative efficiency of the U.S. health care system. *New England Journal of Medicine, 324* (May 2), 1253–1258.

Zimring, Franklin E. (1993). Policy research on firearms and violence. *Health Affairs, 12* (Winter), 109–122.

Hospitals

Derzon, Robert A. (1972). The politics of municipal hospitals. In Douglass Cater & Philip R. Lee (Eds.), *Politics of health.* New York: Medcom Press.

Feder, Judith, & Bruce Spitz. (1979). The politics of hospital payment. *Journal of Health Politics, 4* (Fall), 435–463.

Jaeger, Boi Jon. (1972). Government and hospitals: A perspective on health politics. *Hospital Administration, 17* (Winter), 39–50.

Joskow, Paul L. (1981). *Controlling hospital costs: The role of government regulation.* Cambridge, MA: MIT Press.

Lindsay, Cotton M. (1975). *Veterans administration hospitals: An economic analysis of government enter-*

prise. Washington, D.C.: American Enterprise Institute for Public Policy Research.

Raphaelson, Arnold H., & Charles P. Hall Jr. (1978). Politics and economics of hospital cost containment. *Journal of Health Politics, Policy and Law, 3* (Spring), 87–111.

Rosner, David. (1980). Gaining control: Reform reimbursement and politics in New York's community hospitals, 1890–1915. *American Journal of Public Health, 70* (May), 533–542.

Influenza

Berliner, Howard S., & Warren J. Salmon. (1976). Swine flu, the phantom threat. *Nation, 223* (September 25), 269–272.

Neustadt, Richard E., & Harvey V. Fineberg. (1978). *The swine flu affair: Decision-making on a slippery disease*. Washington, D.C.: U.S. Government Printing Office.

Osborne, June. (1977). *Influenza in America, 1918–1976: History, science, and politics*. New York: Prodist, Neale Watson Academic Publishers.

Silverstein, Arthur M. (1981). *Pure politics and impure science: The swine flu affair*. Baltimore, MD: Johns Hopkins University Press.

Viseltear, Arthur J. (1977). Immunization and public policy: A short political history of the 1976 swine influenza legislation. In June E. Osborne (Ed.), *Influenza in America, 1918–1976: History, science and politics*. New York: Prodist, Neal Watson Academic Publishers.

Long-term Care

Alber, Jens. (1992). Residential care for the elderly. *Journal of Health Politics, Policy and Law, 17* (Winter), 929–958.

Avorn, Jerry. (1984). Benefits and cost analysis in geriatric care: Turning age descrimination into health policy. *New England Journal of Medicine, 310* (May 17), 1294–1301.

Axinn, June, & Mark J. Stern. (1985). Age and dependency: Children and the aged in American social policy. *Milbank Memorial Fund Quarterly, 63* (Fall), 648–670.

Baggett, Sharon A. (1989). *Residential care for the elderly: Critical issues in public policy*. Westport, CT: Greenwood Press.

Barer, Morris L., Clyde Hertzman, Robert Miller, & Marina V. Pascali. (1992). On being old and sick: The burden of health care for the elderly in Canada and the United States. *Journal of Health Politics, Policy and Law, 17* (Winter), 763–782.

Barfield, Claude. (1983). New Federalism and long term care of the elderly. (Update). *Health Affairs, 2* (Spring), 113–125.

Benjamin, A. E. (1993). An historical perspective on home care policy. *Milbank Quarterly, 71* (1), 129–166.

Binney, Elizabeth A., & Carroll L. Estes. (1988). The retreat of the state and transfer of responsibility: The intergenerational war. *International Journal of Health Services, 18* (1), 83–96.

Bishop, Christine E., Joshua M. Wiener, Laurel Hixon Illston, & Raymond J. Hanley. (Eds.). (1995). Sharing the burden: Strategies for public and private long-term care insurance. *Journal of Health Politics, Policy and Law, 20* (Fall), 811–815.

Boerstler, Heidi, Tom Carlough, & Robert E. Schlenker. (1991). Administrative and policy issues in reimbursement for nursing home capital investment. *Journal of Health Politics, Policy and Law, 16* (Fall), 553–572.

Brecher, Charles, & James Knickman. (1985). A reconsideration of long term care policy. *Journal of Health Politics, Policy and Law, 10* (Summer), 245–274.

Brown, Lawrence D., & Catherine McLaughlin. (1990). Constraining costs at the community level: A critique. *Health Affairs, 9* (Winter), 5–28.

Burke, Thomas R. (1988). Long term care: The public role and private initiative. *Health Care Financing Review, Supplement* (December), 1–5.

Cassel, Christine K., Mark A. Rudberg, & S. Jay Ol-shansky. (1992). Price of success: Health care in an aging society. *Health Affairs, 11* (Summer), 87–99.

Clark, Robert L., & John A. Menefee. (1981). Federal expenditures for the elderly: Past and future. *The Gerontologist, 21* (2), 132–137.

Clauser, Steven B., & Brant E. Fries. (1992). Nursing home resident assessment and case-mix classification: Cross-national perspectives. *Health Care Financing Reveiw, 13* (Summer), 135–156.

Cohen, Marc A., Nanda Kumar, Thomas McGuire, & Stanley S. Wallack. (1992). Financing long-term care: A practical mix of public and private. *Journal of Health Politics, Policy and Law, 17* (Fall), 403–424.

Cohen, Marc A., Nanda Kumar, & Stanley S. Wallack. (1994). Long-term care insurance and Medicaid. *Health Affairs, 13* (Fall), 127–139.

Culyer, A. J., & Stephen Birch. (1985). Caring for the elderly: A European perspective on today and tomorrow. *Journal of Health Politics, Policy and Law, 10* (Fall), 469–488.

Doty, Pamela. (1988). Long term care in international perspective. *Health Care Financing Review, Supplement* (December), 145–155.

Eidsdorfer, Carl, David A. Kessler, & Abby N. Spector. (1989). *Caring for the elderly: Reshaping health policy.* Baltimore, MD: Johns Hopkins University Press.

Estes, Carroll L. (1983). Social Security: The social construction of a crisis. *Milbank Memorial Fund Quarterly, 61* (Summer), 445–461.

Estes, Carroll L. (1985). Long term care and public policy in an era of austerity. *Journal of Public Health Policy, 6* (December), 464–475.

Estes, Carroll L., & Elizabeth A. Binney. (1988). Toward a transformation of health and aging policy. *International Journal of Health Services, 18* (1), 69–82.

Etheredge, Lynn. (1984). An aging society and the federal deficit. *Milbank Memorial Fund Quarterly, 62* (Fall), 521–543.

Eustis, Nancy N., Jay N. Greenberg, & Sharon K. Patten. (1984). *Long term care of older persons: A policy perspective.* Monterey, CA: Brooks/Cole Publishing Co.

Freiman, Marc P., Bernard S. Arons, Howard H. Goldman, & Barbara J. Burns. (1990). Nursing home reform and the mentally ill. *Health Affairs, 9* (Winter), 47–60.

Fuchs, Victor R. (1984). Though much is taken: Reflections on aging, health, and medical care. *Milbank Memorial Fund Quarterly, 62* (Spring), 143–166.

Gill, Derek G., & Stanley R. Ingman. (1986). Geriatric care and distributive justice, problems and prospects. *Social Science and Medicine, 23* (12), 1205–1215.

Ginzberg, Eli. (1983). The elderly: An international policy perspective. *Milbank Memorial Fund Quarterly, 61* (Summer), 473–488.

Harrington, Charlene, Robert J. Newcomer, Carroll L. Estes, & Associates. (1985). *Long term care of the elderly: Public policy issues.* Beverly Hills, CA: Sage.

Hollingsworth, J. Rogers, & Ellen Jane Hollingsworth. (1992). Challenges in the provision of care for the chronically ill in the United Kingdom, Germany, and the United States. *Journal of Health Politics, Policy and Law, 17* (Winter), 869–878.

Hudson, Robert B. (1993). Social contingencies, the aged, and public policy. *Milbank Quarterly, 71* (2), 253–278.

Jamieson, Anne. (1992). Home care in old age: A lost cause? *Journal of Health Politics, Policy and Law, 17* (Winter), 879–898.

Jamieson, Anne. (Ed.). (1991). *Home care for older people in Europe: A comparison of policies and practices.* New York: Oxford University Press.

Justice, Diane. (1988). *State long term care reform: Development of community care systems in six states.* Washington, D.C.: National Governors Association.

Kane, Robert L., & Rosalie A. Kane. (1985). *A will and a way: What the United States can learn from Canada about caring for the elderly.* New York: Columbia University Press.

Kane, Robert L., & Rosalie A. Kane. (1994). Implications of the Clinton health reform plan for older persons and long-term care. *Journal of Health Politics, Policy and Law, 19* (Spring), 221–226.

Kane, Rosalie A. (1995). Expanding the home care concept: Blurring distinctions among home care, institutional care, and other long-term care services. *Milbank Quarterly, 73* (2), 161–186.

Kane, Rosalie A., & Robert L. Kane. (1985). The feasibility of universal long term care benefits: Ideas from Canada. *New England Journal of Medicine, 312* (May 23), 1357–1363.

Kane, Rosalie A., & Robert L. Kane. (1987). *Long term care—principles, programs and policies*. Philadelphia, PA: Springer Publishing Co.

Katz, Michael B. (1984). Poorhouses and the origins of the public old age home. *Milbank Memorial Fund Quarterly, 62* (Winter), 110–140.

Leutz, Walter. (1986). Long term care for the elderly: Public dreams and private realities. *Inquiry, 23* (June), 134–140.

Lipson, Debra J. (1988). *State financing of long term care services for the elderly*. Washington, D.C.: Intergovernmental Health Policy Project, George Washington University.

Liu, Korbin, & Genevieve Kenney. (1993). Impact of the catastrophic coverage act and new coverage guidelines on Medicare skilled nursing facility use. *Inquiry, 30* (Spring), 41–53.

Lowe, Beverly F. (1988). Future directions for community based long term care research. *Milbank Memorial Fund Quarterly, 66* (3), 552–571.

Manard, Barbara Bolling. (1986). Doing research for decision makers: Nursing home reimbursement. In Marion Ein Lewin (Ed.), *From research into policy: Improving the link for health services* (pp. 51–71). Washington, D.C.: American Enterprise Institute for Public Policy Research.

McCall, Nelda, James Knickman, & Ellen Jones Bauer. (1991). A new approach to long-term care. *Health Affairs, 10* (Spring), 164–176.

Merrill, Jeffrey. (1992). A test of our society: How and for whom we finance long-term care. *Inquiry, 29* (Summer), 176–187.

Migdail, Karen J. (1992). Nursing home reforms five years later. *Journal of American Health Policy, 1* (September/October), 41–46.

Myles, John F. (1983). Conflict, crisis, and the future of old age security. *Milbank Memorial Fund Quarterly, 61* (Summer), 462–472.

Norton, Edward C., & Joseph P. Newhouse. (1994). Policy options for public long-term care insurance. *Journal of American Medical Association, 271* (May 18), 1520–1524.

Plough, Alonzo L. (1986). *Borrowed time: Artificial organs and the politics of extending lives*. Philadelphia: Temple University Press.

Quadagno, Jill S. (1984). From poor laws to pensions: The evolution of economic support for the aged in England and America. *Milbank Memorial Fund Quarterly, 62* (Summer), 417–466.

Quadagno, Jill S. (1988). *The transformation of old age security: Class and politics in the American welfare state*. Chicago: University of Chicago Press.

Rice, Dorothy P., & Carroll L. Estes. (1984). Health of the elderly: Policy issues and challenges. *Health Affairs, 3* (Winter), 25–49.

Rowland, Diane. (1987). Issues of long-term care. In Carl J. Schramm (Ed.), *Health care and its costs: Can the U.S. afford adequate health care?* (pp. 222–251). New York: W. W. Norton.

Rowland, Diane. (1992). A five-nation perspective on the elderly. *Health Affairs, 11* (Fall), 205–215.

Schechter, Malvin. (1993). *Beyond Medicare: Achieving long-term care security*. San Francisco, CA: Jossey-Bass.

Shaughnessy, Peter W. (1985). Long-term care research and public policy. *Health Services Research, 20* (October), 489–499.

Shaughnessy, Peter W. (1991). *Shaping policy for long-term care*. Ann Arbor, MI: Health Administration Press.

Short Farley, Pamela, Peter Kemper, Llewellyn J. Cornelius, & Daniel C. Walden. (1992). Public and private responsibility for financing nursing-home care: The effect of Medicaid asset spend-down. *Milbank Quarterly, 70* (2), 277–298.

Sloan, Frank A., & May W. Shayne. (1993). Long-term care, Medicaid, and impoverishment of the elderly. *Milbank Quarterly, 71* (4), 575–600.

Smeeding, Timothy M., & Lavonne Straub. (1987). Health care financing among the elderly: Who really pays the bills? *Journal of Health Politics, Policy and Law, 12* (Spring), 35–52.

Somers, Stephen A., & Jeffrey C. Merrill. (1991). Supporting states' efforts for long-term care insurance. *Health Affairs, 10* (Spring), 177–179.

Sparer, Michael S. (1993). States in a reformed health system: Lessons from nursing home policy. *Health Affairs, 12* (Spring), 7–20.

Temkin-Greener, Mark, R. Meiners, E. Petty, & Jill Szydlowski. (1993). Spending-down to Medicaid in the nursing home and in the community. *Medical Care, 31* (8), 663–679.

Tennstedt, Sharon L., Sybil L. Crawford, & John B. McKinlay. (1993). Is family care on the decline? A longitudinal investigation of the substitution of formal long-term care services for informal care. *Milbank Quarterly, 71* (4), 601–624.

Ward, Russell, & Sheldon S. Tobin. (Eds.). (1987). *Health in aging: Sociological issues and policy direction.* New York: Springer Publishing Co.

Weiner, Janet. (1994). Financing long-term care: A proposal by the American College of Physicians and the American Geriatrics Society. *Journal of American Medical Association, 271* (May 18), 1525–1529.

Weissert, William G. (1986). Hard choices: Targeting long term care to the "at-risk" aged. *Journal of Health Politics, Policy and Law, 11* (Fall), 463–481.

Weissert, William G. (1991). A new policy agenda for home care. *Health Affairs, 10* (Summer), 67–77.

Wiener, Joshua M., Raymond J. Hanley, & Laurel Hixon Illston. (1992). Commentary: Financing long-term care: How much public? How much private? *Journal of Health Politics, Policy and Law, 17* (Fall), 425–434.

Wiener, Joshua M., Laurel Hixon Illston, & Raymond J. Hanley. (1994). *Sharing the burden, strategies for public and private long-term insurance.* Washington, D.C.: The Brookings Institution.

Zedlewski Rafferty, Sheila McBride, & Timothy D. McBride. (1992). The changing profile of the elderly: Effects on future long-term care needs and financing. *Milbank Quarterly, 70* (2), 217–276.

Manpower

Dranove, David, & William D. White. (1994). *Clinton's specialist quota: Shaky premise, questionable consequences.* American Enterprise Institue Special Studies in Health Reform. Waldorf, MD: AEI Press.

Ginzberg, Eli, & Miriam Ostow. (1992). Physician supply strategy: The case of the South. *Health Affairs, 11* (Summer), 193–197.

Kohler, Peter O. (1994). Specialists/Primary care professionals: Striking a balance. *Inquiry, 31* (Fall), 289–295.

Moynihan, Daniel Patrick. (1995). The professionalization of reform II. *Public Interest, 121* (Fall), 23–41.

Mullan, Fitzhugh. (1992). Missing: A national medical manpower policy. *Milbank Quarterly, 70* (2), 381–386.

Osterweis, Marion, Christopher J. McLaughlin, Henri R. Manasse, & Cornelius L. Hopper. (Eds.). (1996). *The U.S. health workforce. Power, politics, and policy.* Washington, D.C.: Association of Academic Health Centers.

Medicine and the Medical Profession

Anderson, Odin W. (1976). PSROs: The medical profession and the public interest. *Milbank Memorial Fund Quarterly/Health and Society, 54* (Summer), 379–388.

Berenson, Robert A. (1994). Do physicians recognize their own best interests? *Health Affairs, 13* (Spring), 185–193.

Bonner, T. N. (1953). Social and political attitudes of midwestern physicians. *Journal of the History of Medicine and Allied Sciences, 8* (April), 133–164.

Burrow, James G. (1963). *AMA voice of American medicine.* Baltimore, MD: Johns Hopkins University Press.

Cain, Leonard D., Jr. (1967.). The AMA and the gerontologists: Uses and abuses of "a profile of the aging: USA." In Gideon Sjoberg (Ed.), *Ethics, politics, and social research* (pp. 78–114). Cambridge: Schenkman Publishing Co.

Carter, Richard. (1958). *The doctor business.* New York: Doubleday and Co.

Chase, Edward T. (1961). The politics of medicine. In Marion Sanders (Ed.), *The crisis in American medicine* (pp. 1–19). New York: Harpers.

Colombotos, John. (1969). Physicians and Medicare: A before–after study of the effects of legislation on attitudes. *American Sociological Review, 34* (June), 318–334.

Dodds, Richard W. (1970). A framework for political mapping of conflict in organized medicine—especially pediatrics. *Medical Care Review, 27* (November), 1035–1062.

Eckstein, Harry. (1960). *Pressure groups politics: The case of the British Medical Association.* Palo Alto, CA: Stanford University Press.

Garceau, Oliver. (1941). *The political life of the American Medical Association.* Cambridge, MA: Harvard University Press.

Ginzberg, Eli. (1985.). *American medicine: The power shift.* Totowa, NJ: Rowman and Allanheld.

Ginsberg, Eli. (1990). *The medical triangle: Physicians, politicians and the public.* Cambridge, MA: Harvard University Press.

Ginsberg, Eli. (1990). The politics of the U.S. physicians supply. In Eli Ginsberg (Ed.), *The medical triangle: Physicians, politicians and the public.* Cambridge, MA: Harvard University Press.

Glaser, William A. (1960). Doctors and politics. *American Journal of Sociology, 66* (November), 230–245.

Glaser, William A. (1989). The politics of paying American physicians. *Health Affairs, 8* (Fall), 129– 146.

Glaser, William A. (1994). Doctors and public authorities: The trend toward collaboration. *Journal of Health Politics, Policy and Law, 19* (Winter), 705–728.

Gordon, Gerald, & Selwyn Becker. (1964). Changes in medical practice bring shifts in the patterns of power. *Modern Hospital, 102* (February), 89–91.

Hyde, David R., & Payson Wolff. (1954). The American Medical Association: Power, purpose and politics in organized medicine. *Yale Law Journal, 63* (May), 938–1022.

Iglehart, John K. (1994). Health care reform: The role of physicians. *New England Journal of Medicine, 330* (March 10), 728–731.

Igelhart, John K. (1996). The struggle to reform Medicare. *New England Journal of Medicine, 334* (April 18), 1071–1075.

Johnson, James A., & Walter J. Jones. (1993). *The American Medical Association and organized medicine: A commentary and annotated bibliography.* New York: Garland Publishers.

Lewis, R. (1955). New power at the polls: The doctors. In H. Turner (Ed.), *Politics in the United States: Readings in political parties and pressure groups* (pp. 180–185). New York: McGraw-Hill.

Light, Donald W. (1991). Commentary: Professionalism as a countervailing power. *Journal of Health Politics, Policy and Law, 16* (Fall), 499–506.

Marmor, Theodore R., & David Thomas. (1983). Doctors, politics and pay disputes: Pressure group politics revisited. In Theodore R. Marmor (Ed.), *Political analysis and American medical care* (pp. 107–130). New York: Cambridge University Press.

Means, James Howard. (1953). *Doctors, people, and government.* Boston: Little, Brown.

Mechanic, David. (1984). The transformation of health providers. *Health Affairs, 3* (Spring), 65–72.

Mechanic, David. (1991). Sources of countervailing power in medicine. *Journal of Health Politics, Policy and Law, 16* (Fall), 485–498.

Melicke, Carl A. (1967). *The Saskatchewan medical care dispute of 1962.* Unpublished Ph.D. diss., University of Minnesota, Minneapolis.

Millman, Michael L. (1980). *Politics and the expanding physician supply.* Montclair, NJ: Allanheld, Osmun and Co.

Numbers, Ronald. (1978). *Almost persuaded: American physicians and compulsory health insurance, 1912–1920.* Baltimore, MD: Johns Hopkins University Press.

Osberg, J. Scott. (1994). Changes in positions of authority held by U.S. physicians: A fresh look at existing data. *American Journal of Public Health, 84* (October), 1573–1575.

Painter, Joseph T., Lonnie R. Bristow, & James S. Todd. (1994). Shared sacrifice: The AMA leadership response to the Health Security Act. *Journal of the American Medical Association, 271* (March 9), 786–788.

Rayack, Elton. (1964). The American Medical Association and the supply of physicians: A study of the internal contradictions and the concept of professionalism. Part I. *Medical Care, 2* (October–December), 244–252.

Rayack, Elton. (1965). The American Medical Association and the supply of physicians: A study of the internal contradictions and the concept of professionalism. Part II. *Medical Care, 3* (January–March), 17–25.

Rayack, Elton. (1967a). The American Medical Association and the development of voluntary insurance. Part I. *Social and Economic Administration, 1* (April), 3–25.

Rayack, Elton. (1967b). The American Medical Association and the development of voluntary insurance. Part II. *Social and Economic Administration, 1* (July), 29–55.

Rayack, Elton. (1967c). *Professional power in American medicine: The economics of the American Medical Association.* New York: World Publishing Co.

Rayack, Elton. (1968). Restrictive practices of organized medicine. *Anti-Trust Bulletin, 13* (Summer), 659–719.

Rodwin, Marc A. (1992). The organized American medical profession's response to financial conflicts of interest: 1890–1992. *Milbank Quarterly, 70* (4), 703–742.

Rodwin, Marc A. (1993). *Medicine, money and morals: Physicians' conflicts of interest.* New York: Oxford University Press.

Stevenson, H. Michael, & A. Paul Williams. (1985). Physicians and Medicare: Professional ideology and Canadian health care policy. *Canadian Public Policy, 11* (September 3), 504–521.

Taylor, Malcolm G. (1960). The role of the medical profession in the formulation and execution of public policy. *Canadian Journal of Economic and Political Science, 26* (February), 108–127.

Todd, James S., Steven V. Seekins, John A. Krichbaum, & Lynn K. Harvey. (1991). Health access America—strengthening the U.S. health care system. *Journal of the American Medical Association, 265* (May 15), 2503–2506.

Tollefson, E. A. (1964). *Bitter medicine.* Toronto: University of Toronto Press.

Wilsford, David. (1991). *Doctors and the state: The politics of health care in France and the United States.* Durham, NC: Duke University Press.

Medicare and Medicaid

Medicare

Aaron, Henry, J. (1984). Comment on "alternative Medicare financing sources." *Milbank Memorial Fund Quarterly, 62* (Spring), 349–355.

Aaron, Henry J., & Robert D. Reischauer. (1995). The Medicare reform debate: What is the next step? *Health Affairs, 14* (Winter), 8–30.

Aaronson, William E., Jacqueline S. Zinn, & Michael D. Rosko. (1994). The success and repeal of Medicare catastrophic coverage act: A paradoxical lesson for health care reform. *Journal of Health Politics, Policy and Law, 19* (Winter), 753–772.

Adamache, Killard W., & Louis F. Rossiter. (1986). The entry of HMOs into the Medicare market: Implications for TEFRA's mandate. *Inquiry, 23* (Winter), 349–364.

Aiken, Linda H., & Karl D. Bays. (1984). The Medicare debate—round one. *New England Journal of Medicine, 311* (November 1), 1196–1200.

Anderson, Odin W. (1966a). Compulsory medical care insurance, 1910–1950. In Eugene. Feingold (Ed.), *Medicare: Policy and politics* (pp. 85–156). San Francisco, CA: Chandler Publishing Co.

Anderson, Odin W. (1966b). The Medicare act: The public policy breakthrough, or wheeling, dealing and healing. In Irving. L. Webber (Ed.), *Medical care under Social Security—potentials and problems* (pp. 9–26). Gainsville: University of Florida Press.

Anderson, Odin W. (1968). *The uneasy equilibrium: Private and public financing of health services in the U.S., 1865–1975.* New Haven, CT: College and University Press.

Ball, Robert M. (1992). *Implementation aspects of national health care reform: Reflections on implementing Medicare.* Washington, D.C.: National Academy of Social Insurance.

Ball, Robert M. (1995). Perspectives on Medicare: What Medicare's architects had in mind. *Health Affairs, 14* (Winter), 62–72.

Basu, Joy, Helen C. Lazenby, & Katharine R. Levit. (1995). Data view: Medicare spending by state:

The border-crossing adjustment. *Health Care Financing Review, 17* (Winter), 219–242.

Bayer, Ronald, & Daniel Callahan. (1985). Medicare reform: Social and ethical perspectives. *Journal of Health Politics, Policy and Law, 10* (Fall), 533–547.

Blendon, Robert J., John Benson, Karen Donelan, Robert Leitman, Humphrey Taylor, Christian Koeck, & Daniel G. Herman. (1995). Who has the best health care system? A second look. *Health Affairs, 14* (Winter), 220–230.

Blumenthal, David, Mark Schlesinger, & Pamela Brown Drumheller. (1988). *Renewing the promise: Medicare and its reform.* New York: Oxford University Press.

Brewster, Agness W. (1958). *Health insurance and related proposals for financing personal health services . . . A digest of major legislation and proposals for federal action, 1935–1957.* Washington, D.C.: U.S. Government Printing Office.

Brook, Robert H. (1995). Medicare quality and getting older: A personal essay. *Health Affairs, 14* (Winter), 73–81.

Brown, Lawrence D. (1985). Technocratic corporatism and administrative reform and Medicare. *Journal of Health Politics, Policy and Law, 10* (Fall), 579–599.

Brown, Randall, Dolores Gurnick Clement, Jerrald W. Hill, Sheldon M. Retchin, & Jeanette W. Bergeron. (1993). Do health maintenance organizations work for Medicare? *Health Care Financing Review, 15* (Fall), 7–23.

Burney, Ira, Peter Hickman, Julian Paradise, & George J. Schieber. (1984.). Medicare physician payment, participation and reform. *Health Affairs, 3* (Winter), 5–24.

Butler, Stuart M., & Robert E. Moffit. (1995). The FEHBP as a model for a new Medicare program. *Health Affairs, 14* (Winter), 47–61.

Cafferata, Gail Lee. (1985). Private health insurance of the Medicare population and the Baucus legislation. *Medical Care, 23* (September), 1086–1096.

Christiensen, Sandra. (1991). Did 1980s legislation slow Medicare spending? *Health Affairs, 10* (Summer), 135–142.

Christiensen, Sandra. (1993). *Single-payer and all-payer health insurance systems using Medicare's payment rates.* Washington, D.C.: U.S. Congressional Budget Office.

Christiensen, Sandra, & Rick Kasten. (1988). Covering catastrophic expenses under Medicare. *Health Affairs, 7* (Winter), 79–93.

Chirikos, Thomas N. (1995). Medicare and the Social Security Disability Insurance program. *Health Affairs, 14* (Winter), 244–252.

Chulio, George S., Franklin J. Eppig, Mary O. Hogan, Daniel R. Waldo, & Ross H. Arnett III. (1993). Why more cost-sharing won't slow Medicare spending. *Journal of American Health Policy, 3* (July/August), 15–20.

Cohen, Wilbur. (1985). Reflections on the enactment of Medicare and Medicaid. *Health Care Financing Review, Supplement,* 3–11.

Colby, David C. (1992). Impact of the Medicare physician fee schedule. *Health Affairs, 11* (Fall), 216–226.

Colby, David C., Thomas Rice, Jill Bernstein, & Lyle Nelson. (1995). Balancing billing under Medicare: Protecting beneficiaries and preserving physician participation. *Journal of Health Politics, Policy and Law, 20* (Spring), 49–74.

Corning, Peter A. (1969). *The evolution of Medicare . . . From idea to law* (Office of Research and Statistics, No. 29). Washington, D.C.: U.S. Government Printing Office.

Coster, John M. (1989). The political development of the outpatient prescription drug benefit under the Medicare Catastrophic Converage Act of 1988. Unpublished Ph.D. diss., University of Maryland.

Cromwell, Jerry, & Margo L. Rosenbach. (1988). Reforming anesthesia payment under Medicare. *Health Affairs, 7* (Fall), 5–19.

Cromwell, Jerry, Brooke Harrow, Thomas G. McGuire, & Randall P. Ellis. (1991). Medicare payment to psychiatric facilities. *Health Affairs, 10* (Summer), 124–134.

Culbertson, Richard A. (1991). The Medicare assignment controversy: The construction of public–professional conflict. *Journal of Aging and Social Policy, 3* (4), 47–68.

David, Sheri I. (1985). *With dignity: The search for Medicare and Medicaid.* Westport, CT: Greenwood Press.

Davis, Feather Ann. (1988). Medicare hospice benefit: Early program experiences. *Health Care Financing Review, 9* (Summer), 99–111.

Davis, Karen. (1987). Medicare financing reform: A new Medicare premium. *Milbank Memorial Fund Quarterly, 62* (Spring), 300–316.

Davis, Karen, & Diane Rowland. (1985). *Medicare policy: New directions for health and long term care.* Baltimore, MD: Johns Hopkins University Press.

Davis, Karen, & Cathy Schoen. (1994). Universal coverage: Building on Medicare and employer financing. *Health Affairs, 13* (Spring, II), 7–20.

Davis, Margaret H., & Sally T. Burner. (1995). Three decades of Medicare: What the numbers tell us. *Health Affairs, 14* (Winter), 231–243.

DeLissovoy, Gregory. (1988). Medicare and heart transplants. *Health Affairs, 7* (Fall), 61–72.

Dobson, Allen, John C. Langenbrunner, Steven A. Plovitz, & Judith B. Willis. (1986). The future of Medicare policy reform: Priorities for research and demonstration. *Health Care Financing Review, Annual Supplement* (December), 1–8.

Dodds, Greg, & Lynn Etheredge. (1989). Trends in laboratory testing under Medicare Part B. *Health Affairs, 8* (Summer), 111–115.

Dowd, Bryan, Jon Christianson, Roger Feldman, Catherine Wisner, & John Klein. (1992). Issues regarding health plan payments under Medicare and recommendations for reform. *Milbank Quarterly, 70* (3), 423–454.

Epstein, Arnold M., & David Blumenthal. (1993). Physician payment reform: Past and future. *Milbank Quarterly, 71* (2), 193–216.

Feder, Judith M. (1977). *Medicare: The politics of federal medical insurance.* Lexington, MA: D. C. Heath and Lexington Books.

Feder, Judith, Marilyn Moon, & William Scanlon. (1987). Medicare reform: Nibbling at catastrophic costs. *Health Affairs, 6* (Winter), 5–19.

Fein, Rashi. (1995). Assessing the proposed Medicare reforms. *New England Journal of Medicine, 333* (December 28), 1777–1780.

Feingold, Eugene. (1966). *Medicare: Policy and politics.* San Francisco, CA: Chandler Publishing Co.

Filerman, Gary L. (1962). *The legislative campaign for the passage of a medical care for the aged bill.* Unpublished master's thesis, University of Minnesota, Minneapolis.

Fisher, Charles R. (1987). Impact of the prospective payment system on physician charges under Medicare. *Health Care Financing Review, 8* (Summer), 101–104.

Fraser, Irene, Theodore Koontz, & William C. Moran. (1986). Medicare reimbursement for hospice care: An approach for analyzing cost consequences. *Inquiry, 23* (Summer), 141–153.

Frech, H. E., III. (Ed.). (1991). *Regulating doctor's fees: Competition, benefits, and controls under Medicare.* Waldorf, MD: AEI Press.

Friedman, Emily. (1995). The compromise and the afterthought: Medicare and Medicaid after 30 years. *Journal of the American Medical Association, 274* (July 19), 278–282.

Garfinkel, Steven A., Arthur J. Bonito, & Kenneth R. McLeroy. (1987). Socioeconomic factors and Medicare supplemental health insurance. *Health Care Financing Review, 9* (Fall), 21–30.

Ginsberg, Eli. (1984). Comment on Medicare benefits: A reassessment. *Milbank Memorial Fund Quarterly, 62* (Spring), 230–236.

Ginsburg, Paul B. (1993). Refining Medicare volume performance standards: Commentary. *Inquiry, 30* (Fall), 260–264.

Ginsburg, Paul B., Lauren B. LeRoy, & Glenn T. Hammons. (1990). Medicare physician payment reform. *Health Affairs, 9* (Spring), 178–188.

Ginsburg, Paul B., & Marilyn Moon. (1984). An introduction to the Medicare financing problem. *Milbank Memorial Fund Quarterly, 62* (Spring), 167–182.

Gornick, Marian. (1993). Physician payment reform under medicare: Monitoring utilization and access. *Health Care Financing Review, 14* (Spring), 77–96.

Gornick, Marian, Jay N. Greenberg, Paul W. Eggers, & Allen Dobson. (1985). Twenty years of Medicare and Medicaid: Covered population, use of benefits, and program expenditures. *Health Care Financing Review, Annual Supplement* (December), 13–59.

Gornick, Marian, Alma McMillan, & James Lubitz. (1993). A longitudinal perspective on patterns of Medicare payments. *Health Affairs, 12* (Summer), 140–150.

Gutterman, Stuart, Paul W. Eggers, Gerald Riley, Timothy F. Greene, & Sherry A. Terrell. (1988). The first three years of Medicare prospective payment: An overview. *Health Care Financing Review, 9* (Spring), 67–82.

Hadley, Jack. (1984). How should Medicare pay physicians? *Milbank Memorial Fund Quarterly, 62* (Spring), 279–299.

Hadley, Jack. (1988). Medicare spending and mortality rates of the elderly. *Inquiry, 25* (Winter), 485–493.

Hadley, Jack. (1993). Early evidence from the Medicare fee schedule: The sky isn't falling. *Inquiry, 30* (Fall), 226–227.

Harris, Richard. (1966a). Annals of legislation: Medicare—a sacred trust. *New Yorker, 42* (July 23), 35–63.

Harris, Richard. (1966b). Annals of legislation: Medicare—all very Hegelian. *New Yorker, 42* (July 2), 29–62.

Harris, Richard. (1966). Annals of legislation: Medicare—we do not compromise. *New Yorker, 42* (July 16), 35–91.

Harris, Richard. (1967). *A sacred trust.* New York: New American Library.

Havighurst, Craig. (1995). Medicare: Should it—can it—be reformed? *Medicine and Health Perspectives* (January 16), 1–4.

Haynes, Pamela L. (1985). *Evaluating state Medicaid reforms.* Washington, D.C.: American Enterprise Institute.

Held, Philip J., & John Holohan. (1985). Containing Medicaid costs in an era of growing physican supply. *Health Care Financing Review, 7* (Fall), 49–60.

Hemesath, Michael, & Gregory C. Pope. (1989). Medicare capital payments and hospital occupancy. *Health Affairs, 8* (Fall), 104–116.

Hirshfield, Daniel S. (1970). *The lost reform: The campaign for compulsory health insurance in the United States from 1932–1943.* Cambridge, MA: Harvard University Press.

Holahan, John, Robert A. Berenson, & Peter G. Kachavos. (1990). Area variations in selected Medicare procedures. *Health Affairs, 9* (Winter), 166–175.

Holahan, John, & Lynn Etheredge. (1986). *Medicare physician payment reform.* Washington, D.C.: Urban Institute.

Holahan, John, & John L. Palmer. (1988). Medicare's fiscal problems: An imperative for reform. *Journal of Health Politics, Policy and Law, 13* (Spring), 53–82.

Holahan, John, & Stephen Zuckerman. (1989). Medicare mandatory assignment: An unnecessary risk? *Health Affairs, 8* (Spring), 65–79.

Holahan, John, & Stephen Zuckerman. (1993). The future of Medicare volume performance standards. *Inquiry, 30* (Fall), 235–248.

Holstein, Martha, & Meredith Minkler. (1992). The short life and painful death of the Medicare catastrophic protection act. In Meredith Minkler & Carroll L. Estes (Eds.), *Critical perspectives on aging: The political and moral economy of growing old.* Amityville, NY: Baywood Publishing Co., Inc.

Hsiao, William C., & Nancy L. Kelly. (1984). Medicare benefits: A reassessment. *Millbank Memorial Fund Quarterly, 62* (Spring), 207–229.

Iglehart, John K. (1988). Payment of physicians under Medicare. *New England Journal of Medicine, 318* (March 31), 863–868.

Iglehart, John K. (1989). Medicare's new benefits: Catastrophic health insurance. *New England Journal of Medicine, 320* (February 2), 329–335.

Iglehart, John K. (1996). The struggle to reform Medicare. *New England Journal of Medicine, 334* (April 18), 1071–1075.

Intrator, Orna, Vince Mor, Marilyn A. Hines, Tony Lancaster, Linda L. Laliberte, & Walter Freiberger. (1996). Effect of the Medicare Catastrophic Coverage Act on payer source changes among nursing home residents. *Inquiry, 33* (Spring), 42–52.

Kalison, Michael J., & Richard F. Averill. (1986). The challenge of "real" competition in Medicare. *Health Affairs, 5* (Fall), 47–57.

Kenney, Genevieve M. (1993). Rural and urban differentials in Medicare home health use. *Health Care Financing Review, 14* (Summer), 39–57.

Kent, Christina. (1995). Medicare: Should it—can it—be reformed? *Medicine and Health Perspectives* (January 16).

King, Guy. (1994). Healthcare reform and the Medicare program. *Health Affairs, 13* (Winter), 39–43.

Kingson, Eric R., & Edward D. Berkowitz. (1993). *Social Security and Medicare: A policy primer.* Westport, CT: Auburn House.

Kinkead, Brian M. (1984.). Medicare payment and hospital capital: The evolution of policy. *Health Affairs, 3* (Fall), 49–74.

Langwell, Kathryn M., & James P. Hadley. (1986.). Capitation and the Medicare program: History, issues and evidence. *Health Care Financing Review, Annual Supplement* (December), 9–20.

Langwell, Kathryn, & James P. Hadley. (1990). Insights from the Medicare HMO demonstrations. *Health Affairs, 9* (Spring), 74–84.

Lave, Judith R. (1984). Hospital reimbursement under Medicare. *Milbank Memorial Fund Quarterly, 62* (Spring), 251–268.

Lave, Judith R., Richard G. Frank, Carl Taube, Howard Goldman, & Agnes Rupp. (1988). The early effects of Medicare's prospective payment system on psychiatry. *Inquiry, 25* (Fall), 354–363.

Lave, Judith R., & Howard H. Goldman. (1990). Medicare financing for mental health care. *Health Affairs, 9* (Spring), 19–30.

Leader, Shelah, & Marilyn Moon. (1989). Medicare trends in ambulatory surgery. *Health Affairs, 8* (Spring), 158–170.

Lee, David W., & Kurt D. Gillis. (1993). Physician responses to Medicare physician payment reform: Preliminary results on access to care. *Inquiry, 30* (Winter), 417–428.

Lee, David W., & Kurt D. Gillis. (1994). Physician responses to Medicare payment reform: An update on access to care. *Inquiry, 31* (Fall), 346–353.

Levinsky, N. G. (1993). The organization of medical care—lessons from the Medicare end stage renal disease program. *New England Journal of Medicine, 329* (November 4), 1395–1399.

Long, Stephen H., & Timothy M. Smeedings. (1984). Alternative Medicare financing sources. *Milbank Memorial Fund Quarterly, 26* (Spring), 325–348.

Long, Stephen H., & Russell F. Settle. (1984). Medicare and the disadvantaged elderly: Objectives and outcomes. *Milbank Memorial Fund Quarterly, 62* (Fall), 609–656.

Luft, Harold S. (1984). On the use of vouchers for Medicare. *Milbank Memorial Fund Quarterly, 62* (Spring), 237–250.

Marmor, Theodore R. (1973). *The politics of Medicare* (rev. American ed.). Chicago: Aldine Publishing Co.

McCall, Nancy Taplin. (1993). Monitoring access following Medicare price changes: Physician perspective. *Health Care Financing Review, 14* (Spring), 97–118.

McCall, Nelda, Thomas Rice, & Arden Hall. (1987). The effect of state regulations on the quality and sale of insurance policies to Medicare beneficiaries. *Journal of Health Politics, Policy and Law, 12* (Spring), 53–76.

McMenamin, Peter. (1987). Medicare's Part B rising assignment rates: Rising costs. *Inquiry, 24* (Winter), 344–356.

McMenamin, Peter. (1988). A crime story from Medicare Part B. *Health Affairs, 7* (Winter), 94–101.

McMillan, Alma, & James Lubitz. (1987). Medicare enrollment in health maintenance organizations. *Health Care Financing Review, 8* (Spring), 87–93.

McMillan, Alma. (1993). Trends in Medicare: Health maintenance organization enrollment: 1986–1993. *Health Care Financing Review, 14* (Fall), 135–146.

Meyer, Jack A. (1984). Comments on Medicare financing reform: A new Medicare premium. *Milbank Memorial Fund Quarterly, 62* (Spring), 317–324.

Miller, Mark E., & Margaret B. Sulvetta. (1995). Growth in Medicare's hospital outpatient care: Implications for prospective payment. *Inquiry, 32* (Summer), 155–163.

Miller, Mark E., & W. Pete Welch. (1993). Growth in Medicare inpatient physician charges per admission. *Inquiry, 30* (Fall), 249–259.

Miller, Mark E., Stephen Zuckerman, & Michael Gates. (1993). How do Medicare physician fees compare with private payers? *Health Care Financing Review, 14* (Spring), 25–39.

Minkler, Meredith, & Carroll L. Estes. (1992). *Critical perspectives on aging: The political and moral economy of growing old.* Amityville, NY: Baywood Publishing Co., Inc.

Mitchell, James B., & Stephen M. Davidson. (1989). Geographic variation in Medicare surgical fees. *Health Affairs, 8* (Winter), 113–124.

Mitchell, Janet B. (1992). Area variation in Medicare physician spending. *Health Affairs, 11* (Spring), 224–234.

Mitchell, Janet B., et al. (1987). Packaging physician services: Alternative approaches to Medicare Part B reimbursement. *Inquiry, 24* (Winter), 324–343.

Mitchell, Janet B., Margo L. Rosenbach, & Jerry Cromwell. (1988). To sign or not to sign: Physician participation in Medicare, 1984. *Health Care Financing Review, 10* (Fall), 17–26.

Mitchell, Janet B., Gerard Wedig, & Jerry Cromwell. (1989). The Medicare physician fee freeze. *Health Affairs, 8* (Spring), 21–33.

Moon, Marilyn. (1993). *Medicare now and in the future.* Washington, D.C.: Urban Institute Press.

Moon, Marilyn, & Karen Davis. (1995). Preserving and strengthening Medicare. *Health Affairs, 14* (Winter), 31–46.

Morrisey, Michael A., Frank A. Sloan, & Joseph Valvona. (1988). Shifting Medicare patients out of the hospital. *Health Affairs, 7* (Winter), 52–64.

Munnell, Alicia H. (1985). Paying for the Medicare program. *Journal of Health Politics, Policy and Law, 10* (Fall), 489–512.

Oliver, Thomas R. (1993). Analysis, advice, and congressional leadership: The physician payment review commission and the politics of Medicare. *Journal of Health Politics, Policy and Law, 18* (Spring), 113–174.

Pauly, Mark V., & William B. Kissick. (Eds.). (1988). *Lessons from the first twenty years of Medicare.* Philadelphia: University of Pennsylvania Press.

Pauly, Mark V., & Kathryn M. Langwell. (1986). Physician payment reform—who shall be paid? *Medical Care Review, 43* (Spring), 101–132.

Poetz, Lisa, & Thomas Buchberger. (1985). Medicare's transition to national payment rates: Effects on hospitals. *Health Affairs, 4* (Winter), 62–69.

Reilly, Thomas. (1995). Medicare physician payment reform: Its effect on access to care. *Health Care Financing Review, 17* (Winter), 179–194.

Reinhardt, Uwe E. (1995). Demagoguery and debate over Medicare reform. *Health Affairs, 14* (Winter), 101–103.

Rettig, Paul C., Glenn R. Markus, James Bentley, et al. (1987). Medicare's prospective payment system: The expectations and the realities. *Inquiry, 24* (Summer), 173–188.

Rice, Thomas, Katherine Desmond, & Jon Gabel. (1990). Medicare Catastrophic Coverage Act: A post-mortem. *Health Affairs, 9* (Fall), 75–86.

Rose, Arnold M. (1967). The passage of legislation: The politics of financing medical care for the aging. In Arnold M. Rose (Ed.), *The power structure* (pp. 400–455). New York: Oxford University Press.

Rosenbach, Margo, Killard W. Adamache, & Rezaul K. Khandker. (1995). Variations in Medicare access and satisfaction by health status: 1991–93. *Health Care Financing Review, 17* (Winter), 29–50.

Rosenblum, Robert W. (1985). Medicare reversed: A look through the past to the future. *Journal of Health Politics, Policy and Law, 9* (Winter), 669–682.

Rossiter, Louis F., & Kathryn Langwell. (1988). Medicare's two systems for paying providers. *Health Affairs, 7* (Summer), 120–132.

Ruby, Gloria H., David Banta, & Anne Kesselman Burns. (1985). Medicare coverage, Medicare costs, and medical technology. *Journal of Health Politics, Policy and Law, 10* (Spring), 141–156.

Russell, Louise B. (1989). *Medicare's new hospital payment system: Is it working?* Washington, D.C.: The Brookings Institution.

Russell, Louise B., & Carrie Lynn Manning. (1989). The effect of prospective payment on Medicare expenditures. *New England Journal of Medicine, 320* (February 16), 439–443.

Sager, Mark A., Douglas V. Easterling, David Kindig, & Odin W. Anderson. (1989). Changes in the location of death after passage of Medicare's prospective payment system : A national study. *New England Journal of Medicine, 320* (February 16), 433–438.

Schechter, Malvin. (1993). *Beyond Medicare: Achieving long-term care security.* San Francisco, CA: Jossey-Bass.

Sheingold, Steven H. (1986). Unintended results of Medicare's national prospective payment rates. *Health Affairs, 5* (Winter), 5–21.

Sheingold, Steven H. (1989). The first three years of PPS: Impact on Medicare costs. *Health Affairs, 8* (Fall), 191–204.

Sheingold, Steven H., & Thomas Buchberger. (1986). Implications of Medicare's prospective payment system for the provision of uncompensated hospital care. *Inquiry, 23* (Winter), 371–381.

Short, Pamela Farley, & Alan C. Monheit. (1988). Employers and Medicare as partners in financing health care for the elderly. In Mark. V. Pauly & William B. Kissick (Eds.), *Lessons from the first twenty years of Medicare.* University of Pennsylvania Press.

Sisk, Jane E., Peter McMenamin, Gloria Ruby, & Ellen S. Smith. (1987). An analysis of methods to reform Medicare payment for physician services. *Inquiry, 24* (Spring), 36–47.

Skidmore, Max J. (1970). *Medicare and the American rhetoric of reconciliation.* Tuscaloosa: University of Alabama Press.

Sloan, Frank, & Joel W. Hay. (1986). Medicare pricing mechanisms for physician services: An overview of alternative approaches. *Medical Care Review, 43* (Spring), 59–100.

Smith, David G. (1992). *Paying for Medicare: The politics of reform.* Hawthorne, NY: Aldine deGruyter.

Vladeck, Bruce C. (1984). Comment on "hospital reimbursement under Medicare." *Milbank Memorial Fund Quarterly, 62* (Spring), 269–278.

Vladeck, Bruce C. (1985). Reforming Medicare provider payment. *Journal of Health Politics, Policy and Law, 10* (Fall), 513–532.

Vladeck, Bruce C. (1991). Medicare's prospective payment system at age eight: Mature success or midlife crisis? *Journal of Puget Sound Law Review, 14* (3), 453–482.

Vladeck, Bruce C., & Genrose J. Alfano (Eds.). (1987). *Medicare and extended care: Issues, problems and prospects.* Owings Mills, MD: National Health Publishing (Rynd Communications).

Vladeck, Bruce C., & Kathleen M. King. (1995). The first 30 years of Medicare and Medicaid. *Journal of American Medical Association, 274* (July 19), 259–262.

Vouri, Hannu. (1968). Ideology versus interest: The case of Medicare. *Social Science and Medicine, 2* (September), 355–363.

Walker, Georgia K. (1986). Reforming Medicare: The limited framework of political discourse on equity and economy. *Social Science and Medicine, 23* (12), 1237–1250.

Welch, W. Pete, Steven J. Katz, & Stephen Zuckerman. (1993). Physician fee levels: Medicare versus Canada. *Health Care Financing Review, 14* (Spring), 41–54.

Wilensky, Gail R., & Louis F. Rossiter. (1986). Alternative units of payment for physician services: An overview of the issues. *Medical Care Review, 43* (Spring), 133–156.

Wing, Kenneth. (1985). Medicare and President Reagan's second term. *American Journal of Public Health, 75* (July), 782–784.

Wolkstein, Irwin. (1984). Medicare's financial status: How did we get here? *Milbank Memorial Fund Quarterly, 62* (Spring), 183–206.

Medicaid

Adams, E. Kathleen, David H. Kreling, & Kathleen Gondek. (1994). State Medicaid pharmacy payments and their relation to estimated costs. *Health Care Financing Review, 15* (Spring), 25–42.

Anderson, Maren, & Peter D. Fox. (1987). Lessons learned from Medicaid managed care approaches. *Health Affairs, 6* (Spring), 71–86.

Bachman, Sara S., Dennis F. Beatrice, & Stuart H. Altman. (1987). Implementing change: Lessons for Medicaid reform. *Journal of Health Politics, Policy and Law, 12* (Summer), 237–252.

Bachman, Sara S., Stuart H. Altman, & Dennis F. Beatrice. (1988). What influences a state's approach to Medicaid reform? *Inquiry, 25* (Summer), 243–250.

Bernard, Sydney E., & Eugene Feingold. (1970). The impact of Medicaid. *Wisconsin Law Review, 1970* (3), 726–755.

Bernstein, Betty J. (1969.). *The politics of the New York State Medicaid law of 1966: An analysis.* Unpublished Ph.D. diss., New York University, NY.

Bernstein, Betty J. (1970). Public health—inside or outside the mainstream of the political process? Lessons from the passage of Medicaid. *American Journal of Public Health, 60* (September), 1690–1700.

Bind, Truman. (1996). Medicaid crowd out and the inverse. *Inquiry, 33* (Spring), 5–8.

Blendon, Robert J., Karen Donelan, Craig Hill, Ann Scheck, Woody Carter, Dennis Beatrice, & Drew Altman. (1993). Medicaid beneficiaries and health reform. *Health Affairs, 12* (Spring), 132–143.

Buck, Jeffrey A. (1993). Response to "Medicaid: Taking stock." *Journal of Health Politics, Policy and Law, 18* (Spring), 67–70.

Buck, Jeffrey A., & Mark S. Kamlet. (1993). Problems with expanding Medicaid for the uninsured. *Journal of Health Politics, Policy and Law, 18* (Spring), 1–26.

Chang, Deborah, & John Holahan. (1990). *Medicaid spending in the 1980s: The access-cost containment trade-off revisited* (Urban Institute Report 90-2). Washington, D.C.: Urban Institute.

Cohen, Joel W. (1993). Medicaid physician fees and use of physician and hospital services. *Inquiry, 30* (Winter), 281–292.

Cohen, Joel W., & Peter J. Cunningham. (1995). Medicaid physician fee levels and children's access to care. *Health Affairs, 14* (Spring), 255–262.

Cohen, Marc A., Nanda Kumar, & Stanley S. Wallack. (1994). Long-term care insurance and Medicaid. *Health Affairs, 13* (Fall), 127–139.

Colby, David C. (1994). Medicaid physicians fees, 1993. *Health Affairs, 13* (Spring, 2), 255–263.

Coughlin, Teresa A., Leighton Ku, & John Holahan. (1994). *Medicaid since 1980: Costs, coverage, and the shifting alliance between the federal government and the states.* Washington, D.C.: Urban Institute.

Coughlin, Teresa A., Leighton Ku, John Holahan, David Heslam, & Colin Winterbottom. (1994). State responses to the Medicaid spending crisis: 1988 to 1992. *Journal of Health Politics, Policy and Law, 19* (Winter), 837–864.

Cromwell, Jerry, Sylvia Hurdle, & Rachel Schurman. (1987). Defederalizing Medicaid: Fair to the poor, fair to the taxpayers? *Journal of Health Politics, Policy and Law, 12* (Spring), 1–34.

Curtis, Richard, & Ian Hill. (Eds.). (1986). *Affording access to quality care: Strategies for state Medicaid cost management.* Washington, D.C.: National Governors Association Center for Policy Research.

Davidson, Stephen M. (1993). Commentary—Medicaid: Taking stock. *Journal of Health Politics, Policy and Law, 18* (Spring), 43–66.

Davidson, Stephen M., Jerry Cromwell, & Rachel Schurman. (1986). Medicaid myths: Trends in Medicaid expenditures and the prospects for reform. *Journal of Health Politics, Policy and Law, 10* (Winter), 699–728.

Dubay, Lisa C., Stephen A. Norton, & Marilyn Moon. (1995). Medicaid expansions for pregnant women and infants: Easing hospitals' uncompensated care burdens. *Inquiry, 32* (Fall), 332–344.

Eddy, David M. (1991). Oregon's methods: Did cost-effectiveness analysis fail? *Journal of American Medical Association, 266* (October 16), 2135–2141.

Ehrenhaft, Polly M., & Marie Hackbarth. (1984). *Medicaid reform: Four studies of case management.* Washington, D.C.: American Enterprise Institute.

Ellwood, Marilyn Rymer, & Genevieve Kenny. (1995). Medicaid and pregnant women: Who is being enrolled and when? *Health Care Financing Review, 17* (Winter), 7–28.

Fanning, Thomas, & Martin de Alteriis. (1993). The limits of marginal economic incentive in the Medicaid program: Concerns and cautions. *Journal of Health Politics, Policy and Law, 18* (Spring), 27–42.

Fanning, Thomas, & Martin de Alteriis. (1993). Response to "Medicaid: Taking stock." *Journal of Health Politics, Policy and Law, 18* (Spring), 71–74.

Feldman, Penny H., & Margaret Gerteis. (1987). Private insurance for Medicaid recipients: The Texas experience. *Journal of Health Politics, Policy and Law, 12* (Summer), 271–298.

Foltz, Anne-Marie. (1982). *An ounce of prevention: Child health politics under Medicaid.* Cambridge, MA: MIT Press.

Fossett, James W. (1993). Medicaid and health reform: The case of New York. *Health Affairs, 12* (Fall), 81–94.

Fossett, James W., & James H. Wyckoff. (1996). Has Medicaid growth crowded out state educational spending? *Journal of Health Politics, Policy and Law, 21* (Fall), 409–432.

Fox, Michael H., Jonathan P. Weiner, & Kai Phua. (1992). Effect of Medicaid payment levels on access to obstetrical care. *Health Affairs, 11* (Winter), 150–161.

Freund, Deborah A., Polly M. Ehrenhaft, & Marie Hackbarth. (1984). *Medicaid reform: Four studies of case management.* Washington, D.C.: American Enterprise Institute for Public Policy.

Freund, Deborah A., Louis F. Rossiter, Peter D. Fox, Jack A. Meyer, Robert E. Hurley, Timothy S. Carey, & John E. Paul. (1989). Evaluation of the Medicaid competition demonstrations. *Health Care Financing Review, 11* (Winter), 81–97.

Gardiner, John A., & Theodore R. Lyman. (1984). *The fraud control game: State responses to fraud and abuse in the AFDC and Medicaid programs.* Bloomington: Indiana University Press.

Gentry, John T., & Morris Schaefer. (1969). The impact of state and federal policy planning decisions on the implementation and functional adequacy of Title XIX health care programs. *Medical Care, 7* (January), 92–104.

Grabowski, Henry. (1988). Medicaid patients' access to new drugs. *Health Affairs, 7* (Winter), 102–114.

Harrington, Charlene, Carroll L. Estes, Philip R. Lee, & Robert J. Newcomer. (1986.). Effects of state Medicaid policies on the aged. *The Gerontologist, 26* (August), 437–443.

Harrington, Charlene, & James H. Swan. (1987). The impact of state Medicaid nursing home policies on utilization and expenditures. *Inquiry, 24* (Summer), 159–172.

Hoffman, Catherine. (1994). Medicaid payment for nonphysician practitioners. *Health Affairs, 13* (Fall), 140–152.

Holahan, John. (1985). *The effects of the 1981 Omnibus Budget Reconciliation Act on Medicaid.* Washington, D.C.: Urban Institute.

Holahan, John, & Joel Cohen. (1986). *Medicaid: The tradeoff between cost containment and access to care.* Washington, D.C.: Urban Institute.

Holahan, John, Teresa Coughlin, Leighton Ku, Debra J. Lipson, & Shruti Rajan. (1995). Insuring the poor through Section 115 Medicaid waivers. *Health Affairs, 14* (Spring), 199–216.

Holahan, John, Maureen Lewis, & Marsha Silverberg. (1988). Controlling Medicaid costs in hospitals. *Health Affairs, 7* (Fall), 132–141.

Holahan, John, & David Liska. (1995). *State variations in Medicaid: Implications for block grants and expenditure growth caps.* Washington, D.C.: Kaiser Commission of the Future of Medicaid.

Holahan, John, Diane Rowland, Judith Feder, & David Heslam. (1993). Explaining recent growth in Medicaid spending. *Health Affairs, 12,* 177–193.

Holahan, John, Marcia Wade, Michael Gates, & Lynn Tsoflias. (1993). The impact of Medicaid adoption of the Medicare fee schedule. *Health Care Financing Review, 14* (Spring), 11–24.

Holahan, John, & Sheila Zedlewski. (1991). Expanding Medicaid to cover uninsured Americans. *Health Affairs, 10* (Spring), 45–61.

Iglehart, John K. (1995). Medicaid and managed care. *New England Journal of Medicine, 332* (June 22), 1727–1731.

Jesilow, Paul, Henry M. Pontell, & Gilbert Geis. (1993). *Prescription for profit: How doctors defraud Medicaid.* Berkeley: University of California Press.

Johns, Lucy, & Gerald Adler. (1989). Evaluation of recent changes in Medicaid. *Health Affairs, 8* (Spring), 171–181.

Kaiser Commission on the Future of Medicaid. (1995). *The Medicaid program at a glance: Medicaid facts: A report of the Kaiser Commission on the Future of Medicaid.* Washington, D.C.: Kaiser Commission on the Future of Medicaid.

Kern, Rosemary, & Susan R. Windham. (1986). *Medicaid and other experiments in state health policy.* Washington, D.C.: American Enterprise Institute.

McDevitt, Roland, William Buczko, Josephine Mauskopf, et al. (1985). Medicaid program characteristics: Effects on health care expenditures and utilization. *Health Care Financing Review, 7* (Winter), 1–29.

Miller, Nancy A. (1992). Medicaid 2176 home and community-based care waivers: The first ten years. *Health Affairs, 11* (Winter), 162–177.

Moffit, Robert, & Barbara L. Wolfe. (1993). Medicaid, welfare dependency, and work: Is there a causal link? *Health Care Financing Review, 15* (Fall), 123–133.

Newacheck, Paul W., Dana C. Hughes, Abigail English, Harriette B. Fox, James Perrin, & Neal Halfon. (1995). The effect on children of curtailing Medicaid spending. *Journal of American Medical Association, 274* (November 8), 1468–1471.

Nye, Christine H. (1991). Incompatible goals. *Health Management Quarterly, 13* (4), 25–28.

Oberg, Charles N., & Cynthia L Polich. (1988). Medicaid: Entering the third decade. *Health Affairs, 7* (Fall), 83–96.

Omenn, Gilbert S. (1987). Lessons from a fourteen state study of Medicaid. *Health Affairs, 6* (Spring), 118–122.

Perloff, Janet D., Phillip R. Kletke, & Kathryn M. Neckerman. (1987). Physicians' decision to limit Medicaid participation: Determinants and policy implications. *Journal of Health Politics, Policy and Law, 12* (Summer), 221–236.

Pollard, Michael R., & John M. Coster. (1991). Savings for Medicaid drug spending. *Health Affairs, 10* (Summer), 196–206.

Reschovsky, James D. (1996). Demand for and access to institutional long-term care: The role of Medi-caid in nursing home markets. *Inquiry, 33* (Spring), 18–29.

Rosenbaum, Sara, & Kay Johnson. (1986.). Providing health care for low-income children: Reconciling child health goals with child health financing realities. *Milbank Memorial Fund Quarterly, 64* (3), 442–478.

Rurley, Robert E., Deborah A. Freund, & John E. Paul. (1993). *Managed care in Medicaid: Lessons for policy and program design.* Ann Arbor, MI: Health Administration Press.

Rymer, Marilyn P., & Gerald S. Alder. (1987.). Children and Medicaid: The experience in four states. *Health Care Financing Review, 9* (Fall), 1–20.

Schneider, Saundra K. (1988.). Intergovernmental influences on Medicaid program expenditures. *Public Administration Review, 48* (July/August), 756–763.

Schwartz, Anne, David C. Colby, & Anne Lemhard Reisinger. (1991). Variation in Medicaid physician fees. *Health Affairs, 10* (Spring), 131–139.

Short, Pamela Farley, Joel C. Cantor, & Alan C. Monheit. (1988). The dynamics of Medicaid enrollment. *Inquiry, 25* (Winter), 504–516.

Short, Pamela Farley, Peter Kemper, Llewellyn J. Cornelius, & Daniel C. Walden. (1992). Public and private responsibility for financing nursing-home care: The effect of Medicaid asset spend-down. *Milbank Quarterly, 70* (2), 277–298.

Sloan, Frank A., & May W. Shayne. (1993). Long-term care, Medicaid, and impoverishment of the elderly. *Milbank Quarterly, 71* (4), 575–600.

Sparer, Michael S. (1996). Medicaid managed care and the health reform debate: Lessons from New York and California. *Journal of Health Politics, Policy and Law, 21* (Fall), 433–460.

Spence, Denise A., & Joshua M. Wiener. (1990). Estimating the extent of Medicaid spend-down in nursing homes. *Journal of Health Politics, Policy and Law, 15* (Fall), 607–626.

Spitz, Bruce. (1987). A national survey of Medicaid case-management programs. *Health Affairs, 6* (Spring), 61–70.

Stevens, Robert, & Rosemary Stevens. (1974). *Welfare medicine in America: A case study of Medicaid*. New York: The Free Press.

Stevens, Rosemary, & Robert Stevens. (1970). Medicaid: Anatomy of a dilemma. *Law and Contemporary Problems, 1970* (Spring), 348–425.

Stuart, Bruce, Edward Reutzel, & Thomas Reutzel. (1985.). Medicaid reform: Programming solutions to the equity problem. *Journal of Health Politics, Policy and Law, 10* (Spring), 93–118.

Swan, James H., Charlene Harrington, & Leslie A. Grant. (1988). State Medicaid reimbursement for nursing homes, 1978–1986. *Health Care Financing Review, 9* (Spring), 33–50.

Tallon, James R., Jr., & Diane Rowland. (1995). Federal dollars and state flexibility: The debate over Medicaid's future. *Inquiry, 32* (Fall), 235–240.

Taube, Carl A., Howard H. Goldman, & David Salkever. (1990). Medicaid coverage for mental illness. *Health Affairs, 9* (Spring), 5–18.

Taube, Carl A., & Agnes Rupp. (1986). The effect of Medicaid on access to ambulatory mental health care for the poor and near poor under 65. *Medical Care, 24* (August), 677–686.

Thorpe, Kenneth E. (1989). Costs and distributional impacts of employer health insurance mandates and Medicaid expansion. *Inquiry, 26* (Fall), 335–344.

Vladeck, Bruce C. (1995). Medicaid 1115 demonstration: Progress through partnership. *Health Affairs, 14* (Spring), 217–220.

Weikel, M. K. (1979). *A decade of Medicaid: Some state and federal perspectives on Medicaid*. Washington, D.C.: Health Care Financing Administration.

Welch, W. Pete, & Marcia Wade. (1995). Relative cost of Medicaid enrollees and commercially insured in HMOs. *Health Affairs, 14* (Summer), 212–223.

Wilensky, Gail R., & Marc L. Berk. (1982). Health care, the poor, and the role of Medicaid: Datawatch. *Health Affairs, 1* (Fall), 93–100.

Wing, Kenneth. (1983). The impact of Reagan-era politics on the federal Medicaid program. *Catholic University Law Review, 33* (Fall), 1–93.

Zuckerman, Stephen. (1987). Medicaid hospital spending: Effects of reimbursement and utilization control policies. *Health Care Financing Review, 9* (Winter), 65–78.

Mental Health

Applebaum, Paul. (1994). *Almost a revolution: Mental health law and the limits of change*. New York: Oxford University Press.

Bardach, Eugene. (1972). *The skill factor in politics: Repealing the mental commitment laws in California*. Berkeley: University of California Press.

Bloche, M. Gregg, & Francine Cournos. (1990). Mental health policy for the 1990s: Tinkering in the interstices. *Journal of Health Politics, Policy and Law, 15* (Summer), 387–412.

Borinstein, Andrew B. (1992). Public attitudes toward persons with mental illness. *Health Affairs, 11* (Fall), 186–196.

Boyer, Carol A., & David Mechanic. (1994). Psychiatric reimbursement reform in New York State: Lessons in implementing change. *Milbank Quarterly, 72* (4), 621–652.

Boyle, Philip J., & Daniel Callahan. (1995). Managed care in mental health: The ethical issues. *Health Affairs, 14* (Fall), 7–22.

Boyle, Philip J., & Daniel Callahan. (Eds.). (1995). *What price mental health? The ethics and politics of setting priorities*. Washington, D.C.: Georgetown University Press.

Brown, Phil. (Ed.). (1985). *Mental health care and social policy*. Boston: Routledge and Kegan Paul.

Callahan, Daniel. (1994). Setting mental health priorities: Problems and possibilities. *Milbank Quarterly, 72* (3), 451–470.

Chu, Franklin D., & Sharland Trotter. (1974). *The madness establishment: Ralph Nader's study group report on the National Institute of Mental Health*. New York: Grossman.

Clark, Robin E., Robert A. Dorwart, & Sherrie S. Epstein. (1994). Managing competition in public and private mental health agencies: Implications for services and policy. *Milbank Quarterly, 72* (4), 653–678.

Connery, Robert H. (1968). *The politics of mental health*. New York: Columbia University Press.

Dorwart, Robert A., & Sherrie S. Epstein. (1993). *Privatization and mental health care: A fragile balance.* Westport, CT: Auburn House.

Falkson, Joseph L. (1976). Minor skirmish in a monumental struggle: HEW's analysis of mental health services. *Policy Analysis, 2* (Winter), 93–119.

Felicetti, Daniel A. (1975). *Mental health and retardation politics: The mind lobbies in Congress.* New York: Praeger.

Fogel, Barry S., Antonio Furino, & Gary L. Gottlieb. (Eds.). (1990). *Mental health policy for older Americans: Protecting minds at risk.* Washington, D.C.: American Psychiatric Press.

Foley, Henry A. (1975). *Community mental health legislation: The formative process.* Lexington, MA: Lexington Books.

Foley, Henry A. (1983). *Madness and government.* Washington, D.C.: American Psychiatric Press.

Frank, Richard G., Howard H. Goldman, & Thomas G. McGuire. (1992). A model mental health benefit in private health insurance. *Health Affairs, 11* (Fall), 98–117.

Frank, Richard G., & William G. Manning Jr. (Eds.). (1992). *Economics and mental health.* Baltimore, MD: Johns Hopkins University Press.

Frank, Richard G., & Thomas G. McGuire. (1990). Mandating employer coverage of mental health care. *Health Affairs, 9* (Spring), 31–42.

Frank, Richard G., Thomas G. McGuire, Darrel A. Regier, Ronald Manderscheid, & Albert Woodward. (1994). Paying for mental health and substance abuse care. *Health Affairs, 13* (Spring), 337–342.

Frank, Richard G., David S. Salkever, & Steven S. Sharfstein. (1991). A look at rising mental health insurance costs. *Health Affairs, 10* (Summer), 116–123.

Freeman, Hugh L., Thomas Fryers, & John H. Henderson. (1985). *Mental health services in Europe: Ten years on.* Copenhagen: World Health Organization.

Gilbert, Richard C. (1986). Gramm–Rudman: What it means to mental health and domestic spending. *Administration in Mental Health, 13* (Summer), 249–259.

Goldman, Howard, & Joseph Morrissey. (1985). The alchemy of mental health policy: Homelessness and the fourth cycle of reform. *American Journal of Public Health, 75* (July), 727–731.

Goldman, Howard H., & Antoinette A. Gattozzi. (1988). Balance of powers: Social Security and the mentally disabled, 1980–1985. *Milbank Memorial Fund Quarterly, 66* (3), 531–551.

Goldman, Howard H., & Antoinette A. Gattozzi. (1988). Murder in the cathedral revisited: President Reagan and the mentally disabled. *Hospital and Community Psychiatry, 39* (May), 505–509.

Grob, Gerald N. (1991). *From asylum to community: Mental health policy in modern America.* Princeton, NJ: Princeton University Press.

Grob, Gerald N. (1992). Mental health policy in America: Myths and realities. *Health Affairs, 11* (Fall), 7–22.

Grob, Gerald N. (1994). Government and mental health policy: A structural analysis. *Milbank Quarterly, 72* (3), 471–500.

Gronfein, William. (1985). Incentives and intentions in mental health policy: A comparison of the Medicaid and community mental health programs. *Journal of Health and Social Behavior, 26* (September), 192–206.

Hogan, Michael F. (1992). New futures for mental health care: The case of Ohio. *Health Affairs, 11* (Fall), 69–83.

Hollingsworth, Ellen Jane. (1992). The mentally ill: Falling through the cracks. *Journal of Health Politics, Policy and Law, 17* (Winter), 899–928.

Immergut, Ellen M. (1992). *Health politics: Interests and institutions in Western Europe.* New York: Cambridge University Press.

Isaac, Rael Jean, & Virgin C. Armat. (1990). *Madness in the streets: How psychiatry and the law abandoned the mentally ill.* New York: The Free Press.

Kanaan, Susan Baird. (1991). Financing policy for mental health services. *Health Affairs, 10* (Summer), 207–211.

Kemp, Donna R. (1993). *International handbook in mental health policy.* Westport, CT: Greenwood Press.

Kemp, Donna R. (1994). *Biomedical policy and mental health.* Westport, CT: Praeger.

Kiesler, Charles A., et al. (1983). Federal mental health policy making: An assessment of deinstitutionalization. *American Psychologist, 38* (December), 1292–1297.

Lave, Judith R., & Howard H. Goldman. (1990). Medicare financing for mental health care. *Health Affairs, 9* (Spring), 19–30.

Levine, Murray. (1981). *The history and politics of mental health.* New York: Oxford University Press.

Logan, Bruce M., David A. Rochefort, & Ernest W. Cook. (1985). Block grants for mental health: Elements of the state responses. *Journal of Public Health Policy, 6* (December), 476–492.

Mechanic, David. (1987). Correcting misconceptions in mental health policy: Strategies for improved care of the seriously mentally ill. *Milbank Memorial Quarterly, 65* (2), 203–230.

Mechanic, David. (1993). Mental health services in the context of health insurance reform. *Milbank Quarterly, 71* (3), 349–364.

Mechanic, David. (1994). Establishing mental health priorities. *Milbank Quarterly, 72* (3), 501–514.

Mechanic, David, & David A. Rochefort. (1992). A policy of inclusion for the mentally ill. *Health Affairs, 11* (Spring), 128–150.

Mechanic, David, & Richard C. Surles. (1992). Challenges in state mental health policy and administration. *Health Affairs, 11* (Fall), 34–50.

Merwin, Mary R., & Frank M. Ochberg. (1983). The long voyage: Policies for progress in mental health. *Health Affairs, 2* (Winter), 96–127.

Olfson, Mark, & Harold Alan Pincus. (1994). Measuring outpatient mental health care in the United States. *Health Affairs, 13* (Winter), 172–180.

Rochefort, David A. (1987). The political context of mental health care. In David Mechanic (Ed.), *Improving mental health services: What the social sciences can tell us. New directions for mental health services* (No. 36., pp. 93–105). San Francisco: Jossey-Bass.

Rochefort, David A. (1988). Policymaking cycles in mental health: Critical evaluation of a conceptual model. *Journal of Health Politics, Policy and Law, 13* (Spring), 129–152.

Rochefort, David A. (1992). More lessons of a different kind: Canadian mental health policy in comparative perspective. *Hospital and Community Psychiatry, 43* (November), 1083–1090.

Rochefort, David A. (1993). *From poorhouse to homelessness: Policy analysis and mental health care.* Westport, CT: Auburn House.

Rumer, Richard. (1978). Community mental health centers: Politics and therapy. *Journal of Health Politics, Policy and Law, 2* (Winter), 531–559.

Sardell, Alice. (1988). *The U.S. experiment in social medicine: The community health center program, 1965–1986.* Pittsburgh: University of Pittsburgh Press.

Scallet, Leslie J. (1990). Paying for public mental health care: Crucial questions. *Health Affairs, 9* (Spring), 117–124.

Scheffler, Richard M., Stephen Earl Foreman, Brian J. Cuffel, & Carter Mackley. (1994). Mental health benefits in the Clinton plan. *Health Affairs, 13* (Spring, 2), 201–210.

Sharfstein, Steven S., & Anne M. Stoline. (1992). Reform issues for insuring mental health care. *Health Affairs, 11* (Fall), 84–97.

Sundram, Clarence J. (1986). Mental illness and health care policy. *Journal of Public Health Policy, 7* (Summer), 174–182.

Taube, Carl A., Howard H. Goldman, & David Salkever. (1990). Medicaid coverage for mental illness. *Health Affairs, 9* (Spring), 5–18.

Torrey, E. Fuller. (1988). *Nowhere to go: The tragic odyssey of the homeless mentally ill.* New York: Harper & Row.

National Health Insurance and Health Care Reform

National Health Insurance

Anderson, Odin W. (1966). Compulsory medical care insurance, 1910–1950. In Eugene Feingold (Ed.), *Medicare: Policy and politics* (pp. 85–156). San Francisco, CA: Chandler Publishing Co.

Anderson, Odin W. (1972). The politics of universal health insurance in the United States: An interpretation. *International Journal of Health Services, 2* (4), 577–582.

Anlyan, William G. Jr., & Joseph Lipscomb. (1985). The national health care trust plan: A blueprint for market and long term care reform. *Health Affairs, 4* (Fall), 5–31.

Battistella, Roger M., & Thomas P. Weil. (1989). National health insurance reconsidered: Dilemmas and opportunities. *Hospital and Health Service Administration, 342* (Summer), 139–156.

Cairl, Richard E., & Allen W. Imershein. (1977). National health insurance policy in the United States—a case of non-decision making. *International Journal of Health Services, 7* (2), 167–178.

Enthoven, Alain, & Richard Kronick. (1989). A consumer choice health plan for the 1990s: Universal health insurance in a system designed to promote quality and economy. *New England Journal of Medicine, 320* (January 5), 29–37; (January 12), 94–101.

Evang, Karl. (1973). The politics of developing a national health policy. *International Journal of Health Services, 3* (3), 331–340.

Falk, I. S. (1977). Proposals for national health insurance in the USA: Origins and evolution, and some perceptions for the future. *Milbank Memorial Fund Quarterly/Health and Society, 55* (Spring), 161–192.

Fuchs, Victor R. (1991). National health insurance revisited. *Health Affairs, 10* (Winter), 7–17.

Goodman, Louis J., & Steven R. Steiber. (1981). Public support for national health insurance. *American Journal of Public Health, 71* (October), 1105–1108.

Gordon, Jeoffry B. (1969). The politics of community medicine projects: A conflict analysis. *Medical Care, 7* (November/December), 419–428.

Grey, Michael R. (1994). The medical care programs of the Farm Security Administration, 1932 through 1947: A rehearsal for national health insurance? *American Journal of Public Health, 84* (October), 1678–1687.

Himmelstein, David U., & Steffie Woolhandler. (1986). Socialized medicine: A solution to the cost crisis in health care in the United States. *International Journal of Health Services, 16* (3), 339–354.

Himmelstein, David U., Steffie Woolhandler, & the Writing Committee of the Working Group on Program Design. (1989). A national health program for the United States: A physician's proposal. *New England Journal of Medicine, 320* (January 12), 102–108.

Hirshfield, Daniel S. (1970). *The lost reform: The campaign for compulsory health insurance in the United States, 1932–1943.* Cambridge, MA: Harvard University Press.

Laham, Nicholas. (1993). *Why the United States lacks a national health insurance program.* Westport, CT: Greenwood Press.

Lubove, Roy. (1977). The New Deal and national health. *Current History, 72* (May/June), 198–199, 224–227.

Marmor, Theodore R. (1977). Politics of national health insurance: Analysis and prescription. *Policy Analysis, 3* (Winter), 25–48.

Marmor, Theodore R. (1978). NHI in crisis: Politics, predictions, proposals. *Hospital Progress, 59* (January), 68–72.

Maloni, Antonia. (1995). Nothing succeeds like the right kind of failure: Postwar national health insurance initiatives in Canada and the United States. *Journal of Health Politics, Policy and Law, 20* (Spring), 5–30.

Morone, James A., & Andrew B. Dunham. (1986). Slouching toward national health insurance: The unanticipated politics of DRGs. *Bulletin of the New York Academy of Medicine, 62* (July/August), 646–662.

Navarro, Vicente. (1988a). The arguments against a national health program: Science or ideology. *International Journal of Health Services, 18* (2), 179–189.

Navarro, Vicente. (1988b). Refuting arguments against a national health program. *Health/PAC Bulletin* (Summer), 15–19.

Navarro, Vicente. (1989). The rediscovery of the national health program by the Democratic Party of the United States: A chronicle of the Jesse Jackson 1988 campaign. *International Journal of Health Services, 19* (1), 1–18.

Navarro, Vicente, David U. Himmelstein, & Steffie Woolhandler. (1989). The Jackson national health program. *International Journal of Health Services, 19* (1), 19–44.

Numbers, Ronald L. (1978). *Almost persuaded: American physicians and compulsory health insurance, 1912–1920*. Baltimore, MD: Johns Hopkins University Press.

Numbers, Ronald L. (1982). *Compulsory health insurance, the continuing debate*. Westport, CT: Greenwood Press.

Pauly, Mark, Patricia Danzon, Paul J. Feldstein, & John Hoff. (1991). A plan for "responsible national health insurance." *Health Affairs, 10* (Spring), 5–25.

Pauly, Mark V. Patricia Danzon, Paul J. Feldstein, & John Hoff. (1992). *Responsible national health insurance*. Waldorf, MD: AEI Press.

Pollack, Ronald, & Phyllis Torda. (1992). The pragmatic road toward national health insurance. *American Prospect, 6* (Summer), 92–100.

Prussin, Jeffrey A. (1976). National health insurance: Anatomy of a political issue. *Medical Group Management, 23* (March/April), 22–25.

Relman, Arnold. (1989). Universal health insurance: Its time has come. *New England Journal of Medicine, 320* (January 12), 117–118.

Semmel, Herb. (1987). National health is back on the agenda. *Health/PAC Bulletin* (Fall), 4–6.

Steiber, Steven R., & Leonard A. Ferber. (1981). Support for national health insurance: Intercohort differentials. *Public Opinion Quarterly, 45* (Summer), 179–198.

Stern, Lawrence, Louis F. Rossiter, & Gail R. Wilensky. (1982). Ethics, health care, and the Enthoven proposal. *Health Affairs, 1* (Summer), 48–64.

Westerfield, Donald L. (1993). *National health care: Law, policy, strategy*. Westport, CT: Praeger.

Woolhandler, Steffie, & David U. Himmelstein. (1988). Free care: A quantitative analysis of health and cost effects of a national health program in the United States. *International Journal of Health Services, 18* (3), 393–400.

Health Care Reform

Aaron, Henry J. (1994). Sowing the seeds of reform in 1994. *Health Affairs, 13* (Spring), 57–68.

Aaron, Henry J. (Ed.). (1996). *The problem that won't go away: Reforming U.S. health care financing*. Washington, D.C.: The Brookings Institution.

Altman, Stuart. (1994). Health system reform: Let's not miss our chance. *Health Affairs, 13* (Spring), 69–80.

Angell, Marcia. (1993). The beginning of health care reform: The Clinton plan. *Journal of the American Medical Association, 329* (November 18), 1569–1570.

Antos, Joseph R. (1993). Waivers, research, and health system reform. *Health Affairs, 12* (Spring), 178–182.

Arnould, Richard J., Robert F. Rich, & William D. White. (Eds.). (1993). *Competitive approaches to health care reform*. Washington, D.C.: Urban Institute Press.

Barer, Morris L. (1995). So near, and yet so far: A Canadian perspective on U.S. health care reform. *Journal of Health Politics, Policy and Law, 20* (Summer), 463–476.

Barer, Morris L., Robert G. Evans, Matthew Holt, & J. Ian Morrison. (1994). It ain't necessarily so: The cost implications of health care reform. *Health Affairs, 13* (Fall), 88–99.

Batavia, Andrew I. (1993). Health care reform and people with disabilities. *Health Affairs, 12* (Spring), 40–57.

Battistella, Roger M., & John M. Kuder. (1993). Making health reform work without employer mandates. *Journal of American Health Policy, 3* (May/June), 18–22.

Baumgartner, Frank R., & Jeffrey C. Talbert. (1995). From setting a national agenda on health care to making decisions in Congress. *Journal of Health Politics, Policy and Law, 20* (Summer), 437–445.

Beatrice, Dennis F. (1993). The role of philanthropy in health care reform. *Health Affairs, 12* (Summer), 185–192.

Beauchamp, Dan E. (1993). Waiting for the big one: Confessions of a policy surfer looking for the universal health care wave. *Journal of Health Politics, Policy and Law, 18* (Spring), 203–228.

Bennett, Arnold, & Orville Adams. (Eds.). (1993). *Looking north for health: What we can learn from*

Canada's health care system. San Francisco, CA: Jossey-Bass.

Bilheimer, Linda T., & Robert D. Reischauer. (1995). Confessions of the estimators: Numbers and health reform. *Health Affairs, 14* (Spring), 37–55.

Birenbaum, Arnold. (1995). *Putting health care on the national agenda* (rev. ed.). Westport, CT: Praeger.

Blendon, Robert J., et al. (1992). The implications of the 1992 presidential election for health care reform. *Journal of the American Medical Association, 268* (December 16), 3371–3375.

Blendon, Robert J., Drew E. Altman, John M. Benson, Mollyann Brodie, Matt James, & Larry Hugick. (1994). How much does the public know about health reform? *Journal of American Health Policy, 4* (January/February), 26–31.

Blendon, Robert J., John Benson, Mollyann Brodie, & Larry Hugick. (1994). Channel surfing through health reform. *Journal of American Health Care, 4* (September/October), 41–46.

Blendon, Robert J., & Mollyann Brodie. (Eds.). (1994). *Transforming the system: Building a new structure for a new century* (Vol. 4). Future of American Health Care Series. New York: Faulkner & Gray, Inc.

Blendon, Robert J., Mollyann Brodie, Tracey Stelzer Hyams, & John Benson. (1994). The American public and the critical choices for health system reform. *Journal of the American Medical Association, 271* (May 18), 1539–1544.

Blendon, Robert J., Mollyann Brodie, & John Benson. (1995). What happened to support for the Clinton plan? *Health Affairs, 14* (Summer), 7–23.

Blendon, Robert J., & Jennifer N. Edwards. (1991). Caring for the uninsured: Choices for reform. *Journal of the American Medical Association, 265* (May 15), 2563–2565.

Blendon, Robert J., & Jennifer N. Edwards. (Eds.). (1991). *System in crisis: The case for health care reform* (Vol. 1). Future of American Health Care Series. Washington, D.C.: Faulkner & Gray, Inc.

Blendon, Robert J., & Tracey Hyams. (1992). *Reforming the system: Containing health care costs in an era of universal coverage.* Washington, D.C.: Faulkner & Gray, Inc.

Blendon, Robert J., Karen Donelan, Craig Hill, Ann Scheck, Woody Carter, Dennis Beatrice, & Drew Altman. (1993). Medicaid beneficiaries and health reform. *Health Affairs, 12* (Spring), 132–143.

Blendon, Robert J., John Martilla, John M. Benson, Matthew C. Shelter, Francis J. Connolly, & Tom Kiley. (1994). The beliefs and values shaping today's health reform debate. *Health Affairs, 13* (Spring), 274–284.

Bloch, Robert E., & Donald M. Falk. (1994). Antitrust, competition, and health care reform. *Health Affairs, 13* (Spring), 206–223.

Blumenthal, David. (1991). The timing and course of health care reform. *New England Journal of Medicine, 325* (July 18), 198–200.

Blumenthal, David. (1995). Health care reform—past and future. *New England Journal of Medicine, 332* (February 16), 465–468.

Blumenthal, David, & Gregg S. Meyer. (1993). The future of the academic medical center under health care reform. *New England Journal of Medicine, 329* (December), 1812–1814.

Blumstein, James F. (1994). The Clinton administration health care reform plan: Some preliminary thoughts. *Journal of Health Politics, Policy and Law, 19* (Spring), 201–206.

Bodenheimer, Thomas, & Kevin Grumbach. (1992). Financing universal health insurance: Taxes, premiums, and the lessons of social insurance. *Journal of Health Politics, Policy and Law, 17* (Fall), 435–438.

Bovbjerg, Randall R. (1992). Reform of financing for health coverage: What can reinsurance accomplish? *Inquiry, 29* (Summer), 158–175.

Bovbjerg, Randall R. (1994). Promoting quality and preventing malpractice: Assessing the Health Security Act. *Journal of Health Politics, Policy and Law, 19* (Spring), 207–216.

Bowman, Karlyn H. (1994). *Public attitudes on health care reform: Are the polls misleading the policy makers?* Waldorf, MD: AEI Press.

Bowman, Karlyn H. (1995). Learning from the imperfect debate. *Health Affairs, 14* (Spring), 27–29.

Brady, David W., & Kara M. Buckley. (1995). Health care reform in the 103rd Congress: A predictable failure. *Journal of Health Politics, Policy and Law, 20* (Summer), 447–454.

Brock, Dan W. (1994). The role of ethics in the Clinton reform proposal. *Journal of Health Politics, Policy and Law, 19* (Spring), 217–220.

Brown, E. Richard. (1994). Should single-payer advocates support President Clinton's proposal for health care reform? *American Journal of Public Health, 84* (February), 182–185.

Brown, Lawrence D. (1992). Policy reform as creative destruction: Political and administrative challenges in preserving the public–private mix. *Inquiry, 29* (Summer), 188–202.

Brown, Lawrence D. (1993a). Commissions, clubs, and consensus: Florida reorganizes for health reform. *Health Affairs, 12* (Summer), 7–26.

Brown, Lawrence D. (1993b). Dogmatic slumbers: American business and health policy. *Journal of Health Politics, Policy and Law, 18* (Summer), 339–358.

Brown, Lawrence D. (1994a). The Clinton reform plan's administrative structure: The reach and the grasp. *Journal of Health Politics, Policy and Law, 19* (Spring), 193–200.

Brown, Lawrence D. (1994b). Dogmatic slumbers: American business and health policy. In James Morone & Gary Belkin (Eds.), *The politics of health care reform: Lessons from the past, prospects for the future.* Durham, NC: Duke University Press.

Brown, Lawrence D. (1994c). Politics, money and health care reform. *Health Affairs, 13* (Spring, 2), 175–184.

Bulger, Roger J. (1994). Institutional obstacles to educational reform. *Inquiry, 31* (Fall), 303–309.

Butler, Henry N. (1994). *Unhealthy alliances: Bureaucrats, interest groups, and politicians in health reform.* Waldorf, MD: AEI Press.

Butler, Stuart M. (1995). The conservative agenda for incremental reform. *Health Affairs, 14* (Spring), 150–160.

Campion, Daniel M., W. David Helms, & Nancy L. Barrand. (1993). Perspective: Health reform in rural areas. *Health Affairs, 12* (Fall), 76–80.

Cantor, Joel C., Ian Morrison, Thomas Moloney, & Christian Koeck. (1993). Health reform lessons learned from physicians in three nations. *Health Affairs, 12* (Fall), 194–203.

Cappella, Joseph N., & Kathleen Jamison Hall. (1994). Tuned into "To your health." *Journal of American Health Care, 4* (September/October), 37–40.

The Center for Public Integrity. (1995a). Well-healed: Inside lobbying for health care reform. Part I. *International Journal of Health Services, 25* (3), 411–454.

The Center for Public Integrity. (1995b). Well-healed: Inside lobbying for health care reform. Part II. *International Journal of Health Services, 25* (4), 593–632.

The Center for Public Integrity. (1996). Well-healed: Inside lobbying for health care reform. Part III. *International Journal of Health Services, 26* (1), 19–46.

Chapman, Audrey R. (Ed.). (1994). *Health care reform: A human rights approach.* Washington, D.C.: Georgetown University Press.

Chernichovsky, Dov. (1995). Health system reforms in industrialized democracies: An emerging paradigm. *Milbank Quarterly, 73* (3), 339–372.

Chirba-Martin, Mary Ann, & Troyen A. Brennan. (1994). The critical role of ERISA in state health reform. *Health Affairs, 13* (Spring, 2), 142–156.

Chisman, Forrest P., Lawrence D. Brown, & Pamela J. Larson. (Eds.). (1994). *National health reform: What should the state's role be?* Washington, D.C.: National Academy of Social Insurance.

Chollet, Deborah. (1995). Why the Pauly/Goodman proposal won't work. *Health Affairs, 14* (Summer), 273–274.

Christianson, Jon, & Ira Moscovice. (1993). Health care reform and rural health networks. *Health Affairs, 12* (Fall), 58–75.

Churchill, Larry R. (1994). *Self-interest and universal health care: Why well insured Americans should support coverage for everyone.* Cambridge, MA: Harvard University Press.

Cohen, Jordan. (1993). Sounding board—transforming composition of the physician work force to meet the demands of health care reform. *New England Journal of Medicine, 329* (December 9), 1810–1812.

Crittendon, Robert A. (1993). Managed care competition and premium caps in Washington State. *Health Affairs, 12* (Summer), 82–88.

Cutler, David M. (1995). Cutting costs and improving health: Making reform work. *Health Affairs, 14* (Spring), 161–172.

Dandoy, Suzanne. (1994). Filling the gaps: The role of public Health Departments under health care reform. *Journal of American Health Policy, 4* (May/June), 6–13.

Davis, Karen. (1991). Expanding Medicare and employer plans to achieve universal health insurance. *Journal of the American Medical Association, 265* (May 15), 2525–2528.

Davis, Karen, & Cathy Schoen. (1994). Universal coverage: Building on Medicare and employer financing. *Health Affairs, 13* (Spring, 2), 7–20.

DiIulio, John J. Jr., & Richard P. Nathan. (Eds.). (1994). *Making health reform work: The view from the states.* Washington, D.C.: The Brookings Institution.

Dodson, Anthony L., & Keith J. Mueller. (1993). National health care reform: Whither state government? *Policy Currents, 3* (November), 5–7.

Dowd, Bryan, Jon Christianson, Roger Feldman, Catherine Wisner, & John Klein. (1992). Issues regarding health plan payments under Medicare and recommedations for reform. *Milbank Quarterly, 70* (3), 423–454.

Dowd, Bryan, & Roger Feldman. (1992). Insurer competition and protection from risk redefinintion in the individual and small group health insurance market. *Inquiry, 29* (Summer), 148–157.

Duesterberg, Thomas J., David J. Weinschrott, & David C. Murray. (1994). *Health care reform, regulation, and innovations in the medical device industry.* Washington, D.C.: The Brookings Institution.

Dukakis, Michael L. (1995). Health care reform: Where do we go from here? *Journal of Health Politics, Policy and Law, 20* (Fall), 787–794.

Eckholm, Erik. (Ed.). (1993). *Solving America's health-care crisis.* New York: New York Times Books.

Edwards, Jennifer N., Robert J. Blendon, Robert Leitman, Ellen Morrison, Ian Morrison, & Humphrey Taylor. (1992). Small business and the national health care reform debate. *Health Affairs, 11* (Spring), 164–173.

Ellwood, Paul M., & Alain C. Enthoven. (1995). Responsible choices: The Jackson Hole plan. *Health Affairs, 14* (Summer), 24–39.

Enthoven, Alain, & Richard Kronick. (1989). A consumer choice health plan for the 1990s: Universal health insurance in a system designed to promote quality and economy. *New England Journal of Medicine, 320*, Part I (January 5), 29–37; Part II (January 12), 94–101.

Enthoven, Alain C., & Richard Kronick. (1991). Universal health insurance through incentives reform. *Journal of the American Medical Association, 265* (May 15), 2532–2536.

Enthoven, Alain C., & Sara J. Singer. (1994). A single-payer system in Jackson Hole Clothing. *Health Affairs, 13* (Spring), 81–95.

Enthoven, Alain C., & Sara J. Singer. (1995). Market-based reform: What to regulate and by when. *Health Affairs, 14* (Spring), 105–119.

Epstein, Arnold M. (1993). Change in the delivery of care under comprehensive health care reform. *Journal of the American Medical Association, 329* (November 25), 1672–1676.

Etheredge, Lynn. (1991). Negotiating national health insurance. *Journal of Health Politics, Policy and Law, 16* (Spring), 157–168.

Fallows, James. (1995). A triumph of misinformation. *Atlantic Monthly* (January), 26–37.

Feder, Judith, & Larry Levitt. (1995). Steps toward universal coverage. *Health Affairs, 14* (Spring), 140–149.

Fein, Rashi. (1992). Health care reform. *Scientific American, 267* (5), 46–53.

Feingold, Eugene. (1994). Health care reform—more than cost containment and universal access. *American Journal of Public Health, 84* (May), 727–728.

Feldstein, Paul J. (1994). *Health policy issues: An economic perspective on health reform.* Ann Arbor, MI: AUPHA Press/Health Administration Press.

Fihn, Stephan. (1995). Uninsured children: An unintended consequence of health care system reform efforts. *Journal of the American Medical Association, 274* (November 8), 1472–1474.

Firshein, Janet, & Christina Kent. (1995). 1994: A year of dashed hopes. *Medicine and Health Perspectives* (January 2), 1–7.

Fox, Daniel M., & Howard M. Leichter. (1993). The ups and downs of Oregon's rationing plan. *Health Affairs, 12* (Summer), 66–70.

Fox, Peter D., Thomas Rice, & Lisa Alecxih. (1995). Medigap regulation: Lessons for health care reform. *Journal of Health Politics, Policy and Law, 20* (Spring), 31–48.

Freeman, Phyllis, & Anthony Robbins. (1994). National health care reform minus public health: A formula for failure. *Journal of Public Health Policy, 15* (Autumn), 261–282.

Friedman, Emily. (1994). Getting a head start: The states and health care reform. *Journal of the American Medical Association, 271* (March 16), 875–878.

Fuchs, Victor R. (1994). The Clinton plan: A researcher examines reform. *Health Affairs, 13* (Spring), 102–114.

Gabel, Jon R., & Gail A. Jensen. (1992). Can a universal coverage system temper the underwriting cycle? *Inquiry, 29* (Summer), 249–262.

Garland, Michael J. (1992). Light on the black box of basic health care: Oregon's contribution to the national movement toward universal health insurance. *Yale Law and Policy Review, 10* (2), 409–430.

Ginzberg, Eli. (1992). Health care reform—where are we and where should we be going? *New England Journal of Medicine, 327* (October 29), 1310–1312.

Ginzberg, Eli. (1994a). Improving health care for the poor: Lessons from the 1980s. *Journal of the American Medical Association, 271* (February 9), 464–467.

Ginzberg, Eli. (1994b). *Medical gridlock and health reform.* Boulder, CO: Westview Press.

Ginzberg, Eli. (Ed.). (1994c). *Critical issues in U.S. health reforms.* Boulder, CO: Westview Press.

Glaser, William A. (1993). Universal health insurance that really works: Foreign lessons for the United States. *Journal of Health Politics, Policy and Law, 18* (Fall), 695–722.

Glaudemans, Jon. (1994). The case for local budgeting. *Health Affairs, 13* (Spring), 243–246.

Goldberg, Mark A. (1995). Public judgment and the prospects for reform. *Health Affairs, 14* (Spring), 30–32.

Goldsmith, Jeff. (1993). Hospital/physician relationships: A constraint to health reform. *Health Affairs, 12* (Fall), 160–169.

Gostin, Lawrence. (1993). Foreward: Health care reform in the United States—the presidential task force. *American Journal of Law and Medicine, 19* (1/2), 1–20.

Grabowski, Henry G. (1994). *Health reform and pharmaceutical innovation.* Waldorf, MD: AEI Press.

Graig, Laurence A. (1993). *Health of nations: An international perspective on U.S. health care reform* (2nd ed.). Washington, D.C.: Congressional Quarterly Books.

Gray, Bradford H. (1993). Ownership matters: Health reform and the future of nonprofit health care. *Inquiry, 30* (Winter), 352–361.

Grey, Michael R. (1994). The medical care programs of the Farm Security Administration, 1932 through 1947: A rehearsal for national health insurance? *American Journal of Public Health, 84* (October), 1678–1687.

Grossman, Edward G. (1994). Comparing the options for universal coverage. *Health Affairs, 13* (Spring, 2), 84–100.

Group, The Health Care Study. (1994). Understanding the choices in health care reform. *Journal of Health Politics, Policy and Law, 19* (Fall), 499–542.

Hadley, Jack. (1993). Checking it once, checking it twice. *Inquiry, 30* (Winter), 345–351.

Hadley, Jack. (1994). Workforce policies: Physicians and nurses in health care reform. *Inquiry, 31* (Fall), 342–345.

Hadley, Jack. (1994–95). The view from here: Future issues in health care reform. *Inquiry, 31* (Winter), 363–364.

Hadley, Jack, & Stephen Zuckerman. (1994). The good, the bad, and the bottom line. *Health Affairs, 13* (Spring), 115–131.

Hall, Mark A. (1995). Managed competition meets tax-neutrality. *Health Affairs, 14* (Summer), 274.

Ham, Chris, & Mats Brommels. (1994). Health care reform in the Netherlands, Sweden, and the United Kingdom. *Health Affairs, 13* (Winter), 106–119.

Havighurst, Craig. (1994a). "Gotcha" journalism and the fate of health reform. *Journal of American Health Care, 4* (September/October), 3–4.

Havighurst, Clark C. (1994b). *Health care choices: Private contracts as instruments of health reform.* Waldorf, MD: AEI Press.

The Health Care Study Group. (1994). Understanding the crisis in health care reform. *Journal of Health Politics, Policy and Law, 19* (Fall), 488–542.

Heclo, Hugh. (1995). The Clinton health plan: Historical perspective. *Health Affairs, 14* (Spring), 86–98.

Helms, Robert A. (1993). *Health policy reform: Competition and controls.* Waldorf, MD: AEI Press.

Helms, Robert B. (Ed.). (1993). *American health policy: Critical issue for reform.* Waldorf, MD: AEI Press.

Holahan, John, & Sheila Zedlewski. (1992). Who pays for health care in the United States? Implications for health system reform. *Inquiry, 29* (Summer), 231–248.

Holahan, Marilyn Moon, W. Pete Welch, & Stephen Zuckerman. (1991). *Balancing access, costs and politics: The American context in health system reform* (Report No. 91-6). Washington, D.C.: Urban Institute Press.

Holland, Walter W., & Clifford Graham. (1994). Commentary: Recent reforms in the British National Health Service—lessons for the United States. *American Journal of Public Health, 84* (February), 186–189.

Hughes, Robert G., Tania L. Davis, & Richard C. Reynolds. (1995). Assuring children's health as the basis for reform. *Health Affairs, 14* (Summer), 158–167.

Hurst, Jeremy W. (1991). Reforming health care in seven European nations. *Health Affairs, 10* (Fall), 721.

Hutton, John, Michael Borowitz, Inga Oleksy, & Bryan R. Luce. (1994). The pharmaceutical industry and health reform: Lessons from Europe. *Health Affairs, 13* (Summer), 98–111.

Iglehart, John K. (1993). Health care reform—the labryinths of Congress. *New England Journal of Medicine, 329* (November), 1593–1596.

Iglehart, John K. (1994a). Health care reform—the states. *New England Journal of Medicine, 30* (January 6), 75–79.

Iglehart, John K. (1994b). Health care reform: The role of physicians. *New England Journal of Medicine, 330* (March 10), 728–731.

Intergovernmental Health Policy Project. (1995). *Health care reform: 50 state profiles.* Washington, D.C.: Intergovernmental Health Policy Project.

Jacobs, Lawrence R. (1993). Health reform impasse: The politics of American ambivalence toward government. *Journal of Health Politics, Policy and Law, 18* (Fall), 629–656.

Jacobs, Lawrence R., & Robert Y. Shapiro. (1995). Don't blame the public for failed health care reform. *Journal of Health Politics, Policy and Law, 20* (Summer), 411–423.

Jeppson, David H. (1990). Perspective: Focus on health system reform. *Health Affairs, 9* (Spring), 114–116.

Jones, Stanley B. (1992). Employer-based private health insurance needs structural reform. *Inquiry, 29* (Summer), 120–127.

Kane, Robert L., & Rosalie A. Kane. (1994). Implications of the Clinton health reform plan for older persons and long-term care. *Journal of Health Politics, Policy and Law, 19* (Spring), 221–226.

Karpatkin, Rhoda H., & Gail E. Shearer. (1995). A short-term consumer agenda for health care reform. *American Journal of Public Health, 85* (October), 1852–1855.

Kent, Christina. (Ed.). (1993). The grand old party and health reform. *Medicine and Health Perspectives* (October 4).

Kindig, David A., & Robert B. Sullivan. (Eds.). (1992). *Understanding universal health programs: Issues and options.* Ann Arbor, MI: Health Administration Press.

King, Guy. (1994). Health care reform and the Medicare program. *Health Affairs, 13* (Winter), 39–43.

Koyanagi, Chris, & Joseph Manes. (1995). What did the health care reform debate mean for mental health policy? *Health Affairs, 14* (Fall), 124–130.

Kronick, Richard. (1992). Empowering the demand side: From regulation to purchasing. *Inquiry, 29* (Summer), 213–230.

Kronick, Richard. (1994a). Perspective: A helping hand for the invisible hand. *Health Affairs, 13* (Spring), 96–101.

Kronick, Richard. (1994b). Redistributing health care resources without redistributing income. *Journal of Health Politics, Policy and Law, 19* (Fall), 543–554.

Kronick, Richard, David C. Goodman, John Wennberg, & Edward Wagner. (1993). The marketplace in health care reform—the demographic limitations of managed competition. *New England Journal of Medicine, 328* (January 14), 148–152.

Krueger, Alan B., & Uwe E. Reinhardt. (1994). Economics of employer versus individual mandates. *Health Affairs, 13* (Spring, 2), 34–53.

Laham, Nicholas. (1993). *Why the United States lacks a national health insurance program.* Westport, CT: Praeger.

Lane, James A. (1994). A workable framework for health reform. *Health Affairs, 13* (Spring), 248–249.

Lee, Philip, Denise Softel, & Harold S. Luft. (1992). Special series—costs and coverage: Pressures toward health care reform. *Western Journal of Medicine, 157* (November), 576–583.

Leichter, Howard M. (1993). Minnesota: The trip from acrimony to accommodation. *Health Affairs, 12* (Summer), 48–58.

Leichter, Howard M. (1994). Health care reform in Vermont: The next chapter. *Health Affairs, 13* (Winter), 78–103.

Leichter, Howard M. (Ed.). (1992). *Health policy reform in America.* Armonk, NY: M. E. Sharpe.

Lemco, Jonathan. (1994). *National health care: Lessons for the United States and Canada.* Ann Arbor: University of Michigan Press.

Lewin, Marion Ein, Catherine E. McDermott, & Mary C. Barkley. (1994). Special report: Health care reform and grantmakers. *Health Affairs, 13* (Fall), 186–188.

Lipson, Debra. (1992). *From rhetoric to reality: Federal health reform will be hard—but state reforms may guide the way* (Research Report No. 92-4). Washington, D.C.: Faulkner & Gray, Inc.

Lubin Finkel, Madelon. (1993). Commentary—managed care is not the answer. *Journal of Health Politics, Policy and Law, 18* (Spring), 105–112.

Lundberg, George D. (1992). National health care reform: The aura of inevitability intensifies. *Journal of the American Medical Association, 267* (May 13), 2521–2524.

Lundberg, George D. (1994). United States health care reform: An era of shared sacrifice and responsibility begins. *Journal of the American Medical Association, 271* (May 18), 1530–1533.

Marmor, Theodore R. (1993). Lessons from the frozen North. *Journal of Health Politics, Policy and Law, 18* (Fall), 763–770.

Marmor, Theodore R. (1994). *Understanding health care reform.* New Haven, CT: Yale University Press.

Marmor, Theodore R. (1995). A summer of discontent: Press coverage of murder and medical care reform. *Journal of Health Politics, Policy and Law, 20* (Summer), 495–502.

Marmor, Theodore R., & Michael S. Barr. (1992). Making sense of the national health insurance reform debate. *Yale Law and Policy Review, 10* (2), 228–282.

Marmor, Theodore R., & Mark A. Goldberg. (1995). Reform redux. *Journal of Health Politics, Policy and Law, 20* (Summer), 491–494.

Martin, Cathie Jo. (1995). Stuck in neutral: Big business and the politics of national health reform. *Journal of Health Politics, Policy and Law, 20* (Summer), 430–436.

McArdle, Frank B. (1994). How would business react to employer mandate? *Health Affairs, 13* (Spring, 2), 69–83.

McArdle, Frank B. (1995). Opening up the FEHBP. *Health Affairs, 14* (Summer), 40–50.

McLaughlin, Catherine G., Wendy K. Zellers, & Kevin D. Frick. (1994). Small-business winners and losers under health care reform. *Health Affairs, 13* (Spring, 2), 221–233.

Mechanic, David. (1993a). *Inescapable decisions: The imperatives of health reform*. New Brunswick, NJ: Transaction Publishers.

Mechanic, David. (1993b). Mental health services in the context of health insurance reform. *Milbank Quarterly, 71* (3), 349–364.

Mendelson, Daniel N., & Judith Arnold. (1992). Evaluating the cost of heath-care reform plans. *Yale Law and Policy Review, 10* (2), 283–301.

Merrill, Jeffrey C. (1994). *The road to health care reform: Designing a system that works*. New York: Plenum.

Miller, Velvet G., & Janis L. Curtis. (1993). Health care reform and race-specific policies. *Journal of Health Politics, Policy and Law, 18* (Fall), 747–754.

Mills, Miriam K., & Robert H. Blank. (Eds.). (1992). *Health insurance and public policy: Risk, allocation, and equity*. Westport, CT: Greenwood Press.

Moeller, John F. (1995). Gainers and losers under a tax-based health care reform plan. *Inquiry, 32* (Fall), 285–299.

Moffit, Robert E. (1994). Perspectives on mandates: Personal freedom, responsibility and mandates. *Health Affairs, 13* (Spring, 2), 101–104.

Mongan, James J. (1995). Perspectives: Anatomy and physiology of health reform's failure. *Health Affairs, 14* (Spring), 99–101.

Morone, James A. (1994). The administration of health care reform. *Journal of Health Politics, Policy and Law, 19* (Spring), 233–238.

Morone, James A. (1995). Nativism, hollow corporations, and managed competition: Why the Clinton health care reform failed. *Journal of Health Politics, Policy and Law, 20* (Summer), 391–398.

Morone, James A., & Gary S. Belkin. (Eds.). (1994). *The politics of health care reform: Lessons from the past, prospects for the future*. Durham, NC: Duke University Press.

Navarro, Vicente. (1994). The need to mobilize support for the Wellstone–McDermott–Conyers single-payer proposal. *American Journal of Public Health, 84* (February), 178–179.

Navarro, Vicente. (1995). Why Congress did not enact health care reform. *Journal of Health Politics, Policy and Law, 20* (Summer), 455–462.

Navarro, Vicente. (Ed.). (1992). *Why the United States does not have a national health program*. Amityville, NY: Baywood Publishing Co.

Neubauer, Deanne. (1993). Hawaii: A pioneer in health system reform. *Health Affairs, 12* (Summer), 31–39.

Newhouse, Joseph P. (1994). Patients at risk: Reform and risk adjustment. *Health Affairs, 13* (Spring), 132–146.

Newhouse, Joseph P. (1995). Economists, policy entrepreneurs, and health care reform. *Health Affairs, 14* (Spring), 182–198.

Newhouse, Joseph P., & The Insurance Experiment Group. (1993). *Free for all? Lessons from the Rand Health Insurance Experiment*. Cambridge, MA: Harvard University Press.

Nichols, Len M. (1995a). MSAs and risk segmentation. *Health Affairs, 14* (Summer), 275.

Nichols, Len M. (1995b). Perspectives: Numerical estimates and the policy debate. *Health Affairs, 14* (Spring), 56–59.

Nutter, Donald O., Charles M. Helms, Michael E. Whitcomb, & W. Donald Weston. (1991). Restructuring health care in the United States: A proposal for the 1990s. *Journal of the American Medical Association, 265* (May 15), 2516–2520.

Oliver, Thomas R., & Emery B. Dowell. (1994). Interest groups and reform: Lessons from California. *Health Affairs, 13* (Spring, 2), 123–141.

O'Neill, James E., & Dave M. O'Neill. (1994). *The employment and distributional effects of mandated benefits*. Waldorf, MD: AEI Press.

Organization for Economic Cooperation and Development. (1992). *U.S. health care at the cross roads*. Washington, DC: Organization for Economic Cooperation and Development Publications and Information Center.

Pauly, Mark V. (1992). Risk variation and fazeback insurers in universal coverage insurance plans. *Inquiry, 29* (Summer), 137–147.

Pauly, Mark V. (1994a). A case for employer-enforced individual mandates. *Health Affairs, 13* (Spring, 2), 21–33.

Pauly, Mark V. (1994b). What happened to the tough choices? *Health Affairs, 13* (Spring), 147–160.

Pauly, Mark V., Patricia Danzon, Paul Feldstein, & John Hoff. (1991). A plan for "responsible national health insurance." *Health Affairs, 10* (Spring), 5–25.

Pauly, Mark V., Patricia Danzon, Paul J. Feldstein, & John Hoff. (1992). *Responsible national health insurance.* Waldorf, MD: AEI Press.

Pauly, Mark V., & John C. Goodman. (1995a). Medical savings accounts: The authors respond. *Health Affairs, 14* (Summer), 277–279.

Pauly, Mark V., & John C. Goodman. (1995b). Tax credits for insurance and medical savings accounts. *Health Affairs, 14* (Spring), 125–139.

Peterson, Mark A. (1992). Momentum toward health care reform in the U.S. Senate. *Journal of Health Politics, Policy and Law, 17* (Fall), 553–574.

Peterson, Mark A. (1993). Political influence in the 1990s: From iron triangles to policy networks. *Journal of Health Politics, Policy and Law, 18* (Summer), 395–438.

Peterson, Mark A. (1994). Clinton's plan goes to Congress—now what? *Journal of Health Politics, Policy and Law, 19* (Spring), 261–264.

Peterson, Mark A. (1995). The health care debate: All heat and no light. *Journal of Health Politics, Policy and Law, 20* (Summer), 425–430.

Priester, Reinhard. (1992). A values framework for health system reform. *Health Affairs, 11* (Spring), 84–107.

Reagan, Michael D. (1992). *Curing the crisis: Options for America's health.* New Brunswick, NJ: Westview Press.

Regenstein, Marsha, & Sharon Silow-Carroll. (1994). *Market reforms and regulation: Lessons from Europe's health care systems.* Washington, D.C.: Economic and Social Research Institute.

Reinhardt, Uwe E. (1993a). An "all-American" health reform proposal. *Journal of American Health Policy, 3* (May/June), 11–17.

Reinhardt, Uwe E. (1993b). Reforming the health care system: The universal dilemma. *American Journal of Law and Medicine, 19* (1/2), 21–36.

Reinhardt, Uwe E. (1994). The Clinton plan: A salute to American pluralism. *Health Affairs, 13* (Spring), 161–178.

Reinhardt, Uwe E. (1995). Turning our gaze from bread and circus games. *Health Affairs, 14* (Spring), 33–36.

Relman, Arnold W. (1993). Medical practice under the Clinton reforms—avoiding domination by business. *New England Journal of Medicine, 329* (November 18), 1574–1576.

Rice, Thomas. (1992). Including an all-payer reimbursement system in a universal health insurance program. *Inquiry, 29* (Summer), 203–212.

Rivlin, Alice M., David M. Cutler, & Len M. Nichols. (1994). Financing, estimation, and economic effects. *Health Affairs, 13* (Spring), 30–49.

Roberts, Marc J., & Alexander T. Clyde. (1993). *Your money or your life: The health care crisis explained.* New York: Doubleday.

Robinson, Ray, & Julian Legrand. (1994). *Evaluating the National Health Service reforms.* New Brunswick, NJ: Transaction Publishers.

Rochefort, David A. (1993). Commentary—the pragmatic appeal of employment-based health care reform. *Journal of Health Politics, Policy and Law, 18* (Fall), 683–694.

Rockman, Bert A. (1995). The Clinton presidency and health care reform. *Journal of Health Politics, Policy and Law, 20* (Summer), 399–402.

Rogal, Deborah L., Anne K. Gauthier, & Nancy L. Barrand. (1993). Managing the health care system under a global expenditure limit: A workshop summary. *Inquiry, 30* (Fall), 318–327.

Rogal, Deborah L., & W. David Helms. (1993). State models: Tracking states' efforts to reform their health systems. *Health Affairs, 12* (Summer), 27–30.

Rosenau, Pauline Vaillancourt. (1993). Reforming health care in the U.S. *American Behavioral Scientist, 36* (July).

Rosenau, Pauline Vaillancourt. (Ed.). (1994). *Health care reforms in the nineties.* Thousand Oaks, CA: Sage.

Rothman, David J. (1993). A century of failure: Health care reform in America. *Journal of Health Politics, Policy and Law, 18* (Summer), 271–286.

Rothman, David. (1994). A century of failure: Class barriers to reform. In James A. Morone & Gary Belkin (Eds.), *The politics of health care reform: Les-*

sons from the past, prospects for the future. Durham, NC: Duke University Press.

Rottenberg, Linda D. (1992). America's health care: Which road to reform? *Yale Law and Policy Review, 10* (2).

Saltman, Richard. (1994). A conceptual overview of recent health care reforms. *European Journal of Public Health, 4* (4), 287–293.

Scheffer, Richard M., Stephen Earl Foreman, Brian J. Cuffel, & Carter Mackley. (1994). Mental health benefits in the Clinton plan. *Health Affairs, 13* (Spring, 2), 201–210.

Schieber, Sylvester J. (1994). Employer coolness toward Clinton plan mandates. *Health Affairs, 13* (Spring, 2), 105–107.

Schlesinger, Mark J., & Leon Eisenberg. (Eds.). (1990). *Children in a changing health system: Assessments and proposals for reforms.* Baltimore, MD: Johns Hopkins University Press.

Schramm, Carl J. (1992). Government, private health insurance, and the goal of universal health care coverage. *Inquiry, 29* (Summer), 263–268.

Sharfstein, Steven S., & Anne M. Stoline. (1992). Reform issues for insuring mental health care. *Health Affairs, 11* (Fall), 84–97.

Sheils, John F. (1995). Need for continued refinement in cost estimations. *Health Affairs, 14* (Spring), 60–62.

Sheils, John F., Raymond J. Baxter, & Randall A. Haught. (1995). Data Watch: The public cost of expanding coverage. *Health Affairs, 14* (Spring), 226–233.

Sheils, John F., & Laurence S. Lewin. (1994). Perspective: Alternative estimate: No pain, no gain. *Health Affairs, 13* (Spring), 50–55.

Short, Pamela Farley, & Tamara J. Lair. (1994–95). Health insurance and health status: Implications for financing health care reform. *Inquiry, 31* (Winter), 425–437.

Shortell, Stephen M. (1992). A model for state health care reform. *Health Affairs, 11* (Spring), 108–127.

Silver, George. (1995). Topics of our times: Clausewitz vs. Sun Tzu—the art of health reform. *American Journal of Public Health, 85* (March), 307–308.

Sisk, Jane E., & Sherry A. Glied. (1994). Innovation under federal health care reform. *Health Affairs, 13* (Summer), 82–97.

Skocpol, Theda. (1993). Is the time finally ripe? Health insurance reforms in the 1990s. *Journal of Health Politics, Policy and Law, 18* (Fall), 531–550.

Skocpol, Theda. (1994a). From Social Security to health security? *Journal of Health Politics, Policy and Law, 19* (Spring), 239–242.

Skocpol, Theda. (1994b). Is the time finally right? Health insurance reforms in the 1990s. In James Morone & Gary Belkin (Eds.), *The politics of health care reform.* Durham, NC: Duke University Press.

Skocpol, Theda. (1995a). The aftermath of defeat. *Journal of Health Politics, Policy and Law, 20* (Summer), 485–490.

Skocpol, Theda. (1995b). The rise and resounding demise of the Clinton plan. *Health Affairs, 14* (Spring), 66–85.

Skocpol, Theda. (1996). *Boomerang: Clinton's health security effort and the turn against government in U.S. politics.* New York: W. W. Norton.

Smith, David G. (1992). *Paying for Medicare: The politics of reform.* Hawthorne, NY: Walter de Gruyter.

Smith, Mark D., Drew E. Altman, Robert Leitman, Thomas W. Moloney, & Humphrey Taylor. (1992). Taking the public's pulse on health reform. *Health Affairs, 11* (Summer), 125–133.

Sorian, Richard M., & The Editors of The Health Care Information Center. (Eds.). (1993). *A new deal for American health care: How reform will reshape health care delivery and payment for a new century* (Vol. 1). New York: Faulkner & Gray, Inc.

Sparer, Michael S. (1993). States in a reformed health system: Lessons from nursing home policy. *Health Affairs, 12* (Spring), 7–20.

Sparer, Michael S. (1996). Medicaid managed care and the health reform debate: Lessons from New York and California. *Journal of Health Politics, Policy and Law, 21* (Fall), 433–460.

Starr, Paul. (1991). The middle class and national health reform. *American Prospects, 20* (Summer), 5–12.

Starr, Paul. (1993). Health compromise: Universal coverage and organized competition under a cap. *American Prospect, 12* (Winter), 44–52.

Steinmo, Sven, & Jon Watts. (1995). It's the institutions, stupid! Why comprehensive national health insurance always fails in the United States. *Journal of Health Politics, Policy and Law, 20* (2), 330–372.

Steuerle, C. Eugene. (1994a). *Economic effects of health care reforms.* Waldorf, MD: AEI Press.

Steuerle, C. Eugene. (1994b). Implementing employer and individual mandates. *Health Affairs, 13* (Spring, 2), 54–68.

Steuerle, C. Eugene. (1995). Designing a nondiscriminatory tax credit. *Health Affairs, 14* (Summer), 276.

Susser, Mervyn. (1994). Health care reform and public health: Weighing the proposals. *American Journal of Public Health, 84* (February), 173–175.

Tallon, James R. Jr., & Richard P. Nathan. (1992). Federal/state partnership for health system reform. *Health Affairs, 11* (Winter), 7–16.

Taylor, Humphrey. (1993). And the mother of all political battles has not even begun. *Inquiry, 30* (Fall), 228–234.

Thompson, Richard E. (1993). *Health care reform as social change.* Tampa, FL: American College of Physician Executives.

Thorpe, Kenneth E. (1992). Expanding employment-based health insurance: Is small group reform the answer? *Inquiry, 29* (Summer), 128–136.

Thorpe, Kenneth E. (1995). A call for health services researchers. *Health Affairs, 14* (Spring), 63–65.

Tuohy, Carolyn. (1994). Response to the Clinton proposal: A comparative perspective. *Journal of Health Politics, Policy and Law, 19* (Spring), 249–254.

Tresnowski, Bernard R. (1992). Building a foundation for universal access. *Inquiry, 29* (Summer), 269–273.

Trevino, Fernando, & Jeff P. Jacobs. (1994). Public health and health care reform: The American Public Health Association's perspective. *Journal of Public Health Policy, 15* (Winter), 397–406.

U.S. Congress Office of Technology Assessment. (1994). *Understanding estimates of national health expenditures under health care reform.* Washington, D.C.: U.S. Government Printing Office.

Volpp, Kevin G., & Bruce Siegel. (1993). New Jersey: Long-term experience with all-payer state rate setting. *Health Affairs, 12* (Summer), 59–65.

Weiner, Jonathan P. (1994). Forecasting the effects of health reform on U.S. physician workforce requirement: Evidence from HMO staffing patterns. *Journal of the American Medical Association, 272* (July 20), 222–230.

Weiner, Jonathan P., & Gregory de Lissovoy. (1993). Razing a Tower of Babel: A taxonomy for managed care and health insurance plans. *Journal of Health Politics, Policy and Law, 18* (Spring), 75–104.

Weir, Margaret. (1995). Institutional and political obstacles to reform. *Health Affairs, 14* (Spring), 102–104.

Weissman, Joel S., & Arnold M. Epstein. (1994). *Falling through the safety net: Insurance status and access to health care.* Baltimore, MD: Johns Hopkins University Press.

Wennberg, John A. (1992). Perspective: AHCPR and the strategy for health care reform. *Health Affairs, 11* (Winter), 67–71.

Wennberg, John E. (1994). Health care reform and professionalism. *Inquiry, 31* (Fall), 296–302.

Westerfield, Donald L. (1993). *National health care: Law, policy, strategy.* Westport, CT: Praeger.

White, Joseph. (1995a). *Competing solutions: American health care proposals and international experience.* Washington, D.C.: The Brookings Institution.

White, Joseph. (1995b). The horses and the jumps: Comments on the health law reform steeplechase. *Journal of Health Politics, Policy and Law, 20* (Summer), 373–383.

White, Joseph. (1995c). *Medical savings accounts: Fact versus fiction.* Washington, D.C.: The Brookings Institution.

Wilensky, Gail R. (1994). Health reform: What will it take to pass? *Health Affairs, 13* (Spring), 179–191.

Wilensky, Gail R. (1995). Incremental health system reform: Where Medicare fits in. *Health Affairs, 14* (Spring), 173–181.

Wolfe, Barbara. (1993). Why changing the U.S. health care system is so difficult. *Social Science and Medicine, 36* (3), iii–vi.

Yankelovich, Daniel. (1995). The debate that wasn't: The public and the Clinton plan. *Health Affairs, 14* (Spring), 7–23.

Zedlewski, Sheila, John Holahan, & Colin Winterbottom. (1994). *The Health Security Act: Who would pay?* Washington, D.C.: Urban Institute.

Zelman, Walter A. (1994). Rationale behind the Clinton health reform plan. *Health Affairs, 13* (Spring), 9–29.

The Poor and Disadvantaged (see also Un- and Underinsured)

Blendon, Robert J., Linda H. Aiken, et al. (1986). Uncompensated care by hospitals or public insurance for the poor: Does it make a difference? *New England Journal of Medicine, 314* (May 1), 1160–1163.

Brown, E. Richard, & Michael R. Cousineau. (1984). Effectiveness of state mandates to maintain local government health services for the poor. *Journal of Health Politics, Policy and Law, 9* (Summer), 223–236.

Brown, Lawrence D. (Ed.). (1991). *Health policy and the disadvantaged.* Durham, NC: Duke University Press.

Coute, Richard A. (1975). *Poverty, politics and health care: An Appalachian experience.* New York: Praeger.

Cromwell, Jerry, Sylvia Hurdle, & Rachel Schurman. (1987). Defederalizing Medicaid: Fair to the poor, fair to taxpayers? *Journal of Health Politics, Policy and Law, 12* (Spring), 1–34.

Dans, Peter E., & Samuel Johnson. (1975). Politics in the development of a migrant health center. *New England Journal of Medicine, 292* (April 24), 890–895.

Davis, Karen. (1977). A decade of policy developments in providing health care for low-income families. In R. H. Haveman (Ed.), *A decade of federal antipoverty programs: Achievements, failures and lessons* (pp. 197–231). New York: Academic Press.

Davis, Karen. (1991). Inequality and access to health care. *Milbank Quarterly, 69* (2), 253–274.

Desonia, Randolph, & Kathleen M. King. (1985). *State programs of assistance for the medically indigent.* Washington, D.C.: George Washington University.

Feder, Judith. (1990). Health care of the disadvantaged: The elderly. *Journal of Health Politics, Policy and Law, 15* (Summer), 259–270.

Ginzberg, Eli. (1994). Improving health care for the poor: Lessons from the 1980s. *Journal of the American Medical Association, 271* (February 9), 464–467.

Kinzer, David M. (1984). Care of the poor revisited. *Inquiry, 21* (Spring), 5–16.

Lewin, Lawrence S., & Marion Ein Lewin. (1987). Financing charity care in an era of competition. *Health Affairs, 6* (Spring), 47–60.

Mundinger, Mary O'Neil. (1985). Health service funding cuts and the declining health of the poor. *New England Journal of Medicine, 313* (July 4), 44–47.

Rose, Marilyn G. (1975). Federal regulation of services to the poor under the Hill–Burton Act: Realities and pitfalls. *Northwestern University Law Review, 70* (March/April), 168–201.

Schlesinger, Mark, & Karl Kronebusch. (1990). The failure of prenatal care policy for the poor. *Health Affairs, 9* (Winter), 91–111.

Shenkin, Budd N. (1974). *Health care for migrant workers: Policies and politics.* Cambridge, MA: Ballinger.

Smith, Ellen M. (1987). Health care for Native Americans: Who will pay? *Health Affairs, 6* (Spring), 123–128.

Stevens, Robert, & Rosemary Stevens. (1974). *Welfare medicine in America: A case study of Medicaid.* New York: The Free Press

Stone, Deborah A. (1979). Diagnosis and the dole: The function of illness in American distributive politics. *Journal of Health Politics, Policy and Law, 4* (Fall), 507–521.

Stone, Deborah A., & Theodore R. Marmor. (Eds.). (1990). Special issue on health policy and the disadvantaged—introduction. *Journal of Health Politics, Policy and Law, 15* (Summer), 253–258.

Turnquist, Trude Held. (1987). *An examination of the changing nature of charity care in hospitals: The response of Minnesota hospitals and health care facilities to the Hill–Burton uncompensated care obligation, 1980–1981.* Unpublished Ph.D. diss., University of Minnesota.

Wilensky, Gail R. (1984). Solving uncompensated hospital care: Targeting the indigent and the uninsured. *Health Affairs, 3* (Winter), 50–62.

Public Health (see also Environmental and Occupational Health)

Andrulus, Dennis P., Katherine L. Acuff, Kevin B. Weiss, & Ron J. Anderson. (1996). Public hospitals and health care reform: Choices and challenges. *American Journal of Public Health, 86* (February), 162–165.

Bayer, Ronald. (1994). Commentary—public health policy and tuberculosis. *Journal of Health Politics, Policy and Law, 19* (Spring), 149–154.

Bellin, Lowell E. (1969). Medicaid in New York: Utopianism and bare knuckles in public health, 3. Realpolitik in the health care arena: Standard setting of professional services. *American Journal of Public Health, 59* (May), 820–825.

Bellin, Lowell E. (1970). The new left and American public health—attempted radicalization of the A.P.H.A. through dialectic. *American Journal of Public Health, 60* (June), 973–981.

Bernstein, Betty J. (1970). Public health—inside or outside the mainstream of the political process? Lessons from the passage of Medicaid. *American Journal of Public Health, 60* (September), 1690– 1700.

Cahill, Kevin M. (Ed.). (1992). *Imminent peril: Public health in a declining economy.* Washington, D.C.: The Brookings Institution.

Conant, Ralph W. (1968). *The politics of community health.* Washington, D.C.: Public Affairs Press.

Courtwright, David T. (1980). Public health and public wealth: Social cost as a basis for restrictive policies. *Milbank Memorial Fund Quarterly/Health and Society, 58* (Spring), 268–282.

Dandoy, Suzanne. (1994). Filling the gaps: The role of Public Health Departments under health care reform. *Journal of American Health Policy, 4* (May/June), 6–13.

Fishman, Roslyn U. (1992). What is APHA's future in public health? *Journal of Public Health Policy, 13* (Spring), 14–17.

Foreman, Chrisopher H. (1994). *Plagues, products and politics: Emergent public health hazards and national policymaking.* Washington, D.C.: The Brookings Institution.

Francis, Donald. (1994). Insulating public health from extremist politics—do we need boards of health? *American Journal of Public Health, 84* (May), 720–721.

Gilbert, Benjamin, Merry K. Moos, & C. Arden Miller. (1982). State-level decision making for public health: The status of boards of health. *Journal of Public Health Policy, 3* (March), 51–63.

Gittler, Josephine. (1994). Controlling resurgent tuberculosis: Public health agencies, public policy and law. *Journal of Health Politics, Policy and Law, 19* (Spring), 107–148.

Gordon, Jeoffry B. (1969). The politics of community medicine projects: A conflict analysis. *Medical Care, 7* (November/December), 419–428.

Greenberg, George D. (1975). Reorganization—reconsidered: The U.S. public health service, 1960–1973. *Public Policy, 23* (Fall), 483–522.

Institute of Medicine Committee to Study the Future of Public Health. (1988). *The future of public health.* Washington, D.C.: National Academy Press.

Kaufman, Herbert. (1966). The political ingredient of public health services: A neglected area of research. *Milbank Memorial Fund Quarterly/Health and Society, 44* (October), Part 2, 13–34.

Klaus, Alisa. (1993). *Every child a lion: The origins of maternal and infant health policy in the United States and France, 1880–1920.* Ithaca, NY: Cornell University Press.

Krieger, Nancy. (1992). The making of public health data: Paradigms, politics and policy. *Journal of Public Health Policy, 13* (Winter), 412–427.

Levine, Adeline G. (1982). *Love Canal: Science, politics and people.* Lexington, MA: Lexington Books.

McFarlane, Deborah R., & Larry J. Gordon. (1992). Teaching health policy and politics in U.S. schools of public health. *Journal of Public Health Policy, 13* (Winter), 428–434.

McKinlay, John B. (1979). Epidemiological and political determinants of social policies regarding the public health. *Social Science and Medicine, 13A* (August), 541–558.

Mercy, James A., Mark L. Rosenberg, Kenneth E. Powell, Claire V. Broome, & William L. Roper. (1993). Public health policy for preventive violence. *Health Affairs, 12* (Winter), 7–29.

Meyer, Jack A., & Marion Ein Lewin. (Eds.). (1987). *Charting the future of health care: Policy, politics and public health*. Washington, D.C.: American Enterprise Institute for Public Policy Research.

Mullan, Fitzhugh. (1989). *Plagues and politics: The story of the United States public health service*. New York: Basic Books.

Pauly, Philip J. (1994). Is liquor intoxicating? Scientists, prohibition, and the normalization of drinking. *American Journal of Public Health, 84* (February), 305–313.

Roemer, Milton I. (1984) The politics of public health in the United States. In Theodor J. Litman & Leonard Robins (Eds.), *Health politics and policy* (1st ed., pp. 261–273). New York: John Wiley & Sons.

Roemer, Milton I. (1993). Joseph W. Mountain: Architect of modern public health. *Public Health Reports, 108* (November/December), 727–735.

Roper, William L., Jeffrey P. Kaplan, & Aaron A. Stinnett. (1994). Public health in the new American health system. *Frontiers of Health Services Management, 10* (Summer), 32–36.

Russell, Louise B. (1985). *Is prevention better than cure?* Washington, D.C.: The Brookings Institution.

Scott, H. Denman, John T. Tierney, & William J. Waters Jr. (1990). The future of public health: A survey of the states. *Journal of Public Health Policy, 11* (Fall), 296–304.

Snoke, Albert W. (1982). What good is legislation—or planning—if we can't make it work? Need for comprehensive approach to health and welfare. *American Journal of Public Health, 72* (September), 1028–1033.

Stone, Deborah A. (1986). The resistible rise of preventative medicine. *Journal of Health Politics, Policy and Law, 11* (4), 671–695.

Susser, Mervyn. (1993). Health as a human right: An epidemiologist's perspective on the public health. *American Journal of Public Health, 83* (March), 418–426.

Terris, Milton. (1990). Public health policy for the 1990s. *Journal of Public Health Policy, 11* (Autumn), 281–295.

Turshen, Meredeth. (1989). *The politics of public health*. New Brunswick, NJ: Rutgers University Press.

Rationing

Aaron, Henry J., & William B. Schwartz. (1984). *The painful prescription: Rationing hospital care*. Washington, D.C.: The Brookings Institution.

Blank, Robert H. (1988). *Rationing medicine*. New York: Columbia University Press.

Blumstein, James F. (1983). Rationing medical resources: A constitutional, legal and policy analysis. In President's Commission for the Study of Ethical Problems in Medical and Biomedical and Behavioral Research. *Securing access to health care* (Vol. 3, pp. 349–394). Washington, D.C.: U.S. Government Printing Office.

Brown, Lawrence D. (1991). The national politics of Oregon's rationing plan. *Health Affairs, 10* (Summer), 28–51.

Callahan, Daniel. (1988). *Setting limits: Medical goals in an aging society*. New York: Simon & Schuster.

Etzioni, Amitai. (1991). Health care rationing: A critical evaluation. *Health Affairs, 10* (Summer), 88–95.

Fox, Daniel M., & Howard M. Leichter. (1991). Rationing care in Oregon: The new accountability. *Health Affairs, 10* (Summer), 7–27.

Goold, Susan D. (1996). Allocating health care: Cost-utility analysis, informed democratic decision making, or the veil of ignorance? *Journal of Health Politics, Policy and Law, 21* (Spring), 69–98.

Hall, Mark A. (1993). Informed consent to rationing decisions. *Milbank Quarterly, 71* (4), 645–668.

Mariner, Wendy K. (1995). Rationing health care and the need for credible scarcity: Why Americans can't say no. *American Journal of Public Health, 95* (October), 1439–1445.

Mechanic, David. (1985). Cost containment and the quality of medical care: Rationing strategies in an era of constrained resources. *Milbank Memorial Fund Quarterly, 63* (Summer), 453–475.

Merrill, Jeffrey C., & Alan B. Cohen. (1987). The emperor's new clothes: Unraveling the myths about rationing. *Inquiry, 24* (Summer), 105–109.

Reagan, Michael D. (1988). Health care rationing: What does it mean? *New England Journal of Medicine, 319* (October 27), 1149–1151.

Strosberg, Martin, Joshua M. Wiener, & Robert Baker. (Eds.). (1992). *Rationing America's medical care. The Oregon plan and beyond.* Washington, D.C.: The Brookings Institution.

Smoking and Tobacco

Altman, David G., et al. (1992). Policy alternatives for reducing tobacco sales to minors: Results from a national survey of retail chain and franchise stores. *Journal of Public Health, 13* (Autumn), 318–331.

Barnes, Deborah E., & Lisa A. Bero. (1996). Industry funded research and conflict of interest: An analysis of research sponsored by the tobacco industry through the Center for Indoor Air Research. *Journal of Health Politics, Policy and Law, 21* (Fall), 515–542.

Breslow, Lester, & Michael Johnson. (1993). California's Proposition 99 on tobacco and its impact. *Annual Review of Public Health, 14,* 585–604.

Brumback, Clarence L. (1980). The politics of smoking prevention: A report from the field. *Journal of Public Health Policy, 2* (March), 36–41.

Califano, Joseph A. Jr. (1994). Editorial—revealing the link between campaign financing and deaths caused by tobacco. *Journal of the American Medical Association, 272* (October 19), 1217–1218.

Flewelling, Robert L., Erin Kenney, John Pierce, Michael Johnson, et al. (1992). First-year impact of the 1989 California cigarette tax increase on cigarette consumption. *American Journal of Public Health, 82* (June), 867–869.

Fritschler, A. Lee. (1975). *Smoking and politics: Policymaking and the federal bureaucracy.* Englewood Cliffs, NJ: Prentice-Hall.

Glantz, Stanton A., & Michael E. Begay. (1994). Tobacco industry campaign contributions are affect-

ing tobacco control policymaking in California. *Journal of the American Medical Association, 272* (October 19), 1176–1182.

Glantz, Stanton, A., John Slade, Lisa A. Bero, Peter Hamauer, & Deborah Barnes. (1996). *The cigarette papers.* Berkeley: University of California Press.

Jacobson, Peter D., Jeffrey Wasserman, & Kristina Raube. (1993). The politics of antismoking legislation. *Journal of Health Politics, Policy and Law, 18* (Winter), 787–820.

Joseph, Anne M. (1994). Is Congress blowing smoke at the VA? *Journal of the American Medical Association, 272* (October 19), 1215–1216.

Koplin, Allen N. (1981). Anti-smoking legislation: The New Jersey experience. *Journal of Public Health Policy, 2* (September), 247–255.

Lewitt, Eugene M., & Douglas Coate. (1982). The potential for using excise taxes to reduce smoking. *Journal of Health Economics, 1* (August), 121–145.

Lupton, Deborah. (1995). *The imperative of health: Public health and the regulated body.* Thousand Oaks, CA: Sage.

McGowan, Richard. (1995). *Business, politics and cigarettes: Multiple levels, multiple agendas.* Westport, CT: Greenwood Publishing.

Meyer, John A. (1992). Cigarette century. *American Heritage, 43* (December), 72–89.

Moon, Robert W., Michael A. Males, & David E. Nelson. (1993). The 1990 Montana initiative to increase cigarette taxes: Lesson for other states and localities. *Journal of Public Health Policy, 14* (Spring), 19–33.

Moore, Stephen, Sidney M. Wolfe, Deborah Lindes, & Clifford E. Douglas. (1994). Epidemiology of failed tobacco control legislation. *Journal of the American Medical Association, 272* (October 19), 1171–1175.

Novotny, Thomas E., et al. (1992). The public health practice of tobacco control—lessons learned and directions for the states in the 1990s. *Annual Review of Public Health, 13,* 287–318.

Novotny. Thomas E., & Michael B. Siegal. (1996). California's tobacco control saga. *Health Affairs, 15* (Spring), 58–72.

Peterson, Dan, Scott Zeger, Patrick Remington, & Henry Anderson. (1992). The effect of state cigarette tax increases on cigarette sales, 1955–1988. *American Journal of Public Health, 82* (January), 94–96.

Rabin, Robert L., & Stephen D. Sugarman. (Eds.). (1993). *Smoking policy: Law, politics and culture.* New York: Oxford University Press.

Taylor, Peter. (1984). *The smoke ring: Tobacco, money and multinational politics.* New York: Pantheon Books.

Traynor, Michael P., & Stanton A. Glantz. (1996). California's tobacco intitiative: The development and passage of Proposition 99. *Journal of Health Politics, Policy and Law, 21* (Fall), 543–586.

Wasserman, Jeffrey. (1992). How effective are excise tax increases in reducing cigarette smoking? *American Journal of Public Health, 82* (January), 19–20.

Wasserman, Jeffrey, William G. Manning, Joseph P. Newhouse, & John D. Winkler. (1991). The effects of excise taxes and regulations on cigarette smoking. *Journal of Health Economics, 10* (May), 43–64.

THE POLITICAL ECONOMY OF HEALTH

Alford, Robert R. (1972). The political economy of health care: Dynamics without change. *Politics and Society, 2* (Winter), 126–164.

Bodenheimer, Thomas S. (1989). The fruits of empire rot on the vine: United States health policy in the austerity era. *Social Science and Medicine, 28* (6), 531–538.

Bowler, M. Kenneth, Robert T. Kudrle, & Theodore R. Marmor. (1977). The political economy of national health insurance: Policy analysis and political evaluation. In Kenneth M. Friedman & Stuart H. Rakoff (Eds.), *Toward a national health policy: Public policy and the control of health care costs.* Lexington, MA: Lexington Books.

Bowler, M. Kenneth, Robert T. Kudrle, Theodore R. Marmor, & Amy Bridges. (1977). Political economy of national health insurance—policy analysis and political evaluation. *Journal of Health Politics, Policy and Law, 2* (Spring), 100–133.

Brenner, M. Harvey. (1977). Health costs and benefits of economic policy. *International Journal of Health Services, 7* (4), 581–623.

Campen, James T. (1986). *Benefit, cost and beyond: The political economy of benefit–cost analysis.* Cambridge, MA: Ballinger.

Dowie, Jack. (1985). The political economy of the NHS: Individualist justifications of collective action. *Social Science and Medicine, 20* (10), 1041–1048.

Doyal, Lesley, with Imogen Pennell. (1991). *The political economy of health.* New Brunswick, NJ: Westview Press.

Eyer, Joseph. (1977). Does unemployment cause the death rate peak in each business cycle? A multifactor model of death rate change. *International Journal of Health Services, 7* (4), 625–662.

Feldman, Roger, & Micheal A. Morresey. (1990). Report from the field—health economics. *Journal of Health Politics, Policy and Law, 15* (Fall), 627–646.

Feldstein, Paul J. (1977). *Health associations and the demand for legislation: The political economy of health.* Cambridge, MA: Ballinger.

Feldstein, Paul J. (1993). *Health care economics* (4th ed.). Albany, NY: Delmar.

Feldstein, Paul J. (1994). *Health policy issues: An economic perspective on health reform.* Ann Arbor, MI: AUPHA Press/Health Administration Press.

Frech, H. E., III. (Ed.). (1988). *Health care in America: The political economy of hospitals and health insurance.* San Francisco: Pacific Research Institute for Public Policy.

Fuchs, Victor R. (1986). *The health economy.* Cambridge, MA: Harvard University Press.

Ginzberg, Eli. (1965). The political economy of health. *Bulletin New York Academy of Medicine, 41* (October), 1015–1036.

Gritzer, Glenn, & Arnold Arluke. (1985). *The making of rehabilitation: A political economy of medical specialization.* Berkeley: University of California Press.

Hall, Mark A. (1992). Political economics of insurance market reform. *Health Affairs, 11* (Summer), 108–124.

Hammerle, Nancy. (1994). *Private choices, social costs and public policy: An economic analysis of public health issues*. Westport, CT: Praeger.

Helt, Eric H. (1973). Economic determinism: A model of the political economy of medical care. *International Journal of Health Services, 3* (3), 475–485.

Himmelstein, David U., Steffie Woolhandler, & David H. Bor. (1988). Will cost effectiveness analysis worsen the cost effectiveness of health care? *International Journal of Health Services, 18* (1), 1–10.

Hollingsworth, J. Rogers. (1986). *A political economy of medicine: Great Britain and the United States*. Baltimore, MD: Johns Hopkins University Press.

Iglehart, John K. (1989). A conversation with William B. Schwartz. *Health Affairs, 8* (Fall), 60–75.

Iglehart John K. (1990). Perspectives of an errant economist: A conversation with Tom Schelling. *Health Affairs, 9* (Summer), 109–121.

Kelman, Sander. (1971). Toward the political economy of medical care. *Inquiry, 8* (September), 30–38.

Kelman, Sander. (1975a). Introduction to the theme: The political economy of health. *International Journal of Health Services, 5* (4), 535–538.

Kelman, Sander. (1975b). Special section on political economy of health. *International Journal of Health Services, 5* (4), 535–693.

Kelman, Sander. (1977). Toward the political economy of medical care. In Lewis E. Weeks & Howard J. Berman (Eds.), *Economics in health care* (pp. 39–48). Germantown, MD: Aspen Systems Corp.

Klein, Rudolph. (1972). The political economy of national health: Report from London. *The Public Interest, 26* (Winter), 112–125.

Krause, Elliot A. (1971). Health and the politics of technology. *Inquiry, 8* (September), 51–59.

Krause, Elliot A. (1977). *Power and illness: The political sociology of health and medical care*. New York: Elsevier North-Holland.

Lichtman, R. (1971). The political economy of medical care. In Hans Peter Dreitzel (Ed.), *The social organization of health*. New York: Macmillan.

Markowitz, Gerald, & David Rosner. (1986). More than economism: The politics of worker's safety and health, 1932–1947. *Milbank Quarterly, 64* (3), 331–354.

Marmor, Theodore R., Amy Bridges, & Wayne L. Hoffman. (1978). Comparative politics and health policies: Notes on benefits, costs and limits. In Douglas E. Ashford (Ed.), *Company public policies: New concepts and methods* (pp. 59–80). Beverly Hills, CA: Sage.

Marmor, Theodore R., & Jon B. Christianson. (1982). *Health care policy: A political economy approach*. Beverly Hills, CA: Sage.

Maynard, Alan. (1986). Public and private sector interactions: An economic perspective. *Social Science and Medicine, 22* (11), 1161–1166.

McGuire, A. (1986). Ethics and resource allocation: An economist's view. *Social Science and Medicine, 22* (11), 1167–1174.

McKinlay, John B. (1979). A case for refocusing upstream: The political economy of illness. In E. Gartly Jaco (Ed.), *Patients, physicians and illness* (3rd ed., pp. 9–26). New York: The Free Press.

McKinlay, John B. (1984). *Issues in the political economy of health care*. New York: Tavistock Publications in association with Methuen, Inc.

Mendelson, Mary A., & David Hapgood. (1974). Political economy of nursing homes. *Annals of the American Academy of Political and Social Science, 415* (September), 95–105.

Morrisey, Michael A. (1994). *Cost shifting in health care: Separating evidence from rhetoric*. Washington, D.C.: AEI Press.

Navarro, Vicente. (1975). Political economy of medical care: An explanation of the composition, nature and functions of the present health sector of the United States. *International Journal of Health Services, 5* (1), 65–94.

Navarro, Vicente. (1976). The political and economic determinants of health and health care in rural America. *Inquiry, 13* (June), 111–121.

Navarro, Vicente. (1977). Social class, political power, and the state and their implications in medicine. *International Journal of Health Services, 7* (2), 255–292.

Navarro, Vicente. (1978). The crisis of the Western system of medicine in contemporary capitalism. *International Journal of Health Services, 8* (2), 179–211.

Navarro, Vicente. (1985a). The 1980 and 1984 U.S. elections and the new deal: An alternative interpretation. *International Journal of Health Services, 15* (3), 359–394.

Navarro, Vicente. (1985b). U.S. Marxist scholarship in the analysis of health and medicine. *International Journal of Health Services, 15* (4), 525–546.

Renaud, Marc. (1976). *The political economy of the Quebec state interventions in health: Reform or revolution?* Unpublished Ph.D. diss., University of Wisconsin.

Rice, Dorothy P., & Douglas Wilson. (1976). The American medical economy: Problems and perspectives. *Journal of Health Politics, Policy and Law, 1* (Summer), 150–172.

Russell, Louise B. (1992). Opportunity costs in modern medicine. *Health Affairs, 11* (Summer), 162–169.

Russell, Louise B., & Carol S. Burke. (1978). The political economy of federal health programs in the United States: An historical review. *International Journal of Health Services, 8* (1), 55–77.

Schatzkin, Arthur. (1978). Health and labor-power: A theoretical investigation. *International Journal of Health Services, 8* (2), 213–234.

Scitovsky, Anne A. (1988). The economic impact of AIDS in the United States. *Health Affairs, 7* (Fall), 32–45.

Somers, Herman M. (1977). Observations on policy and politics in the health care economy. In Blue Cross Association (Eds.), *Health care in the American economy: Issues and forecasts.* Chicago, IL: Health Services Foundation.

Stevenson, Gelvin. (1978). Profits in medicine: A context and an accounting. *International Journal of Health Services, 8* (1), 41–54.

Waitzkin, Howard B. (1978). How capitalism cares for our coronaries: A preliminary exercise in political economy. In Eugene B. Gallagher (Ed.), *The doctor–patient relationship in the changing health scene* (DHEW Pub. No. [NIH] 78-183, pp. 317–332).

Washington, D.C.: U.S. Government Printing Office.

Windham, Susan R. (1977). *National health insurance as an issue in political economy—The implications of the Kennedy Health Security Act for developing a strategy to effect major reorganization of health care delivery in America.* Unpublished Ph.D. diss., Brandeis University.

GOVERNMENT AND HEALTH

Aday, Lu Ann, Ronald Andersen, & Gretchen V. Fleming. (1980). *Health care in the U.S.: Equitable for whom?* Beverly Hills, CA: Sage.

Amara, Roy, Gregory Schmid, & J. Ian Morrison. (1988). *Looking ahead at American health care.* Washington, D.C.: McGraw-Hill.

American Nursing Home Association, Government Relations Department. (1973). *An analysis and partial legislative history of Title II of Public Law: 92-603 (H.R.I.), The Social Security amendments of 1972.* Washington, D.C.: American Nursing Home Association.

Anderson, Odin W. (1968). *The uneasy equilibrium: Private and public financing of health services in the U.S., 1865–1975.* New Haven, CT: College & University Press.

Anderson, Odin W. (1985.). *The American health services: A growth enterprise since 1875.* Ann Arbor, MI: Health Administration Press.

Anderson, Odin W. (1988). Government health insurance and privatization: An examination of the concept of equality. *International Journal of Health Planning and Management, 3* (1), 35–43.

Bayer, Ronald, & Jonathan D. Moreno. (1986). Health promotion: Ethical and social dilemmas of government policy. *Health Affairs, 5* (Summer), 72–85.

Beauchamp, Dan E. (1988). *The health of the Republic: Epidemic, medicine, and moralism as challenges for democracy.* Philadelphia: Temple University Press.

Becker, Dorothy D., & Ruth R. Johnson. (1980). *Chronology of health professions legislation, 1956–1979* (DHHS Publication No. [HRA] 80-69).

Washington, D.C.: U.S. Government Printing Office.

Blumstein, James F. (1989). Government's role in organ transplantation policy. *Journal of Health Politics, Policy and Law, 14* (Spring), 5–40.

Blumstein, James F., & Michael Zubkoff. (1973). Perspectives on government policy in the health sector. *Milbank Memorial Fund Quarterly/Health and Society, 51* (Summer), 395–431.

Bredder, Roy. (1994). *Federal health laws, 1990–1993.* Washington, D.C.: Faulkner & Gray, Inc.

Brian, Earl W. (1972). Government control of hospital utilization: A California experience. *New England Journal of Medicine, 286* (June 22), 1340–1344.

Burger, Edward J., Jr. (1976). *Protecting the nation's health: The problems of regulation.* Lexington, MA: Lexington Books.

Caplan, Arthur L., Robert H. Blank, & Janna C. Merrick. (Eds.). (1992). *Compelled compassion: Government intervention in the treatment of critically ill newborns.* Totowa, NJ: Humana.

Carey, Sarah C. (1974). A constitutional right to health care: An unlikely development. *Catholic University of America Law Review, 23* (Spring), 492–514.

Carlton, William G. (1977). Government and health before the New Deal. *Current History, 72* (May/June), 196–197, 223–226.

Carnegie Council on Policy Studies in Higher Education. (1976). *Progress and problems in medical and dental education: Federal support versus federal control.* San Francisco: Jossey-Bass.

Chapman, Carleton B., & John M. Talmadge. (1970). Historical and political background of federal health care legislation. *Law and Contemporary Problems, 35* (Spring), 334–347.

Chapman, Carleton B., & John M. Talmadge. (1971). The evolution of the right to health concept in the United States. *Pharos, 35* (January), 30–51.

Clark, Duncan W. (1973). Politics and health services research: A cameo study of policy in the health services in the 1930's. In E. Evelyn Flook & Paul J. Sanazaro (Eds.), *Health services and R&D in perspective* (pp. 109–125). Ann Arbor, MI: Health Research Administration Press.

Clark, Robert L., & John A. Menefee. (1981). Federal expenditures for the elderly: Past and future. *The Gerontologist, 21* (2), 132–137.

Cohen, Elias S. (1973). Integration of health and social services in federally funded programs. *Bulletin of the New York Academy of Medicine, 49* (December), 1038–1050.

Cooper, Barbara S., & Nancy L. Worthington. (1974). *Comparison of cost and benefit incidence of government medical care programs, fiscal years 1966 and 1969.* Office of Research and Statistics (DHEW Pub. No. [SSA] 75-11852, Staff Paper No. 18). Washington, D.C.: U.S. Government Printing Office.

Darling, Helen. (1986). The role of the federal government in assuring access to health care. *Inquiry, 23* (Fall), 286–295.

Davis, Karen, Marsha Lillie-Blanton, Barbara Lyons, Fitzhugh Mullan, et al. (1987). Health care for black Americans: The public sector role. *Milbank Memorial Fund Quarterly, 65* (Suppl.), 213–247.

Densen, Paul M. (1973). Public accountability and reporting systems in Medicare and other health programs. *New England Journal of Medicine, 289* (August 23), 401–406.

Detwiller, Lloyd F. (1971). The right to health. *Hospitals, 45* (February 16), 63–66.

Detwiller, Lloyd F. (1972). *The consequences of health care through government* (Research Publication No. 6, October). Sydney, Australia: The Office of Health Care Finance.

Detwiller, Lloyd F. (1984). Implications and consequences of government involvement in health and health care. In Theodor J. Litman & Leonard S. Robins (Eds.), *Health politics and policy* (pp. 81–96). New York: John Wiley & Sons.

Dougherty, Charles J. (1988). *American health care: Realities, rights, and reforms.* New York: Oxford University Press.

Dowell, Michael A. (1987). Hill–Burton: The unfulfilled promise. *Journal of Health Politics, Policy and Law, 12* (January), 153–175.

Etheredge, Lynn. (1986). Government and health care costs: The influences of research policy. In Marion

E. Lewin (Ed.), *From research into policy: Improving the link from health services* (pp. 7–19). Washington, D.C.: American Enterprise Institute for Public Policy Research.

Evans, Robert G. (1984). *Illusions of necessity: Evading responsibility for choice in health care.* University of British Columbia, Department of Economics.

Evans, Robert G. (1985). Illusions of necessity: Evading responsibility for choice in health care. *Journal of Health Politics, Policy and Law, 10* (Fall), 439–468.

Fenninger, Leonard D. (1973). Health manpower and the education of health personnel. *Inquiry, 10* (March, Suppl.), 56–60; Commentary, 61–73.

Feshbach, Dan. (1979). What's inside the black box: A case study of allocative politics in the Hill–Burton program. *International Journal of Health Services, 9* (2), 313–339.

Foley, Henry A. (1975). *Community mental health legislation: The formative process.* Lexington, MA: Lexington Books.

Fox, Peter D. (1972). Access to medical care for the poor: The federal perspective. *Medical Care, 10* (May/June), 272–277.

Frank, Kenneth D. (1972). Government support of nursing home care. *New England Journal of Medicine, 287* (September 14), 538–545.

Freedman, Benjamin, & Francoise Baylis. (1987). Purpose and function in government-funded health coverage. *Journal of Health Politics, Policy and Law, 12* (Spring), 97–112.

Friedman, Kenneth M., & Stuart H. Rakoff. (1977). *Toward a national health policy: Public policy and the control of health care costs.* Lexington, MA: D. C. Heath.

Ginzberg, Eli. (1965). The political economy of health. *Bulletin of the New York Academy of Medicine, 41* (October), 1015–1036.

Ginzberg, Eli. (1985). The restructuring of U.S. health care. *Inquiry, 22* (Fall), 272–281.

Ginzberg, Eli. (Ed.). (1985). *The U.S. health care system: A look to the 1990's.* Totowa, NJ: Rowman and Allanheld.

Grogan, Colleen M. (1991). *A political theory to explain the variation in state Medicaid policies.* Unpublished Ph.D. diss., University of Minnesota.

Grogan, Colleen M. (1993). Federalism and health care reform. *American Behavioral Scientist, 36* (July), 741–759.

Havighurst, Clark C. (1977). Controlling health care costs: Strengthening the private sector. *Journal of Health Politics, Policy and Law, 1* (Winter), 471–498.

Health Resources Administration. (1977). *Health resources studies: Government controls on the health care system: The Canadian experience* (DHEW Pub. No. [HRA] 77-246). Washington, D.C.: U.S. Government Printing Office.

Himmelstein, David U., & Steffie Woolhandler. (1986). Cost without benefit: Administrative waste in U.S. health care. *New England Journal of Medicine, 314* (February 13), 441–445.

Iglehart, John K. (1978). The Carter administration's health budget: Charting new priorities with limited dollars. *Milbank Memorial Fund Quarterly/Health and Society, 56* (Winter), 53–77.

Jaeger, Boi Jon. (1972). Government and hospitals: A perspective on health politics. *Hospital Administration, 17* (Winter), 39–50.

Jonas, Steven, David Banta, & Michael Enright. (1977). Government in the health care delivery system. In Steven Jonas (Ed.), *Health care delivery in the United States* (pp. 289–328). New York: Springer Publishing Co.

Katz, Daniel, et al. (1975). *Bureaucratic encounters: A pilot study in the evaluation of government services.* Ann Arbor: University of Michigan, Institute for Social Research.

Kennedy, Edward M. (1978). The Congress and national health policy. *American Journal of Public Health, 68* (March), 241–244.

Kennedy, Virginia C. (1976). Interpreting legislative voting patterns on health issues: A method and rationale. *Journal of Community Health, 1* (Spring), 188–195.

Kessel, Reuben A. (1977). *Ethical and economic aspects of governmental intervention in the medical care market.* Washington, D.C.: American Enterprise Institute, Center for Health Policy Research.

Klarman, Herbert E. (1974). Major pubic initiatives in health care. *Public Interest, 34* (Winter), 106–123.

Lally, John J. (1977). Social determinants of differential allocation of resources to disease research: A comparative analysis of crib death and cancer research. *Journal of Health and Social Behavior, 18* (June), 125–138.

Lashof, Joyce C., & Mark H. Lepper. (1976). Federal–state local partnership in health. In Health Resource Administration USPHS (Ed.), *Health in America: 1877–1976* (pp. 122–137). Washington, D.C.: U.S. Government Printing Office.

Lave, Judith, & Lester Lave. (1974). *The Hospital Construction Act: An evaluation of the Hill–Burton program, 1948–1973.* Washington, D.C.: American Enterprise Institute for Public Policy Research.

Leroy, Lauren, & Philip R. Lee. (Eds.). (1977). *Deliberations and compromise: The Health Professions Educational Assistance Act of 1976.* Cambridge, MA: Ballinger.

Lostetter, John C., & John E. Chapman. (1979). The participation of the United States government in providing financial support for medical education. *Health Policy and Education, 1* (1), 27–65.

Marmor, T., & D. Thomas. (1971). The politics of paying physicians: The determinants of government payment methods in England, Sweden and the United States. *International Journal of Health Services, 1* (1), 71–78.

Marmor, Theodore R. (1975). Origins of the government health insurance issue. In David Kotelchuck (Ed.), *Prognosis negative: Crisis in the health care system* (pp. 293–303). New York: Vintage Books.

McEwan, E. D. (1973). A case for government sponsored health care research and development in the formulation of health policy and an account of early experience of government-sponsored health care research in one jurisdiction. *International Journal of Health Services, 3* (1), 45–58.

McFarlane, Deborah R., & Kenneth J. Meier. (1993). Restructuring federalism: The impact of research policies on the family planning program. *Journal of Health Politics, Policy and Law, 18* (Winter), 821–850.

McNeil, Richard Jr., & Robert E. Schlenker. (1975). HMOs, competition and government. *Milbank Memorial Fund Quarterly/Health and Society, 53* (Spring), 195–224.

Meilicke, Carl A. (1967). *The Saskatchewan medical care dispute of 1962: An analytic social history.* Unpublished Ph.D. diss., University of Minnesota.

Monheit, Alan C. (1990). Returns on U.S. health care expenditures. *Journal of Medical Practice Management, 6* (Summer), 7–13.

Mooney, Anne. (1977). The Great Society and health: Policies for narrowing the gaps in health status between the poor and the nonpoor. *Medical Care, 15* (August), 611–619.

Moran, Michael. (1995). Three faces of the health care state. *Journal of Health Politics, Policy and Law, 20* (Fall), 767–783. Commentary: The health care state in global perspective. 783–786.

Morford, Thomas G. (1989). Federal efforts to improve peer review organizations. *Health Affairs, 9* (Summer), 175–178.

Morris, Jonas. (1984). *Searching for a cure.* New York: Pica Press.

Naimark, Arnold. (1978). Ethical questions posed by community and government pressures on medical education in Canada. *Bulletin of the New York Academy of Medicine, 54* (July/August), 687–696.

Neustadt, Richard E., & Harvey V. Fineberg. (1978). *The swine flu affair: Decision-making on a slippery disease.* Washington, D.C.: U.S. Government Printing Office.

Palley, Howard A. (1974). Policy formulation in health, some considerations of governmental constraints on pricing in the health delivery system. *American Behavioral Scientist, 7* (March/April), 572–584.

Parmet, Wendy E. (1993). Regulation and federalism: Legal impediments to state health care reforms. *American Journal of Law and Medicine, 19* (1/2), 121–144.

Phelps, Charles E. (1976). Public sector medicine: History and analysis. In Institute for Contemporary Studies (Ed.), *New directions in public health care:*

An evaluation of proposals for national health insurance. San Francisco, CA: Institute for Contemporary Studies.

Polsky, Andrew J. (1991). *The rise of the therapeutic state.* Princeton, NJ: Princeton University Press.

Raffel, Marshall W., & Norma K. Raffel. (1989). *The U.S. health system: Origins and functions.* Media, PA: Harwal Publishing Co.

Rakoff, Stuart H., & Kenneth M. Friedman. (1989). Health, health costs and the role of government. In Kenneth M. Friedman & Stuart H. Rakoff (Eds.), *Toward a national health policy: Public policy and the control of health care costs.* Lexington, MA: Lexington Books.

Renn, Steven. (1987). The structure and financing of the health care delivery system in the 1980's. In Carl J. Schramm (Ed.), *Health care and its costs: Can the U.S. afford adequate care?* (pp. 8–48). New York: W. W. Norton.

Rhein, Reginald W., & Larry Marion. (1977). *The saccharin controversy: A guide for consumers.* New York: Monarch Press.

Roemer, Milton I., & Mary H. McClanahan. (1960). Impact of government programs on voluntary hospitals. *Public Health Reports, 75* (June), 537–544.

Rohrer, James E. (1977). The political development of the Hill–Burton program: A case study in distributive policy. *Journal of Health Politics, Policy and Law, 12* (Spring), 137–152.

Rudolph, Ronald J. (1976). *Physician care and government programs: Analysis of the distribution of health and health services in New York City and the nation.* Unpublished Ph.D. diss., Rutgers University.

Russell, Louise R. (1976). Inflation and the federal role in health. In Michael Zubkoff (Ed.), *Health: Victim or cause of inflation?* (pp. 225–244). New York: Neale Watson Academic Publishers, Prodist.

Sade, Robert M. (1971). Medical care as a right: A refutation. *New England Journal of Medicine, 285* (December 2), 1288–1292.

Schelling, Thomas C. (1976). Government and health. In Institute for Contemporary Studies (Ed.), *New directions for public health care: An evaluation of proposals for national health insurance.* San Francisco: Institute for Contemporary Studies.

Schlesinger, Edward R. (1974). The impact of federal legislation on maternal and child health services in the United States. *Milbank Memorial Fund Quarterly/Health and Society, 52* (Winter), 1–13.

Schlesinger, Edward R., Martha M. Skoner, Estelle D. Trooskin, Janet R. Markel, & A. Frederick North. (1976). The effects of anticipated funding changes on maternal and child health projects: A case study of uncertainty. *American Journal of Public Health, 66* (April), 385–388.

Schramm, Carl J. (Ed.). (1987). *Health care and its costs: Can the U.S. afford adequate care?* New York: W. W. Norton.

Schwartz, Joshua I. (1977). *Public health: Case studies on the origins of government responsibility for health services in the United States.* New York: Cornell University Program in Urban and Regional Studies.

Shonick, William. (1995). *Government and health services: Government's role in the development of U.S. Health services, 1930–1980.* New York: Oxford University Press.

Shuck, Peter H. (1989). Government funding for organ transplants. *Journal of Health Politics, Policy and Law, 14* (Spring), 169–190.

Snoke, Albert W. (1982). What good is legislation—or planning—if we can't make it work? The need for a comprehensive approach to health and welfare. *American Journal of Public Health, 72* (September), 1028–1033.

Sobel, Lester A. (1976). *Health care: An American crisis.* New York: Facts on File.

Somers, Herman M. (1975). Health and public policy. *Inquiry, 12* (June), 87–96.

Steiner, Gilbert Y. (1976). *The children's cause.* Washington, D.C.: The Brookings Institution.

Stevens, Robert, & Rosemary Stevens. (1974). *Welfare medicine in America: A case study of Medicaid.* New York: The Free Press.

Strickland, Stephen P. (1972). Medical research: Public policy and power politics. In Douglass Cater & Philip R. Lee (Eds.), *Politics of health.* New York: Medcom Press.

Strickland, Stephen P. (1978). *Research and the health of Americans: Improving the policy process.* Lexington, MA: Lexington Books.

Stuart, Bruce C. (1972). Who gains from pubic health programs. *Annals of American Academy of Political and Social Science, 399* (January), 145–150.

Walsh, Margaret E. (1974). *The health profession educational organization and the governmental process.* New York: National League for Nursing.

Wikler, Daniel I. (1978). Persuasion and coercion for health: Ethical issues in government efforts to change life-styles. *Milbank Memorial Fund Quarterly/Health and Society, 56* (Summer), 303–338.

Williams, A. P. Jr., et al. (1976). *Policy analysis for federal biomedical research* (Rand Report No. R-1945-PBRPJRC). Santa Monica, CA: Rand Corporation.

Wilson, Florence, & Duncan Neuhauser. (1985). *Health services in the United States.* Cambridge, MA: Ballinger.

Wilson, Walter A. (1973). The future role of government in dental practice and education. *Journal of the American College of Dentists, 40* (April), 111–116.

Wing, Kenneth R. (1976). *The law and the public's health.* St. Louis, MO: Mosby Co.

Zubkoff, Michael, & James Blumstein. (1976). *Framework for government intervention in the health sector.* Lexington, MA: D. C. Heath.

Some Foreign Comparisons

General

Abel-Smith, Brian. (1976). *Value for money in health services: A comparative study.* New York: St. Martin's.

Abel-Smith, Brian. (1984). *Cost containment in health care: A study of 12 European countries 1977–1983* (Occassional Papers on Social Administration No. 73). Bedford, UK: London Square Press.

Abel-Smith, Brian. (1985). Global perspective on health service financing. *Social Science and Medicine, 21* (9), 957–963.

Altenstetter, Christa. (1974a). *Health policy making and administration in West Germany and the United States.* Beverly Hills, CA: Sage.

Altenstetter, Christa. (1974b). Medical interests and the public interest: A comparison of West Germany and the United States. *International Journal of Health Services, 4* (Winter), 29–48.

Anderson, Gerard F., Jordi Alonzo, Linda T. Kohn, & Charles Black. (1994). Analyzing health outcomes through international comparisons. *Medical Care, 32* (May), 521–534.

Anderson, Odin W. (1989). *The health services continuum in democratic states: An inquiry into solvable problems.* Ann Arbor, MI: Health Administration Press.

Arnould, Richard J., Robert F. Rich, & William K. White. (1993). *Comparative approaches to health care reform.* Washington, D.C.: Urban Institute Press.

Banta, H. David, & Bryan R. Luce. (1993). *Health care technology and its assessment: An international perspective.* New York: Oxford University Press.

Barer, Morris, Amiram Gafni, & Jonathan Lomas. (1989). Accommodating rapid growth in physician supply: Lessons from Israel, warnings for Canada. *International Journal of Health Services, 19* (1), 95–116.

Barer, Morris L., W. Pete Welch, & Laurie Antioch. (1991). Canadian/U.S. health care: Reflections on the HIAA's analysis. *Health Affairs, 10* (Fall), 229–236.

Bates, Erica. (1983). *Health systems and public scrutiny: Australia, Britain and the United States.* New York: St. Martin's Press.

Berlant, Jeffrey L. (1975). *Profession and monopoly: A study of medicine in the United States and Great Britain.* Berkeley: University of California Press.

Blanpain, Jan. (1978). *National health insurance and health resources: The European experience.* Cambridge, MA: Harvard University Press.

Blendon, Robert J. (1989). Three systems: A comparative survey. *Health Management Quarterly, 11* (1), 2–10.

Blendon, Robert J., Robert Leitman, Ian Morrison, & Karen Donelan. (1990). Satisfaction with health systems in ten nations. *Health Affairs, 9* (Summer), 185–192.

Blendon, Robert J., & Humphrey Taylor. (1989). Views on health care: Public opinion in three nations. *Health Affairs, 8* (Spring), 149–157.

Boyle, Torrey, Barbara Jacobs, & Eva Jacobs. (1993). More than loose change: Household health spending in the United States and Canada. *Health Affairs, 12* (Spring), 126–131.

Chernichovsky, Dov. (1995). Health system reforms in industrialized democracies: An emerging paradigm. *Milbank Quarterly, 73* (3), 339–372.

Clauser, Steven B., & Brant E. Fries. (1992). Nursing home resident assessment and case-mix classification: Cross-national perspectives. *Health Care Financing Review, 13* (Summer), 135–156.

Conrad, Peter, & Eugene Gallagher (Eds.). (1993). *Health and health care in developing countries: Sociological perspectives.* Philadelphia: Temple University Press.

Crichton, Anne. (1980). *Health policy making.* Ann Arbor, MI: Health Administration Press.

Cumper, George E. (1991). *Evaluation of national health systems.* Cary, NC: Oxford University Press.

Cuyler, A. J., & Bengt Jonsson. (Eds.). (1987). *Public and private health services.* London: Basil Blackwell.

deKervasdóue, Jean, John R. Kimberly, & Victor Rodin. (Eds.). (1984). *The end of an illusion: The future of health policy in western industrialized nations.* Berkeley: University of California Press.

deSwaan, Abram. (1989). *In care of the state: Health care education and welfare in Europe and the U.S.A. in the modern era.* New York: Oxford University Press.

Elling, Ray H. (1980). *Cross-national study of health systems: Concepts, methods and data sources: A guide to information sources.* Detroit, MI: Gale Research Co.

Elling, Ray H. (1980). *Cross-national study of health systems: Political economics and health care.* New Brunswick, NJ: Transaction Books.

Fee, Elizabeth, & Roy M. Acheson. (Eds.). (1991). *A history of education and public health: Health that mocks the doctors' rules.* New York: Oxford University Press.

Field, Mark. (Ed.). (1989). *Success and crisis in national health systems: A comparative approach.* New York: Routledge.

Fox, Daniel M. (1986). *Health policies, health politics: The British and American experience, 1911–1965.* Princeton, NJ: Princeton University Press.

Freddi, Giorgio, & James W. Bjorkman. (Eds.). (1989). *Controlling medical professionals: The comparative politics of health governance.* Newbury Park, CA: Sage.

Fry, John, & W. A. J. Farndale. (Eds.). (1972). *International medical care: A comparison and evaluation of medical care services throughout the world.* Wallingsford, PA: Washington Square East Publishers.

Gerdtham, Ulf-G, & Bengt Jönsson. (1991). Price and quantity in international comparisons of health care expenditure. *Applied Economics, 23* (September), 1519–1528.

Gertler, Paul, & Jacques Van Der Gaag. (1991). *The willingness to pay for medical care: Evidence from two developing countries.* Baltimore, MD: Johns Hopkins University Press.

Glaser, William A. (1983). Paying the hospital: Foreign lessons for the United States. *Health Care Financing Review, 4* (Summer), 99–110.

Glaser, William A. (1984a). Health politics: Lessons from abroad. In Theodor J. Litman & Leonard S. Robins (Eds.), *Health politics and policy* (pp. 305–340). New York: John Wiley & Sons.

Glaser, William A. (1984b). Hospital rate regulation: American and foreign comparisons. *Journal of Health Politics, Policy and Law, 8* (Winter), 702–731.

Glaser, William A. (1984c). Juggling multiple payer: American problems and foreign solutions. *Inquiry, 21* (Summer), 178–188.

Glaser, William A. (1991). *Health insurance in practice: International variations in financing: Benefits, and problems.* San Francisco, CA: Jossey-Bass.

Glaser, William A. (1993a). *Comparative research methods: International comparisons of social security systems and policies.* Geneva: International Social Security Association.

Glaser, William A. (1993b). Universal health insurance that really works: Foreign lessons for the United States. *Journal of Health Politics, Policy and Law, 18* (Fall), 695–722.

Godt, Paul J. (1987). Confrontation, consent and corporatism: State strategies and the medical profession in France, Great Britain and West Germany. *Journal of Health Politics, Policy and Law, 12* (Fall), 459–480.

Goggin, Janice M. (1995). Commentary: The health care state in global perspective. *Journal of Health Politics, Policy and Law, 20* (Fall), 783–786.

Graig, Laurence A. (1993). *Health of nations: An international perspective on U.S. health care reform.* Washington, D.C.: Congressional Quarterly Books.

Greenberg, Linda G. (1991). International health grant making. *Health Affairs, 10* (Fall), 246–250.

Gross, David, Jonathan Ratner, James Perez, & Sarah L. Glavin. (1994). International pharmaceutical spending controls: France, Germany, Sweden, and the United Kingdom. *Health Care Financing Review, 15* (Spring), 127–140.

Grumbach, Kevin, & Thomas Bodenheimer. (1995). The organization of health care. *Journal of the American Medical Association, 273* (January 11), 160–167.

Hafferty, Frederic W. & John B. McKinlay. (Eds.). (1993). *The changing medical profession: An international perspective.* New York: Oxford University Press.

Ham, Chris, & Mats Brommers. (1994). Health care reform in the Netherlands, Sweden and the United Kingdom. *Health Affairs, 13* (Winter), 106–119.

Hayes, Gregory J., Steven C. Hayes, & Thane Dykstra. (1993). Physicians who have practiced in both the United States and Canada compare systems. *American Journal of Public Health, 83* (November), 1544–1548.

Helms, Robert B. (Ed.). (1993). *Health care policy and politics: Lessons from four countries.* Waldorf, MD: AEI Press.

Himmelstein, David U., James P. Lewontin, & Steffie Woolhandler. (1996). Who administers? Who cares? Medical administrative and clinical employment in the United States and Canada. *American Journal of Public Health, 86* (February), 172–178.

Hollingsworth, J. Rogers. (1986). *A political economy of medicine: Great Britain and the United States.* Baltimore, MD: Johns Hopkins University Press.

Hollingsworth, J. Rogers, Jerald Hage, & Robert A. Hanneman. (1990). *State intervention in medical care: Consequences for Britain, France, Sweden and the United States, 1890–1970.* Ithaca, NY: Cornell University Press.

Hollingsworth, J. Rogers, & Ellen Jane Hollingsworth. (1992). Challenges in the provision of care for the chronically ill in the United Kingdom, Germany, and the United States. *Journal of Health Politics, Policy and Law, 17* (Winter), 869–878.

Hollingsworth, J. Rogers, & Ellen Jane Hollingsworth. (1994). *Care of the chronically and severely ill: Comparative social policies.* Hawthorne, NY: Aldine de Gruyter.

Hsiao, William C. (1992). What nations can learn from one another. *Journal of Health Politics, Policy and Law, 17* (Winter), 613–636.

Hsiao, William C., & James A. Morone. (Eds.). (1992). Comparative health policy. *Journal of Health Politics, Policy and Law, 17* (Winter).

Hurst, Jeremy W. (1991). Reforming health care in seven European nations. *Health Affairs, 10* (Fall), 7–21.

Hutton, John, Michael Borowitz, Inga Oleksy, & Bryan R. Luce. (1994). The pharmaceutical industry and health reform: Lessons from Europe. *Health Affairs, 13* (Summer), 98–111.

Iglehart, John K. (1991). Conference report: Health systems in three nations. *Health Affairs, 10* (Fall), 254–261.

Jacobs, Lawrence R. (1994). *The health of nations: Public opinion and the making of American and British health policy.* Ithaca, NY: Cornell University Press.

James, John H. (1995). Reforming the British National Health Service: Implementation problems in London. *Journal of Health Politics, Policy and Law, 20* (Spring), 191–210.

Kane, Robert L., et al. (1990). *Improving the health of older people: A world view.* New York: Oxford University Press.

Katz, Steven, Timothy P. Hofer, & Willard G. Manning. (1996). Physician use in Ontario and the United States: The impact of socioeconomic status and health status. *American Journal of Public Health, 86* (August), 520–524.

Klein, Rudolph. (1991). Risks and benefits of comparative studies: Notes from another shore. *Milbank Quarterly, 69* (2), 275–292.

Kohn, Robert, & Susan Radius. (1974). Two roads to health care: U.S. and Canadian policies, 1945–1975. *Medical Care, 12* (March), 189–201.

Kraam, R. J., J. Baldock, B. Davies, A. Evers, L. Johansson, M. Knaden, M. Thorslund, & C. Tunissen. (1991). *Care for the elderly: Significant innovations in three European countries.* Boulder, CO: Westview Press.

Lazenby, Helen C., Katharine R. Levit, Daniel R. Waldo, Gerald S. Adler, Suzanne W. Letsch, & Cathy A. Cowan. (1992). National health accounts: Lessons from the U.S. experience. *Health Care Financing Review, 13* (Summer), 89–104.

Leichter, Howard M. (1979). *Comparative approach to policy analysis: Health care policy in four nations.* New York: Cambridge University Press.

Leichter, Howard M. (1991). *Free to be foolish: Politics and health promotion in the United States and Great Britain.* Princeton, NJ: Princeton University Press.

Lemco, Jonathan. (Ed). (1995). *National health care: Lessons for the United States and Canada.* Ann Arbor: University of Michigan Press.

Litman, Theodor J. (1976). National health care systems. In Theodor J. Litman (Ed.), *The sociology of medicine and health care: A bibliography* (Chapter 10, pp. 556–581). San Francisco, CA: Boyd and Fraser Publications.

Litman, Theodor J., & Leonard Robins. (1971). Comparative analysis of health care systems—a sociopolitical approach. *Social Science and Medicine, 5* (December), 573–581.

Liu, Korbin, Marilyn Moon, Margaret Sulvetta, & Jutti Chawla. (1992). International infant mortality rankings: A look behind the numbers. *Health Care Financing Review, 13* (Summer), 105–118.

Lohr, Kathleen N., Karl Yordy, Patty F. Harrison, & Annetine C. Gelyns. (1992). Health care systems: Lessons from international comparisons. *Health Affairs, 11* (Winter), 239–241.

Lomas, Jonathan, Jane E. Sisk, & Barbara Stocking. (1993). From evidence to practice in the United States, the United Kingdom, and Canada. *Milbank Quarterly, 71* (3), 405–410.

Luft, Harold S. (1991). Translating U.S. HMO experience to other systems. *Health Affairs, 10* (Fall), 172–186.

MacLeod, Gordon K. (1994). International report: Health care financing reform in New Zealand. *Health Affairs, 13* (Fall), 210–215.

Marmor, Theodore R., Amy Bridges, & Wayne L. Hoffman. (1983). Comparative politics and health policies: Notes on benefits, costs, limits. In Theodore R. Marmor (Ed.), *Political analysis and American medical care* (pp. 45–60). New York: Cambridge University Press.

Maxwell, Robert J. (1981). *Health and wealth: An international study of health care spending.* Lexington, MA: Lexington Books, D. C. Heath and Co.

Mills, Anne, & Kenneth Lee. (Eds.). (1993). *Health economics research in developing countries.* New York: Oxford University Press.

Misztal, Barbara A., & David Moss. (Eds.). (1990). *Action on AIDS: National policies in comparative perspective.* Westport, CT: Greenwood Press.

Morone, James A. (1990). American political culture and the search for lessons from abroad. *Journal of Health Politics, Policy and Law, 15* (Spring), 129–143.

Navarro, Vicente. (1985). The public/private mix in the funding and delivery of health services: An international survey. *American Journal of Public Health, 75* (November), 1318–1320.

Newhouse, Joseph P., Geoffrey Anderson, & Leslie L. Roos. (1988). Hospital spending in the U.S. and Canada. *Health Affairs, 7* (Winter), 6–16.

Organization for Economic Cooperation and Development. (1992a). *The reform of health care: A comparative analysis of seven OECD countries.* Health Policy Studies No. 2. Washington, D.C.: Organization for Economic Cooperation and Development Publications and Information Center.

Organization for Economic Cooperation and Development. (1992b). *U.S. health care at the cross roads.* Health Policy Studies No. 1. Washington, D.C.: Organization for Economic Cooperation and Development Publications and Information Center.

Organization for Economic Cooperation and Development. (1995a). *Internal markets in the making: Health systems in Canada, Iceland and the United Kingdom.* Washington, D.C.: Organization for Economic Cooperation and Development Publications and Information Center.

Organization for Economic Cooperation and Development. (1995b). *New orientations in health care policies: Improving cost control and effectiveness.* Washington, D.C.: Organization for Economic Cooperation and Development Publications and Information Center.

Payer, Lynn. (1988). *Medicine and Culture: Varieties of treatment in the United States, England, West Germany, and France.* New York: Henry Holt and Co.

Pescosolido, Bernice, Carol A. Boyer, & Wai-Ying Tsui. (1985). Medical care in the welfare state: A cross-national study of public evaluations. *Journal of Health and Social Behavior, 26* (December), 276–297.

Poullier, Jean-Pierre. (1992). Administrative costs in selected industrialized countries. *Health Care Financing Review, 13* (Summer), 167–172.

Raffel, Marshall W. (1984). *Comparative health systems: Descriptive analyses of fourteen national health systems.* University Park: Pennsylvania State University Press.

Rakich, Jonathan. (1991). The Canadian and U.S. health care systems: Profiles and policies. *Hospital and Health Services Administration, 36* (Spring), 25–42.

Redelmeier, Donald A., & Victor R. Fuchs. (1993). Hospital expenditures in the United States and Canada. *New England Journal of Medicine, 328* (March 8), 772–778.

Regenstein, Marsha, & Sharon Silow-Carroll. (1994). *Market reforms and regulation: Lessons from Europe's health care systems.* Washington, D.C.: Economic and Social Research Institute.

Rodwin, Victor G. (1984). *The health planning predicament: France, Quebec, England, and the United States.* Berkeley, CA: University of California Press.

Rodwin, Victor G. (1987). American exceptionalism in the health sector: The advantages of "backwardness" in learning from abroad. *Medical Care Review, 44* (Spring), 119–154.

Roemer, Milton I. (1977). *Comparative national policies on health care.* New York: Marcel Dekker.

Roemer, Milton I. (1985). *National strategies for health care organization: A world overview.* Ann Arbor, MI: Health Administration Press.

Roemer, Milton I. (1993a). *National health systems of the world,* vol. 2: *The issues.* New York: Oxford University Press.

Roemer, Milton I. (1993b). National health systems throughout the world. *Annual Review of Public Health, 14* (May), 335–354.

Roemer, Milton I. (Ed.). (1976). *Health care systems in world perspective.* Ann Arbor, MI: Health Administration Press.

Roemer, Milton I., & Ruth J. Roemer. (1981). *Health care systems and comparative manpower policies.* New York: Marcel Dekker.

Roemer, Milton I., & Ruth Roemer. (1990). Global health, national development and the role of government. *American Journal of Public Health, 80* (October), 1188–1192.

Ron, Aviva. (1986). Sharing in the financing of health care: Government, insurance and the patient. *Health Policy, 6* (1), 87–101.

Roos, Leslie L., Elliot S. Fisher, Ruth Brazanskas, Sandra M. Shard, & Evelyn Shapiro. (1992). Health and surgical outcomes in Canada and the United States. *Health Affairs, 11* (Summer), 56–72.

Rosenthal, Marilynn M. (1988). *Dealing with medical malpractice: The British and Swedish experience.* Durham, NC: Duke University Press.

Rosenthal, Marilynn, & Deborah Frederick. (1984). Physician maldistribution in cross-cultural perspective: United States, United Kingdom, and Sweden. *Inquiry, 21* (Spring), 60–74.

Rosenthal, Marilyn M., & Marcel Frenkel. (Eds.). (1992). *Health care systems and their patients: An international perspective.* Boulder, CO: Westview Press.

Rowland, Diane. (1992). A five-nation perspective on the elderly. *Health Affairs, 11* (Fall), 205–215.

Rublee, Dale A. (1989). Medical technology in Canada, Germany and the U.S. *Health Affairs, 8* (Fall), 178–181.

Rublee, Dale A. (1994). Medical technology in Canada, Germany, and the United States: An update. *Health Affairs, 13* (Fall), 113–117.

Rublee, Dale A., Markus Schneider, George J. Schieber, & Jean-Pierre Poullier. (1991). International spending: Comparisons with OECD. *Health Affairs, 10* (Fall), 187–201.

Saltman, Richard, & Casten Van Otter. (1992). *Planned markets and public competition: Strategic reform in Northern European health systems.* Bristol, PA: Open University Press.

Sass, Hans-Martin, & Robert U. Massey. (Eds.). (1988). *Health care systems: Moral conflicts in European and American public policy.* Hingham, MA: Kluwer Academic Publishers.

Scarpaci, Joseph L. (Ed.). (1989). *Health service privatization in industrial societies.* New Brunswick, NJ: Rutgers University Press.

Scheiber, George J., & Jean-Pierre Poullier. (1987). Recent trends in international health care spending. *Health Affairs, 6* (Fall), 105–112.

Schieber, George J., & Jean-Pierre Poullier. (1988). International health spending and utilization trends. *Health Affairs, 7* (Fall), 105–112.

Schieber, George J., & Jean-Pierre Poullier. (1989). International health care expenditures trends: 1987. *Health Affairs, 8* (Fall). 169–177.

Schieber, George J., & Jean-Pierre Poullier. (1991). International health spending: Issues and trends. *Health Affairs, 10* (Spring), 106–117.

Schieber, George J., Jean-Pierre Poullier, & Leslie M. Greenwald. (1991). Health care systems in twenty-four countries. *Health Affairs, 10* (Fall), 22–38.

Schieber, George J., Jean-Pierre Poullier, & Leslie M. Greenwald. (1992). U.S. health expenditure performance: An international comparison and data update. *Health Care Financing Review, 13* (Summer), 1–88.

Schieber, George J., Jean-Pierre Poullier, & Leslie M. Greenwald. (1994). Health system performance in OECD countries, 1980–1992. *Health Affairs, 13* (Fall), 100–112.

Silverman, Milton, Mia Lydecker, & Philip R. Lee. (1992). *Bad medicine: The prescription drug industry in the third world.* Stanford, CA: Stanford University Press.

Thorpe, Kenneth E. (1993). The American States and Canada: A comparative analysis of health care spending. *Journal of Health Politics, Policy and Law, 18* (Summer), 477–490.

U.S. Congress, Office of Technology Assessment. (1993). *International health statistics: What the numbers mean for the United States.* Washington, D.C.: U.S. Government Printing Office.

U.S. Congress, Office of Technology Assessment. (1994). *International comparisons of administrative costs in health care.* Washington, D.C.: U.S. Government Printing Office.

U.S. General Accounting Office. (1991). *Health care spending control: The experience of France, Germany, and Japan* (GA0/HRD-92-9). Washington, D.C.: U.S. Government Printing Office.

Van Atteveld, Lettie, Corine Broeders, & Ruud Lapré. (1987). International comparative research in health care: A study of the literature. *Health Policy, 18* (1), 105–136.

Waldo, Daniel R., & Sally T. Sonnefeld. (1991). U.S./Canadian health spending: Methods and assumptions. *Health Affairs, 10* (Summer), 159–165.

Weil, Connie, & Joseph L. Scarpaci. (Eds.). (1992). *Health and health care in Latin America during the lost decade: Insights for the 1990s.* Minneapolis: University of Minnesota.

Weiner, Jonathan P. (1987). Primary care delivery in the United States and four northwest European countries: Comparing the "corporatized" with the "socialized." *Milbank Memorial Fund Quarterly, 65* (3), 426–461.

Weller, Geoffry R., & Pranal Manga. (1983). The push for reprivatization of health care in Canada, Britain and the United States. *Journal of Health Politics, Policy and Law, 8* (Fall), 495–517.

Welsh, William W. (1983). Modeling budgetary strategies in health policy, east and west. *Journal of Health Politics, Policy and Law, 8* (Fall), 519–553.

White, Joseph. (1995). *Competing solutions: American health care proposals and international experience.* Washington, D.C.: The Brookings Institution.

Wiley, Miriam M. (1992). Hospital financing reform and case-mix measurement: An international review. *Health Care Financing Review, 13* (Summer), 119–134.

Wilsford, David. (1987). The cohesion and fragmentation of organized medicine in France and the United States. *Journal of Health Politics, Policy and Law, 12* (Fall), 481–503.

Wilsford, David. (1990). *The politics of health in France and the United States.* Durham, NC: Duke University Press.

Wilsford, David. (1991). *Doctors and the state: The politics of health care in France and the United States.* Durham, NC: Duke University Press.

Wilsford, David. (1995). States facing interests: Struggles over health care policy in advanced industrial democracies. *Journal of Health Politics, Policy and Law, 20* (Fall), 571–614.

Wolfe, Patrice R., & Donald W. Moran. (1993). Global budgeting in the OECD countries. *Health Care Financing Review, 14* (Spring), 55–76.

World Health Organization Study Group. (1993). *Evaluation of recent changes in the financing of health services* (Technical Report Series No. 829). Geneva, Switzerland: World Health Organization.

Canada

Andrepolous, Spyros. (1975). *National health insurance: Can we learn from Canada?* New York: John Wiley & Sons.

Atkinson, Michael A., & Marsha A. Chandler. (Eds.). (1983). *The politics of Canadian public policy.* Toronto: University of Toronto Press.

Barer, Morris L. (1988). Regulating physician supply: The evolution of British Columbia's Bill 41. *Journal of Health Politics, Policy and Law, 13* (Spring), 1–26.

Barer, Morris L., & Robert G. Evans. (1992). Interpreting Canada: Models, mind-sets, myths. *Health Affairs, 11* (Spring), 44–61.

Barer, Morris L., Clyde Hertzman, Robert Miller, & Marina V. Pascali. (1992). On being old and sick: The burden of health care for the elderly in Canada and the United States. *Journal of Health Politics, Policy and Law, 17* (Winter), 763–782.

Barer, Morris L., W. Pete Welch, & Laurie Antioch. (1991). Canadian/U.S. health care. Reflections on the HIAA's analysis. *Health Affairs, 10* (Fall), 229–236.

Bennett, Arnold, & Orvill Adams. (Eds.). (1993). *Looking north for health: What we can learn from Canada's health care system.* San Francisco, CA: Jossey-Bass.

Boyle, Torrey, Barbara Jacobs, & Eva Jacobs. (1993). More than loose change: Household health spending in the United States and Canada. *Health Affairs, 12* (Spring), 126–131.

Bryant, Bertha E. (1981). Issues on the distribution of health care: Some lessons from Canada. *Public Health Reports, 96* (September/October), 442–447.

Coburn, David B., George M. Torrance, & Joseph M. Kaufert. (1983). Medical dominance in Canada in historical perspective: The rise and fall of Canadian medicine? *International Journal of Health Services, 13* (3), 407–432.

Contandriopoulos, André-Pierre. (1986). Cost containment through payment mechanisms: The Quebec experience. *Journal of Public Health Policy, 7* (Summer), 224–238.

Conway, J. F. (1988). It's time for Canada to finish Medicare's job. *Journal of Health Policy, 10* (Summer), 157–160.

Coyte, Peter C. (1990). Current trends in Canadian health care: Myths and misconceptions in health economics. *Journal of Public Health Policy, 11* (Summer), 169–188.

Crichton, Anne. (1976). The shift from entrepreneurial to political power in the Canadian health system. *Social Science and Medicine, 10* (January), 59–66.

Crichton, Anne. (1994). Health insurance and medical practice organization in Canada: Findings from a literature review. *Medical Care Review, 51* (Summer), 149–177.

Cuyler, A. J. (1988). *Health expenditures in Canada: Myth and reality, past and future.* Toronto: Canadian Tax Foundation.

Danzon, Patricia M. (1992). Hidden overhead costs: Is Canada's system really less expensive? *Health Affairs, 11* (Spring), 21–43.

Deber, Raisa B. (1993). Canadian Medicare: Can it work in the United States? Will it survive in Canada? *American Journal of Law and Medicine, 19* (1/2), 75–94.

Deber, Raisa B. (Ed.). (1992). *Case studies in Canadian health policy and management* (Vols.1–2). Ottawa, Ontario: Canadian Hospital Association Press.

Deber, Raisa B., John E. F. Hastings, & Gail G. Thompson. (1991). Health care in Canada: Current trends and issues. *Journal of Public Health Policy, 12* (Spring), 72–82.

Evans, Robert G. (1983). Health care in Canada: Patterns of funding and regulation. *Journal of Health Politics, Policy and Law, 8* (Spring), 1–43.

Evans, Robert G. (1984). *Strained mercy: The economics of Canadian health care*. Toronto: Butterworths.

Evans, Robert G. (1986). Finding the levers, finding the courage: Lessons from cost containment in North America. *Journal of Health Politics, Policy and Law, 11* (4), 565–615.

Evans, Robert G. (1988). Perspectives: Canada. *Health Affairs, 7* (Winter), 17–24.

Evans, Robert G. (1992a). Canada: The real issues. *Journal of Health Politics, Policy and Law, 17* (Winter), 739–762.

Evans, Robert G. (1992b). The Canadian health-care financing and delivery system: Its experience and lessons for other nations. *Yale Law and Policy Review, 10* (2), 362–396.

Evans, Robert G., et al. (1989). Controlling health expenditures—the Canadian reality. *New England Journal of Medicine, 320* (March 2), 571–577.

Evans, Robert G., & Greg L. Stoddart. (Eds.). (1986). *Medicare at maturity: Achievements, lessons and challenges*. Calgary, Alberta: University of Calgary Press.

Eve, Susan Brown, Betty Havens, & Stanley R. Ingman. (1995). *The Canadian health care system. Lessons for the United States*. Lanham, MD: University Press of America.

Eyles, John, Stephen Birch, & K. Bruce Newbold. (1995). Delivering the goods? Access to family physician services in Canada: A comparison of 1985–1991. *Journal of Health and Social Behavior, 36* (December), 322–332.

Fried, Bruce J., Raisa B. Deber, & Peggy Leatt. (1987). Corporatization and deprivation of health services in Canada. *International Journal of Health Services, 17* (4), 567–584.

Fuchs, Victor R., & James S. Hahn. (1990). How does Canada do it? A comparison of expenditures for physicians' service in the United States and Canada. *New England Journal of Medicine, 323* (September 27), 884–890.

Fulton, Jane. (1993). *Canada's health system: Bordering on the possible*. New York: Faulkner & Gray, Inc., Health Care Information Center.

Hamowy, Ronald. (1984). *Canadian medicine: A study of restricted entry*. Vancouver, BC: Fraser Institute.

Heiber, S., & R. Deber. (1987). Banning extra-billing in Canada: Just what the doctor didn't order. *Canadian Public Policy, 13* (March), 62–74.

Iglehart, John K. (1986). Canada's health care systems. *New England Journal of Medicine, 315* (July 17), 202–208; (September 18), 778–784; (December 18), 1623–1628.

Kane, Robert L., & Rosalie A. Kane. (1985). *A will and a way: What the United States can learn from Canada about caring for the elderly*. New York: Columbia University Press.

Kaufman, Caroline. (1994). Rights and the provision of health care: A comparison of Canada, Great Britain, and the United States. In Howard S. Schwartz (Ed.), *Dominant issues in medical sociology* (3rd ed., pp. 376–396) New York: McGraw-Hill.

Kohn, Robert, & Susan Radius. (1974). Two roads to health care: U.S. and Canadian policies; 1945–1975. *Medical Care, 12* (March), 189–199.

Krasny, Jacques, & Ian R. Ferrier. (1991). A closer look at health care in Canada. *Health Affairs, 10* (Summer), 152–158.

Laframboise, Hubert. (1990). Non-participative policy development: The genesis of a new perspective on the health of Canadians. *Journal of Public Health Policy, 11* (Autumn), 316–322.

Lave, Judith. (1992). Transitional funding: Changing Ontario's global budgeting system. *Health Care Financing Review, 13* (Spring), 77–96.

Lemco, Jonathan (Ed). (1995). *National health care: Lessons for the United States and Canada.* Ann Arbor: University of Michigan Press.

Lomas, Jonathan. (1990). Finding audiences, changing beliefs: The structure of research use in Canadian health policy. *Journal of Health Politics, Policy and Law, 15* (Fall), 525–542.

Lomas, Jonathan, Catherine Fooks, Thomas Rice, & Roberta J. LaBelle. (1989). Paying physicians in Canada: Minding our Ps and Qs. *Health Affairs, 8* (Spring), 80–102.

Maioni, Antonia. (1995). Nothing succeeds like the right kind of failure: Post-war national health insurance initiatives in Canada and the United States. *Journal of Health Politics, Policy and Law, 20* (Spring), 5–30.

Marmor, Theodore R. (1985). Canada's path, America's choices: Lessons from the Canadian experience with national health insurance. In Peter Conrad & Rochelle Kerr (Eds.), *Sociology of health and illness, critical perspectives* (2nd. ed., pp. 443–467). New York: St. Martin's.

Marmor, Theodore R. (1993). Lessons from the frozen North. *Journal of Health Politics, Policy and Law, 18* (Fall), 763–770.

Marmor, Theodore R., & Jerry L. Mashaw. (1990). Canada's health insurance and ours: The real lessons, big choices. *American Prospect, 3* (Fall), 18–29.

Moloney, Thomas W., & Barbara Paul. (1989). A new financial framework: Lessons from Canada. *Health Affairs, 8* (Summer), 148–159.

Naylor, C. David. (1986). *Private practice, public payment: Canadian medicine and the politics of health insurance, 1911–1966.* Kingston and Montreal: McGill-Queens University Press.

Naylor, C. David. (1991). A different view of queues in Ontario. *Health Affairs, 10* (Fall), 110–128.

Palley, Howard A. (1987). Canadian federalism and the Canadian health care program: A comparison of Ontario and Quebec. *International Journal of Health Services, 17* (4), 595–616.

Pineault, Raynald, André-Pierre Contandriopoulos, & Richard Lessard. (1985). The Quebec health system: Care objectives or health objectives. *Journal of Public Health Policy, 6* (September), 394–409.

Rachlis, Michael, & Carol Kushner. (1989). *Second opinions: What's wrong with Canada's health-care system and how to fix it.* Toronto, Ontario: Collins Publishers.

Rakich, Jonathan. (1991). The Canadian and U.S. health care systems: Profiles and policies. *Hospital and Health Services Administration, 36* (Spring), 25–42.

Redelmeier, Donald A., & Victor R. Fuchs. (1993). Hospital expenditures in the United States and Canada. *New England Journal of Medicine, 328* (March 18), 772–778.

Robinson, Geoffrey C., et al. (1993). *Children, politics, and Medicare: Experience in a Canadian province.* Calgary, Alberta: University of Calgary Press.

Rochefort, David A. (1992). More lessons of a different kind: Canadian mental health policy in comparative perspective. *Hospital and Community Psychiatry, 43* (November), 1083–1090.

Roos, Leslie L., Elliot S. Fisher, Ruth Brazauskas, Sandra M. Sharp, & Evelyn Shapiro. (1992). Health and surgical outcomes in Canada and the United States. *Health Affairs, 11* (Summer), 56–72.

Rublee, Dale A. (1989). Medical technology in Canada, Germany, and the U.S. *Health Affairs, 8* (Fall), 178–181.

Rublee, Dale A. (1994). Medical technology in Canada, Germany, and the United States: An update. *Health Affairs, 13* (Fall), 113–117.

Sheils, John F., Gary J. Yaing, & Robert J. Rubin. (1992). O Canada: Do we expect too much from its health system? *Health Affairs, 11* (Spring), 7–20.

Spasoff, Robert A. (1990). Current trends in Canadian health care: Disease prevention and health promotion. *Journal of Public Health Policy, 11* (Summer), 161–168.

Stevenson, H. Michael, & A. Paul Williams. (1985). Physicians and Medicare: Professional ideology and Canadian health care policy. *Canadian Public Policy, 11* (September), 504–521.

Stevenson, H. Michael, A. Paul Williams, & Eugene Vayda. (1988). Medical politics and Canadian Medicare: Professional response to the Canada health act. *Milbank Quarterly, 66* (1), 65–104.

Sutherland, Ralph, & Jane Fulton. (1994). *Spending smarter and spending less: Policies and partnerships for health care in Canada*. Ottawa, Ontario: The Health Group.

Taylor, C. David. (1986). *Private practice, public payment: Canadian medicine and the politics of health insurance, 1911–1966*. Kingston and Montreal: McGill-Queen's University Press.

Taylor, Malcolm G. (1978). *Health insurance and Canadian public policy: The seven decisions that created the Canadian health insurance system and their outcomes*. Montreal: McGill-Queen's University Press.

Terris, Milton. (1990). Lessons from Canada's health program. *Journal of Public Health Policy, 11* (Summer), 151–160.

Tuohy, C. J. (1976). Medical politics after Medicare: The Ontario case. *Canadian Public Policy, 2* (2), 192–210.

U.S. General Accounting Office. (June 1991). *Canadian health insurance: Lessons for the United States* (GAO/HRD-91-90). Washington, D.C.: U.S. Government Printing Office.

Vayda, Eugene. (1983). Aspects of medical manpower under national health insurance in Canada. *Journal of Public Health Policy, 4* (December), 504–513.

Vayda, Eugene, & Raisa B. Deber. (1984). The Canadian health care system: An overview. *Social Science and Medicine, 18* (3), 191–197.

Waldo, Daniel R., & Sally T. Sonnefeld. (1991). U.S./Canadian health spending: Methods and assumptions. *Health Affairs, 10* (Summer), 159–165.

Welch, W. Pete, Steven J. Katz, & Stephen Zuckerman. (1993). Physician fee levels: Medicare versus Canada. *Health Care Financing Review, 14* (Spring), 41–54.

Weller, Geoffrey R. (1986). Common problems, alternative solutions: A comparison of the Canadian and American health systems. *Policy Studies Journal, 14* (June), 604–620.

Weller, Geoffrey R., & Pranal Manga. (1983a). The development of health policy in Canada. In Michael A. Atkinson & Marsha A. Chandler (Eds.), *The politics of Canadian public policy* (pp. 223–246). Toronto: University of Toronto Press.

Weller, Geoffrey R., & Pranal Manga. (1983b). The push for reprivatization in health care services in Canada, Britain, and the United States. *Journal of Health Politics, Policy and Law, 8* (Fall), 495–517.

Williams, A. Paul, Eugene Vayda, May L. Cohen, Christel A. Woodward, & Barbara H. Ferrier. (1995). Medicare and the Canadian state: From the politics of conflict to the politics of accommodation. *Journal of Health and Social Behavior, 36* (December), 303–321.

Wolfe, Samuel, & Robin Badgley. (1974). How much is enough? The payment of doctors—implications for health policy in Canada. *International Journal of Health Services, 4* (Spring), 245–264.

Wolfe, Samuel, & Robin Badgley. (1981). Immigration, emigration and opting out by Canadian physicians under national Medicare. *Journal of Public Health Policy, 2* (1), 80–86.

York, Geoffrey. (1992). Fee-for-service: Cashing in on the Canadian medical care system. *Journal of Public Health Policy, 13* (Summer), 140–145.

Great Britain, the United Kingdom, and the National Health Service

Allen, David. (1984). Perspectives in NHS management: Are there lessons from abroad for the NHS? *British Medical Journal, 289* (July 28), 265–268.

Baggott, Rob. (1994). *Health and health care in Britain*. New York: St. Martin's.

Barnard, Keith, & Kenneth Lee. (Eds.). (1977). *Conflicts in the National Health Service*. New York: Prodist: Neale Watson Academic Publication.

Birch, Stephen. (1988). DRGs U.K. style: A comparison of U.K. and U.S. policies for hospital cost containment and their implications for health status. *Health Policy, 10* (2), 143–154.

Black, Douglas. (1992). Change in the NHS. *Journal of Public Health Policy, 13* (Summer), 156–164.

Blendon, Robert J., & Karen Donelan. (1989). British public opinion on NHS reform. *Health Affairs, 8* (Winter), 52–62.

Butler, John R., & Michael S. B. Vaile. (1984). *Health and health services: An introduction to health care in Britain.* Boston: Routledge and Kegan Paul.

Culyer, A. J., & Andrew Meads. (1992). The United Kingdom: Effective, efficient, equitable? *Journal of Health Politics, Policy and Law, 17* (Winter), 667–688.

Day, Patricia. (1992). The state, the NHS and general practice. *Journal of Health Policy, 13* (Summer), 165–179.

Day, Patricia, & Rudolf Klein. (1991). Britain's health care experiment. *Health Affairs, 10* (Fall), 39–59.

Draper, Peter, & Tony Smart. (1974). Social science and health policy in the United Kingdom: Some contributions of the social sciences to the bureaucratization of the National Health Service. *International Journal of Health Services, 4* (Summer), 453–470.

Enthoven, Alain C. (1985). *Reflections on the management of the National Health Service.* London: Nuffield Provincial Hospitals Trust.

Enthoven, Alain C. (1991). Internal market reform of the British NHS. *Health Affairs, 10* (Fall), 60–70.

Freeman, Richard. (1995). Prevention and government: Health policy making in the United Kingdom and Germany. *Journal of Health Politics, Policy and Law, 20* (Fall), 745–766.

Halper, Thomas. (1985). Life and death in a welfare state: End-stage renal disease in the United Kingdom. *Milbank Memorial Fund Quarterly, 63* (Winter), 52–93.

Ham, Christopher. (1985). *Health policy in Britain: The politics and organization of the National Health Service.* London: Macmillan.

Ham, Chrisopher, & Mats Brommers. (1994). Health-care reform in the Netherlands, Sweden and the United Kingdom. *Health Affairs, 13* (Winter), 106–119.

Harrison, Stephen. (1994). The dynamics of health care organization in Britain. *Journal of Public Health Policy, 15* (Autumn), 283–297.

Higgins, Joan. (1990). American hospitals in the British health care market. *Medical Care Review, 47* (Spring), 105–130.

Holland, Walter W., & Clifford Graham. (1994). Commentary: Recent reforms in the British National Health Service—lessons for the United States. *American Journal of Public Health, 84* (February), 186–189.

Hollingsworth, J. Rogers. (1986.). *A political economy of medicine: Great Britain and the United States.* Baltimore, MD: Johns Hopkins University Press.

Iglehart, John. (1983). The British National Health Service under the conservatives. *New England Journal of Medicine, 309* (November 17), Part I, 1264–1268.

Iglehart, John. (1984). The British National Health Service under the conservatives. *New England Journal of Medicine, 310* (January 5), Part II, 63–67.

Jacobs, Lawrence R. (1993). *The health of nations: Public opinion and the making of American and British health policy.* Ithaca, NY: Cornell University Press.

James, John H. (1995). Reforming the British National Health Service: Implementation problems in London. *Journal of Health Politics, Policy and Law, 20* (Spring), 191–210.

Jonas, Steven, & David Banta. (1975). The 1974 reorganization of the British National Health Service: An analysis. *Journal of Community Health, 1* (Winter), 91–105.

Kavanagh, Shane, & Martin Knapp. (1995). International report: Market rationales, rationing, and rationality: Mental health care reform in the United Kingdom. *Health Affairs, 14* (Fall), 260–268.

Klein, Rudolf. (1976). The rise and decline of policy analysis: The strange case of health policy-making in Britain. *Policy Analysis, 2* (Summer), 459–475.

Klein, Rudolf. (1979). Ideology, class and the National Health Service. *Journal of Health Politics, Policy and Law, 4* (Fall), 464–490.

Klein, Rudolf. (1983). *The politics of the National Health Service.* London and New York: Longman.

Klein, Rudolf. (1984). The politics of ideology versus the reality of politics: The case of Britain's National

Health Service in the 1980's. *Milbank Memorial Fund Quarterly, 62* (Winter), 82–109.

Klein, Rudolf. (1985). Why Britain's conservatives support a socialist health care system. *Health Affairs, 4* (Spring), 41–58.

Klein, Rudolf. (1990). Research, policy, and the National Health Service. *Journal of Health Politics, Policy and Law, 15* (Fall), 501–524.

Klein, Rudolf. (1995). Big bang health care reform—does it work? The case of Britain's 1991 National Health Service reforms. *Milbank Quarterly, 73* (3), 299–338.

Klein, Rudolf, Ray Robinson, & Julian LeGrand. (Eds.). (1995). Evaluating the NHS reforms. *Journal of Health Politics, Policy and Law, 20* (Fall), 802–806.

Kushnick, Louis. (1988). Racism, the National Health Service, and the health of black people. *International Journal of Health Services, 18* (3), 457–470.

The Labour Party. (1996). Renewing the National Health Service: Labour's agenda for a healthier Britain. *International Journal of Health Services, 26* (2), 269–308.

Lee, Philip R., & Lynne Etheredge. (1989). Clinical freedom: Two lessons for the U.K. from U.S. experience with privatization of health care. *Lancet, 1* (February 4), 263–266.

Levitt, Ruth, & Andrew Hall. (1984). *The reorganized National Health Service* (3rd ed.). London: Croom-Helm.

Light, Donald W. (1992). The radical experiment: Transforming Britain's national health system to interlocking markets. *Journal of Public Health Policy, 13* (Summer), 146–155.

Lister, John. (1986). The politics of medicine in Britain and the United States. *New England Journal of Medicine, 315* (July 17), 168–173.

Lister, John. (1989). Proposals for reform of the British National Health Service. *New England Journal of Medicine, 320* (March 30), 877–880.

Loveridge, Ray, & Ken Starkey (Eds.). (1992). *Continuity and crisis in the NHS.* Philadelphia, PA: Open University Press.

MacKenzie, W. J. M. (1979). *Power and responsibility in health care: The National Health Service as a political institution.* New York: Oxford University Press.

MacMillan, Donald, et al. (Eds.). (1975). *NHS reorganization: Issues and prospects.* Leeds: Nuffield Centre for Health Services Studies.

Maynard, Alan. (1986). Financing the U.K. National Health Services. *Health Policy, 6* (4), 329–340.

Maynard, Alan. (1994). Can competition enhance efficiency in health care? Lessons from the reform of the UK National Health Service. *Social Science and Medicine, 39* (10), 1433–1446.

McLachlan, Gordon. (1990). *What price quality? The NHS in review.* London: Nuffield Provincial Hospitals Trust.

Mechanic, David. (1995). Americanization of the British National Health Service. *Health Affairs, 14* (Summer), 51–67.

Mohan, John, & Kevin J. Woods. (1985). Restructuring health care: The social geography of public and private health care under the British conservative government. *International Journal of Health Services, 15* (2), 197–216.

Pollitt, Christopher. (1993). The politics of medical quality: Auditing doctors in the UK and the USA. *Health Services Management Research, 6* (February), 24–34.

Powell, Martina A. (1996). The ghost of health services past: Comparing British health policy of the 1930s with the 1980s and 1990s. *International Journal of Health Services, 26* (2), 253–268.

Rainier, Geoffrey. (1987). Lessons from America? Commercialization and growth of private medicine in Britain. *International Journal of health services, 17* (2), 197–216.

Robinson, Ray, & Julian LeGrand. (Eds.). (1994). *Evaluating the NHS reforms.* London: Kings Fund Institute.

Scheffler, Richard M. (1992). Culture versus competition: The reforms of the British National Health Service. *Jounal of Public Health Policy, 13* (Summer), 180–185.

Schulz, Rockwell, & Steve Harrison. (1984). Consensus management in the British National Health Service:

Implications for the United States? *Milbank Memorial Fund Quarterly, 62* (Fall), 657– 681.

Schwartz, William B., & Henry J. Aaron. (1984). Rationing hospital care: Lessons from Britain. *New England Journal of Medicine, 310* (January 5), 52– 56.

Stocking, Barbara. (1993). Implementing the findings of effective care in pregnancy and childbirth in the United Kingdom. *Milbank Quarterly, 71* (3), 497–522.

Susser, Mervyn. (1993). Health as a human right: An epidemiologist's perspective on the public health. *American Journal of Public Health, 83* (March), 418–426.

Germany

Altenstetter, Christa. (1974a). *Health policy making and administration in West Germany and the United States*. Beverly Hills, CA: Sage.

Altenstetter, Christa. (1974b). Medical interests and the public interest: A comparison of West Germany and the United States. *International Journal of Health Services, 4* (Winter), 29–48.

Altenstetter, Christa. (1987). An end to a consensus on health care in the Federal Republic of Germany? *Journal of Health Politics, Policy and Law, 12* (Fall), 505–536.

Brenner, Gerhard, & Dale A. Rublee. (1991). The 1987 revision of physician fees in Germany. *Health Affairs, 10* (Fall), 147–156.

Files, Ashley, & Margaret Murray. (1995). German risk structure compensation: Enhancing equity and effectiveness. *Inquiry, 32* (Fall), 300–309.

Freeman, Richard. (1995). Prevention and government: Health policy making in the United Kingdom and Germany. *Journal of Health Politics, Policy and Law, 20* (Fall), 745–766.

Glaser, William. (1983). Lessons from Germany: Some reflections occasioned by Schulenberg's report. *Journal of Health Politics, Policy and Law, 8* (Summer), 352–365.

Henke, Klaus-Dirk. (1986). A "concerted" approach to health care financing in the Federal Republic of Germany. *Health Policy, 6* (4), 341–351.

Henke, Klaus-Dirk, Margaret A. Murray, & Claudia Ade. (1994). Global budgeting in Germany: Lessons for the United States. *Health Affairs, 13* (Fall), 7–21.

Hinrichs, Karl. (1995). The impact of German health insurance reforms on redistribution and the cuture of solidarity. *Journal of Health Politics, Policy and Law, 20* (Fall), 653–688.

Hurst, Jeremy. (1991). Reform of health care in Germany. *Health Care Financing Review, 12* (Spring), 73–86.

Iglehart, John K. (1991). Germany's health care system. *New England Journal of Medicine, 324* (February 14), Part I, 503–505; (June 13), Part II, 1750–1756.

Katz, Eric M. (1994). Pharmaceutical spending and German reunification: Parity comes quickly to Berlin. *Health Care Financing Review, 15* (Spring), 141–156.

Knox, Richard. (1993). *Germany's health system: One nation united with health care for all*. Washington, D.C.: Faulkner & Gray, Inc.

LaBisch, Alfons. (1987). The role of the hospital in the health policy of the German social democratic movement before World War I. *International Journal of Health Services, 17* (2), 279–294.

Light, Donald W. (1985a). Comparing health care systems: Lessons from East and West Germany. In Peter Conrad & Rochelle Kern (Eds.), *Sociology of health and illness: Critical perspectives*. New York: St. Martin's.

Light, Donald W. (1985b). Values and structure in the German health care systems. *Milbank Memorial Fund Quarterly, 63* (Fall), 615–647.

Light, Donald W., Stephan Liebfried, & Florian Tennstedt. (1986). Social medicine vs. professional dominance: The German experience. *American Journal of Public Health, 76* (January), 78–83.

Light, Donald W., & Alexander Schuller. (1986). *The impact of political values and health care: The German experience*. Cambridge, MA: MIT Press.

Nippert, R. Peter. (1992). Back to direct payment: German dentists lobby to leave the national sickness fund scheme. *Journal of Public Health Policy, 13* (Winter), 491–500.

Powell, Francis D. (1994). Government participation in physician negotiations in German economic policy as applied to universal health care coverage in the United States. *Social Science and Medicine, 38* (1), 35–43.

Reinhardt, Uwe E. (1994). Perspective on the German health care system. *Health Affairs, 13* (Fall), 22–24.

Rublee, Dale A. (1989). Medical technology in Canada, Germany and the U.S. *Health Affairs, 8* (Fall), 178–181.

Rublee, Dale A. (1994). Medical technology in Canada, Germany and the United States: An update. *Health Affairs, 13* (Fall), 113–117.

Schulenburg, J-Matthias Graf. (1983). Report from Germany: Current conditions and controversies in health care systems. *Journal of Health Politics, Policy and Law, 8* (Summer), 320–351.

Schulenburg, J-Matthias Graf. (1992). Germany: Solidarity at a price. *Journal of Health Politics, Policy and Law, 17* (Winter), 715–738.

Stone, Deborah A. (1980). *The limits of professional power: National health care in the Federal Republic of Germany.* Chicago: University of Chicago Press.

Stone, Deborah A. (1995). Commentary: The durability of social capital. *Journal of Health Politics, Policy and Law, 20* (Fall), 689–694.

U.S. General Accounting Office. (1994). *German health reforms: Changes result in lower costs in 1993* (GAO/HRD-95-27). Washington, D.C.: U.S. Government Printing Office.

Wysong, Jere A., & Thomas Abel. (1990). Universal health insurance and high-risk groups in West Germany: Implications for U.S. health policy. *Milbank Quarterly, 68* (4), 527–560.

Sweden and Norway

Anton, Thomas J. (1995). Commentary: Scandinavian realism. *Journal of Health Politics, Policy and Law, 20* (Fall), 739–744.

Erichsen, Vibeke. (1995). Health care reform in Norway: The end of the "Profession state"? *Journal of Health Politics, Policy and Law, 20* (Fall), 719–738.

Gardner, Elizabeth. (1994). Swedes test capitalist waivers in new health systems reforms. *Journal of American Health Policy, 6* (March/April), 43–49.

Garpenby, Peter. (1995). Health care reform in Sweden in the 1990s: Local pluralism versus national coordination. *Journal of Health Politics, Policy and Law, 20* (Fall), 695–718; Thomas J. Anton, Commentary: Scandinavian realism, 739–744.

Gerdtham, Ulf-G, & Bengt Jönsson. (1991). Health care expenditure in Sweden—an international comparison. *Health Policy, 19* (December), 211–228.

Gustafsson, Rolf A. (1989). Origins of authority: The organization of medical care in Sweden. *International Journal of Health Services, 19* (1), 121–133.

Ham, Christopher, & Mats Brommers. (1994). Health care reform in the Netherlands, Sweden and the United Kingdom. *Health Affairs, 13* (Winter), 106–119.

Heidenheimer, Arnold, & Nils Elvander. (Eds.). (1980). *The shaping of the Swedish health system.* New York: St. Martin's.

Heidenheimer, Arnold, & Lars N. Johansen. (1985). Organized medicine and Scandinavian professional unionism: Hospital policies and exit options in Denmark and Sweden. *Journal of Health Politics, Policy and Law, 10* (Summer), 347–370.

Hessler, Richard M., & Andrew C. Twaddle. (1982). Sweden's crisis in medical care: Political and legal changes. *Journal of Health Politics, Policy and Law, 7* (Summer), 440–459.

Rahkonen, Ossi, Eero La Helma, Antti Karisto, & Kristina Manderbacka. (1993). Persisting health inequalities: Social class differentials in illness in the Scandinavian countries. *Journal of Public Health Policy, 14* (Spring), 66–81.

Rosenthal, Marilynn M. (1986). Beyond equity: Swedish health policy and the private sector. *Milbank Quarterly, 64* (4), 592–621.

Saltman, Richard B. (1990). Competition and reform in the Swedish health system. *Milbank Quarterly, 68* (4), 597–618.

Saltman, Richard B. (1992). Recent health policy initiatives in Nordic countries. *Health Care Financing Review, 13* (Summer), 157–166.

Shenkin, Budd N. (1973). Politics and medical care in Sweden: The seven crowns reform. *New England Journal of Medicine, 288* (March 15), 555–559.

Twaddle, Andrew C., & Richard M. Hessler. (1986). Power and change: The case of the Swedish commission of inquiry on health and sickness care. *Journal of Health Politics, Policy and Law, 11* (Spring), 19–40.

Western Europe

Abel-Smith, Brian. (1992). Cost containment and new priorities in the European community. *Milbank Quarterly, 70* (3), 393–416.

Abel-Smith, Brian, & Elias Mossialos. (1994). Cost containment and health care reform: A study of the European union. *Health Policy, 28* (May), 89–132.

Altenstetter, Christa. (1992). Health policy regimes and the single European market. *Journal of Health Politics, Policy and Law, 17* (Winter), 813–846.

Burstall, M. L. (1991). Europe after 1992: Implications for pharmaceuticals. *Health Affairs, 10* (Fall), 157–171.

Elola, Javier. (1996). Health care system reforms in Western European countries: The relevance of health care organization. *International Journal of Health Services, 26* (2), 239–252.

Elola, Javier, Antonio Daponte, & Vicente Navarro. (1995). Health indicators and the organization of health care systems in Western Europe. *American Journal of Public Health, 85* (October), 1397–1401.

Ferrera, Maurizio. (1995). The rise and fall of democratic universalism: Health care reform in Italy, 1978–1994. *Journal of Health Politics, Policy and Law, 20* (Summer), 275–302.

Ham, Christopher, & Mats Brommers. (1994). Health care reform in the Netherlands, Sweden and the United Kingdom. *Health Affairs, 13* (Winter), 106–119.

Immergut, Ellen M. (1992). *Health politics: Interests and institutions in Western Europe.* New York: Cambridge University Press.

Jamieson, Anne. (Ed.). (1991). *Home care for older people in Europe: A comparison of policies and practices.* New York: Oxford University Press.

Kabcenell, Andrea I., Alan B. Cohen, & Jeffrey Merrill. (1991). Importing a model of hospital quality from the Netherlands. *Health Affairs, 10* (Fall), 240–245.

Kent, George D. (1989). Socializing health services in Greece. *Journal of Public Health Policy, 10* (Summer), 222–245.

McCarthy, Mark, & Sian Rees. (1992). *Health systems and public medicine in the European community.* London, UK: Royal College of Physicians.

Morone, James A., & Janice M. Goggin. (1995). Introduction—health policies in Europe: Welfare states in a market era. *Journal of Health Politics, Policy and Law, 20* (Fall), 557–570.

Morone, James A., & Janice M. Goggin. (Eds.). (1995). European health policies: Welfare states in a market era. *Journal of Health Politics, Policy and Law, 20* (Fall), 557–594.

Orzack, Louis H., Kenneth I. Kaitin, & Louis Lasagna. (1992). Pharmaceutical regulation in the European community: Barriers to single market integration. *Journal of Health Politics, Policy and Law, 17* (Winter), 847–868.

Regenstein, Marsha, & Sharon Silow-Carroll. (1994). *Market reforms and regulation: Lessons from Europe's health care systems.* Washington, D.C.: Economic and Social Research Institute.

Saltman, Richard, & Casten Von Otter. (1992). *Planned markets and public competition: Strategic reform in Northern European health systems.* Bristol, PA: Open University Press.

Taylor-Gooby, Peter. (1996). The future of health care in six European countries: The views of policy elites. *International Journal of Health Services, 26* (2), 203–220.

Thompson, Lawrence H. (1992). Observations on "cost containment and new priorities in the European community" by Brian Abel-Smith. *Milbank Quarterly, 70* (3), 417–422.

Wilsford, David. (1995). States facing interests: Struggles over health care policy in advanced, industrial democracies. *Journal of Health Politics, Policy and Law, 20* (Fall), 571–614.

FEDERALISM, THE FEDERAL GOVERNMENT, AND HEALTH AND HEALTH CARE

Altenstetter, Christa, & James W. Bjorkman. (1976). The rediscovery of federalism: The impact of federal child health programs in Connecticut state health policy formation and service delivery. In R. Thomas & C. O. Jones (Eds.), *Public policy-making in a federal system* (pp. 217–237). Beverly Hills, CA: Sage.

Altenstetter, Christa, & James W. Bjorkman. (1978). Policy, politics and child health: Four decades of federal initiative and state response. *Journal of Health Politics, Policy and Law, 3* (Summer), 196–234.

Altman, Stuart, H., & Harvey M. Sapolsky. (Eds.). (1981). *Federal health programs: Problems and prospects*. Cambridge, MA: Lexington Books.

Anderson, Odin, & David Banta. (1977). The federal legislative process and health care. In Steven Jonas (Ed.), *Health care delivery in the United States* (pp. 329–345). New York: Springer Publishing Co.

Barfield, Claude. (1983). New Federalism and long term care of the elderly: Update. *Health Affairs, 2* (Spring), 113–125.

Baydin, Lynda D. (1977). The end-stage renal disease networks: An attempt through federal regulation to regionalize health care delivery. *Medical Care, 15* (July), 586–598.

Berkowitz, Edward D. (1980). *Rehabilitation: The federal government's response to disability, 1935–1954*. Unpublished Ph.D. diss., Northwestern University. (Also New York: Arno Press, 1980).

Bloom, Bernard S., & Samuel P. Martin. (1976). The role of the federal government in financing health and medical services. *Journal of Medical Education, 51* (March), 161–169.

Blumenthal, David. (1983). Federal policy toward health care technology: The case of the national center. *Milbank Memorial Fund Quarterly, 61* (Fall), 584–613.

Blumstein, James F. (1974). Foundations of federal fertility policy. *Milbank Memorial Fund Quarterly/Health and Society, 52* (Spring), 131–168.

Bonnen, James T. (1984). Federal statistical coordination today: A disaster or a disgrace? *Milbank Memorial Fund Quarterly, 62* (Winter), 1–41; Comments, 42–52.

Bredder, Roy. (1994). *Federal health laws, 1990–1993*. Washington, D.C.: Faulkner & Gray, Inc.

Brown, Lawrence D. (1978). The formulation of federal health care policy. *Bulletin of the New York Academy of Medicine, 54* (January), 45–58.

Brown, Lawrence D. (1984). The politics of devolution in Nixon's New Federalism. In Lawrence D. Brown, James W. Fossett, & Kenneth T. Palmer (Eds.), *The changing politics of federal grants* (pp. 54–107). Washington, D.C.: The Brookings Institution.

Bryant, John H., Myron E. Wegman, Reuel A. Stallones, Lester Breslow, & Cecil G. Sheps. (1973). The impact of the New Federalism on schools of public health. *Milbank Memorial Fund Quarterly/Health and Society, 51* (Fall), 435–472.

Budetti, Peter P., John Butler, & Peggy McManus. (1982). Federal health program reform: Implications for child health. *Milbank Memorial Fund Quarterly/Health and Society, 60* (Winter), 155–181.

Buntz, C. Gregory, Theodore F. Macaluso, & Jay A. Azarow. (1978). Federal influence on state health policy. *Journal of Health Politics, Policy and Law, 3* (Spring), 71–86.

Carter, G. M., D. Schu, J. E. Koehler, R. L. Slighton, & A. P. Williams Jr. (1974). *Federal manpower legislation and the academic health centers: An interim report* (Rand Report No. 4-1464-HEW). Santa Monica, CA: Rand Corporation.

Chapman, Carleton B., & John M. Talmadge. (1970). Historical and political background of federal health care legislation. *Law and contemporary problems, 35* (Spring), 334–347.

Clark, Robert L., & John A. Menefee.(1981). Federal expenditures for the elderly: Past and future. *The Gerontologist, 21* (2), 132–137.

Darling, Helen. (1986). The role of the federal government in assuring access to health care. *Inquiry, 23* (Fall), 286–295.

Decker, Barry. (1977). Federal strategies and the quality of local health care. In Arthur Levin (Ed.), *Health services: The local perspective, Proceedings of the Academy of Political Science* (Vol. 32, No. 3, pp. 200–214). New York: Academy of Political Science.

Derzon, Robert A. (1979). *A legitimate role of government in the private health services system, 1979.* Chicago: University of Chicago Center for Health Administration Studies, Graduate School of Business.

Drew, David E., John G. Wirt, F. W. Finnegan, M. C. Fujisake, & A. L. Laniear. (1976). *The effects of federal funds upon selected health-related disciplines* (Rand Report No. R-1944-PBRP). Santa Monica, CA: Rand Corporation.

Dunham, Andrew B., & Theodore Marmor. (1978). Federal policy and health: Recent trends and different perspectives. In Theodore J. Lowi & Alan Stone (Eds.), *Nationalizing government: Public policies in America.* Beverly Hills, CA: Sage.

Edwards, Charles C. (1975). The federal involvement in health: A personal view of current problems and future needs. *New England Journal of Medicine, 292* (March 13), 559–562.

Etheredge, Lynn. (1984). An aging society and the federal deficit. *Milbank Memorial Fund Quarterly, 62* (Fall), 521–543.

Feingold, Eugene, & George D. Greenberg. (1984). Health policy and the federal executive. In Theodor J. Litman & Leonard S. Robins (Eds.), *Health politics and policy* (1st ed., pp. 114–125). New York: John Wiley & Sons.

Foltz, Anne-Marie. (1975). The development of ambiguous federal policy: Early and periodic screening, diagnosis and treatment (EPSTD). *Milbank Memorial Fund Quarterly, 53* (Winter), 35–64.

Foltz, Anne-Marie. (1978). *Uncertainties of federal child health politics: Impact in two states.* (DHEW Pub. No. [PHS] 78-3190). Hyattsville, MD: National Center for Health Services Research.

Fox, Peter D. (1972). Access to medical care for the poor: The federal perspective. *Medical Care, 10* (May/June), 272–277.

Fritschler, A. Lee. (1975). *Smoking and politics: Policymaking and the federal bureaucracy.* Englewood Cliffs, NJ: Prentice-Hall.

Glaser, William A. (1977). *Federalism in Canadian health services—lessons for the United States.* Preprint Series, New York: Center for the Social Sciences, Columbia University.

Gold, Byron D. (1974). Role of the federal government in the provision of social services to older persons. *Annals of the American Academy of Political and Social Science, 415* (September), 55–69.

Grogan, Colleen M. (1991). *A political theory to explain the variation in state Medicaid policies.* Unpublished Ph.D. diss., University of Minnesota.

Grogan, Colleen M. (1993). Federalism and health care reform. *American Behavioral Scientist, 36* (July), 741–759.

Hageboeck, Helen E. (1978). *An analysis of the impact of federal legislation on community based health services to functionally dependent adults.* Unpublished Ph.D. diss., University of Iowa.

Jaeger, Boi Jon. (1971). *Hospitals and the federal government: A study of the development and outcomes of public policy.* Unpublished Ph.D. diss., Duke University.

Jones, E. Terrence. (1974). The impact of federal aid on the quality of life: The case of infant health. *Social Indicators Research, 1* (September), 209–216.

Judd, Leda R. (1977). Federal involvement in health care after 1945. *Current History, 12* (May/June), 201–206, 227–228.

Klerman, Lorraine V. (1984). Intergovernmental relationships: A delicate balance (editorial). *American Journal of Public Health, 74* (September), 965–967.

Komaroff, Anthony L., & Paul J. Duffell. (1976). An evaluation of selected federal categorical health programs for the poor. *American Journal of Public Health, 66* (March), 255–261.

Lee, Philip R., & Caroll L. Estes. (1983). New federalism and health policy. *Annals of the American Acad-*

emy of Political and Social Science, 468 (July), 88–102.

Lockett, Betty A. (1984). Setting the federal agenda in health research: The case of the National Institute on Aging. *Journal of Health Politics, Policy and Law, 9* (Spring), 63–79.

Logan, Bruce M., David A. Rochefort, & Ernest W. Cook. (1985). Block grants for mental health: Elements of the state response. *Journal of Public Health Policy, 6* (December), 476–492.

Lostetter, John O., & John E. Chapman. (1979). The participation of the United States government in providing financial support for medical education. *Health Policy and Education, 1* (1), 27–65.

Martin, Edward D. (1975). Federal initiative in rural health. *Public Health Reports, 90* (July/August), 291–297.

McFarlane, Deborah R., & Kenneth J. Meier. (1993). Restructuring federalism: The impact of Reagan policies on the family planning program. *Journal of Health Politics, Policy and Law, 18* (Winter), 821–850.

Monheit, Alan C. (1990). Returns on U.S. health care expenditures. *Journal of Medical Practice Management, 6* (Summer), 7–13.

Mooney, Anne. (1977). The great society and health: Policies for narrowing the gaps in health status between the poor and the nonpoor. *Medical Care, 15* (August), 611–619.

Morford, Thomas G. (1989). Federal efforts to improve peer review organizations. *Health Affairs, 8* (Summer), 175–178.

Navarro, Vicente. (1987). Federal health policies in the United States: An alternative explanation. *Milbank Memorial Fund Quarterly, 65* (1), 81–111.

Parmet, Wendy E. (1993). Regulation and federalism: Legal impediments to state health care reform. *American Journal of Law and Medicine, 19* (1/2), 121–144.

Penchansky, Roy, & Elizabeth Axelson. (1974). Old values, New Federalism and program evaluation. *Medical Care, 12* (November), 893–905.

Perkoff, Gerald. (1976). The impact of federal programs, long-term dialysis programs: New selection criteria, new problems. *Hastings Center Report, 6* (June), 8–13.

Prussin, Jeffrey A. (1976). The nursing home administrator as an effective political advocate: An overview of the federal arena. *Journal of Long Term Care Administration, 4* (4), 1–13.

Rabe, Barry G. (1987). The refederalization of American health care. *Medical Care Review, 44* (Spring), 37–63.

Raskin, Ira E. (1975). Conceptual framework for research on the cost-effective allocation of federal resources. *Socio-Economic Planning Sciences, 9* (February), 1–10.

Rich, Robert F. (1975). Selective utilization of social sciences related information by federal policymakers. *Inquiry, 12* (September), 239–245.

Roemer, Milton I., & Mary H. McClanahan. (1960). Impact of government programs on voluntary hospitals. *Public Health Reports, 75* (June), 537–544.

Russell, Louise B. (1975). Effects of inflation on federal health spending. *Medical Care, 13* (September), 713–721.

Russell, Louise B. (1976). Inflation and the federal role in health. In Michael Zubkoff (Ed.), *Health: A victim or cause of inflation?* (pp. 225–244). New York: Prodist, Neale Watson Academic Publishers.

Russell, Louise B., Blair Bourque, Daniel Bourque, & Carol Burke. (1974). *Federal health spending, 1969–1974.* Washington, D.C.: Center for Health Policy Studies, National Planning Association

Russell, Louise B., & Carol S. Burke. (1978). The political economy of federal health programs in the United States: An historical review. *International Journal of Health Services, 8* (1), 55–77.

Schlesinger, Edward R. (1974). The impact of federal legislation on maternal and child health services in the United States. *Milbank Memorial Fund Quarterly/Health and Society, 52* (Winter), 1–14.

Scotch, Richard K. (1984). *From good will to civil rights: Transforming federal disability policy.* Philadelphia: Temple University Press.

Shannon, James A. (1976). Federal support of biomedical sciences, development and academic impact.

Journal of Medical Education, 51 (July, Suppl.), 1–98.

Shonick, William. (1995). *Government and health services: Government's role in the development of U.S. health services 1930–1980.* New York: Oxford University Press.

Smith, David G. (1971). Emerging patterns of federalism: The case of public health. In Mary F. Arnold, Mary L. Vaughn Blankenship, & John M. Hess (Eds.), *Administering health systems, issues and perspectives* (pp. 131–142). Chicago, IL: Aldine Publishing Co.

Stone, Deborah. (1980). The problem of monopoly power in federal health policy. *Milbank Memorial Fund Quarterly/Health and Society, 58* (Winter), 50–53.

Thompson, Frank J. (1986). New Federalism and health care policy: States and the old questions. *Journal of Health Politics, Policy and Law, 11* (1), 647–669.

Vladeck, Bruce C. (1979). The design of failure: Health policy and the structure of federalism. *Journal of Health Politics, Policy and Law, 4* (Fall), 522–535.

Warner, Judith S. (1976). Trends in the federal regulation of physician fees. *Inquiry, 13* (December), 364–370.

Warren, B. S. (1975). Coordination and expansion of federal health activities. *Public Health Reports, 9* (May/June), 270–277.

White, Ben B. (1977). *Falling arches: The case against federal intervention in the practice of medicine.* Hicksville, NY: Exposition Press.

Williams, A. P., et al. (1976). *The effect of federal biomedical research programs on academic medical centers* (Rand Report No. R-1943-PBRP). Santa Monica, CA: Rand Corporation.

Wilson, Florence A., & Duncan Neuhauser. (1985). The federal government and health. In Florence A. Wilson & Duncan Neuhauser (Eds.), *Health services in the United States* (2nd ed., pp. 130–225). Cambridge, MA: Ballinger.

Zwick, Daniel I., & Clyde J. Behney. (1976). Federal health services grants, 1965–1975. *Public Health Reports, 91* (November/December), 493–495.

Congress and the Legislative Process

Baumgartner, Frank R., & Jeffrey C. Talbert. (1995). From setting a national agenda on health care to making decisions in Congress. *Journal of Health Politics, Policy and Law, 20* (Summer), 437–445.

Bradley, John P. (1980). Shaping administrative policy with the aid of congressional oversight: The senate finance committee and medicare. *Western Political Quarterly, 33* (December), 492–501.

Common Cause. (1992). The medical-industry complex and its PAC contributions to congressional candidates, January 1, 1981 through June 30, 1991: A Common Cause study. *Journal of Public Health Policy, 13* (Summer), 224–241.

Davis, Raymond G. (1985). Congress and the emergence of public health policy. *Health Care Management Review, 10* (Winter), 61–74.

Feldstein, Paul J. (1988). *The politics of health legislation: An economic perspective.* Ann Arbor, MI: Health Administration Press.

Fuchs, Beth C., & John F. Hoadley. (1987). Reflections from inside the Beltway: How Congress and the president grapple with health policy. *PS, 20* (Spring), 212–220.

Ginsburg, Paul B. (1989). Physician payment policy in the 101st Congress. *Health Affairs, 8* (Spring), 5–20.

Gray, Bradford H. (1992). The legislative battle over health services research. *Health Affairs, 11* (Winter), 38–66.

Jones, Woodrow, Jr., & K. Robert Keiser. (1986). U.S. Senate voting on health and safety regulation: The effects of ideology and interest-group orientations. *Health Policy, 6* (1), 33–44.

Iglehart, John K. (1993). Health care reform: The labyrinth of Congress. *New England Journal of Medicine, 329* (November 18), 1593–1596.

Mann, Thomas E., & Norman J. Ornstein. (Eds.). (1995). *Intensive care: How Congress shapes health policy.* Washington, D.C.: The Brookings Institution.

Mariner, Wendy K. (1992). Legislative report: The national vaccine injury compensation program. *Health Affairs, 11* (Spring), 255–265.

Mueller, Keith J. (1986). An analysis of congressional health policy voting in the 1970's. *Journal of Health Politics, Policy and Law, 11* (Spring), 117–135.

Nexon, David. (1987). The politics of congressional health policy in the second half of the 1980's. *Medical Care Review, 44* (Spring), 65–88.

Rabe, Barry G. (1990). Legislative incapacity: The congressional role in environmental policy-making and the case of Superfund. *Journal of Health Politics, Policy and Law, 15* (Fall), 571–590.

Redman, Eric (1973). *The dance of legislation.* New York: Simon & Schuster.

Talbert, Jeffrey. (1995). Congressional partisanship and the failure of moderate health care reforms. *Journal of Health Politics, Policy and Law, 20* (Winter), 1033–1050.

Whiteman, David. (1987). What do they know and when do they know it? Health staff on the Hill. *PS, 20* (Spring), 221–225.

Federal Bureaucracy (see also Regulation)

Chu, Franklin D., & Sharland Trotter. (1974). *The madness establishment: Ralph Nader's study group report on the National Institute of Mental Health.* New York: Grossman Publishers.

Falkson, Joseph L. (1976). Minor skirmish in a monumental struggle: HEW's analysis of mental health services. *Policy Analysis, 2* (Winter), 93–119.

Feder, Judith M. (1976). The Social Security Administration and Medicare: A strategy of implementation. In Kenneth M. Friedman & Stuart H. Rakoff (Eds.), *Toward a national health policy: Public policy and the control of health care cost.* Lexington, MA: Lexington Books.

Fredrickson, Donald S. (1978). The National Institute of Health: Yesterday, today and tomorrow. *Public Health Reports, 93* (November/December), 642–647.

Greenberg, George D. (1975). Reorganization reconsidered: The U.S. public health service, 1960–1973. *Public Policy, 23* (Fall), 483–522.

Greenberg, George D. (1980). Constraints on management and secretarial behavior at HEW. *Polity, 13* (Fall), 57–79.

Harden, Victoria A. (1986). *Inventing the NIH: Federal biomedical research policy, 1887–1937.* Baltimore, MD: Johns Hopkins University Press.

Miles, Rufus E., Jr. (1974). *The Department of Health, Education, and Welfare.* New York: Praeger.

Sherman, John F. (1977). The organization and structure of the National Institutes of Health. *New England Journal of Medicine, 297* (July), 18–26.

Sparer, Michael, & Lawrence D. Brown. (1993). Between a rock and a hard place: How public managers manage Medicaid. In Frank J. Thompson (Ed.), *Revitalizing state and local public service* (pp. 279–306). San Francisco, CA: Jossey Bass.

Thompson, Frank J. (1981). *Health policy and the bureaucracy: Politics and implementation.* Cambridge, MA: MIT Press.

Federal–State Relations in Health and Health Care

Altenstetter, Christa, & James Bjorkman. (1975). *Federal impacts on state health policy: Lessons from Connecticut and Vermont.* New Haven: Yale Health Policy Project.

Altenstetter, Christa, & James Bjorkman. (1976). The impact of federal child health programs in Connecticut state health policy formation and service delivery: The rediscovery of federalism. In R. Thomas & C. O. Jones (Eds.), *Public policy making in a federal system* (Vol. 3, pp. 217–237). Beverly Hills, CA: Sage.

Altenstetter, Christa, & James Bjorkman. (1978). *Federal–state health policies and impacts: The politics of implementation.* Washington, D.C.: University Press of America.

Brown, Lawrence D. (1992). Political evolution of federal health care regulation. *Health Affairs, 11* (Winter), 17–37.

Buntz, C. Gregory, Theodore F. Macaluso, & Jay A. Azarow. (1978). Federal influence on state health policy. *Journal of Health Politics, Policy and Law, 3* (Spring), 71–86.

Dobson, Allen, Donald Moran, & Gary Young. (1992). Role of federal waivers in the health policy process. *Health Affairs, 11* (Winter), 72–94.

Foltz, Anne-Marie. (1978). *Uncertainties of federal child health politics: Impact in two states* (DHEW Pub. No. [PHS] 78-3190). Washington, D.C.: National Center for Health Services Research.

Foltz, Anne-Marie, & Donna Brown. (1975). State response to federal policy: Children, EPSTD and the Medicaid muddle. *Medical Care, 13* (August), 630–642.

Lashof, Joyce C., & Mark H. Lepper. (1976). Federal-state-local partnership in health. In United States Public Health Service, Health Resources Administration (Ed.), *Health in America, 1776–1976* (DHEW Pub. No. [HRA] 76–616, pp. 122–137). Washington, D.C.: U.S. Government Printing Office.

Passel, Petter, & Leonard Ross. (1978). *State policies and federal programs: Priorities and constraints.* New York: Praeger.

Potter, Margaret A., & Beaufort B. Longest Jr. (1994). The divergence of federal and state policies on the charitable tax exemption of nonprofit hospitals. *Journal of Health Politics, Policy and Law, 19* (Summer), 393–419. (Commentary: Paul M. Rosenberg, pp. 421–422).

Price, Isabel. (1978). What's happening to federally aided health programs under state departments of human resources. *Public Health Reports, 93* (May/June), 221–231.

Robins, Leonard. (1972). The impact of decategorizing federal programs: Before and after 314(d). *American Journal of Public Health, 62* (January), 24–29.

Robins, Leonard. (1975). The impact of converting categorical into block grants: The lessons from the 314(d) block grants in the Partnership for Health Act. *Publius, 6* (Winter), 49–70.

Scherr, Lawrence. (1978). Coping with intrusions by state and federal government agencies. *Federal Bulletin, 65* (3), 69–80.

Schneider, Saundra K. (1988). Intergovernmental influences on Medicaid program expenditures. *Public Administration Review, 48* (July/August), 756–763.

Snoke, Albert W., & Parnie S. Snoke. (1976). Linking private, public energies in health and welfare planning. *Hospitals, 50* (August), 53–58.

Tallon James R., Jr., & Richard P. Nathan. (1992). Federal/state partnership for health system reform. *Health Affairs, 11* (Winter), 7–16.

Webb, Bruce J. (1974). Impact of revenue sharing on local health centers. *Black Scholar, 5* (May), 10–15.

Role of the States in Health and Health Care

Altenstetter, Christa, & James Bjorkman. (1978). *Federal–state health policies and impacts: The politics of implementation.* Washington, D.C.: University Press of America.

Altman, Drew E., & Douglas H. Morgan. (1983). The role of state and local government in health. *Heath Affairs, 2* (Winter), 7–31.

Anderson, Gerard, Patrick Chaulk, & Elizabeth Fowler. (1993). Maryland: A regulatory approach to health system reform. *Health Affairs, 12* (Summer), 40–47.

Bachman, Sara, Stuart H. Altman, & Dennis F. Beatrice. (1988). What influences a state's approach to Medicaid reform? *Inquiry, 25* (Summer), 243–250.

Barrand, Nancy L., & Steven A. Schroeder. (1994). Lessons from the states. *Inquiry, 31* (Spring), 10–13.

Barrilleaux, Charles J., & Mark E. Miller. (1988). The political economy of state Medicaid policy. *American Political Science Review, 82*, 1089–1108.

Bentak, J. M. (Ed.). (1973). *A digest of state laws affecting prepayment of medical care, group practice and HMO's.* Germantown, MD: Aspen Systems Corporation.

Blendon, Robert J. (1981). The prospects for state and local governments playing a broader role in health care in the 1980's. *American Journal of Public Health, 71* (January, Suppl.), 9–14.

Blewett, Lynn A. (1994). State report: Reforms in Minnesota: Forging the path. *Health Affairs, 13* (Fall), 200–209.

Bovbjerg, Randall R. (1991). Commentary: Lessons for tort reform from Indiana. *Journal of Health Politics, Policy and Law, 16* (Fall), 465–484.

Bovbjerg, Randall R., & Barbara A. Davis. (1983). State's responses to federal health care "block grants": The first year. *Milbank Memorial Fund Quarterly, 61* (Fall), 523–560.

Bovbjerg, Randall R., & Christopher F. Koller. (1986). State health insurance pools: Current performance, future prospects. *Inquiry, 23* (Summer), 111–121.

Brown, E. Richard. (1990). State approaches to financing health care for the poor. *Annual Review of Public Health, 11,* 377–400.

Brown, E. Richard, & Michael R. Cousineau. (1984). Effectiveness of state mandates to maintain local government health services for the poor. *Journal of Health Politics, Policy and Law, 9* (Summer), 223–236.

Brown, Lawrence D. (1991). The national politics of Oregon's rationing plan. *Health Affairs, 10* (Summer), 28–51.

Brown, Lawrence D. (1993). Commissions, clubs, and consensus: Florida reorganizes for health reform. *Health Affairs, 12* (Summer), 7–26.

Butter, Irene H., & Bonnie J. Kay. (1988). State laws and the practice of midwifery. *American Journal of Public Health, 78* (September), 1161–1169.

Callahan, Daniel. (1991). Ethics and priority setting in Oregon. *Health Affairs, 10* (Summer), 78–87.

Cantor, Joel C. (Ed.). (1995). Health reform in the states. *Advances in Health Economics and Health Services Research, 15.*

Cantor, Joel C., Stephen H. Long, & M. Susan Marquis. (1995). Private employment-based insurance in ten states. *Health Affairs, 14* (Summer), 199–211.

Chirba-Martin, Mary Ann, & Troyen A. Brennan. (1994). The critical role of ERISA in state health reform. *Health Affairs, 13* (Spring, 2), 142–156.

Chirikos, Thomas N. (1977). State health manpower policy: An appraisal. *Journal of Community Health, 2* (Spring), 163–177.

Christianson, Jon B., & Diane G. Hillman. (1986). *Health care for the indigent and competitive contracts: The Arizona experience.* Ann Arbor, MI: Health Administration Press.

Christianson, Jon B., Diane Hillman, & Kenneth R. Smith. (1983). The Arizona experience: Competitive bidding for indigent medical care. *Health Affairs, 2* (Fall), 87–103.

Christianson, Jon B., Douglas R. Wholey, & Susan M. Sanchez. (1991). State responses to HMO failures. *Health Affairs, 19* (Winter), 78–91.

Clarke, Gary J. (1975). *Health programs in the states: A survey.* New Brunswick, NJ: Rutgers University, Eagleton Institute of Politics.

Clarke, Gary J. (1976). *Health expenditures by state governments.* Washington, D.C.: Georgetown University Health Policy Center.

Clarke, Gary J. (1981). The role of the state in the delivery of health services. *American Journal of Public Health, 71* (January, Suppl.), 59–61.

Colner, Alan N. (1977). The impact of state government rate setting on hospital management. *Health Care Management Review, 2* (Winter), 37–49.

Connor, Gerald R. (1976). State government financing of health planning. *American Journal of Health Planning, 1* (October), 48–49, 51.

Cooper, Paul P., III, & Kylanne Green. (1991). The impact of state laws on managed care. *Health Affairs, 10* (Winter), 161–169.

Coughlin, Teresa A., Leighton Ku, John Holahan, David Heslam, & Colin Winterbottom. (1994). State responses to the Medicaid spending crisis: 1988 to 1992. *Journal of Health Politics, Policy and Law, 19* (Winter), 837–864.

Crittenden, Robert A. (1993). Managed competition and premium caps in Washington State. *Health Affairs, 12* (Summer), 82–88.

Crittenden, Robert A. (1995). State report: Recent action in Washington and Oregon. *Health Affairs, 14* (Summer), 302–305.

Cromwell, Jerry. (1987). Impact of state hospital rate setting on capital formation. *Health Care Financing Review, 8* (Spring), 57–67.

Curtis, Rick. (1986). The role of state governments in assuring access to care. *Inquiry, 23* (Fall), 277–285.

Davidson, Stephen M. (1978). Variations in state Medicaid programs. *Journal of Health Politics, Policy and Law, 3* (Spring), 54–70.

Dean, Howard M. (1993). New rules and roles for states. *Health Affairs, 12* (Spring), 183–184.

Desonia, Randolph, & Kathleen M. King. (1985). *State programs of assistance for the medically indigent.* Washington, D.C.: Intergovernmental Health Policy Project, George Washington University.

Dick, Andrew W. (1994). State report: Will employer mandates really work? Another look at Hawaii. *Health Affairs, 13* (Spring), 343–349.

DiIulio, John J., & Richard P. Nathan. (Eds.). (1994). *Making health reform work: The view from the states.* Washington, D.C.: The Brookings Institution.

Dowell, Emery B., & Thomas R. Oliver. (1994). Small-employer health alliance in California. *Health Affairs, 13* (Spring), 350–351.

Dranove, David, & Kenneth Kone. (1985). Do states' rate setting regulations really lower hospital expenses? *Journal of Health Economics, 4* (June), 159–165.

Dukakis, Michael S. (1992a). Hawaii and Massachusetts: Lessons from the states. *Yale Law and Policy Review, 10* (2), 397–408.

Dukakis, Michael. (1992b). The states and health care reform. *New England Journal of Medicine, 327* (October 8), 1090–1092.

Eddy, David M. (1991). Oregon's methods: Did cost-effectiveness analysis fail? *Journal of American Medical Association, 266* (October 16), 2135–2141.

Ellet, T. Van. (1980a). *Medigap: State responses to problems with the sale of health insurance to the elderly.* Washington, D.C.: George Washington University, Intergovernmental Health Policy Project.

Ellet, T. Van. (1980b). *State comprehensive and catastrophic health insurance plans: An overview.* Washington, D.C.: George Washington University, Intergovernmental Health Project.

Ernst & Young. (1994). *Not waiting for Washington: State health care reform.* Washington, D.C.: Ernst & Young.

Essock, Susan M., & Howard H. Goldman. (1995). States' embrace of managed mental health care. *Health Affairs, 14* (Fall), 34–44.

Feldman, Penny, Marsha Gold, & Karyen Chu. (1994). Enhancing information for state health policy. *Health Affairs, 13* (Summer), 236–250.

Finkler, Merton D. (1987). State rate setting revisited. *Health Affairs, 6* (Winter), 82–89.

Fossett, James W. (1993). Medicaid and health reform: The case of New York. *Health Affairs, 12* (Fall), 81–94.

Fox, Daniel M., & Howard M. Leichter. (1991). Rationing care in Oregon: The new accountability. *Health Affairs, 10* (Summer), 7–27.

Fox, Daniel M., & Howard M. Leichter. (1993). The ups and downs of Oregon's rationing plan. *Health Affairs, 12* (Summer), 66–70.

Fraley, Collette. (1995). States guard their borders as Medicaid talks begin. *Congressional Quarterly, 54* (223), 1637–1641.

Freedman, Ben. (1975). Cost of fragmentation of state government operated health services. *Inquiry, 12* (September), 216–227.

Friedman, Emily. (1994). Getting a head start: The states and health care reform. *Journal of American Medical Association, 271* (March 16), 875–878.

Gabel, Jon R., & Gail A. Jensen. (1989). The price of state mandated benefits. *Inquiry, 26* (Winter), 419–431.

Gardner, Annette, & Deane Neubauer. (1995). Update: State report: Hawaii's health quest. *Health Affairs, 14* (Spring), 300–303.

Gardiner, John A., & Theodore R. Lyman. (1984). *The fraud control game: State responses to fraud and abuse in the AFDC and Medicaid programs.* Bloomington: Indiana University Press.

Garland, Michael J. (1992). Light on the black box of basic health care: Oregon's contribution to the national movement toward universal health insurance. *Yale Law and Policy Review, 10* (2), 409–430.

Gartland, Jenifer D. C., & Beth K. Yudkowsky. (1993). State estimates of uninsured children. *Health Affairs, 12* (Spring), 144–151.

Gilbert, Benjamin, Merry-K Moos, & C. Arden Miller. (1982). State level decision making for public health: The status of boards of health. *Journal of Public Health Policy, 3* (March), 51–63.

Ginzberg, Eli, Edith Davis, & Miriam Ostow. (1985). *Local health policy in action: The municipal health services program.* Savage, MD: Rowman & Littlefield Publishers, Inc.

Glantz, Leonard H. (1985). Mandating health insurance benefits in the private sector: A decision for state legislatures. *American Journal of Public Health, 75* (November), 1344–1346.

Glied, Sherry, Michael Sparer, & Lawrence Brown. (1991). Comment: Containing state health care expenditures—the competition versus regulation debate. *American Journal of Public Health, 85* (October), 1347–1349.

Goddeeris, John H., & Andrew J. Hogan. (Eds.). (1992). *Improving access to health care: What can the states do?* Kalamazoo, MI: W. E. Upjohn Institute.

Goggin, Malcolm L. (1987). *Policy design and the politics of implementation: The case of child care in the American states.* Knoxville: University of Tennessee Press.

Gold, Steven D. (1992). One approach to tracking state and local health spending. *Health Affairs, 11* (Winter), 135–144.

Grogan, Colleen M. (1995). Hope in federalism? What can the states do and what are they likely to do? *Journal of Health Politics, Policy and Law, 20* (Summer), 477–484.

Grossman, Bob, & Jim Shon. (Eds.). (1994). *The unfinished health agenda: Lessons from Hawaii.* Honolulu: University of Hawaii Press.

Hackey, Robert B. (1992). Trapped between state and market: Regulating hospital reimbursement in the Northeastern states. *Medical Care Review, 49* (Fall), 355–388.

Hackey, Robert B. (1993). Commentary: Regulatory regimes and state cost containment programs. *Journal of Health Politics, Policy and Law, 18* (Summer), 491–502.

Hanson, Russell L. (1993). Defining a role for states in a federal health care system. *American Behavioral Scientist, 36* (July), 760–781.

Harrington, Charlene, et al. (1986). Effects of state Medicaid policies on the aged. *The Gerontologist, 26* (September), 437–443.

Harrington, Charlene, & James H. Swan. (1987). The impact of state Medicaid nursing home policies on utilization and expectations. *Inquiry, 24* (Summer), 157–172.

Haynes, Pamela L. (1985). *Evaluating state Medicaid reforms.* Washington, D.C.: American Enterprise Institute.

Hillman, Diane G., & Jon B. Christianson. (1985). Health care expenditure containment in the United States: Strategies at the state and local levels. *Social Science and Medicine, 20* (12), 1319–1330.

Hoadley, John F., & Donald F. Cox. (1994). Measuring state health spending: Another look. *Health Affairs, 13* (Winter), 202–207.

Hoare, Geoffrey, Marilyn Mayers, & Carolyn Madden. (1992). Lessons from implementation of Washington's basic health plan. *Health Affairs, 11* (Summer), 212–218.

Holahan, John. (1985). State rate setting and its effects on the cost of nursing home care. *Journal of Health Politics, Policy and Law, 9* (Winter), 647–668.

Iglehart, John K. (1994). Health care reform—the states. *New England Journal of Medicine, 330* (January 6), 75–79.

Jain, Sager. (Ed.). (1981a). Role of state and local governments in relation to personal health services. *American Journal of Public Health, 71* (January, Suppl.).

Jain, Sager. (Ed.). (1981b). *Role of state and local governments in relation to personal health services.* Washington, D.C.: American Public Health Association.

Justice, Diane. (1988). *State long term care and reform: Development of community care systems in six states.* Washington, D.C.: National Governors Association.

Kaplan, Sherrie H., & Sheldon Greenfield. (1994). Evaluation of new statewide health reform initiatives. *Milbank Quarterly, 72* (4), 695–700.

Kennedy, Virginia C., Stephen H. Linder, & William D. Spears. (1987). Estimating the impact of state manpower policy: A case study of reducing medical school enrollments. *Journal of Health Politics, Policy and Law, 12* (Summer), 299–312.

Kern, Rosemary Gibson, & Susan R. Windham. (1986). *Medicaid and other experiments in state health policy.* Washington, D.C.: American Enterprise Institute.

Kiel, Joan M. (1993). How state policy affects rural hospital consortia: The rural health care delivery system. *Milbank Quarterly, 71* (4), 625–644.

Kindig, David A., & Donald L. Libby. (1994). Setting state health spending limits. *Health Affairs, 13* (Spring, 2), 288–289.

Kovner, Anthony R., & Edward J. Lusk. (1975). State regulation of health care costs. *Medical Care, 13* (August), 619–629.

Kronick, Richard. (1991). Can Massachusetts pay for health care for all? *Health Affairs, 10* (Spring), 26–44.

Laird, Maureen. (1976). State roles in financing medical education. *Journal of Medical Education, 51* (March), 206–209.

Laudicina, Susan S. (1988). State health risk pools: Insuring the "uninsurable." *Health Affairs, 7* (Fall), 97–104.

Laumann, Edward O., David Knoke, & Yong-Hak Kim. (1985). An organizational approach to state policy formation: A comparative study of energy and health domains. *American Sociological Review, 50* (February), 1–19.

Leichter, Howard M. (1992). The states and health care policy: Taking the lead. In Howard M. Leichter (Ed.), *Health policy reform in America.* Armonk, NY: M. E. Sharpe.

Leichter, Howard M. (1993a). Health care reform in Vermont: A work in progress. *Health Affairs, 12* (Summer), 71–81.

Leichter, Howard M. (1993b). Minnesota: The trip from acrimony to accommodation. *Health Affairs, 12* (Summer), 48–58.

Leichter, Howard M. (1994). Healthcare reform in Vermont: The next chapter. *Health Affairs, 13* (Winter), 78–103.

Levine, Peter. (1984). An overview of the state role in the United States health scene. In Theodor J. Litman & Leonard S. Robins (Eds.), *Health politics and policy* (1st ed., pp. 194–220). New York: John Wiley & Sons.

Levit, Katharine R. (1985). Personal health care expenditures, by state: 1966–1982. *Health Care Financing Review, 6* (Summer), 1–49.

Levit, Katharine R. (1994). Use of state-specific data for policy: The author responds. *Health Affairs, 13* (Winter), 214–219.

Levit, Katharine R., Helen C. Lazenby, Cathy A. Cowan, & Suzanne W. Letsch. (1993). Health spending by state: New estimates for policy making. *Health Affairs, 12* (Fall), 7–26.

Lewin, John C., & Peter A. Sybinsky. (1994). State health spending estimates: Concerns from a small state. *Health Affairs, 13* (Winter), 208–213.

Lewin, Lawrence S., & Robert A. Derzon. (1982). Health professions education: State responsibilities under the New Federalism. *Health Affairs, 1* (Spring), 69–85.

Lipson, Debra J. (1988a). *Major changes in state Medicaid and independent care programs.* Washington, D.C.: Intergovernmental Health Policy Project, George Washington University.

Lipson, Debra J. (1988b). Massachusetts legislation: A model for other states or a costly mistake? *Business and Health, 5* (August), 48–49.

Lipson, Debra J. (1992). *From rhetoric to reality: Federal health reform will be hard—but state reforms may guide the way.* (Faulkner & Gray Research Report No. 92–4). Washington, D.C.: Faulkner & Gray, Inc.

Lipson, Debra J., & Elizabeth Donohoe. (1988). *State financing of long term care services for the elderly.* Washington, D.C.: George Washington University, Intergovernmental Health Policy Project.

Logan, Bruce M., David A. Rochefort, & Ernest W. Cook. (1985). Block grants for mental health: Elements of the state response. *Journal of Public Health Policy, 6* (December), 476–494.

Long, Stephen H., & M. Susan Marquis. (1996). Some pitfalls in making cost estimates of state health insurance coverage expansions. *Inquiry, 33* (Spring), 85–91.

Madden, Carolyn W., Geoffrey Hoare, Marilyn Mayers, & William J. Hagens. (1992). Washington State's basic health plan: Choices and challenges. *Journal of Public Health Policy, 13* (Spring), 81–96.

Manning, Bayless, & Bruce C. Vladeck. (1983). The role of state and local government in health: Update. *Health Affairs, 2* (Winter), 134–140.

McCall, Nelda. (1983). *Medigap—study of comparative effectiveness of various state regulations.* Menlo Park, CA: SRI International.

McCall, Nelda, Thomas Rice, & Arden Hall. (1987). The effect of state regulations on the quality and sale of insurance policies to Medicare beneficiaries. *Journal of Health Politics, Policy and Law, 12* (Spring), 53–76.

McCall, Nelda, C. William Wrightson, Lynne Parringer, & Gordon Trapnell. (1994). Managing Medicaid cost savings: The Arizona experience. *Health Affairs, 13* (Spring, 2), 234–245.

McCloskey, Amanda, Jennifer Woolwich, & Danielle Holahan. (1995). *Reforming the health care system: State profiles 1995.* Washington, D.C.: American Association of Retired Persons Public Policy Institute.

McCombs, Jeffrey S., & Jon B. Christianson. (1987). Applying competitive bidding to health care. *Journal of Health Politics, Policy and Law, 12* (Winter), 703–722.

Mechanic, David, & Richard C. Surles. (1992). Challenges in state mental health policy and administration. *Health Affairs, 11* (Fall), 34–50.

Melnick, Glenn, & Jack Zwanziger. (1995). State health care expenditures under competition and regulation, 1980 through 1991. *American Journal of Public Health, 85* (October), 1391–1396.

Mendelson, Daniel N., Richard G. Abramson, & Robert J. Rubin. (1995). State involvement in technology assessment. *Health Affairs, 14* (Summer), 83–98.

Merritt, Richard, & Susan Mertes. (1980). *State innovations in health.* Washington, D.C.: George Washington University, Intergovernmental Health Policy Project.

Milne, Thomas L. (1990). A separate Department of Health in Washington State: Four years before the mast. *Journal of Public Health Policy, 11* (Autumn), 305–315.

Morrisey, Michael A., Frank A. Sloan, & Samuel A. Mitchell. (1983). State rate setting: An analysis of some unresolved issues. *Health Affairs, 2* (Summer), 36–47.

Moscovice, Ira. (1986). Health services research and the policy making process: State response to federal cutbacks in programs affecting child health. In Marion Ein Lewin (Ed.), *From research into policy: Improving the link for health services* (pp. 34–50). Washington, D.C.: American Enterprise Institute for Public Policy Research.

Neubauer, Deane. (1993). Hawaii: A pioneer in health system reform. *Health Affairs, 12* (Summer), 31–39.

O'Kane, Margaret. (1984). State implementation of health block grants. *Focus On . . . No. 5.* Washington, D.C.: George Washington University, Intergovernmental Health Policy Project.

Omenn, Gilbert S. (1987). Lessons from a fourteen state study of Medicaid. *Health Affairs, 6* (Spring), 118–122.

Parmet, Wendy. (1993). Regulation and federalism: Legal impediments to state health care reform. *American Journal of Law and Medicine, 19* (1/2), 121–144.

Paul, Rebecca R. (1995). *From payer to purchaser: State strategies to purchase health benefits.* Washington, D.C.: Alpha Center.

Peterson, George E., Randall R. Bovbjerg, & Barbara A. Davis. (1986). *The Reagan block grants: What have we learned?* Washington, D.C.: Urban Institute Press.

Polich, Cynthia L., & Laura H. Iversen. (1987). State preadmission screening programs for controlling utilization of long term care. *Health Care Financing Review, 8* (Fall), 43–48.

Pollack, David A., Bentson H. McFarland, Robert A. George, & Richard H. Angell. (1994). Prioritization of mental health services in Oregon. *Milbank Quarterly, 72* (3), 515–550.

Potter, Margaret A., & Beaufort B. Longest Jr. (1994). The divergence of federal and state policies on the charitable tax exemption of nonprofit hospitals. *Journal of Health Politics, Policy and Law, 19* (Summer), 393–420.

Renaud, Marc. (1975). On the structural constraints to state intervention in health. *International Journal of Health Services, 5* (4), 559–572.

Rivo, Marc, Tim M. Henderson, & Debbie M. Jackson. (1995). State legislative strategies to improve supply and distribution of generalist physicians, 1985–1992. *American Journal of Public Health, 85* (March), 405–407.

Rogal, Deborah L., & W. David Helms. (1993). State models: Tracking states' efforts to reform their health systems. *Health Affairs, 12* (Summer), 27–30.

Rosenbaum, Sara, & Kay Johnson. (1986). Providing health care for low income children: Reconciling child health goals with child health financing realities. *Milbank Quarterly, 64* (3), 442–478.

Rosenberg, Paul M. (1994). Federal and state policies on the charitable tax exemption of nonprofit hospitals. *Journal of Health Politics, Policy and Law, 19* (Summer), 421–422.

Rosenkrantz, Barbara G. (1972). *Public health and the state: Changing views in Massachusetts, 1842–1936.* Cambridge, MA: Harvard University Press.

Schramm, Carl J. (1978). Regulatory hospital labor costs: A case study in the politics of state rate commissions. *Journal of Health Politics, Policy and Law, 3* (Fall), 364–374.

Schramm, Carl J. (1986). State hospital cost containment: An analysis of legislative initiatives. *Indiana Law Review, 19* (4), 919–954.

Schwartz, Jerome L. (1979). Strategies for monitoring the effects of Proposition 13 on health services. *Journal of Health Politics, Policy and Law, 4* (Summer), 142–154.

Shortell, Stephen M. (1992). A model for state health care reform. *Health Affairs, 11* (Spring), 108–127.

Shultz, James M., Michael E. Moen, Terry F. Pechacek, et al. (1986). The Minnesota plan for nonsmoking and health: The legislative experience. *Journal of Public Health Policy, 7* (Autumn), 300–313.

Sloan, Frank A. (1985). State responses to the malpractice insurance "crisis" of the 1970's: An empirical assessment. *Journal of Health Politics, Policy and Law, 9* (Winter), 629–646.

Smith, David W., Stephanie L. McFall, & Michael B. Pine. (1993). State rate regulation and inpatient mortality rates. *Inquiry, 30* (Spring), 23–33.

Snoke, Parnie S., & Albert W. Snoke. (1975). State role in the regulation of the health delivery system. *University of Toledo Law Review, 6* (Spring), 617–646.

Somers, Stephen A., & Jeffrey C. Merrill. (1991). Supporting states' efforts for long-term care insurance. *Health Affairs, 10* (Spring), 177–179.

Soumerai, Stephen B., & Dennis Ross-Degman. (1990). Experience of state drug benefit programs. *Health Affairs, 9* (Fall), 36–54.

Soumerai, Stephen B., Dennis Ross-Degman, Eric E. Fortess, & Julia Abelson. (1993). A critical analysis of studies of state drug reimbursement policies: Research in need of discipline. *Milbank Quarterly, 71* (2), 217–252.

Sparer, Michael S. (1993a). Commentary: States in a reformed health system: Lessons from nursing home policy. *Health Affairs, 12* (Spring), 7–20.

Sparer, Michael S. (1993b). States and the health care crisis. *Journal of Health Politics, Policy and Law, 18* (Summer), 503–514.

Sparer, Michael S. (1995). Great expectations: The limits of state health care reform. *Health Affairs, 14* (Winter), 191–202.

Stearns, Sally C., & Rebecca T. Slifkin. (1995). State risk pools and mental health care use. *Health Affairs, 14* (Fall), 220–231.

Stone, Deborah A. (1992). Why the states can't solve the health care crisis. *The American Prospect, 12* (Spring), 51–60.

Strosberg, Martin A., Joshua M. Wiener, & Robert Baker with I. Alan Fein. (Eds.). (1992). *Rationing America's medical care: The Oregon plan and beyond.* Washington, D.C.: The Brookings Institution.

Swan, James H., Charlene Harrington, & Leslie A. Grant. (1988). State Medicaid reimbursement for nursing homes, 1978–1986. *Health Care Financing Review, 9* (Spring), 33–50.

Teevans, James W., & Daniel M. Campion. (1995). *State-action immunity? Immunizing health care cooperative agreements.* Washington, D.C.: Alpha Center.

Thomas, Constance S., Thomas M. Henderson, Linda R. Lipson, & Peter A. Dibiaso. (1995). *A review of state legislation related to increasing the training, supply, recruitment and retention of generalist physicians, 1985–1991.* Prepared by the Intergovernmental Health Policy project at the George Washington University. Publication No. HRSA-HC-PC-94-2. Health Resources and Services Administration. Washington, D.C.: U.S. Government Printing Office.

Volpp, Kevin G., & Bruce Siegel. (1993). New Jersey: Long-term experience with all-payer state rate setting. *Health Affairs, 12* (Summer), 59–65.

Weissert, Carol S., Jack H. Knott, & Blair E. Stieber. (1994). Education and the health professions: Expanding policy choices among the states. *Journal of Health Politics, Policy and Law, 19* (Summer), 361–392.

Williams-Crowe, Sharon M., & Terry V. Aultman. (1994). State health agencies and the legislative policy process. *American Journal of Public Health, 109* (May/June), 361–367.

Winterbottom, David, W. Liska, & Karen M. Obermaier. (1995). *State-level databook on health care access and financing* (2nd ed.). Washington, D.C.: Urban Institute Press.

Yawn, Barbara P., William E. Jacott, & Roy A. Yawn. (1993). MinnesotaCare (HealthRight): Myths and miracles. *Journal of the American Medical Association, 269* (January 21), 511–515.

Ziegler, Andrew. (1987). *States address shortage, distribution of health professionals.* Washington, D.C.: George Washington University, Intergovernmental Health Policy Project.

Zwanziger, Jack, Geoffrey M. Anderson, Susan G. Haber, Kenneth E. Thorpe, & Joseph P. Newhouse. (1993). Comparison of hospital costs in California, New York and Canada. *Health Affairs, 12* (Summer), 130–139.

State–Local Relationships

Berger, Stephen. (1977). The interplay of state and local government in health care. In Arthur Levin (Ed.), *Health services: The local perspective* (Vol. 32, No. 3, pp. 63–67). New York: Academy of Political Science.

Fowinkle, Eugene. (1977). The state role in the delivery of local health services. In Arthur Levin (Ed.), *Health services: The local perspective* (Vol. 32, No. 3, pp. 53–62). New York: Academy of Political Science.

Gayer, David. (1972). The effects of medicaid on state and local government finances. *National Tax Journal, 25* (December), 511–519.

Local Government

Bellin, Lowell E. (1977). Local Health Departments: A prescription against obsolescence. In Arthur Levin (Ed.), *Health services: The local perspective* (Vol. 32, No. 3, pp. 42–52). New York: Academy of Political Science.

Glaudemans, Jon. (1994). The case for local budgeting. *Health Affairs, 13* (Spring), 243–246.

Hahn, Alan J. (1994). *The politics of caring.* New Brunswick, NJ: Westview Press.

Ingraham, Norman R. (1961). Formulation of public policy in medical care: Dynamics of community action at local level. *American Journal of Public Health, 51* (August), 1144–1151.

Koppel, J., & J. Clark. (1976). *The role of county government in Medicaid.* Washington, D.C.: National Association of Counties.

Levin, Arthur. (1977). *Health services: The local perspective.* Paper presented at the Proceedings of the Academy of Political Science (Vol. 32, No. 3). New York: Academy of Political Science.

Miller, C. Arden. (1975). Issues of health policy: Local government and the public's health. *American Journal of Public Health, 65* (December), 1330–1334.

Millman, Michael. (1981). The role of city government in personal health services. *American Journal of Public Health, 71* (January, Suppl.), 47–57.

Mytinger, Robert E. (1967). Barriers to adoption of new programs as perceived by local health officers. *Public Health Reports, 82* (February), 108–114.

Piore, Nora, Purlaine Lieberman, & James Linane. (1977a). Financing local health services. In Arthur Levin (Ed.), *Health services: The local perspective* (Vol. 32, No. 3, pp. 15–28). New York: Academy of Political Science.

Piore, Nora, Purlaine Lieberman, & James Linane. (1977b). Public expenditures and private control? Health care dilemma in New York City. *Milbank Memorial Fund Quarterly/Health and Society, 55* (Winter), 79–116.

Robins, Leonard. (1977). Controlling health care costs. In Arthur Levin (Ed.), *Health services: The local perspective* (Vol. 32, No. 3, pp. 215–226). New York: Academy of Political Science.

Schwartz, Jerome L. (1979). Strategies for monitoring the effects of Proposition 13 on health services. *Journal of Health Politics, Policy and Law, 4* (Summer), 142–154.

Shonick, William, & Walter Price. (1977). Reorganizations of health agencies by local government in American urban centers: What do they portend for "public health." *Milbank Memorial Fund Quarterly/Health and Society, 55* (Spring), 233–271.

Shonick, William, & Walter Price. (1978). Organizational milieus of local public health units: Analysis of response to questionnaire. *Public Health Reports, 93* (November/December), 648–665.

PARTICIPATORY DEMOCRACY

Public Opinion

Altman, Drew E. (1995). The realities behind the polls. *Health Affairs, 14* (Spring), 24–26.

Berk, Marc L. (1994). Perspective: Should we rely on polls? *Health Affairs, 13* (Spring), 299–300.

Blendon, Robert J. (1988). The public's view of the future of health care. *Journal of the American Medical Association, 259* (June 24), 3587–3593.

Blendon, Robert J., & Drew E. Altman. (1984). Public attitudes about health care costs: A lesson in national schizophrenia. *New England Journal of Medicine, 311* (August), 613–616.

Blendon, Robert J., & Drew E. Altman. (1987). Public opinion and health care costs. In Carl J. Schramm (Ed.), *Health care and its cost: Can the U.S. afford adequate care?* (pp. 49–63). New York: W. W. Norton.

Blendon, Robert J., Drew E. Altman, John M. Benson, Mollyann Brodie, Matt James, & Larry Hugick. (1994). How much does the public know about health reform? *Journal of American Health Policy, 4* (January/February), 26–31.

Blendon, Robert J., Mollyann Brodie, & John M. Benson. (1995). What happened to American's support for the Clinton plan? *Health Affairs, 14* (Summer), 7–23.

Blendon, Robert J., Mollyann Brodie, Tracey Stelzer Hyams, & John M. Benson. (1994). The American public and the critical choices for health system reform. *Journal of the American Medical Association, 271* (May 18), 1539–1544.

Blendon, Robert J., & Karen Donelan. (1991). Interpreting public opinion surveys. *Health Affairs, 10* (Summer), 166–169.

Blendon, Robert J., Karen Donelan, Craig Hill, Ann Scheck, Woody Carter, Dennis Beatrice, & Drew Altman. (1993). Medicaid beneficiaries and health reform. *Health Affairs, 12* (Spring), 132–143.

Blendon, Robert J., Karen Donelan, Albert J. Jonell, Laura Pellisé, & Enrique Costas Lombardia. (1991). Spain's citizens assess their health care system. *Health Affairs, 10* (Fall), 216–228.

Blendon, Robert J., Jennifer N. Edwards, & Ulrike S. Szalay. (1991). Perspectives: Future of private health insurance, health insurance industry in the year 2001. *Health Affairs, 10* (Winter), 170–177.

Blendon, Robert J., & Tracey Hyams. (1992). Reforming the system: *Containing health care costs in an era of universal coverage.* Washington, D.C.: Faulkner & Gray, Inc.

Blendon, Robert J., Robert Leitman, Ian Morrison, & Karen Donelan. (1990). Satisfaction with health systems in ten nations. *Health Affairs, 9* (Summer), 185–192.

Blendon, Robert J., John Mattila, John M. Benson, Matthew C. Shelter, Francis J. Connolly, & Tom Kney. (1994). The beliefs and values shaping today's health reform debate. *Health Affairs, 13* (Spring), 274–284.

Blendon, Robert J., & Humphrey Taylor. (1989). Views on health care: Public opinion in three nations. *Health Affairs, 8* (Spring), 149–157.

Bowman, Karlyn H. (1994). *Public attitudes on health care reform: Are the polls misleading the policy makers?* American Enterprise Institute Special Studies in Health Reform. Waldorf, MD: AEI Press.

Brodie, Mollyann, & Robert J. Blendon. (1995). The public's contribution to congressional gridlock on health care reform. *Journal of Health Politics, Policy and Law, 20* (Summer), 403–410.

Cantor, Joel C., Nancy L. Barrand, Randolph A. Desonia, Alan B. Cohen, & Jeffrey C. Merrill. (1991). Business leader's views on American health care. *Health Affairs, 10* (Spring), 98–105.

Cappella, Joseph N., & Kathleen Hall Jamieson. (1994). Tuned into "to your health." *Journal of American Health Care, 4* (September/October), 37–40.

Erskine, Hazel. (1975). The polls: Health insurance. *Public Opinion Quarterly, 39* (Spring), 128–143.

Gabel, Jon, Howard Cohen, & Stephen Fink. (1989). Americans' views on health care. *Health Affairs, 8* (Spring), 103–118.

Harvey, Lynn, & Stephanie Shubat. (1986). *AMA surveys of physician and public opinion: 1986.* Chicago: American Medical Association.

Iglehart, John R. (1984). Opinion polls on health care. *New England Journal of Medicine, 310* (June 14), 1616–1620.

Jacobs, Lawrence R. (1993). *The health of nations: Public opinion and the making of American and British health policy.* Ithaca, NY: Cornell University Press.

Jacobs, Lawrence R., & Robert Y. Shapiro. (1994). Public opinion's tilt against private enterprise. *Health Affairs, 13* (Spring), 285–298.

Jacobs, Lawrence R., & Robert Y. Shapiro. (1995). Don't blame the public for failed health care reform. *Journal of Health Politics, Policy and Law, 20* (Summer), 411–423.

Jacobs, Lawrence R., Robert Shapiro, & Eli Schulman. (1993). Poll trends: Medical care in the United States—an update. *Public Opinion Quarterly, 57* (Fall), 394–427.

Jajich-Toth, Cindy, & Burns W. Roper. (1990). Views on health care: A study in contradictions. *Health Affairs, 9* (Winter), 149–157.

Jeffe, Douglas, & Sherry Bebitch Jeffe. (1984). Losing patience with doctors: Physicians versus the public on health care costs. *Public Opinion, 7* (February/March), 45–55.

Mick, Stephen S., & John D. Thompson. (1984). Public attitudes towards health planning under the Health Systems Agencies. *Journal of Health Politics, Policy and Law, 8* (Winter), 782–800.

Perlstadt, Harry, & Russell E. Holmes. (1987). The role of public opinion polling in health legislation. *American Journal of Public Health, 77* (May), 612–614.

Rochefort, David A., & Carol A. Boyer. (1988). Use of public opinion data in public administration: Health care polls. *Public Administration Review, 48* (March/April), 649–660.

Rogers, David E., & Eli Ginzberg. (Eds.). (1989). *Public and professional attitudes toward AIDS patients: A national dilemma.* Boulder, CO: Westview Press.

Shapiro, Robert, & John Young. (1986). The polls: Medical care in the United States. *Public Opinion Quarterly, 50* (Fall), 418–428.

Singer, Eleanor, Theresa F. Rogers, & Mary Corcoran. (1987). The polls—a report: AIDS. *Public Opinion Quarterly, 51* (Winter), 580–595.

Smith, Mark D., Drew E. Altman, Robert Leitman, Thomas W. Moloney, & Humphrey Taylor. (1992). Taking the public's pulse on health reform. *Health Affairs, 11* (Summer), 125–133.

Steiber, Steven R., & Leonard A. Ferber. (1981). Support for national health insurance: Intercohort differentials. *Public Opinion Quarterly, 45* (Summer), 179–198.

Taylor, Humphrey. (1985). Healing the health care system. *Public Opinion Quarterly, 8* (August/September), 16–20, 60.

Vernick, Jon S., Stephen P. Teret, Kim Ammann Howard, Michael D. Teret, & Caren J. Wintemute.

(1993). Public opinion polling on gun policy. *Health Affairs, 12* (Winter), 198–208.

Wagenaar, Alexander C., & Fredrick M. Steff. (1990). Public opinion on alcohol policies. *Journal of Public Health Policy, 11* (Summer), 189–205.

Yankelovich, Daniel. (1995). The debate that wasn't: The public and the Clinton plan. *Health Affairs, 14* (Spring), 7–23.

Yankelovich, Daniel, & John Immerwahr. (1991). The gap between public perception of a problem and expert perceptions must be narrowed before solutions can be found. *Health Management Quarterly, 13* (3), 11–14.

Political Parties and Health

Goldsmith, Seth B. (1973). Political party platform planks: A mechanism for participation and prediction? *American Journal of Public Health, 63* (July), 594–601.

Silver, George A. (1976). Medical politics, health policy, party health platforms, promise and performance. *International Journal of Health Services, 6* (2), 331–343.

Interest Group Politics and Health (see also Medicine and the Medical Profession)

Alford, Robert R. (1975). *Health care politics: Ideological and interest group barriers to reform.* Chicago: University of Chicago Press.

Binstock, Robert H. (1972). Interest-group liberalism and the politics of aging. *Gerontologist, 12* (Fall), Part 1, 265–280.

Butler, Henry N. (1994). *Unhealthy alliances: Bureaucrats, interest groups, and politicians in health reform.* American Enterprise Institute Special Studies in Health Reform. Waldorf, MD: AEI Press.

The Center for Public Integrity. (1995). Well-healed: Inside lobbying for health care reform. *International Journal of Health Services, 25* (3), Part I, 411–454; Part II, *25* (4), 593–632.

The Center for Public Integrity. (1996). Well-healed: Inside lobbying for health care reform. *International Journal of Health Services, 26* (1), Part III, 19–46.

Common Cause. (1992). The medical-industry complex and its PAC contributions to congressional candidates, January 1, 1981 through June 30, 1991: A Common Cause study. *Journal of Public Health Policy, 13* (Summer), 224–241.

Congressional Quarterly. (May, 1968). *Legislators and lobbyists: Medicare over the years.* Washington, D.C.: Congressional Quarterly.

Drew, Elizabeth. (1967). The health syndicate—Washington's noble conspirators. *Atlantic Monthly, 220* (December), 75–82.

Feldstein, Paul J. (1977). *Health associations and the demand for legislation: The political economy of health.* Cambridge, MA: Ballinger.

Feldstein, Paul J. (1982). *Health associations and the legislative process.* Ann Arbor: University of Michigan Press.

Feldstein, Paul J. (1988). *The politics of health legislation: An economic perspective.* Ann Arbor, MI: Health Administration Press.

Felicetti, Daniel A. (1975). *Mental health and retardation politics: The mind lobbies in Congress.* New York: Praeger.

Flash, William, Milton Roemer, & Sander Kelman. (1976). Stalking the politics of health care reform: Three critical perspectives on Robert Alford's "health care politics ideological and interest group barriers to reform." *Journal of Health Politics, Policy and Law, 1* (Spring), 112–129.

Fox, Daniel M., & Daniel C. Schaffer. (1989). Health policy and ERISA: Interest groups and semi-preemption. *Journal of Health Politics, Policy and Law, 14* (Summer), 239–268.

Graddy, Elizabeth. (1991). Interest groups or the public interest—Why do we regulate health occupations? *Journal of Health Politics, Policy and Law, 16* (Spring), 25–50.

Hoffman, Lilly M. (1989). *The politics of knowledge: Activist movements in medicine and planning.* New York: State University of New York Press.

Hutton, John, Michael Borowitz, Inga Oleksy, & Bryan R. Luce. (1994). The pharmaceutical industry and health reform: Lessons from Europe. *Health Affairs, 13* (Summer), 98–111.

Iglehart, John K. (1994). Health care reform: The role of physicians. *New England Journal of Medicine, 330* (March 10), 728–731.

Jones, Woodrow, Jr., & K. Robert Keiser. (1986). U.S. Senate voting on health and safety regulations: The effects of ideology and interest-group orientations. *Health Policy, 6* (1), 33–44.

Makinson, Larry. (1992). Political contributions from the health and insurance industries. *Health Affairs, 11* (Winter), 119–134.

Marmor, Theodore R., & David Thomas. (1972). Doctors, politics and pay disputes: Pressure group politics revisited. *British Journal of Political Science, 2* (October), 421–442.

Marmor, Theodore R., & David Thomas. (1983). Doctors, politics and pay disputes: Pressure group politics revisited. In T. Marmor (Ed.), *Political analysis and American medical care.* New York: Cambridge University Press.

Novello, Dorothy J. (1976). People, power and politics for health care. In National League for Nursing (Ed.), *People, power, politics for health care* (pp. 1–8). New York: National League of Nursing.

Oliver, Thomas R., & Emery B. Dowell. (1994). Interest groups and reform: Lessons from California. *Health Affairs, 13* (Spring, 2), 123–141.

Podhorzer, Michael. (1995). Unhealthy money: Health reform and the 1994 elections. *International Journal of Health Sciences, 25* (3), 393–402.

Poen, Monte M. (1979). *Harry S. Truman versus the medical lobby: The genesis of medicare.* Columbia: University of Missouri Press.

Pond, M. Allen. (1971). Politics of social change: Abortion reform, the role of health professionals in the legislative process. *American Journal of Public Health, 61* (May), 904–909.

Reinhardt, Uwe E. (1991). Breaking American health policy gridlock. *Health Affairs, 10* (Summer), 36–102.

Rodwin, Marc A. (1992). The organized American medical profession's response to financial conflicts of interest: 1890–1992. *Milbank Quarterly, 70* (4), 703–742.

Rosen, George. (1972). The committee of one hundred on national health and the campaign for a national health department, 1906–1912. *American Journal of Public Health, 62* (February), 261–263.

Tierney, John T. (1972). Organized interests in health politics and policy making. *Medical Care Review, 44* (Spring), 89–118.

Wagner, Lynn, & Eric Weissenstein. (1992). As health-care groups help fill campaign coffers, the question is: What is the money buying? *Modern Healthcare* (November 2), 38–40.

Ward, Paul D. (1972). Health lobbies: Vested interests and pressure politics. In Douglass Cater & Philip R. Lee (Eds.), *Politics of health.* New York: Medcom Press.

Waltzman, Nancy, & Patrick Woodall. (1995). Managed health care companies' lobbying frenzy. *International Journal of Health Services, 25* (3), 402–410.

Weller, G. R. (1977). From "pressure group politics" to "medical-industrial complex": The development of approaches to the politics of health. *Journal of Health Politics, Policy and Law, 1* (Winter), 444–470.

Wier, Richard A. (1970). *Patterns of interaction between interest groups and the Canadian political system: The case of the Canadian Medical Association.* Unpublished Ph.D. diss., Georgetown University, Washington, D.C.

Wilsford, David. (1987). The cohesion and fragmentation of organized medicine in France and the United States. *Journal of Health Politics, Policy and Law, 12* (Fall), 481–503.

Wysong, Earl. (1992). *High risk and high stakes: Health professionals, politics, and policy.* Westport, CT: Greenwood Press.

Community Power Structure and Health

Arnold, Mary F., & Isabel M. Welsh. (1971). Community politics and health planning. In Mary F. Arnold, L. Vaughn Blankenship, & John M. Hess (Eds.), *Administering health systems: Issues and perspectives* (pp. 154–175). Chicago: Aldine-Atherton.

Belknap, Ivan, & John G. Steinle. (1963). *The community and its hospitals: A comparative analysis.* Syracuse, NY: Syracuse University Press.

Berg, Robert L. (1977). "Movers" and "statics" refine political strategies in HSAs. *Hospital Progress, 58* (September), 64–69.

Blankenship, L. Vaughn. (1962). *Organizational support and community leadership in two New York state communities.* Unpublished Ph.D. diss., Cornell University.

Blankenship, L. Vaughn, & Ray H. Elling. (1962). Organizational support and community power structure: The hospital. *Journal of Health and Human Behavior, 3* (Winter), 257–269.

Blankenship, L.Vaughn, & Ray H. Elling. (1971). Effects of community power on hospital organization. In Mary F. Arnold, L. Vaughn Blankenship, & John M. Hess (Eds.), *Administering health systems: Issues and perspectives* (pp. 176–196). Chicago: Aldine Publishing Co.

Elling, Ray H. (1963). The hospital support game in urban center. In Elliot Friedson (Ed.), *The hospital in modern society* (pp. 73–111). New York: The Free Press.

Elling, Ray H. (1968). The shifting power structure in health. *Milbank Memorial Fund Quarterly, 46* (January), Part 2, 119–144.

Elling, Ray H., & Sandor Halebsky. (1961). Organizational differentiation and support: A conceptual framework. *Administrative Science Quarterly, 6* (September), 185–209.

Elling, Ray H., & Ollie J. Lee. (1966). Formal connections of community leadership to the health system. *Milbank Memorial Fund Quarterly, 44* (July), Part 1, 294–306.

Elling, Ray H., & Milton I. Roemer. (1961). Determinants of community support. *Hospital Administration, 6* (Summer), 17–34.

Freeborn, Donald K., & Benjamin J. Darsky. (1974). A study of the power structure of the medical community. *Medical Care, 12* (January), 1–12.

Gossert, Daniel J., & C. Arden Miller. (1973). State boards of health, their members and commitments. *American Journal of Public Health, 63* (June), 486–493.

Hanson, Robert C. (1962). The systemic linkage hypothesis and role consensus patterns in hospital-community relations. *American Sociological Review, 27* (June), 304–313.

Holloway, Robert G., Jay H. Artis, & Walter E. Freeman. (1963). The participation patterns of "economic influentials" and their control of a hospital board of trustees. *Journal of Health and Human Behavior, 4* (Summer), 88–98.

Hunter, Floyd, Ruth C. Schaffer, & Cecil G. Sheps. (1956). *Community organization: Action and inaction.* Chapel Hill: University of North Carolina Press.

Kupst, Mary Jo, Phil Reidda, & Thomas F. McGee. (1975). Community mental health boards: A comparison of their development, functions, and powers by board members and mental health center staff. *Community Mental Health Journal, 11* (Fall), 249–256.

Laur, Robert J. (1969). *A study of the extramural sector of governing board responsibility in non-profit general hospitals: Trustee interest in interorganizational relations.* Unpublished Ph.D. diss., University of Minnesota.

Miller, Paul A. (1952). The process of decision-making within the context of community organization. *Rural Sociology, 17* (June), 153–161.

Perrow, Charles. (1961). Organizational prestige: Some functions and dysfunctions. *American Journal of Sociology, 66* (January), 335–341.

Saunders, J. V. D., & J. H. Bruehing. (1959). Hospital–community relations in Mississippi. *Rural Sociology, 24* (March), 48–51.

Smith, David B., & Carl G. Homer. (1977). The hospital support group revisited. *Journal of Health Politics, Policy and Law, 2* (Summer), 257–265.

Smith, Richard A. (1976). Community power and decision making: A replication and extension of Hawley. *American Sociological Review, 41* (August), 691–705.

Thacker, Stephen B., Carolee Osborne, & Eva J. Salber. (1978). Health care decision making in a southern county. *Journal of Community Health, 3* (Summer), 347–356.

Warnecke, Richard B., Saxon Graham, William Mosher, & Erwin B. Montgomery. (1976). Health guides as influentials in Central Buffalo. *Journal of Health and Social Behavior, 17* (March), 22–34.

White, Marjorie A. (1976). *Attitudes of influentials toward health and illness care delivery.* Unpublished Ph.D. diss., Case Western Reserve University.

Initiative and Referenda in Health (see also Smoking and Tobacco)

General

Breslow, Lester, & Michael Johnson. (1993). California's Proposition 99 on tobacco and its impact. *Annual Review of Public Health, 14*, 585–604.

Fenton, Joshua, Ralph Catalano, & William A. Hargraves. (1996). Effect of Proposition 187 on mental health service use in California: A case study. *Health Affairs, 15* (Spring), 182–190.

Moon, Robert W., Michael A. Males, & David E. Nelson. (1993). The 1990 Montana initiative to increase cigarette taxes: Lessons for other states and localities. *Journal of Public Health Policy, 14* (Spring), 19–33.

Traynor, Michael P., & Stanton A. Glantz. (1996). California's tobacco initiative: The development and passage of Proposition 99. *Journal of Health Politics, Policy and Law, 21* (Fall), 543–586.

Ziv, Tai Ann, & Bernard Lo. (1995). Denial of care to illegal immigrants: Proposition 187 in California. *New England Journal of Medicine, 332* (April 20), 1095–1098.

The Fluoridation Controversy

Abelson, Robert P., & Alex Bernstein. (1963). A computer simulation model of community referendum controversies. *Public Opinion Quarterly, 27* (Spring), 93–122.

Burns, James MacGregor. (1953). The crazy politics of flourine. *New Republic, 128* (July 13), 14–15.

Burt, B. A., P. D. Bristow, & T. B. Dowell. (1973). Influencing community decisions on fluoridation. *British Dental Journal, 135* (July), 75–77.

Christoffel, Tom. (1985). Fluorides, facts and fanatics: Public health advocacy shouldn't stop at the court house door. *American Journal of Public Health, 75* (August), 888–891.

Conant, Ralph W. (1966). Bibliography of social-scientific studies in the fluoridation controversy. *Journal of Oral Therapeutics and Pharmacology, 3* (November), 203–211.

Crain, Robert L. (1966). Fluoridation: The diffusion of an innovation among cities. *Social Forces, 44* (June), 467–476.

Crain, Robert L., Elihu Katz, & Donald B. Rosenthal. (1969). *The politics of community conflict: The fluoridation decision.* Indianapolis: Bobbs-Merrill Co.

Dalzell-Ward, A. J. (1959). Fluoridation and public opinion. *Health Education Journal, 17* (November), 247–258.

Davis, Morris. (1960). Community attitudes toward fluoridation. *Public Opinion Quarterly, 23* (Winter), 474–482.

Dickson, S. (1969). Class attitudes to fluoridation. *Health Education Journal, 28* (September), 139–149.

Douglass, Chester W., & Dennis C. Stacey. (1972). Demographical characteristics and social factors related to public opinion on fluoridation. *Journal of Public Health Dentistry, 32* (Spring), 128–134.

Dwore, Richard B. (1978). A case study of the 1976 referendum in Utah on fluoridation. *Public Health Reports, 93* (January/February), 73–78.

Evans, Caswell A., Jr., & Tomm Pickles. (1978). Statewide antifluoridation initiatives: A new challenge to health workers. *American Journal of Public Health, 68* (January), 59–62.

Eveland, Charles L. (1969). *The political significance of dental health orientations in the fluoridation controversy: A post-referendum assessment.* Unpublished Ph.D. diss., University of Michigan.

Fish, D. G., E. S. Hirabayashi, & G. K. Hirabayashi. (1965). Voting turnout on a fluoridation plebiscite. *Journal of the Canadian Medical Association, 31* (February), 88–93.

Flanders, Raymond A. (1981). The denturism initiative. *Public Health Reports, 96* (September/October), 410–418.

Frankel, John M., & Myron Allukian. (1973). Sixteen referenda on fluoridation in Massachusetts: An analysis. *Journal of Public Health Dentistry, 33* (Spring), 96–103.

Gamson, William A. (1961a). The flouridation dialogue: Is it an ideological conflict? *Public Opinion Quarterly, 25* (Winter), 526–537.

Gamson, William A. (1961b). Public information in a fluoridation referendum: A summary of research. *Health Education Journal, 19* (March), 47–54.

Gamson, William A. (1961). Social science aspects of fluoridation: A summary of research. *Health Education Journal, 19* (September), 159–169.

Gamson, William A. (1965). Social science aspects of fluoridation: A supplement. *Health Education Journal, 24* (September), 135–143.

Gamson, William A., & Carolyn G. Lindberg. (1961). An annotated bibliography of social science aspects of fluoridation. *Health Education Journal, 19* (November), 209–230.

Gamson, William A., & Peter H. Orons. (1961). Community characteristics and fluoridation outcome. *Journal of Social Issues, 17* (4), 66–74.

Green, Arnold L. (1961). The ideology of anti-fluoridation leaders. *Journal of Social Issues, 17* (4), 13–25.

Grossman, J. (1966). Problems in the translation of social science theory to field action: An example in the case of fluoridation. *Journal of Dental Research, 45* (November/December, Suppl.), 1595–1601.

Hahn, Harlan. (1965). Voting behavior on fluoridation referendums: A reevaluation. *Journal of American Dental Association, 71* (November), 1138–1144.

Hahn, Harlan. (1969). Health concerns and attitudes regarding fluoridation. *Public Health Reports, 84* (July), 655–659.

Hutchison, John A. (1953). A small-town fluoridation fight. *Scientific Monthly, 77* (5), 240–243.

Isman, Robert. (1981). Fluoridation: Strategies for success. *American Journal of Public Health, 71* (July), 717–721.

Jackson, D. (1972). Attitudes to fluoridation: A survey of British housewives. *British Dental Journal, 132* (March 21), 219–222.

Kegeles, S. Stephen. (1961). Some unanswered questions and action implications of social research in fluoridation. *Journal of Social Issues, 17* (4), 75–81.

Kegeles, S. Stephen, & Gloria Latter. (1962). *Population characteristics and fluoridation referendums.*

Unpublished paper. U.S. Public Health Service, Division of Dental Health.

Kimball, Solon T., & Marion Pearsall. (1954). The health inventory at work: The fluoridation project. In Solon Kimball & Marion Pearsall (Eds.), *The Talladega story: A study in community process* (pp. 100–115). Tuscaloosa: University of Alabama Press.

Kirscht, John P. (1961). Attitude research on the fluoridation controversy. *Health Education Monographs, 10,* 16–28.

Kirscht, John P., & Andie L. Knutson. (1961). Science and fluoridation: An attitude study. *Journal of Social Issues, 17* (4), 37–44.

Kirscht, John P., & Andie L. Knutson. (1963). Fluoridation and the "threat" of science. *Journal of Health and Human Behavior, 4* (Summer), 129–135.

Lantos, Joseph, Lois A. Marsh, & Ronald P. Schultz. (1973). Small communities and fluoridation; Three case-studies. *Journal of Public Health Dentistry, 33* (Summer), 149–159.

Linn, E.L. (1969a). An appraisal of sociological research on the public's attitudes toward fluoridation. *Journal of Public Health Dentistry, 29* (Winter), 36–45.

Linn, E. L. (1969b). Effect of community leaders and organizations on public attitudes toward fluoridation. *Journal of Public Health Dentistry, 29* (Spring), 108–117.

MacRae, P., C. R. Castaldi, & W. Zacherl. (1964). Dental health, socioeconomic level, interest response to polio vaccination program, and voting in a fluoridation plebiscite. *Journal of Dental Research, 43* (October, Suppl.), 898–899.

Markle, Gerald E., James C. Peterson, & Morton O. Wagenfeld. (1978). Notes from the cancer underground: Participation in the laetrile movement. *Social Science and Medicine, 12* (1), 31–37.

Marmor, Judd, Viola W. Bernard, & Perry Ottenberg. (1978). Psychodynamics of group opposition to health programs. *American Journal of Orthopsychiatry, 30* (April), 330–345.

Masterton, G. (1963). A study of responses to a questionnaire on fluoridation. *American Journal of Public Health, 53* (August), 1243–1251.

Mausner, Bernard. (1957). The fluoridation controversy: A study in the acceptance of scientific authority. *Journal of American College of Dentists, 24* (September), 202–205.

Mausner, Bernard, & J. Mausner. (1955). A study of the anti-scientific attitude. *Scientific American, 192* (February), 35–39.

Mazur, Allan. (1981). *The Dynamics of technical controversy.* Washington, D.C.: Communications Press.

McNeil, Donald R. (1962a). *The fight for fluoridation.* New York: Oxford University Press.

McNeil, Donald R. (1962b). Political aspects of fluoridation. *Journal of the American Dental Association, 65* (November), 659–662.

Metz, A. Stafford. (1965). Research directions in fluoridation. In Division of Dental Health, U.S. Public Health Service (Ed.), *Social science research opportunities in dental health* (pp. 31–35). Washington, D.C.: U.S. Government Printing Office.

Metzner, Charles A. (1957). Referenda for fluoridation. *Health Education Journal, 15* (September), 168–177.

Mitchell, Austin. (1960). Fluoridation in Dunedin: A study of pressure groups and public opinion. *Political Science (New Zealand), 12* (March), 71–93.

Mueller, John E. (1966). The politics of fluoridation in seven California cities. *Western Political Quarterly, 19* (March), 54–67.

Mueller, John E. (1968). Fluoridation attitude change. *American Journal of Public Health, 58* (October), 1876–1882.

Murray, J. J. (1974). Water fluoridation: A choice for the community. *Community Health (England), 6* (September/October), 75–83.

O'Meara, B. J. (1960). Observations on a fluoridation plebiscite. *Canadian Journal of Public Health, 51* (May), 207–209.

O'Shea, Robert J., & S. Stephen Kegeles. (1963). An analysis of anti-fluoridation letters. *Journal of Health and Human Behavior, 4* (Summer), 135–140.

O'Shea, Robert M., & Lois K. Cohen. (1969). Social science and dentistry: Public opinions on fluoridation, 1968. *Journal of Public Health Dentistry, 29* (Winter), 57–58.

Paul, Benjamin D. (1959). Synopsis of report on fluoridation. *Massachusetts Dental Society Journal, 8* (January), 19–21.

Paul, Benjamin D. (1961). Fluoridation and the social scientists: A review. *Journal of Social Issues, 17* (4), 1–12.

Paul, Benjamin D., William A. Gamson, S. Stephen Kegeles, et al. (1961). Trigger for community conflict: The case of fluoridation. *Journal of Social Issues, 17* (4).

Peterson, James C., & Gerald E. Markle. (1979). The laetrile controversy. In Dorothy Nelkin (Ed.), *Controversy: Politics of technical decisions* (pp. 159–179). Beverly Hills, CA: Sage.

Petterson, Elof O. (1972). Abolition of the right of local Swedish authorities to fluoridate drinking water. *Journal of Public Health Dentistry, 32* (Fall), 243–247.

Pinard, Maurice. (1963). Structural attachments and political support in urban politics: The case of fluoridation referendums. *American Journal of Sociology, 68* (March), 513–526.

Plaut, Thomas F. A. (1958). Analysis of voting behavior on a fluoridation referendum. *Public Opinion Quarterly, 23* (Summer), 213–222.

Ramirez, A., R. B. Connor, R. M. Gibbs, H. G. Griggs, J. O. Neilsen, & O. W. Reeder. (1969). *Anomie and political powerlessness: Their relationship to attitudes and knowledge concerning fluoridation.* Birmingham: University of Alabama, School of Dentistry.

Raulet, Harry M. (1961). The health professional and the fluoridation issue: A case of role conflict. *Journal of Social Issues, 17* (4), 45–53.

Roemer, Ruth. (1965). Water fluoridation: Public health responsibility and democratic process. *American Journal of Public Health, 55* (September), 1337–1348.

Rosenstein, David I., Robert Isman, Tomm Pickles, & Craig Benben. (1978). Fighting the latest challenge to fluoridation in Oregon. *Public Health Reports, 93* (January/February), 69–72.

Rosenthal, Donald B., & Robert L. Cain. (1966). Executive leadership and community innovation:

The fluoridation experience. *Urban Affairs Quarterly, 1* (March), 39–57.

Sanders, Irwin T. (1961a). *The physician and fluoridation: A summary of research findings* (Document No. 16-S). Cambridge, MA: Harvard University School of Public Health.

Sanders, Irwin T. (1961b). The stages of a community controversy: The case of fluoridation. *Journal of Social Issues, 17* (4), 55–65.

Sanders, Irwin T. (1962). The involvement of health professionals and local officials in fluoridation controversies. *American Journal of Public Health, 52* (August), 1274–1287.

Sapolsky, Harvey M. (1968). Science, voters, and the fluoridation controversy. *Science, 62* (October), 427–433.

Sapolsky, Harvey M. (1969). The fluoridation controversy: An alternative explanation. *Public Opinion Quarterly, 33* (Summer), 240–248.

Scism, Thomas E. (1972). Fluoridation in local politics: Study of the failure of a proposed ordinance in one American city. *American Journal of Public Health, 62* (October), 1340–1345.

Shaw, C. T. (1969). Characteristics of supporters and rejecters of a fluoridation referendum and a guide for other community programs. *Journal of the American Dental Association, 78* (February), 339–341.

Simmel, Arnold G. (1961). A signpost on fluoridation conflicts: The concept of relative deprivation. *Journal of Social Issues, 17* (4), 23–36.

Simmel, Arnold G. (1969). *The structuring of opinion on a controversial topic: Studies and explanations of fluoridation conflicts.* Unpublished Ph.D. diss., Columbia University.

Smith, Richard A. (1976). Community power and decision making: A replication and extension of Hawley. *American Sociological Review, 41* (August), 691–705.

Stephens, Douglas W. (1958). Why fluoridation was defeated in Long Beach, California. *Oral Hygiene, 48* (May), 30–34.

Thomas, C. R. (1966). *The press and fluoridation referenda in selected Wisconsin cities.* Unpublished master's thesis, University of Wisconsin.

Walsh, Diana C. (1977). Fluoridation: Slow diffusion of a proven preventive measure. *New England Journal of Medicine, 296* (May), 1118–1120.

Warner, Morton. (1972). Communication overkill in a fluoridation campaign. *Canadian Journal of Public Health, 63* (May/June), 219–227.

Wilson, Robert N. (1968). *Community structure and health action.* Washington, D.C.: Public Affairs Press.

INDEX

Note: The letter n *following an index page number indicates an entry may be found in a footnote on that page.*

D

I

N